MW01131171

HUMAN CARDIOVASCULAR CONTROL

Human Cardiovascular Control

Loring B. Rowell
Professor of Physiology and Biophysics
Adjunct Professor of Medicine (Cardiology)
University of Washington School of Medicine

New York   Oxford
OXFORD UNIVERSITY PRESS
1993

Oxford University Press

Oxford   New York   Toronto
Delhi   Bombay   Calcutta   Madras   Karachi
Kuala Lumpur   Singapore   Hong Kong   Tokyo
Nairobi   Dar es Salaam   Cape Town
Melbourne   Auckland   Madrid

and associated companies in
Berlin   Ibadan

Library of Congress Cataloging-in-Publication Data
Rowell, Loring B.
Human cardiovascular control/Loring Rowell.
p.   cm.   Includes bibliographical references and index.

ISBN 978-0-19-507362-1

1. Blood—Circulation—Regulation.   2. Blood pressure—Regulation.
I. Title.
[DNLM: 1. Adaptation, Physiological.   2. Cardiovascular System—
–physiology.   3. Exercise.   4. Hemodynamics.   WG 106 R881ha]
QP109.R68   1992   612.1'3–dc20
DNLM/DLC   for Library of Congress   92-16434

Printed in the United States of America
on acid-free paper

This book is dedicated to my family and to my friends,
all of whom make everything worthwhile.
I also dedicate this book to the memory
of two great friends and scientists,
Philip D. Gollnick (1934–1991)
and
Erling Asmussen (1907–1991)

Preface

A few observations and much reasoning leads [*sic*] to error; many observations and a little reasoning [lead to] truth.

———*Alexis Carrell*

In this book, many observations and much reasoning may not lead to "truth," but the hope is that they will reveal the consistency that is a goal of science.

This is a *new* book about the *integrative* aspects of cardiovascular control in humans. It is not a new edition of *Human Circulation: Regulation During Physical Stress* (Rowell, 1986), but rather a fresh approach engendered by ideas and questions generated during the writing of that book and by the readers' responses to it. *Human Cardiovascular Control* attempts to integrate some of the most important features of this control—both neural and humoral—at the whole-body level. A particularly strong stimulus for this effort was the repeated statement in the previous book that "it is as though arterial pressure were the primary variable being regulated." This statement has been critically examined and constitutes one theme that is woven throughout all of the chapters.

The circulatory adjustments to upright posture and dynamic exercise are the two primary topics of *Human Cardiovascular Control* because they provide the most insight about how this system functions. The responses to these two stresses demand the full capabilities of the reflexes that govern cardiovascular function; they also show how the physical properties of the vascular system influence its function, particularly the performance of the heart. A major objective of this book is to pinpoint what is being regulated, and how, during orthostasis and exercise. It examines the variables that are regulated, what the sensors are, and what errors are being corrected by them. It attempts to show how the physical properties of the vasculature force interactions between flow and volume distribution and thus limit the functional range of particular reflex effectors. Reflexes are considered in the context of conventional negative feedback controllers, and the role of feed-forward mechanisms, which sometimes appear to dominate, is also considered.

The first four chapters treat the complex stress of orthostasis, a particular problem for humans. The human circulation was not well "designed" for being positioned upright with its pump high above a system of compliant tubes, which are highly susceptible to effects of gravity. Upright posture requires precise control of blood vessels by the autonomic nervous system. Gravity forces blood volume away from the heart and into the dependent vascular beds, especially into those not equipped with their own *veno*constrictor and/or blood-pumping mechanisms. Small "errors" in vasomotor control precipitate large systemic effects that can cause regulation of cardiac output and arterial pressure to fail. These four chapters deal with the passive effects of gravity on the circulation and with its reflex control, with neural and humoral adjustments and long-term control, and, finally, with some of the mechanisms of orthostatic intolerance.

The second part of the book, Chapters 5 to 12, deals with cardiovascular control during exercise. Humans, relative to some other species, are at a disadvantage; we have a more difficult problem of supplying adequate blood flow to active muscle because of gravitational effects stressed in previous chapters. Furthermore, we have small hearts with only one-half to one-third the pumping capacity of many other animals. An equally serious problem is that skeletal muscle may be a "sleeping giant" with a capacity to vasodilate that far outstrips the pumping capacity of the heart. How, then, do we match the rise in vascular conductance to the rise in total flow? We have learned in recent years that the mechanisms that govern the cardiovascular responses to exercise (so-called "exercise-reflexes") include some successful adjustments to exercise; and there are some that are not. Whereas some reflexes serve to increase blood flow, others may jeopardize even muscle blood flow to raise arterial pressure. This apparent paradox leads one to ask: What do we regulate? Is regulation directed to the correction of mismatches between blood flow and metabolism, called "flow-errors," or is regulation directed toward the correction of mismatches between cardiac output and vascular conductance, called "pressure errors"? Are the highly predictable relationships among the various indices of sympathetic nervous activity and the cardiac and vasomotor responses to exercise a signature of the arterial baroreflex, which corrects the "pressure-errors"?

One chapter deals extensively with how oxygen gets from the mouth to the skeletal muscle mitochondria, and examines both functional and structural limitations to oxygen transfer. It looks in detail at the potentially limiting steps in convective transfer, that is, the transport steps of ventilation and blood flow, and in diffusive transfer of oxygen, which is limited by structural barriers. In showing that there are commonly several specific limitations (both convective and diffusive) to oxygen transfer, a fundamental disagreement is raised with the hypothesis called *symmorphosis*.

The preceding paragraphs reveal something about the flavor of the book. Experimental details are provided to deal with all the questions that have been raised. Although these details are important to the lines of reasoning, it is the questions and the ideas they generate as well as the new hypotheses they stimulate that are the backbone of this book.

Why was the book written, and for whom was it written? First, the book was written because there are new things to say and new ideas to discuss. Also, ideas introduced in the predecessor book have been solidified and expanded and need a fresh treatment. Finally, I wished to have a book on these subjects that is suitable for teaching. Writing this book has been a learning experience that I am anxious to share with students.

Sometimes it may be more important to tell what we *do not* know than what we do know. Many perceive that there is currently a need to point out that some of the most basic aspects of cardiovascular control are still not understood—and cannot be explained at a molecular level. For example, we are still unable to tell students precisely what reflexes cause us to breathe harder and pump more blood when we exercise; yet this is perhaps the most basic question one can ask about the control of the cardiovascular system. Some current ideas about this control seem flawed, and may lead to error. These are criticized. Others seem worth pursuing, but they are still questioned. The process of questioning and putting forward new hypotheses seems to have more appeal to students than an encyclopedic rendition. I hope this book will provide a continuing opportunity to share questions and ideas with others.

The book is written for anyone who is interested in how the cardiovascular system works and who has some basic background in cardiovascular physiology. Some of the subjects are complex; nevertheless, every effort has been made to discuss them as straightforwardly as possible, and to provide clarity without oversimplification, while at the same time directing attention to more difficult and controversial areas. My goal was to strike a balance between discussion of basic principles and controversial ideas so as to foster an appreciation of the problems we still face.

This book has been written for a broad audience that includes medical students and residents, graduate students in the medical sciences and kinesiology, cardiologists, anesthesiologists, specialists in aerospace medicine and gravitational physiology, and any physician or medical professional with an interest in human cardiovascular function. The book should also be useful to physical educators who are concerned with cardiovascular adjustments to exercise.

The findings on which this book is based have been published as original journal articles, and many have appeared as well in review articles and book chapters. References are provided at the end of each chapter in order to give a source for all important points, even if it is sometimes a secondary or a tertiary source, such as a review article or chapter that references the primary sources. Unfortunately, it was not possible to list more than a portion of the primary references used in writing this book, and I apologize to all authors whose important contributions are not specifically listed. This had to be done to keep the size of the book manageable. The book has two types of illustrations to assist in explaining the concepts; one type serves a didactic function and is the schematic drawing designed to explain concepts and ideas. The other type of illustration presents actual experimental data and provides evidence for the concepts.

Although the focus of the book is on humans, the importance of experiments on other species is emphasized. At every step the human physiologist depends on those who can uncover information from animals that is inaccessible to those who study humans. Happily, the converse is sometimes true as well. In short, the ideas put forward in this book are as dependent on good experiments conducted on nonhuman species as they are on good experiments carried out on human subjects.

Seattle   L.B.R.
1992

Acknowledgments

I am deeply grateful to all who have made this book possible, especially Ms. Pamela Stevens and Mrs. Fusako Kusumi. Their superb skills and dedication for more than two decades have been vital. Ms. Stevens also prepared all of the illustrations plus the entire manuscript for this book. Ms. Carol Taylor photographed all of the illustrations.

The constant professional and personal support and friendship from my esteemed colleagues, Dr. John R. Blackmon, Dr. George L. Brengelmann, and Dr. Allen M. Scher, have nourished and sustained me. I find no adequate way to express my gratitude to them. Their contributions are immeasurable.

I am a beneficiary of the skills, curiosity, and enthusiasm of talented graduate students and postdoctoral fellows. They have provided a constant stimulus, a continuing education, and a feeling of reward. I am grateful to them.

I am indebted to Dr. John Krasney, Dr. Jerome Dempsey, Dr. John Johnson, Dr. Douglas Seals, and Dr. Allen Cowley, and also their colleagues and students, for their critical and constructive evaluations of various chapters. Their knowledge and their insight and candor improved the book. I also thank Dr. Wayne Crill, Dr. Allen Scher, and all others who looked over portions of this book and provided helpful comments.

I appreciate the research support provided by the National Institutes of Health and the National Heart, Lung, and Blood Institute over three decades, and also a period of support from the American Heart Association.

I am grateful to those at Oxford University Press who have helped in the production of this book—especially Mr. Jeffrey House, who originally suggested the project, and whose encouragement, assistance, and friendship helped to keep me on track.

Contents

1. Passive Effects of Gravity   3
   History   3
   Hydrostatics and Distribution of Vascular Transmural
   Pressures   6
   Structural Features That Counteract Gravitational
   "Pooling"   20
   Mechanical Adjustments to Orthostasis   28
   Summary   33

2. Reflex Control During Orthostasis   37
   Brief History   37
   Circulatory Responses to Upright Posture   39
   Summary   74

3. Neural-Humoral Adjustments to Orthostasis and Long-Term
   Control   81
   Neural Control   82
   Humoral Control   96

4. Orthostatic Intolerance   118
   Normal Individuals: Maldistribution of Blood Flow and Blood
   Volume   120
   Cardiovascular Dysfunction   139
   Autonomic Dysfunction   153

5. Central Circulatory Adjustments to Dynamic Exercise   162
   Cardiovascular Functional Capacity: The Concept   162
   Determinants of Oxygen Uptake: A Brief Review   167
   Regulation of the Central Circulation   172
   Adjustments to Chronic High Loads: Physical
   Conditioning   190

6. Control of Regional Blood Flow During Dynamic
   Exercise   204
   Splanchnic Circulation   205

Cutaneous Circulation   219
The Renal Circulation   235
Cerebral Circulation   241

7. Control of Blood Flow to Dynamically Active Muscles   255
Control of Blood Flow to the Heart   256
Control of Blood Flow to Respiratory Muscles   265
Control of Blood Flow to Active Skeletal Muscle   268
Peripheral Vascular Adjustments to Physical
Conditioning   288

8. Cardiovascular Adjustments to Isometric
Contractions   302
Blood Flow to Active Muscles   304
Central Circulatory Responses   312
Peripheral Vascular Responses   316
Summary   322

9. Limitations to Oxygen Uptake During Dynamic
Exercise   326
Limitations in the Respiratory System   330
Alveolar to Arterial Oxygen Transfer   339
Cardiac Output as a Limitation to Oxygen Uptake   348
Transfer of Oxygen from Muscle Capillary to
Mitochondria   350
Limitations in Skeletal Muscle Metabolism   360
Summary   366

10. What Signals Govern the Cardiovascular Responses to
Exercise? Role of Central Command   371
What Is Central Command?   372
How Does Central Command Exert Its Effects on the
Cardiovascular System?   382
Is Central Command Exclusively a Feed-Forward
Mechanism?   386
Summary   392

11. What Signals Govern the Cardiovascular Responses to
Exercise? Reflexes from Active Muscles   396
Neurophysiological Evidence for Muscle Chemoreflexes
and Mechanoreflexes   398
Reflex Responses to Voluntary Isometric
Contractions   403

Importance of the Muscle Chemoreflex During
Dynamic Exercise   408
Summary   434

12. Arterial Baroreflexes, Central Command, and Muscle
Chemoreflexes: A Synthesis   441
Overall Assessment of Baroreflex Regulation of Arterial
Pressure During Exercise   443
Functional Characteristics of the Carotid Sinus Reflex
During Exercise   449
Role of Cardiopulmonary Baroreceptors in Dynamic
Exercise   464
Central Command, Muscle Chemoreflexes and Arterial
Baroreflexes: How Do They Operate Together?   465
Summary   478

Index   485

HUMAN CARDIOVASCULAR CONTROL

Passive Effects of Gravity

HISTORY

The great French physician Piorry stated in 1826: "It is in consequence of gravity that when the arms are held down the veins swell and the capillaries are filled, and the reverse occurs when the arms are held up, that varicoceles enlarge on standing up, and diminish in the horizontal position, and that the head and face redden when held down" (from McDowall, 1956).

"When man's subhuman ancestors first dared to rise and walk upon their hind legs, they essayed a physiologic experiment of no mean difficulty" (Amberson, 1943).

The ancients knew that prolonged exposure to upright posture, without weight bearing on the legs, would eventually lead to unconsciousness and death. Death was the consequence of hypotension and cerebral ischemia. Another example of orthostatic hypotension (from the Greek: *orthos* = "straight" or "upright," and *statikos* = "causing to stand") is the familiar sight of the prostrate and unconscious soldier who has stood too long motionless and at attention. Although the brain is the organ most susceptible to ischemia, its location with respect to the heart in upright posture also makes it and the lung the two organs most susceptible to the effects of gravity on blood flow. As soon as cerebral blood flow falls below a critical level, consciousness is lost.

In their discussions of the effects of upright posture on the circulation, McDowall (1956) and Amberson (1943) revealed the high quality of thinking by eighteenth- and nineteenth-century investigators about causes of orthostatic hypotension. These able scientists were aware that most of the quadrupeds in standing position have hearts in a position slightly below the large veins of the trunk. Thus, filling of the heart is normally *assisted* by gravity. They recognized the problems imposed by gravity on upright bipeds. In his beautifully simple experiments, Friedrich Goltz in 1864 shows that the marked reduction in cardiac filling pressure in frogs and snakes held in a vertical, held-up position, could be reversed by submersing the lower half of the animals in water.

The eighteenth- and nineteenth-century pioneers had good insight into the role played by the distensible veins in the reactions to upright posture. Initially, consideration of the compensatory adjustments to upright posture appears to have centered on the importance of the "respiratory pump" on venous return. Antonio Valsalva (1666–1723) observed that the jugular vein collapsed during inspiration and filled during expiration. John Hunter in 1794 referred to "a degree of stagnation" during expiration, whereas "During inspiration, the veins readily empty themselves." Jean L. M. Poiseuille in 1830 demonstrated the importance of negative intrathoracic pressure on venous return. Franklin (1937) emphasized the action of the respiratory pump on venous outflow from the liver acting mainly through compression of the liver and release thereof by the diaphragm during inspiration and expiration. J. Pal in 1888 postulated that hepatic venous outflow is dominated by respiratory movement (cited by Franklin). The important influence of the liver on venous return to the heart during breathing was confirmed in more technically advanced studies in the 1960s. Although Hill and Barnard in 1897 recognized the importance of vascular "tone" of the splanchnic region, they felt that the respiratory pump was almost as important.

The venous valves, which led to Sir William Harvey's discovery of the circulation, were recognized as being important to orthostatic adjustments. Attention was drawn to the importance of movement (muscle pumping) by Hunter in 1794 and by François Magendie in 1830 through their simple demonstrations that swelling of the feet was reduced by muscular movements. R. Burton-Opitz in 1903 emphasized the importance of muscle contractions in preventing edema. Turner in 1927 showed that humans placed in stationary upright position for 20 minutes experience swelling (edema) in the lower limbs. It was previously understood that positioning an animal vertically for long periods led to slow cardiac failure (along with cerebral ischemia), presumably as a consequence of the fluid lost from blood. Edgar Atzler and R. Herbst in 1923 concluded that 500 cm^3 of additional blood volume accumulated in human legs during quiet standing for 1 hour.

In 1885 L. Hermann set out to find the "indifferent point" of the circulatory system in order to eliminate hydrostatic effects on pressure so that the dynamic effects (of the heart) alone could be studied. He found what Hill (1895) called "*the hydrostatic indifferent point*," in which hydrostatic pressure does not change when the circulatory system is rotated around this point. Later Hill (1895) considered the effects of reflex vasoconstriction on the hydrostatic indifferent point.

Although quadrupeds are more ideally suited to withstanding gravity while they stand on all four feet, some species share in part the problems of humans. This prompted the comment from Gauer and Thron (1965) that "it certainly was a bold enterprise of nature to create quadrupeds like man or the giraffe with a predominantly vertical extension, who carry their heads and hearts at a considerable distance above the center of gravity of the body."

Figure 1-1 schematically illustrates the distribution of pressures and venous volume in an upright human (Rowell, 1983). The contrast is with

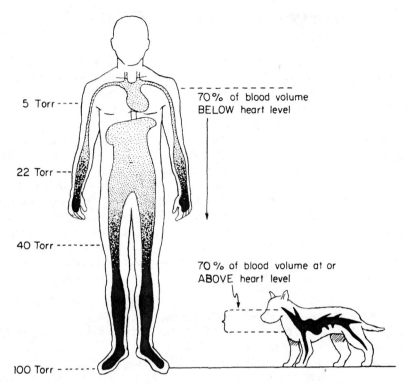

5 Torr - - - -

70% of blood volume
BELOW heart level

22 Torr - - -

40 Torr - - - - - - -

70% of blood volume at or
ABOVE heart level

100 Torr - - - - - -

Figure 1-1   Schematic illustration of gravitationally dependent distribution of blood volume and venous pressures in the upright human compared with that in the dog. (Adapted from Folkow and Neil, 1971, reproduced from Rowell, 1983, with permission from the American Physiological Society.)

other animals in which most of the blood volume is close to heart level along the nearly horizontal axis of the aorta; thus, hydrostatic effects on blood volume distribution are much less than in humans.

The following references contain reviews of cardiovascular adjustments to gravitation stress: Amberson (1943), Gauer and Thron (1965), Blomqvist and Stone (1983), and Rowell (1986).

The objectives of this chapter are first, to explain some physical properties of the vascular system that exacerbate the effects of gravity on the entire cardiovscular system and some properties that ameliorate these effects; second, the importance of some structural features of the system is described; third, the importance of mechanical effects on the circulation is elaborated, showing how these effects help to lessen the fall in ventricular filling pressure. This chapter describes the events occurring primarily in the early moments of being upright, before reflexes can compensate for the shifts in blood volume. The idea is to describe the substrate on which reflexes must act and to provide the basis for understanding where they must act and why.

HYDROSTATICS AND DISTRIBUTION OF VASCULAR TRANSMURAL PRESSURES

Increased gravitational force causes marked redistribution of blood volume in accordance with the changes in transmural pressure. When humans stand up, the heart is about 1.2 to 1.5 m above the feet, and about 75 percent of the blood volume is in compliant veins. Approximately 70 to 75 percent of total blood volume is below the level of the pump and must somehow be driven back to the right atrium. If an engineering analysis of the aeronautical features of the bumblebee could lead to the conclusion that these insects cannot fly, then a hydrodynamic analysis of the human ciculation could also lead to the conclusion that human beings cannot stand up. They do stand, and this chapter discusses the structural and mechanical features of the circulation that aid in this adjustment, as well as the features that oppose it. The critical regulatory problem originates from the displacement of blood volume away from the heart and the consequent fall in ventricular filling pressure and in stroke volume.

Pressures within the blood vessels have three basic components:

1. A static pressure that is related to the volume of blood within the vascular system at zero flow
2. A hydrostatic pressure caused by the force of gravity and referred to as ρgh, where ρ is fluid density, g is the acceleration due to gravity, and h is the height of the hydrostatic column
3. A dynamic pressure generated by the heart and equal to blood flow × resistance

A detailed description of the distribution of vascular transmural pressure is shown in Figure 1-2.

In supine posture, the pressure generated by the heart is approximately 100 mmHg throughout the large arteries (ignoring energy losses as heat associated with blood flow). Venous pressures in the supine position range from approximately 5 mmHg at the right atrium up to 15 to 20 mmHg in the smallest veins. Therefore, *the driving pressure for the entire left ventricular output from the immediate postcapillary vessels back to the right ventricle is only 10 to 15 mmHg.* (Figure 1-2 shows a similar net driving pressure for venous return in upright posture—see venous pressure + ρgh.)

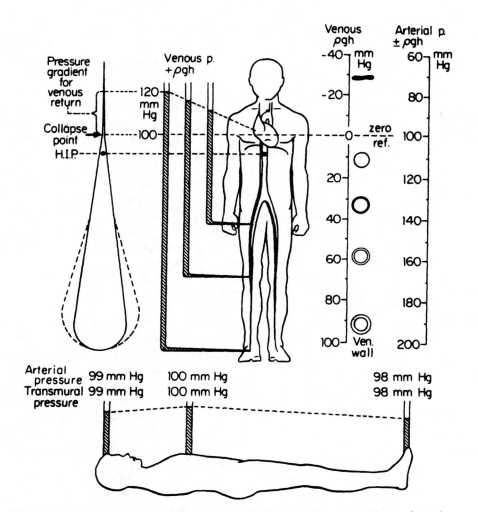

Figure 1-2 Distribution of pressures in upright humans. Pressure scales on the right are arterial pressures, including dynamic pressure generated by the heart plus the hydrostatic pressure (*ρgh*). Venous hydrostatic pressure (*ρgh*) is without additional driving pressure (see below). Ellipse and circles show shape and wall thickness of veins (*Ven. Wall*) relative to distance from the heart. Heart level is the zero pressure reference level (*Zero Ref.*). On the person's left, water-filled tubes show measured venous pressure (driving pressure + *ρgh*), showing a 20-mmHg gradient (120 − 100 mmHg) the *pressure gradient for venous return*. Veins collapse at the zero pressure reference level (*Collapse Point*), as illustrated by the water-filled, thin-walled rubber tube on the left. Note insensitivity of collapse point to added volume (*dashed line around tube*). The hydrostatic indifferent point (*H.I.P.*) is below collapse point—at approximately diaphragmatic level. The supine human below shows distribution of dynamic arterial driving pressure and transmural pressure in this posture. (From Rowell, 1986, with permission from Oxford University Press.)

In upright posture the zero pressure reference level, called "venostatic level," is usually at the right atrium where pressure is zero with respect to atmospheric pressure. Above this level, intravenous pressures become increasingly negative as the height of the hydrostatic column above the heart increases. Veins are collapsed unless they are held open by tethering to the surrounding tissues as, for example, are veins in the cerebral circulation. In the upright posture, the hydrostatic and dynamic components of pressure add in proportion to ρgh below the heart so that, at the feet, arterial transmural pressure equals the sum of the dynamic pressure (100 mmHg) and the hydrostatic pressure (also 100 mmHg in this example). The hydrostatic pressure at any point in the circulation is determined by the height of the continuous column of blood between that point and the heart. The venous transmural pressure is the sum of the dynamic pressure (as high as 20 mmHg in postcapillary venules) and the hydrostatic pressure, which is also 100 mmHg at the feet when all venous valves are open (this condition is represented in Figure 1-2), so that there is an uninterrupted hydrostatic column of venous blood between the right atrium and the feet.

Note that the venous water manometers in Figure 1-2 (centimeters of water are specified in millimeters of mercury) show the pressure gradient for venous return from the feet to be about 20 mmHg with the gradient decreasing in the large veins as blood moves upward and closer to the heart. Again, in this posture the driving pressure for blood flow *to* the capillaries is about 80 mmHg, whereas the pressure driving blood from postcapillary vessels back to the heart is 15 to 20 mmHg. Not only must the entire cardiac output be returned from the microvasculature to the heart by a net driving pressure of only 15 to 20 mmHg, but, to make matters worse, all this blood must return through a distensible venous network. The venous system is highly compliant, and its volume increases markedly with small increases in transmural pressure.

Above venostatic or right atrial level, intravenous pressures are *negative,* and if they fall in proportion to their distance above the heart, mural pressures would reach as low as -40 mmHg at the top of the head. In 1877, Edouard Brissaud and Charles Francois-Frank, and later Hill (1895), measured human intracranial pressure and observed that it became negative when the patient sat upright and then positive in the feet-up position. Cerebral veins are kept partially open by their tethering to surrounding structures; when an open needle is inserted into a cerebral vein, air is sucked into the vein. Two important points to keep in mind: *First,* arterial pressures at the top of the head do not normally fall below the level at which autoregulation of cerebral blood flow is effective. *Second,* the pressure distending the carotid sinus is approximately 15 to 20 mmHg lower than the distending pressure at the aorta in upright posture. During graded head-up tilt, for example, the difference in aortic and carotid sinus distending pressures increases in proportion to the sine of the angle of tilt $\times \rho gh$. Thus, the pressure difference between the two receptor sites provides information about the degree of tilt.

Cerebral vessels are enclosed in a rigid skull so that intra- and extravascular volume are constant. Within this rigid container, the cerebral vessels are surrounded by cerebrospinal fluid, which is in effect a fluid column running from the top of the head to the end of the spine (Figure 1-3). Theoretically, the cerebrospinal fluid could exert a hydrostatic force outside of the cerebral vessels that is similar to the force exerted inside. If so, this gravitationally induced counterpressure would oppose the fall in cerebral venous and arterial transmural pressure, and the hydrostatic effect on cerebral perfusion pressure would be minimized (Rushmer et al., 1947).

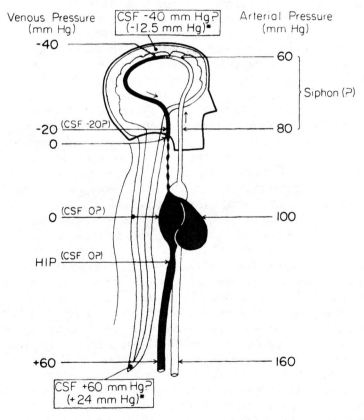

Figure 1-3 Hypothetical and actual distribution of dynamic (arterial) pressure and hydrostatic pressures in arteries, veins, and cerebrospinal fluid (CSF). Reduction in arterial pressure to 60 mmHg would be counteracted if CSF pressure was −40 mmHg; arterial transmural pressure would be 100 mmHg, and venous transmural pressure would be zero. Measured CSF pressure in humans is lower than predicted. A siphon effect on cerebral blood flow has also been proposed. If true, the siphon effect would end when veins leave the skull and collapse to atmospheric pressure (zero transmural pressure). See text.

Cerebrospinal fluid is in constant communication with the cerebral and spinal veins through a series of small pressure-sensitive, one-way valves (Allen 1986). Accordingly, cerebrospinal fluid pressure should match the pressure within these veins, assuming that zero pressure for both cerebrospinal fluid and venous blood is at heart level (as shown in Figure 1-3), so that both pressures should be the same and thus counterbalance each other at all points along this cavity, irrespective of body position. For example, when cats were centrifuged in the longitudinal axis over a range of gravitational forces, from +6 to −6 × gravity, the cerebrospinal fluid and venous pressures measured at the same level along the spinal column, both above and below the heart, varied together and by approximately the same amount—that is, they counterbalanced each other.

Studies on humans have not yielded the near-perfect counterbalancing cerebral spinal and venous pressures observed by Rushmer and colleagues (1947). For example, the rise in lumbar cerebrospinal fluid pressure in humans when they sat upright (90°) was only 40 percent of that predicted from distance below the heart ($\rho g h$) (Davson, 1967). The fall in cerebrospinal fluid pressure in the superior sagittal sinus at the top of the head (at cerebrospinal fluid = −40 mmHg(?) in Figure 1-3) was found to be only −12.5 mmHg or approximately 30 percent of the predicted value (Bradley, 1970). This small negative value for cerebrospinal fluid pressure would mean that effective arterial perfusion pressure at the top of the head is 72.5 mmHg [60 − (−12.5) mmHg] given the pressures listed in Figure 1-3. Postural adjustments in cerebrospinal fluid pressure are complex and tend to occur slowly, over minutes, owing possibly to a somewhat elastic nonrigid nature of the cerebrospinal fluid container; that is, the container may partially collapse and cause resistance to fluid movement (Davson, 1967).

Were cerebrospinal fluid and venous pressures as well counterbalanced in humans as postulated in Figure 1-3, then there should be no gravitational effects on cerebral blood flow. In general, cerebral blood flow is well maintained via autoregulation until arterial perfusion pressure falls below 60 mmHg (there may be a 6 to 7 percent decrease in cerebral blood flow for every 10-mmHg reduction in arterial blood pressure in its autoregulatory range [Heistad and Kontos, 1983]). If cerebral blood flow falls significantly in upright posture as observed by some (see Gauer and Thron, 1965; Heistad and Kontos, 1983), then pressures in the cerebrospinal fluid and venous compartments must not counterbalance each other.

The effects of gravity on perfusion of the lung are different from those of other organs because of the low arterial perfusion pressure of the lung and its position both above and below the heart and venostatic level. The distribution of blood flow throughout the lung is uniquely sensitive to changes in posture. The homogeneously perfused normal lung in supine posture divides into roughly three zones in upright posture as illustrated in Figure 1-4 derived from West (1965). This figure illustrates the principles, which, stated briefly, are that a constant alveolar pressure (PA) surrounds

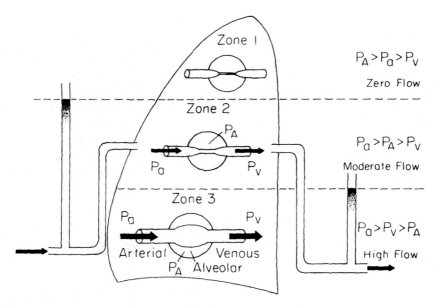

Zone 1

$P_A > P_a > P_V$

Zero Flow

Zone 2

P_A

$P_a > P_A > P_V$

Moderate Flow

P_a P_V

Zone 3

P_a P_V

$P_a > P_V > P_A$

High Flow

Arterial   Venous
P_A Alveolar

Figure 1-4 Blood flow through dependent regions of the lung (below heart level) and above heart level in upright humans is determined by the differences between pressures in pulmonary arteries (Pa), the alveolus (PA) and pulmonary veins (Pv)—and not the usual arteriovenous pressure difference. See text.

pulmonary capillaries from the top (above the heart) to the bottom of the lung (below the heart), but perfusion pressure (arterial pressure or Pa) and venous outflow pressure (Pv) rise or fall in proportion to the distance above or below venostatic level. Thus, in zone 1 above the heart, where alveolar pressure may exceed arterial pressure, flow is zero. In zone 2, where arterial pressure exceeds alveolar pressure, which in turn exceeds venous pressure, blood flow is determined by the difference between Pa and PA. At the bottom of the lung, in zone 3, which is below heart level, Pa exceeds Pv which in turn exceeds PA; therefore, the driving pressure is determined by the difference between arterial and venous pressure, which is common for many (not all) vascular beds.

Figure 1-2 shows on separate scales the pressures within the arterial and venous systems all referenced to zero pressure at heart level. Inasmuch as intravascular pressures above the heart fall, and those below the heart rise on standing up, there is a point in the vasculature at which pressure is independent of posture. It is called the *hydrostatic indifferent point* (HIP), which is a transition zone at which intravascular pressure remains constant and, as such, represents a center of gravity for the vascular system (Hill, 1895; Gauer and Thron, 1965). In humans, the HIP is located close to the level of the diaphragm or 5 to 6 cm below the point of *venous collapse,* which is the upper end of the venous hydrostatic column. The location of HIP is determined by the distribution of compliances in the upper and lower half of the vascular system. The more compliant the legs, for example, the lower the HIP. Anything that would actively reduce compliance, or in some other way reduce pooling in dependent regions (e.g., exercise), would shift HIP headward and restrict the fall in central venous pressure. Conversely, anything that would increase compliance (e.g., heat stress and cutaneous vasodilation) would shift HIP downward and increase the fall in central venous pressure.

Note the collapse point in the thin-walled tube shown on the right of Figure 1-2 and the apparent insensitivity of this point to an increase in volume. The intent is to portray the concept that a substantial increase in volume would be required to raise HIP, the collapse point, and right atrial pressure. Clearly this volume will depend on the compliance of structures below the heart and their blood flow. Bear in mind that expansion of blood volume can reduce the fall in blood pressure in patients with severe orthostatic hypotension; on the other hand, it is probably a poor way to improve exercise performance.

Summary. In summary, upright humans are faced with two problems. First, most of the blood is below venostatic level and most of this blood is contained in distensible veins rather than stiff arteries. Second, blood volume is too small to fill the vascular container in upright posture. Were veins as noncompliant as arteries, the hydrostatic effects of upright posture would be minimal, and one could view the vascular system simply as a rigid container.

Distribution of Resistance and Compliance and Volume

The extent to which gravitational force translocates blood volume into dependent organs will depend on their distensibility or compliance (as defined below). The rate at which veins fill with blood will depend on the resistance to blood flow in the arterioles that precede them in the circuit.

Blood is delivered to the microcirculation at high pressures and in tubes that are 30 to 50 times stiffer than veins. Most of the pressure drop in the circulation occurs across the small arteries and arterioles called resistance vessels. Blood is returned from the microcirculation to the heart at low pressures in highly distensible tubes. It is fundamentally important to recognize that veins also offer some resistance to flow. It is this resistance (albeit small) that explains the pressure gradient of approximately 15 to 20 mmHg between the postcapillary vessels and the heart (see Figure 1-2). *Because of their high compliance, small changes in intravenous pressure, owing to changes in blood flow, will have marked effects on venous volume.* Thus, the distribution of blood volume depends on the distribution of resistance and blood flow. We will return repeatedly to this fundamental point.

Most of the blood in the body is contained in veins, and, at normal venous distending pressures, veins are larger in diameter than their arterial counterparts at comparable branches of the vascular tree. If the entire vascular system is viewed as a single container, venules, small and large veins, liver sinusoids, and the spleen contain approximately 70 percent of its total blood volume. The venous compartment can be considered a reservoir for the cardiovascular system because large changes in volume can occur with small changes in distending pressure, thereby buffering stresses such as hemorrhage. The same properties exacerbate the effects of stresses, such as upright posture.

From rough estimates based on data from nonhuman species, as much as 85 percent of the total blood volume is in the compliant low-pressure compartment, namely, systemic veins, the right atrium, right ventricle, pulmonary circulation, and left atrium. Again, 70 percent of total blood volume is in the systemic veins, and 15 percent is in the heart and lungs, with 10 percent in the systemic arteries, and about 5 percent in the capillaries. Taken together as a single vascular container, the entire systemic circulation has a compliance estimated to be between 2.5 and 3.0 ml $mmHg^{-1} kg^{-1}$ total body weight.

Before proceeding with this discussion, it is necessary to describe some physical characteristics of the venous system. The characteristics of isolated veins with zero flow are described first to reduce the confusion that often stems from trying to apply an understanding of the characteristics of isolated veins to the *distributed* characteristics of the venous system within an entire organ—or entire animal.

Physical Properties of Isolated Veins and Features That Lead to Vascular "Pooling"

Compliance. The flaccidity or stiffness of a hollow elastic tube can be described quantitatively in terms of a relationship between its distending pressure—or transmural pressure: that is, the difference between pressure inside and outside the tube—and its volume. Figure 1-5 shows the characteristics of a typical vein. Compliance of the vein is described as the slope of the volume-pressure relationship $(\Delta V/\Delta P)$. The volume-pressure relationship is nonlinear; therefore, compliance is variable and depends on distending pressure. At low pressures, the curve is steep, meaning that a large change in volume accompanies only a small change in pressure so that compliance is high. At higher pressures the slope is less steep and compliance is relatively low. The venous cross sections shown in Figure 1-5 illustrate that the early phase of expansion of the vein involves no actual stretch of the elastic material in its wall. A small change in distending pressure merely changes the geometry of the vein. Once the vein has assumed a circular cross section, subsequent increases in its transmural pressure are opposed by the development of increased tension in the walls; stiff collagen fibers must be stretched in order to increase volume.

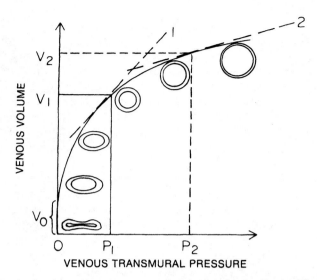

Figure 1-5 Typical volume-pressure curve of an isolated vein. Dashed lines (1 and 2) show the compliance ($\Delta V/\Delta P$) at two venous transmural pressures, P_1 and P_2. Note that compliance varies with pressure, being greatest at the lower pressures (line 1) and decreases as pressure increases (line 2). V_0 is the unstressed volume, which is the volume contained at zero transmural pressure. The change in volume from V_2 to V_1 is the passive effect of changing pressures from P_2 to P_1. Note how changing cross-sectional geometry contributes to *passive* emptying. (From Rowell, 1986, with permission from Oxford University Press.)

Stress-Relaxation, Delayed Compliance, and Creep. The volume contained within a vein at a given distending pressure is time-dependent due to the viscoelastic property called stress-relaxation. Creep refers to the gradual change in volume following a sudden change in distending pressure. When venous pressure is suddenly raised, compliance gradually increases over some given time interval, that is, delayed compliance. Thus, the term compliance includes time-dependent and history-dependent components (Gow, 1980).

Regional Differences in Veins. Venous characteristics vary markedly from region to region. For example, in dependent regions of humans, Figure 1-2 shows a thickening of the walls in veins that are most distant from the heart. The thicker venous walls tend to oppose some of the hydrostatic pressure encountered during upright posture. In contrast, veins near or above heart level are thin-walled and more distensible (Conrad, 1971). The fact that veins are stiff at high transmural pressures and flabby at low transmural pressures has great importance to human adjustments to upright posture and to hemorrhage (see below).

Distributed Venous Properties of an Intact Organ

Compliance. Curves analogous to that shown in Figure 1-5 can be determined from the slope, relating changes in total organ volume to changes in intravascular pressure. As in an isolated vein, compliance can vary with distending pressure so that the value needs to be related to a specific transmural pressure. The volume-pressure curve represents the *distributed* properties of all veins (microvessels to large veins) *and arteries*. Inasmuch as veins are approximtely *30 to 50* times more compliant than arteries, compliance is usually dominated by veins, but sometimes special organ features intervene (see below).

Specific Compliance. Total vascular compliance varies markedly from organ to organ. In order to compare the compliances of different organs, normalization per unit of total body weight or organ weight is necessary; this normalized value is called specific compliance. For example, the compliance of individual vessels in the lung of a small infant and a large adult might be the same, but the volume of blood held at a given distending pressure by the infant lung will be far less than that of the adult lung—that is, lower total compliance. However, the volume of blood per 100 grams, or per kilogram, of lung tissue (i.e., the specific compliance) would be the same for the infant and adult lungs.

Factors other than venous properties can determine the relationship between volume and pressure of an organ. Some organs are encased in rigid capsules that restrict expansion, whereas others have extensive tethering of veins that limit their emptying. The volume-pressure relationship will also be affected by the organ's vascular anatomy, which determines what fraction of its total volume is in the smallest veins as opposed to the largest ones (e.g., the capacious liver sinusoids and cutaneus venous plexes as opposed to the far less compliant and noncapacious networks in the kidneys or in skeletal muscle). A complex and often undefined distribution of compliances also exists within an organ between the smallest venules and the largest veins. Total organ compliance will vary with the size, relative number, and the wall structure of each venous segment.

Regional compliances differ markedly. Actual specific compliances are, of course, not known for individual organs in humans, but some of their special features permit rough comparisons. For example, the brain is encased in a rigid skull so that volume expansion is prevented and venous collapse is prevented by surrounding tissues. Human skin and liver are known to be highly compliant, whereas veins in the dependent limb are thicker walled and would be expected to be less compliant than organs situated closer to or above heart level where hydrostatic forces are less. In short, the distribution of regional organ compliances in humans is probably such that the hydrostatic forces associated with upright posture are partially counteracted.

Specific compliances of different vascular beds in the dog vary widely (Rothe, 1983). Similar values have been estimated for humans (Echt et al., 1974). The most compliant regions in dogs are the spleen, liver, and small intestines; their specific compliances per kilogram of organ tissue weight are 80, 20, and 2.0 to 3.4 ml $mmHg^{-1}$ kg^{-1}, respectively. The entire splanchnic bed has a compliance of about 0.7 ml $mmHg^{-1}$ kg^{-1} of total body weight and thus comprises about 25 percent of total systemic vascular compliance. In contrast, compliance of skeletal muscle was low; hindlimb compliance was only 0.48 ml $mmHg^{-1}$ kg^{-1} of tissue weight. Pulmonary compliance per kilogram of body weight is one-tenth of total systemic compliance, and per kilogram of lung tissue weight, pulmonary compliance is about 12 ml $mmHg^{-1}$. Thus, the distribution of blood volume among various organs is determined by their size and vascular compliance—*and by the fraction of cardiac output they receive.* Sight should not be lost of the fact that in humans, two of the largest vascular beds in terms of the percent of cardiac output they can receive have high compliance (splanchnic and cutaneous), whereas the largest vascular bed (skeletal muscle) has low specific and total compliance.

Capacitance. The capacitance of an organ relates its transmural pressure to the total volume contained within the vasculature (veins plus arteries). The term is drawn from an analogy with electrical circuits in which electrical capacitance is the ratio of stored charge to applied potential difference. It is important to keep in mind *that organ capacitance can change without a measurable change in compliance.* This stems from the distributed nature of venous compliances within the organs. In effect, the measurement of capacitance for an organ is relatively simple, but measurement of compliance requires determination of volume over a range of distending pressures. The apparent dissociation between capacitance and compliance is seen most readily when there is blood flow.

Stress-Relaxation, Delayed Compliance, and Creep. These properties, as defined above for isolated veins, also exist in intact organs. As with the other properties described for whole organs, the surrounding tissue matrix may contribute. Also, in organs with semirigid capsules, distension of the capsule could limit stress-relaxation and creep.

Summary. In summary, the specific compliances of different organs differ markedly. Some are stiff and some are quite flaccid. Organs that have high specific compliance and are a long distance from the heart would be expected to have large volumes per kilogram of tissue in upright posture, owing to their higher vascular transmural pressures. Despite the marked increase in arterial blood pressure with increased distance below the heart, blood flow would be unaffected by posture in a vascular system *lacking valves,* myogenic reactions, nerves, and hormonal influences in which veins and arteries were equally rigid. That is, hydrostatic pressure ($\rho g h$)

would be added equally to both arterial and venous vessels (Figure 1-2) so that net driving pressure is unchanged.

Venous Transmural Pressure
Importance of Extravascular Fluid Pressure

The key to our potential problems in the upright posture lies in the extent to which venous transmural pressure and volume increase. Figure 1-2, which shows the posturally induced increase in venous *mural* pressure in dependent regions of the body (i.e., ρgh), does not take into account any counterpressure exerted by the fluid in the extravascular spaces surrounding the veins. However, extravascular fluid does not form a continuous column; rather, discontinuities in these fluid "spaces" limit its effectiveness as a venous counterpressure. For example, in the simplest model, a long snake held vertically, interstitial fluid pressure does not match the hydrostatic gradient from head to tail (Scholander et al., 1968). This fluid exerts a pressure that is quite variable and not well quantified.

The giraffe provides a unique animal model for investigation of large gravitationally induced alterations in vascular transmural pressure (Figure 1-6). An adult giraffe is 5 to 6 m tall with the heart being more than 2 m above the ground. Venous pressures reach 150 to 180 mmHg in the veins of the lower limbs. Mean pressure near heart level is approximately 250 mmHg; it is approximately 75 mmHg at the level of the brain, nearly 2 m above the heart; and, at the feet, arterial pressures must exceed 400 mmHg. These high vascular transmural pressures were only partially counteracted by an extravascular or interstitial fluid pressure of 40 to 50 mmHg (this was measured in young giraffes only 4 m tall with venous pressures of 150 mmHg at the feet) (Figure 1-6). These high interstitial fluid pressures were supported by the carapace of a very tight and nondistensible skin and fascia surrounding the legs called by Hargens and colleagues (1987) a "giraffe antigravity suit."

Humans also have relatively thick fascial layers around their lower extremities but this and the elastic cutaneous coverings are much looser than the giraffe's. As a consequence, subcutaneous tissue pressures in the legs (outside of the muscle) are only slightly above those measured in supine posture, even after prolonged standing (Gauer and Thron, 1965). Subcutaneous tissue pressures in upright humans are only 2 to 3 mmHg. In short, the specific compliance of a human leg is very much greater than that of a giraffe leg.

An Abdominal "Water Jacket"

Are there extravascular hydrostatic forces in the abdominal cavity that serve as a "water jacket" around the visceral organs that counteract the hydrostatic pooling of blood in them?

The splanchnic region is the most compliant as well as the most capacious vascular bed, and it is below the heart in upright humans. The

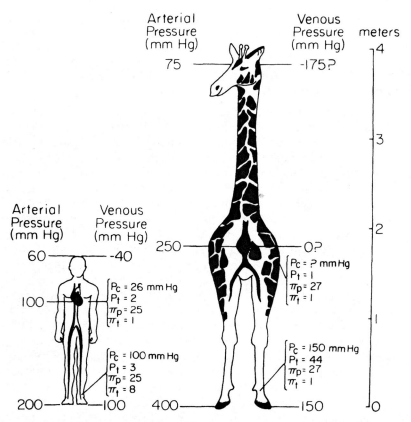

Figure 1-6 Comparison of arterial and hydrostatic pressures in an upright human and young (not full-grown) giraffe. In brackets are pressures (all in millimeters of mercury) inside and outside capillaries at heart level and foot level. (Pc = capillary pressure, Pt = surrounding tissue pressure, π_p = plasma oncotic pressure, π_t = tissue oncotic pressure). Pt in the giraffe helps to counteract filtration and edema. (Adapted from Hargens et al., 1987.)

importance of this region to orthostatic adjustments was recognized by clinical scientists in the last century, in particular by Hill and Barnard (1897). Death of rabbits held in vertical, head-up position could be prevented by binding the abdomen (McDowall, 1956). However, the abdominal wall of the rabbit is probably much more flaccid than that of dogs, cats, or humans (Gauer and Thron, 1965). Nevertheless, Edholm (1942) showed that the liver swells in cats placed in vertical position; when the cats' livers were removed, blood pressure no longer fell. In contrast, measurements in dogs held upright suggest that abdominal viscera are held in place by the rigid muscles of the abdominal wall (Rushmer, 1970; Wood, 1987). Pressures within the abdominal cavity increase linearly with height between the pelvis and diaphragm as though the adomen were a water-filled jacket that could counteract any intravascular hydrostatic pressure gradient and prevent passive pooling of blood in visceral organs. One could argue that anesthesia contributed to the lack of rigidity in the abdominal walls of the cats and rabbits.

More recent evidence discussed later in Chapters 2 and 4 reemphasizes the pivotal importance of the splanchnic region in the maintenance of arterial blood pressure during upright posture in humans. Failure to vasoconstrict visceral organs in upright posture leads to rapid collapse. Apparently the "water jacket" analogy is not applicable to humans and rabbits, who commonly lack the strong and rigid abdominal musculature of dogs.

Is There a Cerebral Siphon Effect?

The mural pressures of veins above the heart are negative if they are held open by surrounding structures, as are some cerebral veins. The veins that descend out from the cranium and down the neck to the heart are collapsible and therefore their mural pressures are not a function of the height of the hydrostatic column above the heart once they exit from the skull.

It has been postulated that the pressure-related work of the heart in driving blood uphill to the brain is reduced by a siphon effect. If a true siphon exists, no work would be done on blood to increase its gravitational potential energy because gravity returns the blood back down to heart level (Hicks and Badeer, 1989). Parenthetically, Hill and Barnard (1897) concluded that application of the siphon principle to the vascular system is "entirely fallacious because veins and arteries have such different distensibility and elasticity." A siphon occurs only in that portion of the circulation in which there is a continuous column of blood in both arterial and venous arms of the loop. For the cerebral circulation, a siphon could exist from the left ventricle to the point where veins leave the cranium and become collapsed, as shown in Figure 1-3. If the veins really collapse, the siphon effect is impossible because there can be no gravitational pressure gradient in them; during flow, the pressure at any point down the vein would be essentially atmospheric.

The giraffe again provides a unique example with its brain more than 2 m ($\rho g h$ = ~150 mmHg) above the heart. Whereas pressures within the arteries to the head match the difference in hydrostatic height above the heart, venous pressures do not. The jugular vein has many valves, especially near the head. Venous pressure is higher, by about 10 mmHg, up near to the head, than down close to the heart in an upright giraffe. This suggests that blood is compartmentalized in the jugular vein and thus a siphonlike mechanism would not be expected to aid jugular venous blood flow (see Seymour and Johansen, 1987).

Parenthetically, Figure 1-3 points to another complication. How would the siphon effect be altered by the tendency for cerebrospinal fluid pressures to counterbalance partially gravitational effects on cerebral veins?

In general (see "Structural Adaptations" below) all animals have arterial pressures that are capable of counteracting normal negative hydrostatic influences on cerebral perfusion without the aid of a siphon effect. In the giraffe, this requires a high aortic mean pressure, which, at 200 to 300 mmHg, is sufficient to provide adequate cerebral perfusion. Among the snakes (described below), some of which climb trees, blood pressure increases in proportion to the distance between the heart and the head (Lillywhite, 1985, 1987). With a true siphon the position of the heart in the vertical axis would be irrelevant.

STRUCTURAL FEATURES THAT COUNTERACT GRAVITATIONAL "POOLING"

What are those anatomical or structural features that restrict the translocation of blood away from the heart and into dependent vessels? The term "pooling" is commonly used to describe the increase in the volume of blood within dependent veins. This volume is not actually "pooled" or stationary in these veins, but its mean transit time through them is increased at a given blood flow because of the increased volume. Thus, return of blood to the heart is delayed. We sometimes speak of a lengthened "time constant" for venous return. The analogy is with electrical circuits containing significant capacitance.

Shape of Venous Volume-Pressure Curve

Inasmuch as most of the blood volume in upright humans is below venostatic level and most of this volume is in distensible tubes rather than stiff ones such as arteries, the volume of blood available to the heart is not adequate unless some active changes in the vascular system occur. On the other hand, if veins were as noncompliant as arteries, the hydrostatic effects of upright posture would be minimal, and one could view the vascular system simply as a rigid container. This prompts an obvious question: inasmuch as humans spend a large fraction of their lives in upright posture, of what evolutionary value is such a compliant venous system? Although the problem of hydrostatic "pooling" would be eliminated if veins were as stiff as arteries, this would also eliminate the capacitance function of veins, that is, the large changes in volume associated with small changes in transmural pressure. This volume *reservoir* function of veins allows substantial loss of blood with only small changes in venous pressure and, consequently, in arterial pressure as well.

The shape of the venous volume-pressure curve represents a *compromise in design* to meet two requirements. Again, the steep or compliant portion of the venous volume-pressure curve, which is the principal culprit in human orthostatic intolerance, is also the feature that permits our adjustment to blood loss. A second requirement is that veins be relatively stiff at high pressures so that further pooling is limited at the highest

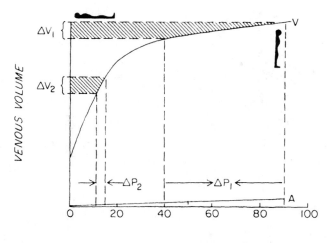

Figure 1-7 Approximate volume-pressure curve for human venous system (V), showing its compliant and stiff characteristics in supine versus upright posture. Line A shows approximate volume-pressure curve for arteries. ΔV_1 and ΔV_2 show equal volumes being passively released from veins by very large pressure drop (ΔP_1) in the stiff (ΔV_1) region of the curve, and small pressure drop (ΔP_2) in the most compliant region (ΔV_2) of the curve. (Adapted from Rowell, 1986.)

transmural pressures, as shown in Figure 1-7. Without this stiff portion of the volume-pressure curve, upright posture without hypotension would be impossible. Figure 1-7 could represent the volume-pressure curve of a human leg. The slope of the curve at the pressure at which it flattens and shows little further volume increase is a function of venous wall thickness.

Venous Valves

When humans suddenly stand up, the hydrostatic column of blood extending from the veins in the foot back up to the heart is broken up by a series of valves. As illustrated in Figure 1-8, the hydrostatic column is short at the onset of upright posture, but as blood continues to flow from the arteries into the dependent veins, they fill up with blood and the valves are forced open in a heartward progression until there is an uninterrupted hydrostatic column between the right atrium and the feet. When all the valves are open, an estimated 600 ml of blood has been displaced from the central circulation into the dependent vessels, mainly veins of the legs (Sjostrand, 1952; Ludbrook, 1966). The rate at which the veins fill up with blood is determined by the rate at which blood flows into them (see Chapter 2). If leg blood flow is normal, the full hydrostatic effects are not seen for approximately 2 minutes (Henry and Gauer, 1950). If blood flow is high,

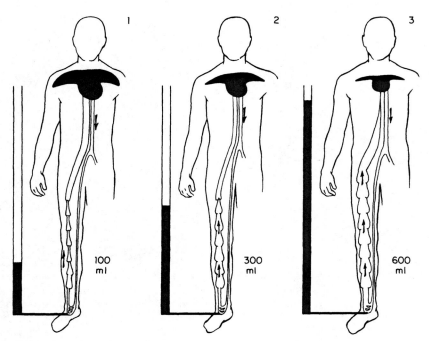

Figure 1-8   Time-dependent effect of venous valves on volume displacement during a sudden shift to upright posture (*left*). Progressive opening of venous valves by inflowing blood with maintained upright posture increases the length of the hydrostatic column and the volume of pooled blood. See text for details. (From Rowell, 1986, with permission from Oxford University Press.)

as in a hot environment, the veins fill within 2 or 3 seconds. Parenthetically, the circulatory effects of actively standing up are different from those of being passively tilted upright (Sprangers, 1990). The muscle contractions associated with standing transiently alter muscle vascular resistance and mechanically reduce muscle venous volume.

Patients whose venous valves are incompetent or are congenitally absent suffer from severe orthostatic intolerance (Bevegård and Lodin, 1962). As soon as they stand up, the uninterrupted hydrostatic column between the heart and the dependent veins causes abrupt pooling of blood in the lower extremities. The sudden loss of ventricular filling pressure and consequent inability to maintain adequate cardiac output leads to abrupt syncope. The mechanism of syncope is discussed later in Chapter 4. These individuals can stand up with ease in water up to the level of the diaphragm as illustrated in Figure 1-9, or when tight leotards counteract the rise in venous transmural pressure. In the water bath, the surrounding fluid medium cancels hydrostatic increases in transmural pressure below the heart (Risch et al., 1978). This is the converse of the situation in the head, as mentioned earlier, where the negativity of cerebrospinal fluid

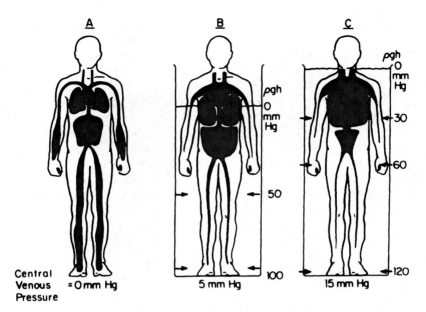

Figure 1-9 **(A)** Central venous pressure and blood volume distribution in upright human in air. **(B)** Immersed in water to level of diaphragm. **(C)** Immersed to chin. Densities of water and blood are similar so that water can counteract gravitational displacement of blood volume (effect of ρgh canceled). In Figure B, water level simulates supine posture (water pressure = venous hydrostatic pressure in legs; water hydrostatic pressures shown beside the tank). Figure C shows additional hydrostatic effects of higher water levels: counterpressure squeezes blood flow from legs and visceral organs into the thorax, raising central venous pressure even higher. Thoracic engorgement with blood causes diuresis. See text and the discussion of vasopressin and water immersion in Chapter 3 in the section "Humoral Control." (From Rowell, 1986, with permission from Oxford University Press.)

pressure tends to counteract partially the negative venous mural pressures that collapse cerebral veins (Rushmer et al., 1947).

Position of the Heart

The closeness of the heart to the head determines how well the brain is perfused in upright posture, whereas the distance from the feet determines the hydrostatic force that causes venous "pooling." Were human hearts repositioned to midabdominal level, ρgh at the feet would decrease from approximately 100 mmHg to 80 mmHg, thereby lessening downward displacement of intravascular volume; however, intra-arterial pressure at the head would be reduced from approximately 60 mmHg down to 40 mmHg (where unconsciousness occurs). The importance of the location of the heart within the body is particularly obvious in snakes in which the long intravascular fluid columns are uniquely susceptible to hydrostatic effects of gravity. Apparently the most consistent morphological adjustment of snakes to environmental gravitational forces is the position of the heart along the long axis of the body (Lillywhite, 1985, 1987). Figure 1-10 reveals the effects of vertical orientation on a tree-climbing or arboreal snake, a nonclimbing terrestrial snake, and a sea snake. The adaptations that protect each type of snake represent compromises in design. The proximity of the heart to the head in arboreal snakes maximizes cerebral perfusion pressure when they are vertical, but it also minimizes hydrostatic pooling—which is counteracted by the slender body. Surprisingly, snakes appear to lack venous valves but have developed instead localized constrictions of vascular smooth muscle that restrict retrograde flow (Lillywhite, 1987). In terrestrial snakes, the heart is closer to the midbody

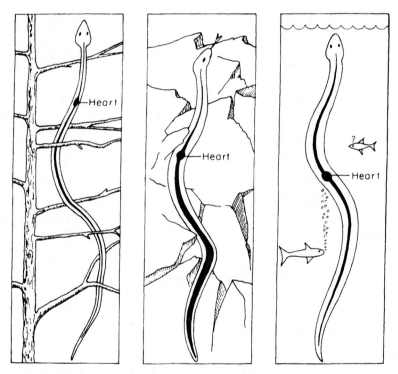

Figure 1-10 Effects of vertical position on the circulatory systems of three types of snake: a climbing (tree) snake (*left*), a terrestrial snake (*middle*), and a sea snake (*right*). The closeness of the heart to the head protects the brain, and the slim body and tight skin minimizes vascular pooling in the tree snake. In the terrestrial snake, shown climbing a vertical rock face, neither the brain nor dependent regions fare well because of the heart's relatively long distance from both regions. The position of the heart in the sea snake is less important, inasmuch as effects of gravity are counteracted by the sea; however, its position in midbody minimizes distances to which the heart must pump blood. (Redrawn from Lillywhite, 1988).

position where energy costs of cardiac pumping to distant tissues are minimized, but the effects of gravity on venous return when the snake is vertical are severe. In the sea snakes, the heart is closest to midbody. They experience no hydrostatic forces when held up vertically in the water.

Microcirculation and Edema Formation

The leakage of fluid out of the capillaries and into the tissue spaces is determined by the hydrostatic pressure and to a much smaller extent by tissue oncotic pressure. Capillary oncotic pressure and tissue hydrostatic pressure oppose filtration. This is still called the Starling-Landis "hypothesis," but it is no longer considered a hypothesis. In tall animals like humans and giraffes, gravitational forces can impose extremely high pressures on the microvasculature. Increased filtration leads to edema, and the eventual rise in hydrostatic pressure of tissues surrounding capillaries will arrest filtration. The customary textbook depiction of the Starling-Landis principle, as shown at the bottom of Figure 1-11, applies to a skeletal muscle capillary at *heart level*. When animals stand up, capillaries are exposed to

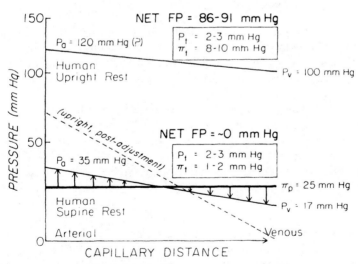

Figure 1-11 Estimated net outward filtration pressures (FP) in human skeletal muscle capillaries at heart (venostatic) level (lower Pa − Pv line, Pv = 17 mmHg) and at foot level (upper line with Pv = 100 mmHg) in an upright human. (Values from Hargens et al., 1981.) Symbols Pa, Pt, π_p, and π_t are defined in Figure 1-6 and text (Pv = postcapillary venous pressure). Pressure at the arterial end of the capillary in upright posture (*top*) assumes a pressure drop from 200 mmHg in the large arteries to 120 mmHg in the small arterioles. The dashed line (upright postadjustment) estimates effects of regional vasoconstriction and the muscle pump on Pa, Pv, and net FP, which, as shown, would still be greater than zero.

drastically altered pressure gradients, shown by the upper line in Figure 1-11, in which outward filtration pressure reaches 91 mmHg. This figure also shows how reflexes can adjust filtration pressure, and this aspect of the figure is covered in Chapter 2.

Above the hydrostatic indifferent point reabsorption is favored, whereas filtration is dominant below this point. When humans become upright, the shifts of volume into peripheral vessels and the surrounding tissue matrix are time-dependent. Volume leaves the vascular compartment rapidly at first so that plasma volume falls by about 10 percent.

The giraffe has unique structural adaptation to upright posture. Arterial pressure can reach 400 mmHg in the feet (Figure 1-6). Capillary pressure is not known but must be close to the venous pressure at 2 to 2.5 m below the heart (150 to 180 mmHg). Direct measurements in the lower limbs of young giraffes (4 m tall, heart 2 m above the feet) reveal the following: (1) venous pressure (Pv) reached 150 mmHg; (2) subcutaneous tissue pressure (Pt) was high at 40 to 50 mmHg; (3) plasma oncotic pressure (π_p) was normal at 27 mmHg; and (4) tissue oncotic pressure (π_t) was low at approximately 1 mmHg. Net filtration pressure (FP) in the lower legs ranged from 88 to 152 mmHg (Hargens et al., 1981).

$$FP = (Pc - Pt) - (\pi_p - \pi_t)$$
$$FP = (150 - 44) - (27 - 1) = 80 \text{ mmHg} \tag{1-1}$$

Capillary pressure (Pc) in Equation 1-1 and Figure 1-6 was assumed to equal Pv, venous pressure. Based on these measurements, net filtration pressure would be approximately 80 mmHg. From the same measurements made above the heart in the neck of the giraffe, a net *reabsorptive* pressure of −7 mmHg was calculated.

Equivalent values for net filtration pressure at the feet in an upright 190-cm human, based on measurements of Hargens and collagues (1981) and shown in Figure 1-11, would be approximately 85 to 90 mmHg. The higher tissue oncotic pressure in humans (π_t = 8 mmHg) stems from "leaky" capillaries. Thus, the giraffe appears to be better protected against edema formation than humans. The giraffe's protection comes from several morphological features referred to as its "antigravity suit" (Hargens et al., 1987). The capillaries of its legs are highly impermeable to protein, owing to thick capillary basement membranes, the thickness of which is two times greater in leg muscles than in neck muscles (the same relative differences also exist in human capillaries, but their permeability to protein is greater in humans). In the giraffe, leg arterial wall hypertrophy provides a potential for greater changes in vascular resistance, and a prominent, valved lymphatic system within a tight carapace of thick skin and fascia force blood upward through one-way valves against the gravitational pressure gradient and prevents "pooling" (Hargens et al., 1987).

Human legs are highly susceptible to edema owing mainly to their relatively high total compliance and "leaky" (relative to the giraffe) capil-

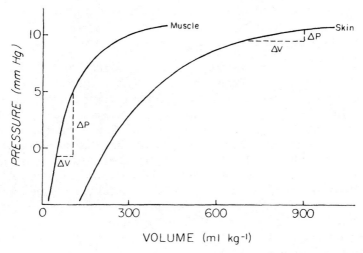

Figure 1-12 Pressure-volume curves showing interstitial compliance of skin and skeletal muscle. This compliance is three times greater in skin than in muscle. (Adapted from Renkin, 1989.)

laries. Nearly one-half of our total mass is in the legs, and their cutaneous and fascial covering is relatively loose and distensible. Also, as much as one-third to one-half of the total limb blood flow passes through skin that has unusually high interstitial compliance (see Figure 1-12) (Renkin, 1989) (as mentioned previously, tissue pressure deep within the muscle during standing can be quite high). Therefore, some of the inability of humans to maintain adequate cardiac output after prolonged head-up tilt with leg muscles relaxed stems from the following:

1. Total vascular compliance of the legs is high so that they accommodate a large volume of blood at elevated hydrostatic pressures.
2. The high transmural pressures cause viscoelastic creep and continued distension of venous walls, meaning that their volume will continue to increase over prolonged periods (delayed compliance).
3. Capillary pressures at high, subcutaneous tissue pressure is low, and its oncotic pressure is high, so that filtration proceeds until the rise in tissue fluid pressure and in plasma oncotic pressure counterbalance the outward filtration force; thus edema represents a self-limiting feature that reduces both filtration and venous transmural pressure, thereby limiting vascular capacitance in the legs.

Usually syncope (discussed in Chapter 4) precedes equilibration of these pressures, particularly when the changes are rapid (Chapter 4).

MECHANICAL ADJUSTMENTS TO ORTHOSTASIS

The Muscle Pump

Totally passive upright posture, as in a head-up tilt, is a potentially lethal stress for many animals. Sequestration of blood continues for long periods due to the slow stress-relaxation or delayed compliance of dependent veins. High capillary transmural pressures cause continued filtration into tissue spaces that vary markedly in their compliance among the species. In the previous section, the compliant human limbs were compared to the highly noncompliant limbs of the giraffe. In humans, the volume of blood eventually sequestered in the dependent veins and the volume of plasma ultrafiltrate lost from vasculature into tissue spaces will reduce ventricular filling pressure to a point where adequate cardiac output can no longer be maintained. The consequent fall in arterial blood pressure will lead to unconsciousness and eventually to the lethal effects of cerebral ischemia is supine posture is not quickly restored.

There are marked differences in human tolerance to upright posture that depend on whether this posture is maintained by standing or by suspension at the crotch in passive head-up tilt. Amberson (1943) stressed that the skeletal muscle tone during upright standing, in the absence of any movement, has critical bearing on the quantity of blood displaced into the legs. Even during quiet standing with all movement consciously stopped, rhythmic changes in the activity of the antigravity muscles act to decrease venous transmural pressure, as illustrated in Figure 1-13. Amberson cited work from the 1930s that revealed a relationship between syncope and intramuscular pressures. Intramuscular pressure was 200 to

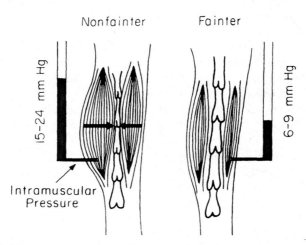

Figure 1-13 Intramuscular pressures in normal nonfainters during quiet standing (*left*) and in patients after surgery or prolonged bed rest (fainters, *right*). Intramuscular pressures reflect muscle tone, which is low in fainters (see Amberson, 1943).

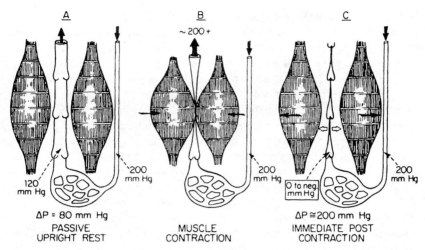

Figure 1-14 Muscle pump—the "second heart." **(A)** Passive upright rest (stable period). Arterial and venous driving pressure plus ρgh are 200 and 120 mmHg with a net driving pressure into veins of 80 mmHg (as shown in Figure 1-2). **(B)** Muscle contraction empties the veins, momentarily blocks arterial inflow, and greatly increases venous driving pressure back toward the heart (ρgh, 120 mmHg + maximal driving pressure; 70 to 90 mmHg). **(C)** Immediately after contraction, pressure in emptied veins falls to zero (valves momentarily prevent back flow and back pressure) and arterial to venous driving pressure is *momentarily* raised to 200 mmHg (200 to 0 mmHg) in *upright* posture. (Adapted from Rowell, 1986.)

320 mmH$_2$O (15 to 24 mmHg) in nonfainters during head-up tilt and only 80 to 120 mmH$_2$O (6 to 9 mmHg) in fainters. Intramuscular pressure is depressed after prolonged bed rest and also after surgery, and similar changes could contribute to the orthostatic intolerance following prolonged weightlessness during space flight (Blomqvist and Stone, 1983).

The Second Heart

Without a second heart on the return or venous side of the circulation, upright humans clearly cannot force enough blood back to the right ventricle to maintain adequate cardiac output. In combination with competent venous valves, the skeletal muscles of the leg serve as an effective pump, driving blood back to the heart. Contracting muscles can generate a driving force of 90 mmHg as illustrated in Figure 1-14 (Shepherd, 1963; Stegall, 1966). Also, muscle-pumping capacity must be similar to that of the left ventricle (see Chapter 7). Ventricular filling pressure and stroke volume are restored rapidly by only modest muscle contractions while standing in stationary position (Wang et al., 1960). In contrast, when venous valves are incompetent, the mucle pump becomes ineffective, and syncope rapidly follows a shift to upright posture. Chapter 5 points out that the overall effectiveness of the muscle pump depends on the proportion of total leg blood flow that passes through extramuscular tissues of the limbs. For example, when cutaneous arterioles are dilated along with those of muscle, the muscle pump acts mainly to empty muscle veins. As a consequence, total venous volume of the leg is increased despite maintained effectiveness of the muscle pump on venous return from muscle (see Figure 6-13).

The muscle pump, in addition to its effects on venous volume in the muscle, also influences muscle blood flow at any given perfusion pressure. Immediately after each muscle contraction, the veins are empty and venous valves prevent any back flow so that venous mural pressure is momentarily near zero (possibly below zero, owing to elastic recoil of relaxed muscles away from empty veins) (Laughlin, 1987). At this instant, the arteriovenous pressure gradient is maximum in upright posture; the hydrostatic and dynamic components of pressure are summed on the arterial side and both are momentarily missing on the venous side. The latter point is fundamental to understanding why patients with atherosclerosis obliterans and restricted leg circulation experience relief from the pain of ischemia when they contract leg muscles in the dependent posture. The increased pressure gradient caused by the combined effects of gravity and the muscle pump increases muscle perfusion (often through collateral vessels). This also explains why peak flows to exercising legs are much higher in upright than in supine posture (Folkow et al., 1971) (see Chapter 7).

In addition to its effect on muscle perfusion, the muscle pump also alters the blood and tissue fluid pressures that govern transcapillary exchange of fluid. Muscle contraction not only lowers local venous pressure (see Figure 1-11) but it also raises extravascular fluid pressure. Direct measurements in the legs of walking giraffes showed striking oscillations in intra-arterial ($+70$ to $+380$ mmHg), venous (-250 to $+240$ mmHg), and tissue fluid pressures (-120 to $+80$ mmHg) (Hargens et al., 1987). These pressure excursions, particularly the extremely large negative values, are probably exaggerated by effects of inertia on pressure gauges during movement. Nevertheless, the muscle pump clearly prevents edema; plasma oncotic pressure does not rise in dependent foot veins when the muscle pump is active.

The Respiratory Pump

The significance of a respiratory pump on venous return was debated for centuries after the early observations of Valsalva (1666–1723). The argument opposing the pump idea was that the negative pressure in the thorax would collapse the veins during inspiration so that the respiratory pump could not increase venous return (see Brecher, 1956; Moreno et al., 1969). Brecher showed this collapse to be a time-dependent phenomenon that would curtail caval blood flow only if the downstream fall in intravascular pressure was too prolonged or unusually deep. Subsequently, Wexler and colleagues (1968) directly measured an acceleration of vena caval blood flow in normal humans during inspiration (and exercise increased this inspiratory acceleration).

Breathing changes transmural pressure in the great veins passing through the thoracic cavity. A deepening of *inspiration* in upright posture lowers intrathoracic pressure and increases the pressure gradient between the right atrium and the point where the inferior vena cava enters the thoracic cavity. Figure 1-15 shows that breathing has considerable effect on venous return (Brecher, 1956; Moreno et al., 1967). Several factors influence the effectiveness of the respiratory pump. The downward descent of the diaphragm with *inspiration* lowers intrathoracic pressure as elastic lung tissue is stretched. Inspiration raises intra-abdominal pressure so that the gradient between the abdomen and the thorax is increased, causing the inferior vena cava to discharge blood centrally. In addition, the inferior vena cava is shortened and the reduction in its volume contributes more blood flow to the thorax. Toward the end of inspiration the increased intra-abdominal pressure temporarily impedes venous flow from the legs into the abdomen.

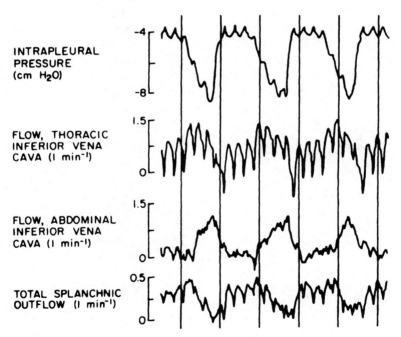

INTRAPLEURAL
PRESSURE
(cm H$_2$O)

FLOW, THORACIC
INFERIOR VENA
CAVA (l min^{-1})

FLOW, ABDOMINAL
INFERIOR VENA
CAVA (l min^{-1})

TOTAL SPLANCHNIC
OUTFLOW (l min^{-1})

Figure 1-15 Respiratory-induced alternation in abdominal caval flow (just below the liver) and hepatic venous outflow (the two flows are 180° out of phase). Inspiration reduced intrapleural pressure, increased abdominal caval flow immediately below the liver, and stopped hepatic outflow; expiration did the opposite so that excursions in thoracic inferior vena caval flow above the liver and also thoracic blood volume and central venous pressure were minimized. (Adapted from Moreno et al., 1967, From Rowell, 1986, with permission from Oxford University Press.)

Expiration lowers intra-abdominal pressure and releases blood flow from the legs as the diaphragm relaxes and ascends. The concomitant rise in intrathoracic pressure toward atmospheric pressure as tension within the inflated lungs is released retards inflow to the heart. Also, expiration elongates the inferior vena cava and increases its volume so that blood flow from the abdomen to the thorax is slowed.

Moreno and colleagues (1967) explained the importance of the liver as a pre-right ventricular sump that smooths out the fluctuations in venous return caused by breathing (see Figures 1-15 and 1-16). The mechanical compression of hepatic veins that occurs as the diaphragm descends onto them during inspiration virtually stops hepatic venous outflow. At the same time, hepatic inflow continues and the liver swells rapidly with blood (hepatic specific compliance is 10 times greater than that of systemic vascular bed [Rothe, 1983]). During expiration, which retards inferior vena caval flow into the thorax, the compression of hepatic veins is relieved by the ascent of the diaphragm. The contents of the liver are rapidly discharged into the right atrium by the elastic recoil of the distended hepatic vasculature. This purely mechanical effect on the liver causes hepatic venous outflow to rise and fall out of phase with the rise and fall in caval flow into the thorax. The result is that the respiratory oscillations in central venous pressure are smoothed out. In patients with noncompliant livers caused by cirrhosis, liver volume varies little during inspiration and expiration with the consequence being large respiratory excursions in venous return and right ventricular filling pressure (Moreno and Burchell, 1982).

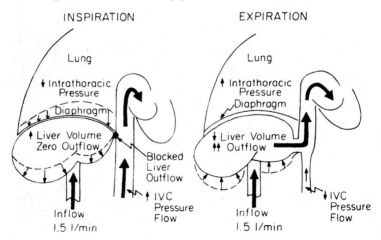

Figure 1-16 Interaction between diaphragm and liver blood volume during inspiration (*left*) and expiration—the *respiratory pump*. Descent of diaphragm in inspiration reduces intrathoracic pressure and mechanically stops hepatic venous outflow while inflow continues and liver swells. Increased inferior vena caval pressure accelerates venous return. Expiration reverses the process, but venous return is partially maintained by passive release (elastic recoil) of hepatic blood back to right atrium (see Moreno and Burchell, 1982).

The effects of breathing on right and left ventricular outputs is treated in more detail in Chapter 2.

SUMMARY

In summary, despite the structural features that counteract gravitational shifts in blood volume, about 500 to 600 ml of blood move into the legs and another 200- to 300-ml shift into the veins of the buttocks and pelvic area during quiet standing. Much of this volume is translocated from the thoracic vessels (Sjostrand, 1952). If total systemic vascular compliance is actually 2.5 ml mmHg^{-1} kg^{-1} body weight, then the commonly observed fall of 5 mmHg in central venous pressure means that, in a human weighing 75 kg, approximately 940 ml of blood would be translocated out of the central circulation (2.5 × 75 kg × 5 mmHg) *if cardiac output were to remain constant*. As discussed later, the fact that cardiac output falls in upright posture means that this volume is probably an underestimate.

The shifts in blood volume into peripheral veins and the surrounding tissue matrix are time-dependent. Volume leaves the vascular compartment slowly at first and plasma volume falls by about 10 to 12 percent due to the increased filtration stemming from the rise in capillary hydrostatic pressure (Sejrsen et al., 1981). This filtration has the effect of a delayed compliance change. As filtration proceeds, the increase in extravascular volume and pressure (i.e., edema) represents a self-limiting feature; the rise in tissue pressure reduces both filtration and venous transmural pressure. In effect, filtration will eventually tend to reduce vascular capacitance in the legs, but at the same time, the "delayed compliance" or viscoelastic properties of the veins cause a slow expansion of their volume at a given transmural pressure (i.e., increased capacitance).

The passive effects of gravity on blood flow are in some cases lessened above the heart (e.g., cerebral blood flow) by the counteracting effects of gravity on surrounding fluid pressures (e.g., cerebrospinal fluid). In some animals, extravascular fluid pressure below heart level also counteracts the effects of increased transmural pressure, as in the legs and abdominal cavities of some species. These adjustments seem not to be important in humans. The most important structural adjustments that counteract gravitational pooling are the shape of the venous pressure-volume curve, the venous valves, and the position of the heart in the body. The most important mechanical adjustments to counteract orthostatic pooling are the muscle and respiratory pumps.

REFRENCES

Allen, R. (1986). Intracranial pressure: a review of clinical problems, measurement techniques and monitoring methods. *J. Med. Eng. Technol. 10,* 299–320.

Amberson, W.R. (1943). Physiologic adjustments to the standing posture. Univ. Md. Sch. Med. Bull. 27, 127–145.

Bevegård, S., and A. Lodin (1962). Postural circulatory changes at rest and during exercise in five patients with congenital absence of valves in the deep veins of the legs. *Acta Med. Scand. 172*, 21–29.

Blomqvist, C.G., and H.L. Stone (1983). Cardiovascular adjustments to gravitational stress. In J.T. Shepherd, F.M. Abboud, and S.R. Geiger, eds. *Handbook of Physiology. The Cardiovascular System: Peripheral Circulation and Organ Blood Flow*, sect. 2, vol. III, part 2, pp. 1025–1063. American Physiological Society, Bethesda, MD.

Bradley, K.C. (1970). Cerebrospinal fluid pressure. *J. Neurol. Neurosurg. Psychiatry 33*, 387–397.

Brecher, G.A. (1956). *Venous Return*. Grune & Stratton, New York.

Conrad, M. (1971). *Functional Anatomy of the Circulation to the Lower Extremities*. Year Book, Chicago.

Davson, H. (1967). The cerebrospinal fluid-pressure. In *Physiology of the Cerebrospinal Fluid*, pp. 337–382. Little, Brown, Boston.

Echt, M., J. Düweling, O.H. Gauer, and L. Lange (1974). Effective compliance of the total vascular bed and the intrathoracic compartment derived from changes in the central venous pressure induced by volume changes in man. *Circ. Res. 34*, 61–68.

Edholm, O.G. (1942). The compensatory mechanism of the splanchnic circulation during changes of posture. *J. Physiol. (Lond.) 101*, 1–10.

Folkow, B., U. Haglund, M. Jodal, and O. Lundgren (1971). Blood flow in the calf muscle of man during heavy rhythmic exercise. *Acta Physiol. Scand. 81*, 157–163.

Franklin, K.J. (1937). *A Monograph on Veins*. C.C. Thomas, Springfield, IL.

Gauer, O.H., and H.L. Thron (1965). Postural changes in the circulation. In W.F. Hamilton and P. Dow, eds. *Handbook of Physiology. Circulation*, sect. 2, vol. III, pp. 2409–2439. American Physiological Society, Washington, D.C.

Gow, B.S. (1980). Circulatory correlates: vascular impedance, resistance, and capacity. In D.F. Bohr, A.P. Somlyo, and H.V. Sparks Jr., eds. *Handbook of Physiology. The Cardiovascular System: Vascular Smooth Muscle*, sect. 2, vol. II, pp. 353–408. American Physiological Society, Bethesda, MD.

Hargens, A.R., J.B. Cologne, F.J. Menninger, J.S. Hogan, B.J. Tucker, and R.M. Peters (1981). Normal transcapillary pressures in human skeletal muscle and subcutaneous tissues. *Microvasc. Res. 22*, 177–189.

Hargens, A.R., R.W. Millard, K. Pettersson, and K. Johansen (1987). Gravitational haemodynamics and oedema prevention in the giraffe. *Nature 329*, 59–60.

Heistad, D.D., and H.A. Kontos (1983). Cerebral circulation. In J.T. Shepherd and F.M. Abboud, eds. *Handbook of Physiology. The Cardiovascular System: Peripheral Circulation and Organ Blood Flow*, sect. 2, vol. III, part 1, pp. 137–182. American Physiological Society, Bethesda, MD.

Henry, J.P., and O.H. Gauer (1950). The influence of temperature upon venous pressure in the foot. *J. Clin. Invest. 29*, 855–861.

Hicks, J.W., and H.S. Badeer (1989). Siphon mechanism in collapsible tubes: application to circulation of the giraffe head. *Am. J. Physiol. 256 (Regulatory Integrative Comp. Physiol. 25)*, R567–R571.

Hill, L. (1895). The influence of the force of gravity on the circulation of the blood. *J. Physiol. (Lond.) 18*, 15–53.

Hill, L., and H. Barnard (1897). The influence of the force of gravity on the circulation. *J. Physiol. (Lond.) 21*, 323–352.

Laughlin, M.H. (1987). Skeletal muscle blood flow capacity: role of muscle pump in exercise hyperemia. *Am. J. Physiol. 253 (Heart Circ. Physiol. 22)*, H993–H1004.

Lillywhite, H.B. (1985). Postural edema and blood pooling in snakes. *Physiol. Zool. 58*, 759–766.

Lillywhite, H.B. (1987). Circulatory adaptations of snakes to gravity. *Am. Zool. 27*, 81–95.

Lillywhite, H.B. (1988). Snakes, blood circulation and gravity. *Sci. Am (Dec.)*, 92–98.

Ludbrook, J. (1966). *Aspects of Venous Function in the Lower Limbs*. C.C. Thomas, Springfield, IL.

McDowall, R.J.S. (1956). *The Control of the Circulation of the Blood*. Dawson, London.

Moreno, A.H., and A.R. Burchell (1982). Respiratory regulation of splanchnic and systemic venous return in normal subjects and in patients with hepatic cirrhosis. *Surg. Gynecol. Obstet. 154*, 257–267.

Moreno, A.H., A.R. Burchell, R. van der Woude, and J.H. Burke (1967). Respiratory regulation of splanchnic and systemic venous return. *Am. J. Physiol. 213*, 455–465.

Moreno, A.H., A.I. Katz, and L.D. Gold (1969). An integrated approach to the study of the venous system with steps toward a detailed model of the dynamics of venous return to the right heart. *IEEE Trans. Bio-Med. Eng. BME-16*, 308–324

Renkin, E.M. (1989). Microcirculation and exchange. In H.D. Patton, A.F. Fuchs, B. Hille, A.M. Scher, and R. Steiner, eds. *Textbook of Physiology. Circulation, Respiration, Body Fluids, Metabolism, and Endocrinology*, 21st ed., vol. 2, pp. 860–878. W.B. Saunders, Philadelphia.

Risch, W.D., H.J. Koubenec, U. Beckmann, S. Lange, and O.H. Gauer (1978). The effect of graded immersion on heart volume, central venous pressure, pulmonary blood distribution, and heart rate in man. *Pflugers Arch. 374*, 115–118.

Rothe, C.F. (1983). Venous system: physiology of the capacitance vessels. In J.T. Shepherd and F.M. Abboud, eds. *Handbook of Physiology. The Cardiovascular System: Peripheral Circulation and Organ Blood Flow*, sect. 2, vol. III, part 1, pp. 397–452. American Physiological Society, Bethesda, MD.

Rowell, L.B. (1983). Cardiovascular adjustments to thermal stress. In J.T. Shepherd, F.M. Abboud, and S.R. Geiger, eds. *Handbook of Physiology. The Cardiovscular System: Peripheral Circulation and Organ Blood Flow*, sect. 2, vol. III, part 2, pp. 927–1023. American Physiological Society, Bethesda, MD.

Rowell, L.B. (1986). *Human Circulation. Regulation During Physical Stress*. Oxford University Press, New York.

Rushmer, R.F. (1970). *Cardiovascular Dynamics*. W.B. Saunders, Philadelphia.

Rushmer, R.F., E.L. Beckman, and D. Lee (1947). Protection of the cerebral circulation by the cerebrospinal fluid under the influence of radial acceleration. *Am. J. Physiol. 151*, 355–365.

Scholander, P.F., A.R. Hargens, and S.L. Miller (1968). Negative pressure in the interstitial fluid of animals. *Science 161*, 321–328.

Sejrsen, P., O. Henriksen, W.P. Paaske, and S.L. Nielsen (1981). Duration of increase in vascular volume during venous stasis. *Acta Physiol. Scand. 111,* 293–298.

Seymour, R.S., and K. Johansen (1987). Blood flow uphill and downhill: does a siphon facilitate circulation above the heart? *Comp. Biochem. Physiol. 88A,* 167–170.

Shepherd, J.T. (1963). *Physiology of the Circulation in Human Limbs in Health and Disease.* W.B. Saunders, Philadelphia.

Sjostrand, T. (1952). The regulation of the blood distribution in man. *Acta Physiol. Scand. 26,* 312–327.

Sprangers, R.L.H. (1990). *On the Role of Cardiopulmonary Receptors at the Onset of Muscular Exercise.* Rodopi, Amsterdam.

Stegall, H.F. (1966). Muscle pumping in the dependent leg. *Circ. Res. 19,* 180–190.

Wang, Y., R.J. Marshall, and J.T. Shepherd (1960). The effect of changes in posture and of graded exercise on stroke volume in man. *J. Clin. Invest. 39,* 1051–1061.

West, J.B. (1965). *Ventilation/Blood Flow and Gas Exchange.* Blackwell, Oxford, UK.

Wexler, L., D.H. Bergel, I.T. Gabe, G.S. Makin, and C.J. Mills (1968). Velocity of blood flow in normal human venae cavae. *Circ. Res. 23,* 349–359.

Wood, E.H. (1987). Some effects of the force environment on the heart, lungs and circulation. *Clin. Invest. Med. 10,* 401–427.

2

Reflex Control During Orthostasis

BRIEF HISTORY

The studies of Hill (1895) and Hill and Barnard (1897) extended beyond hydrostatic effects on the circulation. Even without a knowledge of arterial baroreflexes, their two publications on vasomotor adjustments are nevertheless classics that encourage humility.

Hill (1895) states: "... that pressure falls in the carotid artery under the influence of gravity in the feet-down posture, and rises in the feet-up posture, that compensation takes place more or less in normal animals (that is to say, the hydrostatic moment [which he also called a hydrostatic indifferent point] is compensated for by a dynamic moment), that this compensation takes place by vaso-constriction in the splanchnic area in the feet-down position—within some cases cardiac acceleration—and by cardiac inhibition and by vasodilation in the feet-up position...."

The same importance assigned to the passive dynamic effects of respiration on the volume of the splanchnic reservoir was also assigned to vasomotor control. Hill and Barnard concluded that, if the vasomotor system is intact and people are essentially healthy, arterial blood pressure (mean) does not fall and may even rise on assumption of upright posture. They stated "so long as the vaso-motor mechanism is intact, the splanchnic area forms the resistance box of the circulation and the effect of gravity is of no importance." The importance of vasomotor control in the legs was not recognized until later.

In 1885 L. Hermann observed that when the position of an animal is changed, the consequent changes in pressure will depend on "(a) the altered relationship of level between the given spot and the rest of the vascular system (hydrostatic moment), (b) the altered relation between pressure and resistance produced indirectly by the change in position on the heart beat, the filling of the heart, the vasomotor nerves, etc. (dynamic moment)." Hermann was emphasizing the importance of the position of the "hydrostatic indifferent point" in the vascular system (McDowall, 1956). Hill (1895) recognized that it was impossible to find the true hydrostatic indifferent point on a dead animal "because such indifferent point depends on the coefficient of elasticity which must constantly alter in the living animal with every alteration of the arterioles by vaso-constriction or dilation.... The compensation with individual differences is incomplete in nearly all rabbits, cats, and dogs, but in monkeys it is far more complete." Hill (1895) considered compensation (the adjustments to upright position) to be most complete in humans.

With remarkable insight, Hill and Barnard (1897) considered the manner in which vasomotor adjustments altered the circulation. They disputed the idea of William Bayliss and Ernest Starling that reflexes would act to alter what they termed as "static mean pressure" (later called "mean circulatory pressure" by Guyton). Hill and Barnard also disputed the notion of Bayliss and Starling that contraction of the arterioles raised arterial pressure by diminishing the capacity of the vascular system. Bayliss and Starling used vena cava pressure as an index of the changes in tension produced by reduction of capacity. Hill and Barnard (1897) stated that *"so long as the heart remains constant, which is a sine qua non in such experiments, the pulmonary arterial or venous pressure would afford an equally good index.* We hold that constriction of the arterioles does not cause a rise of pressure by diminishing the capacity of the vascular system because the system as a whole is not filled to distension by the blood it contains because the container is not full" (they thought mean circulatory pressure was essentially zero). Bayliss and Starling provided examples of elevations in vena cava pressure which they felt were due to vasoconstriction causing a diminution in the *"capacity"* of the vascular system. Hill and Barnard felt that the rise in venous pressure could be due either to the *failure of the heart to maintain its output* or to a diminution in the capacity of the *venous* system (they assumed the latter was mechanical). They concluded that the main effect of vasoconstriction was on vascular resistance, in accordance with Ohm's law, and not on vascular capacity. Hill and Barnard may have been the first to realize (or at least to express the idea) that changes in central venous pressure cannot be assigned to any active vascular change unless cardiac output is held constant.

The effect of cardiac output on central venous pressure and the distribution of blood volume is of central importance in cardiovascular physiology. This concept is emphasized in this book because of its pivotal importance in understanding how vascular capacitance, ventricular filling pressure, and the distribution of blood volume are altered by both active and passive mechanisms.

The rise in diastolic pressure during upright posture was assumed very early to indicate that a compensatory vasoconstriction had occurred. From his systematic study of systolic and diastolic pressures in the tibial artery in different postures, Francesco in 1921 concluded that blood vessels of the legs were constricted in upright posture (McDowall, 1956). In 1930, Florkin and colleagues estimated that assumption of upright posture caused a 50 percent decreasein blood flow to the legs, based on changes in venous oxygen saturation.

The effect of posture and gravity in producing edema in dependent parts was also recognized early. In 1887, Klemensiewicz pointed out that the vasoconstriction he observed in the frog's (dependent) web not only served arterial pressure regulation, but it also lowered capillary pressure and prevented edema (McDowall, 1956). Youmans and colleagues (1935) attributed part of the increase in volume of dependent human legs to edema. They observed a rise in the protein concentration of venous blood draining a quiet dependent leg and no change in the contralateral active leg.

Clinical studies during the 1930s and 1940s showed that "orthostatic hypotension" was caused by a failure of the "postural vasoconstrictor reflex" (Amberson, 1943).

The tachycardia associated with upright posture was recognized long ago, but documentation of the effect of gravity on cardiac output proved elusive, owing to the insensitivity of the methods available at that time. The results from a large number of experiments encompassed all three possibilities—cardiac output either increased, decreased, or did not change; on the "average" it appeared to be unaffected (Amberson, 1943; McDowall, 1956), but this appearance later proved to be false.

The basic mechanisms underlying the reflex cardiovascular adjustments to upright posture were not understood until the baroreceptors and their reflexes were discovered. Originally, activation of higher centers in the brain and possibly the vestibular apparatus were suspected (Amberson, 1943). McDowall (1924) described a pressor reflex originating from the right atrium and elicited by a fall in central venous and atrial pressure. Heymans' (1929) final proof that arterial blood pressure is controlled by baroreceptors in the carotid sinus and aortic arch provided a basic underlying mechanism for both cardiac and vasomotor control during orthostasis.

CIRCULATORY RESPONSES TO UPRIGHT POSTURE

The main objective of this chapter, after the initial circulatory adjustments to upright posture are described, is to present the evidence showing which adjustments are essential, which are not, and why. The second objective is to show what reflexes are active and important during orthostasis and to show where they must act in order to optimize the distribution of blood volume and to maintain arterial pressure. The details of sympathetic and humoral vasomotor control are covered in Chapter 3.

It is clear from the brief histories presented at the beginning of Chapter 1 and this chapter that despite the mechanical actions of the respiratory pump, and especially the muscle pump, adequate circulatory adjustment to upright posture requires active participation of the autonomic nervous system. Reflex adjustments mediated by both nerves and hormones would be expected to maintain arterial pressure in the following ways:

1. Increase heart rate and cardiac output
2. Increase peripheral vascular resistance
3. Decrease the rate at which dependent veins fill with blood

    4. Make blood available for filling the right and left ventricles

    5. Reduce fluid loss from the capillaries

One view is that adjustments 2 through 5 above require only constriction of the resistance vessels; others argue that constriction of the veins is required to minimize the fall in ventricular filling pressure. Another argument is that cardiac output cannot be increased during completely *passive* upright posture (orthostasis) because of the low ventricular filling pressure.

Although the importance of most of these adjustments in maintaining arterial blood pressure was recognized in the nineteenth and early twentieth centuries, it has taken us much longer to recognize that constriction of the resistance vessels may be the *only* adjustment that has primary importance.

Before dealing with the reflexes, a distinction between responses to actively standing up and being passively tilted to a vertical head-up position needs to be made. An active change in posture requires sudden vigorous contraction of large muscles. Reflex responses to this brief burst of activity do not keep pace with muscle vasodilation and arterial pressure falls as soon as contractions cease. The muscle vasodilation and initial fall in arterial pressure are not normally seen in passive head-up tilt (Sprangers et al., 1991).

Heart Rate and Cardiac Output

The most important point developed in this section is that because of the dominance of length-tension effects on the ventricle during upright posture (and this includes hemorrhage as well), reflexes have little effect on cardiac output.

The immediate responses to head-up tilt (90°) are summarized in Figure 2-1. The muscle pump is not active and about 500 to 600 ml of blood move into the veins of the legs and another 200 to 300 ml into the buttocks and pelvic area. The immediate downward translocation of blood volume is slowed by the venous valves so that 1 to 2 minutes (Henry and Gauer, 1950) may be required to fill the dependent veins and establish a continuous hydrostatic column of blood up to the heart (see Chapter 1).

Vagal Versus Sympathetic Control

The most rapid circulatory adjustment is the vagally mediated rise in heart rate; it occurs within one beat. For a few beats, tachycardia maintains left ventricular output, but due to the almost immediate fall in right ventricular stroke volume, the volume of blood in the pulmonary vasculature, the volume sump or "reservoir" for the left ventricle, is depleted. If the total pulmonary blood volume were 900 ml and stroke volume 100 ml, this entire reservoir could disappear in nine heartbeats. Clearly any significant imbalance between right and left ventricular output must be brief.

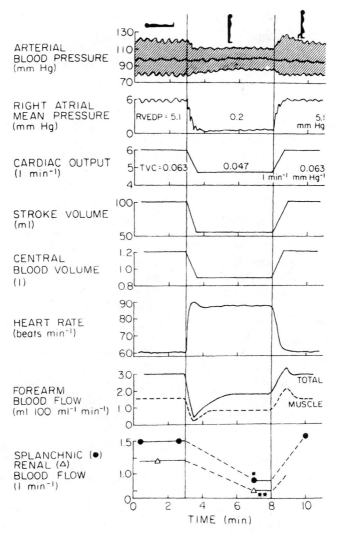

Figure 2-1 Summary of normal cardiovascular responses to upright posture (quiet standing, *middle column*) and activation of muscle pump by gently contracting leg muscles without movement (*right column*). Numbers in panel 2 (right atrial pressure) show right ventricular end-diastolic pressure (RVEDP). Numbers in panel 3 show total vascular conductance (TVC). Time courses for changes in cardiac output and derived variables and for splanchnic and renal flows are approximate. (Compiled from data of Brigden et al., 1950; Culbertson et al., 1951; Poliner et al., 1980; Ring-Larsen et al., 1982; for additional references, see Amberson, 1943; Rowell, 1986; also see Chapter 1). (From Rowell, 1986, with permission of Oxford University Press.)

Figure 2-1 shows the rapid decrease in right atrial mean pressure, stroke volume, and cardiac output and also in central blood volume in response to being tilted upright to 90° (central blood volume includes the volume of blood in the pulmonary vessels and the four chambers of the heart).

The Effects of Breathing

Standing up causes a transient imbalance between right and left ventricular outputs as does breathing, the rate and depth of which increase with upright posture, presumably as a consequence of the small fall in cerebral blood flow (Arieli and Farhi, 1987). Simultaneous recordings from flow meters on the aorta and main pulmonary artery of conscious dogs revealed that the maximal right ventricular stroke volume during inspiration could be as much as 50 percent greater than the minimal stroke volume on expiration, but usually differences were 10 to 20 percent in the dog (Hoffman et al., 1965). Left ventricular stroke volume was less variable because the capacitive properties of the pulmonary circulation buffered the changes in left atrial filling. During inspiration the right ventricle ejected more blood into pulmonary vessels than was removed by left ventricular ejection, whereas during expiration the previously expanded pulmonary blood volume was depleted as stroke volume of the right ventricle fell below that of the left (Figure 2-2).

In humans inspiration *decreases* left ventricular stroke volume, and this persists even when lung volume is kept constant by mouthpiece occlusion and when heart rate is held constant by pacing. This change in stroke volume was minimized in patients with pericardectomy, supporting the view the *left ventricular stroke volume is reduced in humans because the ventricles must compete for space within the pericardium* (Guz et al., 1987). (Note this is our first hint that the pericardium can limit cardiac performance in humans; see Chapter 5.)

When the dogs were held upright for 20 to 30 seconds, right ventricular stroke volume fell immediately, but the fall in left ventricular stroke volume occurred only after six to eight heartbeats, meaning that systemic cardiac output was transiently maintained by depleting the blood volume "stored" in the pulmonary vessels (Figure 2-2) (Hoffman et al., 1965).

Franklin and colleagues (1962) concluded that in dogs, neural factors keep stroke outputs of both ventricles in phase and in balance during postural change. However, the most rapid neural response is vagal and affects primarily heart rate, whereas the sympathetic responses affecting myocardial contractile force are much slower. The 5 to 10 seconds required for a sympathetic response is far too slow to account for the balancing of ventricular outputs in response to breathing and postural change (Hoffman et al., 1965). *This difference in vagal versus sympathetic response times is of fundamental importance.* Finally, the notion that phasic neural outflow modulates ventricular contractility with breathing is refuted by the fact

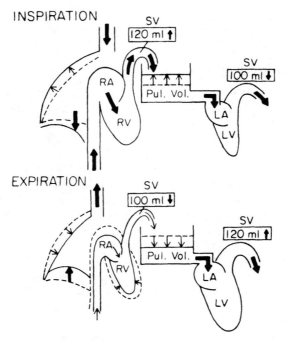

Figure 2-2 Effect of normal breathing on right and left ventricular stroke volume in *humans*. Inspiration increases venous return to the heart (see Figure 1-16) and right ventricular stroke volume increases from 110 to 120 ml. Increased right ventricular output raises pulmonary blood volume providing a sump that can supply the left ventricle so as to maintain its stroke volume and left ventricular output (this happens in dogs). In humans inspiration *decreases* left ventricular stroke volume because space within the pericardium is limited. On expiration, right ventricular stroke volume is reduced by the decline in venous return, but blood stored in the pulmonary vessels provides a sump for left ventricular filling (Hoffman et al., 1965; Guz et al., 1987).

that right and left ventricular effects are 180° out of phase (Guz et al., 1987) (Figuer 2-2).

Frank-Starling or Length-Tension Relationship

The relative slowness of sympathetic nervous responses and the immediate changes in stroke volume within inspiration and expiration, or with standing up, indicates that the Frank-Starling relationship provides the most obvious mechanism for balancing of right and left ventricular outputs. However, positive length-tension effects on stroke volume are limited by pericardial constraints, which may be greater in dogs than in man. In humans and dogs, effects of breathing were unaltered by vagal blockade with atropine. From the length-tension relationship, one would also predict that stroke volume would fall along with right atrial pressure when humans stand up. In upright man, stroke volume is customarily reduced by 40 percent, based on conventional measurements of cardiac output and heart rate and on scintographic nuclear imaging of ventricular size (Poliner, 1980; Rowell, 1986).

Importance of Heart Rate Changes

Tyden (1977) investigated the relative contributions of cardiac output and peripheral vascular resistance on cardiovascular adjustments to orthostasis. Pharmacological isolation of the heart from sympathetic or vagal influences by propranolol and atropine did not affect the constancy of mean arterial pressure in response to a 70° head-up tilt, even though cardiac output fell 26 pecent before autonomic blockade as compared to 51 percent after blockade. Thus, the contribution of peripheral vascular resistance nearly doubled after the blockade. When the gravitational force displacing blood volume was increased threefold by head-to-foot acceleration at three times gravity, mean arterial pressure rose after autonomic blockade of the heart as it did before blockade. *Peripheral vascular rather than cardiac mechanisms are essential to maintaining arterial pressure in upright posture* (Tyden, 1977). This conclusion is easy to understand when the effect of cardiac output on right atrial pressure is considered. Right atrial pressure falls from approximately 5 to 6 mmHg toward 0 mmHg when we stand up. Bear in mind that this right atrial pressure is referenced to atmospheric pressure rather than to intrapleural pressure, which is slightly negative (more during inspiration than expiration). Therefore, when right atrial pressure is 0 mmHg (referred to atmospheric pressure), right atrial transmural pressure and effective right ventricular filling pressure are slightly positive.

Figure 2-1 shows a relatively small rise in heart rate, up to 90 beats min^{-1}, in response to upright posture. What would happen if we could increase heart rate further by ventricular pacing? The answer is that cardiac output would not increase significantly because a rise would further reduce central venous pressure and thus ventricular filling pressure. The consequent reduction in stroke volume (as predicted from the length-tension relationship) introduces a self-limiting control on cardiac output by preventing its further increase. For example, during electrical pacing of the heart in a resting subject, any rise in cardiac output as heart rate is increased is limited by the fall in right atrial pressure and stroke volume (Bevegård et al., 1967). Furthermore, if cardiac output should rise with right atrial pressure so close to zero, the consequent negative pressures would collapse the great veins feeding the right atrium (as predicted by Guyton et al., 1973). For this reason, it is not possible to increase cardiac output in upright posture (or after hemorrhage) when central venous pressure is so close to zero. Keep in mind that the only possible way to increase cardiac output in this setting would be to raise right atrial pressure by activating the muscle pump or by infusing volume.

The preceding points are so fundamental to understanding how cardiac output and its distribution affect the distribution of blood volume and cardiac filling pressure that the underlying principles are reviewed in the next section.

Why Does a Rise in Cardiac Output Reduce Central Venous Pressure?

The corollary question is: why does a fall in cardiac output raise central venous pressure? Guyton's famous experiments on circulatory control were carried out by the investigator pumping (sucking) blood out of the right atrium and the venous system so that the lower the pressure at the atrium, the higher the "venous return" and vice versa. The "venous return curve" demonstrates how the *changes in right atrial pressure can act in a retrograde direction to alter the flow of blood, from the left ventricle, through the systemic circulation, into the right atrium* (Figure 2-3A). We seek here a description of *how right atrial pressure responds, in an anteriograde direction, when cardiac output is varied by the left ventricle* (Figure 2-3B). When we consider what the experimenters' pump did in one type of experiment as opposed to what the left ventricle does in another type of experiment, we change the variable that is dependent and the one that is independent in the relationship beween cardiac output and right atrial pressure (cf. Guyton and colleagues, 1973; Levy, 1979). Often *it is the cardiac output* (and thus venous return as both must be the same, except for transient imbalances) *that determines the central venous pressure.* Nevertheless, the converse can be the case when something

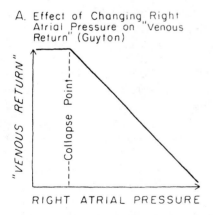
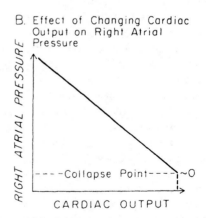

Figure 2-3   Two ways of expressing the interaction between cardiac output and right atrial pressure. In one case (panel A) the investigator manipulates right atrial pressure by pumping blood into it from the animal's venous system and observes the effects on "venous return". Inasmuch as flow was also changed, blood flow as well as right atrial pressure was a determinant of venous return (Guyton et al., 1973; Levy, 1979). A second and entirely different interaction shown in panel B is the effect of raising or lowering cardiac output on right atrial pressure, which is caused, in turn by the effect of blood flow on peripheral vascular volume. See text and Figures 2-4 and 2-7.

suddenly moves blood into (rapid transfusion) or takes blood out of the right atrium (as in standing up).

Figure 2-3 illustrates two types of experiments that demonstrate the interaction between blood flow and right atrial pressure. Figure 2-3A shows the results of Guyton's experiments in which he withdrew blood from the right atrium by an external pump in series with a volume reservoir next to the right atrium. "Venous return" to the atrium could be altered by externally changing the pump rate and the height of the reservoir or the right atrial blood pressure. Figure 2-3B shows the results of an experiment in which the investigator attempts to increase cardiac output by pacing the heart at a faster rate. The ability to raise cardiac output is limited by the fall in right atrial pressure which results from the flow-induced transfer of blood volume into the peripheral vasculature. The following paragraphs explain why volume is transferred.

The reason for the effect of changing cardiac output on central venous pressure originates from the flow-dependency of venous-pressure volume relationships (for brief review, see chapter 3 in Rowell, 1986). As a starting point for this analysis, one can visualize the effect of changing flow through a stiff rubber hose (artery) that feeds directly into a hose made of thin-walled rubber tubing (vein). Figure 2-4 shows the effects of suddenly increasing or decreasing the inflow on the volume of the thin-walled tube and its outflow. As the inflow and distending pressure increase, the volume of the thin-walled tube increases (like charging a capacitor), so that outflow does not rise to equal inflow until a new steady level of volume and wall tension (or transmural pressure) is reached. Conversely, a decrease in inflow shown in the bottom of Figure 2-3 does the opposite.

Krogh (1912) proposed a model for the vascular system that treated *circuits* in which some had tubing that was quite stiff, whereas others had tubing that was "flabby" or compliant. If flow changed through the compliant sections of a closed system, like the cardiovascular system, in which total vascular volume is constant, the increase in volume of the compliant section would decrease the volume somewhere else in the circuit. This concept is discussed in more detail later along with the venous system (see Figure 2-17).

Figure 2-5 illustrates the flow dependency of venous pressure and volume in the cardiovascular system when cardiac output is increased, for example, by pacing, while vascular *resistance remains constant*. The higher flow increases the pressure drop across the veins and lowers central venous pressure. In addition, the rise in arterial pressure raises arterial volume a little (arteries are stiff), further contributing to the decrease in central venous pressure (total volume of the system is constant).

Figure 2-6 shows how vasoconstriction and vasodilation affect central venous pressure or ventricular preload. In both cases, central arterial pressure remains constant owing to a compensatory rise or fall in cardiac output. Dilation of the resistance vessels reduces the pressure gradient across them because of their lower resistance so that their pressure is

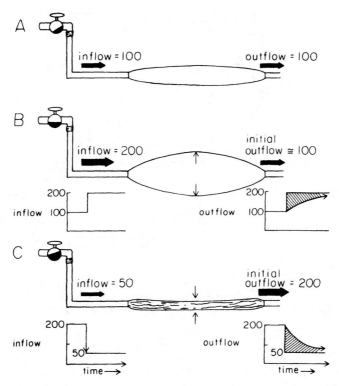

Figure 2-4 **(A)** Hydraulic model showing effects of changing flow through a stiff rubber tube (analogue of arteries, e.g., garden hose) in series with highly compliant thin-walled rubber tubing (analogue of veins). Object is to illustrate effects of flow changes on venous capacitance. **(B)** Flow suddenly increased from 100 to 200 units; outflow slowly increases from 100 to 200 units. Eventually thin-walled tubing reaches stable new wall tension with increased volume; outflow equals inflow. Analogy shows why increased cardiac output increases venous pressure and volume. **(C)** Flow suddenly decreased from 200 to 100 units (analogous to decreased cardiac output and vasoconstriction). Elastic recoil of thin-walled tubing expels volume outward so outflow transiently exceeds inflow until new steady state is reached.

greater than before where they join the capillaries (their increase in volume is small). *The big effect of vasodilation is on venous volume.* The pressure gradient across the veins increases in proportion to blood flow; that is, they have a finite resistance to flow. With vasodilation, the elevated pressure in venules is of crucial importance because they are the most compliant segments of the vascular tree, and the most capacious, as they contain as much as 25 percent of total blood volume. With vasodilation their pressure and volume increase, meaning that central venous volume and pressure must decrease (i.e., total volume is constant). The opposite occurs with vasoconstriction.

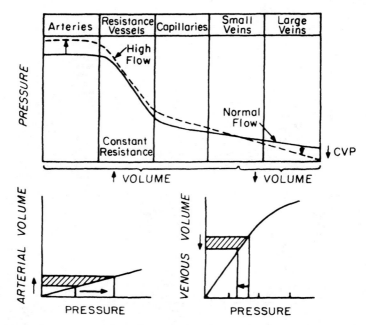

Figure 2-5 Pressure and flow dependency of central venous volume and pressure (CVP). Increased cardiac output with constant vascular resistance increases arterial, arteriolar, and postcapillary venous pressures. Pressure drop across the resistance vessels and across the venous system increases (i.e., higher pressure gradient and higher flow). Arterial volume is increased by higher pressure and therefore venous volume must decrease by the same amount (total vascular volume is constant). The consequence is a fall in CVP. (Adapted from Rowell, 1986.)

The key to understanding why ventricular preload is so sensitive to peripheral blood flow or cardiac output is shown in Figure 2-7, which magnifies the venous portion of the flow-dependent pressure profile shown in Figure 2-6. Although venous resistance is small compared with that of arterioles and has no significant direct influence on total peripheral resistance, it does have major bearing on where blood volume is distributed in the venous system. Figure 2-7 illustrates how flow rate alters the pressure within the various segments of the venous system as blood flows from highly compliant venules, which offer the greatest venous resistance (R_1), down a flow-dependent pressure profile to R_4, the large conduit veins, which offer the least resistance. Each segment of the venous bed also has its own compliance, greatest in venules and lowest in conduit veins, as shown by the volume-pressure curves in Figure 2-7. *It is this pressure gradient from arterioles across the venous segments to large veins that determines the passive effects of blood flow on venous volume and the volume of blood available for ventricular filling.* And it is for this reason that we say: *The performance of the heart is determined primarily by the peripheral circulation.*

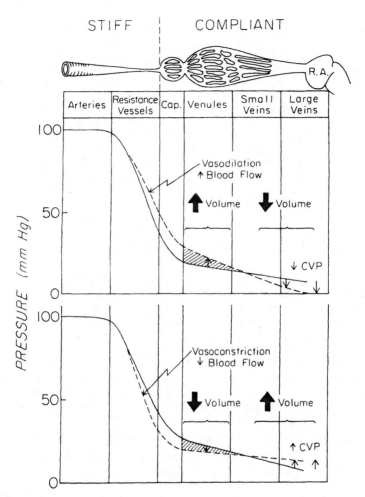

Figure 2-6 (*Top*): Effect on blood volume distribution of generalized vasodilation accompanied by increased cardiac output and constant arterial pressure. Vasodilation reduces pressure drop across resistance vessels and raises arteriolar, capillary, and venular pressures and their volumes. Increased flow steepens pressure gradient across a compliant venous system so that volume shifts into peripheral veins and away from central veins. Thoracic or central venous pressure (CVP) must fall. (*Bottom*): Vasoconstriction accompanied by reduced cardiac output shifts blood volume from small peripheral veins into large central veins, raising CVP. Note reduced flow decreases pressure gradient across the venous system.

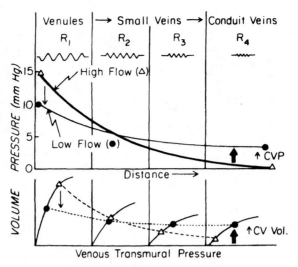

Figure 2-7 *(Top)*: Relationship between pressure and distance along veins at high and low flows. Resistance (R_1 to R_4) symbols show resistance decreasing from venules to conduit veins. Because veins offer finite resistance to flow, a flow-dependent pressure profile exists across them. At high flows *(triangle)* pressure and intravenous volume fall more steeply across venous segments *(top of figure)*. The flow-dependent pressure gradient across the venous system determines the distribution of venous volume. When flow drops, pressure and volume in venules and small veins decrease causing volume to shift toward the heart. *(Bottom)*: Pressures and volumes for each venous segment when flow is high *(triangle)* and low *(solid circle)*. Decreased flow reduces venular pressure and volume and raises central venous (*CV*) volume.

It will be shown later that this highly sensitive pressure-flow-volume relationship in the small veins is what makes it so difficult to decide if blood is actively or passively moved out of veins.

Summary. In summary, when humans stand up, the heart rate rises immediately by vagal withdrawal followed soon after by sympathetic activation. Right atrial pressure and stroke volume fall immediately. Left ventricular output is maintained for only a few heartbeats by depleting the pulmonary reservoir which also serves to buffer imbalances between right ventricular output caused by breathing as well as standing up. The reduction in stroke volume is explained by the fall in preload or the length-tension (Frank-Starling) relationship. After its initial transient effects on cardiac output (before the pulmonary sump is depleted) the rise in heart rate offers no benefit in upright posture. Blockade of autonomic effects on the heart does not disturb the regulation of arterial pressure, which is maintained almost exclusively by increased peripheral vascular resistance. Cardiac output cannot be increased in resting animals and humans without further lowering central venous pressure, which in upright posture is already close to zero. Further lowering of central venous pressure could collapse large veins supplying the atrium and once this happens, cardiac output cannot be increased further. The explanation for why raising or lowering cardiac output lowers or raises central venous pressure, respectively, is to be found in the blood flow-dependent pressure profile across the venous system which has its greatest effects on the postcapillary venules and small veins which are highly sensitive to small changes in transmural pressure. This pressure gradient from resistance vessels across the venules and small veins to large conduit veins determines the passive effects of flow on venous volume; it determines the volume of blood available to fill the heart, and therefore it determines cardiac performance through the length-tension relationship.

Regional Circulations

Where do the regional vasomotor adjustments to upright posture occur? Inasmuch as cardiac output falls 20 percent in upright posture, arterial pressure must be maintained by reduction in total vascular conductance through active vasoconstriction. The vasoconstriction will not only maintain pressure, but will also reduce peripheral blood flow and peripheral venous volume as illustrated in Figure 2-6.

Fortunately, the brain is not actively involved (and owing to its size and position above the heart, would not help if it were). However, despite its autoregulation, cerebral blood flow appears to decline passively in upright posture so that blood flow is reduced by about 6 percent or approximately 45 ml min^{-1} for every 10 mmHg reduction in arterial pressure over the autoregulatory range (Heistad and Kontos, 1983). For example, in one study cerebral blood flow in upright resting humans decreased 20 percent (from 750 to 600 ml min^{-1} at a time when cerebral perfusion pressure fell from 84 to 55 mmHg). This means that cerebral vascular resistance fell from 112 to 92 units rather than to the 73 units needed to maintain constant flow. These findings suggest that the counterpressure exerted by the column of cerebrospinal fluid (Figure 1-3) does not effectively counteract the reduction in driving pressure relative to the distance above the heart.

The most important regions to vasoconstrict are the ones in which the greatest fractions of total vascular conductance are found; that is, splanchnic (25 percent of total conductance), renal (20 percent), and skeletal muscle (~20 percent). Vasoconstriction of these organs will exert the greatest effects on blood pressure. Figure 2-1 shows that blood flow to splanchnic organs (Culbertson et al., 1951), kidneys (Hesse et al., 1978; Ring-Larsen et al., 1982), skeletal muscle (Bridgen et al., 1950), and skin (Amberson, 1943, Johnson et al., 1974a) are all actively reduced.

In response to a 75° head-up tilt, splanchnic blood flow fell by approximately 40 percent, and splanchnic vascular resistance rose by 45 percent, while arterial pulse pressure fell and mean arterial pressure remained constant (Culbertson et al., 1951). As during other stresses, renal vasomotor responses appeared to parallel those in the splanchnic circulation (see

Chapter 6). For example, renal blood flow is reduced by 32 percent in a 60° head-up tilt (Ring-Larsen et al., 1982). When splanchnic vasoconstriction was abolished in chronically hypertensive patients who had undergone splanchnic sympathectomy, they developed severe postural hypotension during head-up tilts (Wilkins et al., 1951) (see Chapter 4 and Figure 4-19).

Shepherd (1963) reviewed the many studies showing marked vasoconstriction of the forearm during head-up tilt. The absence of vasoconstriction in the hand led some to conclude that the cutaneous circulation was not involved in orthostatic reflexes (see Beaconsfield and Ginsberg, 1955; Shepherd, 1963). On the other hand, upright posture in neutral thermal environments consistently produced a fall in skin temperature and a rise in oral temperature, often by 1°C or more, which was caused by a diminished rate of heat loss from the body (see Amberson, 1943). Subsequent experiments showed clearly that cutaneous resistance vessels in nonacral regions constrict in upright posture (Rowell, 1977; Johnson, 1986) (see Figure 4-4).

Reflexes Causing Vasoconstriction

Early thinking turned to both arterial baroreflexes and to reflexes on the low-pressure side of the circuit called cardiopulmonary baroreflexes as the "orthostatic reflexes" that initiate vasoconstriction. There was also a suggestion by H.H. Woollard in 1926 (see Amberson, 1943) that distension of dependent vessels could activate axon "reflexes" (which are not truly reflexes) that might also cause local vasoconstriction (discussed below as sympathetic venoarteriolar "reflexes").

The Nature of the Stimulus

Experimental studies on man's adjustment to large shifts in intravascular volume commonly employed head-up tilts at various angles, quiet standing, which Amberson (1943) called "movement upon a stationary base," and lower body suction. Comparison of these stresses is difficult. Upright standing includes a tonic skeletal muscle contraction not present in a passive tilt. Lower body suction, in contrast to upright posture, applies a uniform increase in transmural pressure to all parts of the lower body (suction is usually applied below the iliac crest). Also, any increased extravascular fluid pressure, which might counteract venous distending pressure (see Chapter 1) is lost in lower body suction. In fact, the suction increases arterial and venous transmural pressures by *decreasing* extravascular pressures. Finally, any local sympathetic axon "reflexes" or purely myogenic vascular responses in the legs would be influenced by the different distribution of transmural pressures in lower body suction as opposed to upright posture.

An advantage of using lower body suction in supine subjects is that it improves our ability to separate central venous and arterial pressure responses. It permits more uniform reduction in transmural pressure of aortic and cardiopulmonary baroreceptors, which are subject to the same hydrostatic forces and transmural pressure in supine posture. In upright posture, pressure distending the carotid sinuses is 15 to 20 mmHg lower than that distending aortic baroreceptors. Thus, during head-up tilts, carotid sinus distending pressure increases in proportion to the sine of the tilt angle times ρgh so that the pressure difference between the two receptor sites provides the central nervous system with additional information about gravitational effects.

Cardiopulmonary Baroreflexes

McDowall (1924) proposed that mechanoreceptors in the atria trigger a pressor reflex in any condition that reduces central venous pressure. During the past two decades, these reflexes have been thoroughly studied. For reviews see Shepherd (1963), Kirchheim (1976), Bishop and colleagues (1983), Mancia and Mark (1983), and Abboud and Thames (1983). The cardiopulmonary or low-pressure baroreceptors are a group of mechanoreceptors lying in the chambers of the heart and the pulmonary artery and veins and their properties are similar to those of the arterial baroreceptors (see below). They decrease their firing with a decrease in transmural pressure in the chambers of vessels in which they lie and vice versa (their putative importance in blood volume control is discussed in Chapter 3). Their afferent impulses travel centrally in the vagus nerve. These receptors alter peripheral vascular resistance but have little effect on heart rate or cardiac output. In dogs, the major target organs of cardiopulmonary baroreflexes are the kidneys and splanchnic organs; skeletal muscle and skin are minimally affected. In contrast, skin and muscle appear to be the major target organs of these reflexes in humans (Johnson et al., 1974b).

The importance of cardiopulmonary baroreceptors is still unclear. There appear to be no obvious deficits in blood pressure regulation in humans with transplanted hearts or in animals with denervated hearts. However, forearm vasoconstriction is blunted, presumably because ventricular receptors are lost (see below). Experimentally the major problem has been the separation of reflexes originating from the high- versus low-pressure parts of the circulation. It is possible even in humans to reduce central venous pressure without also causing a simultaneous reduction in aortic pulse pressure or mean pressure, as shown in Figure 2-8. On the other hand, it is not possible to reduce aortic pulse pressure without altering central venous pressure at the same time.

Figure 2-8 illustrates the reflex adjustments to selective inhibition of human cardiopulmonary baroreceptors (Johnson et al., 1974b) as might occur in response to a slow and progressive increase in the angle of head-up tilt from 0° to 90°. A lower body suction of −45 to −50 mmHg is roughly the equivalent of a 90° head-up tilt in terms of total translocation of blood volume. Figure 2-8 shows that exposure of subjects to a slow ramp of lower body suction (-1 mmHg min^{-1}) gradually reduced right atrial mean pressure from 5 to 0 mmHg without any measurable change in aortic pulse

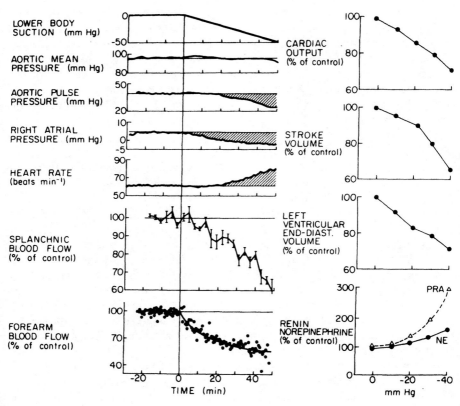

Figure 2-8 Cardiovascular responses to graded lower body suction. Panels on the left show average responses to suction applied at a continuous rate of −1 mmHg min⁻¹ for 50 minutes (Johnson et al., 1974b). Panels on the right show central circulatory responses to 10 mmHg steps in negative pressure down to −40 mmHg (Ahmad et al., 1977). (From Rowell, 1986, with permission of Oxford University Press.)

pressure or mean pressure until suction exceeded −20 mmHg (the constant amplitude, shape, and rate of rise or *dp/dt* of high-fidelity recordings of the aortic pulse waveform were confirmed by computer analysis of individual pulses). The startling result was the "perfect" regulation of aortic pressure variables by peripheral vasoconstriction—in the face of falling cardiac output and stroke volume as shown subsequently by Ahmad and associates (1977). The fall in right atrial pressure was unaccompanied by changes in heart rate, testifying to the weak or nonexistent *Bainbridge reflex* in humans (it is also very weak in monkeys [Vatner and Zimpfer, 1981]).

Figure 2-8 reveals that most of the vasoconstriction in forearm muscle and skin (both tissues were equally engaged) occurred before aortic pulse pressure started to fall at -20 mmHg. Splanchnic blood flow fell only 10 percent during this period. The effect of reduced central venous pressure on renal blood flow in humans is unknown. Parenthetically, when low levels of lower body suction were applied to upright, seated primates, the responses just described for *supine* humans were not seen (Cornish et al., 1988). The reason for the lack of response (in contrast to what the authors proposed) was that central vascular volume was already depleted and ventricular pressures were already near zero in the seated upright primates.

Clearly, the regional vasoconstriction and consequent maintenance of mean arterial pressure accompanying large reductions in central venous pressure is of importance when humans stand up. Our lack of a Bainbridge reflex, which would depress heart rate, is not functionally significant because of the dominant importance of vasoconstriction. A perplexing puzzle is that the primary target of this reflex appears to be skeletal muscle and probably skin. This is contrary to the expectation that the region most affected would be the splanchnic, vasoconstriction of which would cause the greatest transfer of blood toward the heart.

Another puzzle is the apparent role of cardiopulmonary baroreflexes in maintaining *arterial* pressure. Cardiopulmonary baroreceptors are hydraulically isolated from arterial pressure. How could the cardiopulmonary reflex correct changes in a signal that the receptors do not detect? Could left ventricular mechanoreceptors provide a functional link between the high- and low-pressure circuits? Ventricular receptors show little or no response to changes in left ventricular end-diastolic pressure per se. They are active mainly in systole—paradoxically, the frequency of discharge in systole is related mainly to diastolic events (Bishop et al., 1983).

Available information does not yet tell us how reflexes from cardiopulmonary and ventricular receptors might interact. The carotid sinus baroreflex may be more sensitive when cardiopulmonary baroreceptors are inactivated by low central venous pressure (Bevegård et al., 1977).

Some important clues have come from patients who have lost part of their pressure-regulating system. For example, in patients with orthotopically transplanted hearts the new ventricles are without afferent connections (atrial afferents should be intact). Figure 2-9 shows that cardiopulmonary baroreflex control of forearm vascular resistance is markedly impaired, but mean arterial pressure was maintained despite this impairment. Thus ventricular receptors may play a role in these baroreflexes heretofore not recognized (Mohanty et al., 1987).

Observations complementary to those just described were obtained from a patient with bilateral sinoaortic denervation owing to mediastinal radiation and carotid bypass surgery. Arterial baroreflex control of heart rate and arterial pressure in response to drug-induced changes in arterial pressure was lost. Conversely a lowering of cardiac filling pressure by lower body suction markedly raised sympathetic nerve activity. Neverthe-

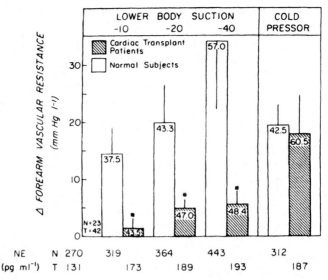

Figure 2-9 Attenuated forearm vascular response to three levels of lower body suction in cardiac transplant patients is contrasted with responses from normal subjects. Baseline resistances were 23 units for normal (N) and 42 units for transplant patients (T). Resistance values during suction are inside bars. Beneath bars are plasma norepinephrine (NE) concentrations during control and lower body suction for groups N and T. Note identical changes in forearm vascular resistance in response to cold pressor test on right. (Adapted from Mohanty et al., 1987.)

less arterial pressure fell at a low level of lower body suction (−10 mmHg), suggesting that arterial baroreflexes are needed to maintain blood pressure during low levels of orthostatic stress (Aksamit et al., 1987).

Arterial Baroreflexes

The baroreflexes originating from mechanoreceptors in the aortic arch and the carotid sinuses are the sine qua non of the cardiovascular reflexes. These are the most important and the best understood reflexes, and they provide the clearest example in physiology of a conventional negative-feedback control system. The efferent arm of the arterial baroreflex differs depending on whether pressure rises or falls. Inasmuch as both adjustments underlie much of the regulation analyzed in this book, both are reviewed here to provide clarity later on.

Responses to a Fall in Pressure. During events that precipitate a fall in arterial pressure, such as vasodilation, loss of blood, or translocation of blood to peripheral veins by gravity, central venous pressure also falls. As explained earlier, the low filling pressure of the heart greatly limits the extent to which cardiac output can be increased by acceleration of rate or by positive inotropic effects on the small ventricular volumes. Therefore, the *rapid* vagal effects on heart rate are of little value; blood pressure must be corrected by the *slower* (5 to 15 seconds) responding sympathetic nervous system. *Thus, initial corrections of hypotension are slow, sympathetically mediated, and directed to the resistance vessels.* The importance of vasoconstriction was illustrated earlier in upright humans with autonomic blockade of the heart (Tyden, 1977). The responses to arterial hypotension are summarized in Figure 2-10.

Response to a Rise in Blood Pressure. The responses to sudden hypertension are *fast—within one heart beat—vagally mediated, and directed mainly to the heart.* The fastest way to reduce blood pressure is to drop heart rate and cardiac output. Speed may be important in sudden, severe hypertension because of the possibility of damage to cerebral vessels and especially the blood-brain barrier (Heistad and Kontos, 1983). Reflex responses to hypertension are summarized in Figure 2-11. Sympathetic vasomotor responses are small because of the lack of tonic sympathetic vasoconstrictor outflow to most organs in humans. That is, the only way

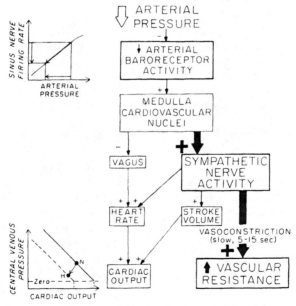

Figure 2-10 Summary of how arterial baroreflex restores blood pressure back toward normal during arterial hypotension. Correction is by relatively *slow* (5 to 15 seconds) vasoconstriction. Increased heart rate has little or no effect if cardiac filling pressure is low and cardiac output cannot be increased for reasons illustrated in small graph next to cardiac output box (central venous pressure versus cardiac output). When normal (N) cardiac output increases, central venous pressure falls. When both cardiac output and central venous pressure are low during hemorrhage (H), output cannot rise much without collapsing central veins as central venous pressure goes to zero.

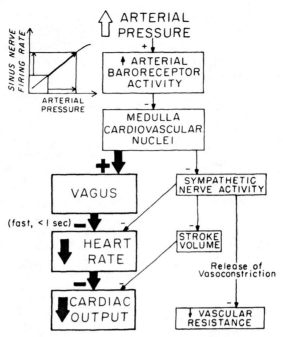

Figure 2-11 Summary of how arterial baroreflex restores blood pressure back toward normal after *sudden* hypertension. Correction is *rapid* and achieved by immediate vagal activation and reduced heart rate and cardiac output. Release of tonic vasoconstriction is slow and has minimal effect because only skeletal muscle has significant tonic vasoconstriction to be withdrawn in resting humans.

to lower peripheral vascular resistance by the sympathetic nervous system is to shut off tonic vasoconstrictor outflow, relaxing vessels already constricted. In humans and other mammals, baroreflexes appear not to activate vasodilator fibers. We lack either sympathetic or parasympathetic vasodilator fibers to most organs (human skin is an important exception). Normally, skeletal muscle appears to be the only major organ receiving significant tonic vasoconstriction. Inasmuch as it represents only 20 percent of total vascular conductance and loss of sympathetic tone raises its blood flow twofold in the legs (Tyden et al., 1979) and forearms (Shepherd, 1963), the effect on blood pressure is not large. Sympathetic cardiac responses are small because heart rate is dominated by vagal influences in resting humans (Robinson et al., 1966).

Selected Stimulation of Human Carotid Sinus. The only means of restricting a change in distending pressure to arterial baroreceptors in humans is to apply positive and negative pressure to the neck in order to alter carotid sinus transmural pressure. However, this stimulus is opposed by the reflexly induced change in blood pressure of the opposite sign at the aortic receptors (that is, systemic arterial pressure falls when carotid sinus transmural pressure rises, and vice versa). These changes occur without any change in central venous pressure. The fall in arterial pressure with increased carotid sinus transmural pressure (neck suction) is due mainly to a fall in cardiac output in resting humans (later its importance to resting sympathetic vasoconstriction when sympathetic activity is increased by stress is described). There is some release of vasoconstrictor tone in muscle and, as expected, none in the splanchnic region (Tyden et al., 1979).

A reduction in carotid sinus transmural pressure causes a rise in blood pressure that stems from peripheral vasoconstriction plus a rise in cardiac output (which in this setting is not initially limited by filling pressure, that is, not until cardiac output has risen some). Autonomic blockade of the heart prevented the rise in cardiac output, but the rise in mean arterial pressure is sustained by greater peripheral vasoconstriction. Thus, despite some opposition by the aortic baroreflex, changes in carotid sinus transmural pressure provide a means for qualitatively assessing the action of arterial baroreflexes (Tyden, 1977).

Eckberg (1980) has carefully analyzed the effects of sudden, brief carotid sinus stimulation on reflex parasympathetic control of heart rate. The rapid vagal response can occur before the fall in blood pressure triggers an opposing aortic baroreflex. Positive and negative pressure at the neck has been used in rapid (a few seconds) upward or downward steps to trace out a stimulus-response curve for the carotid sinus reflex. Inasmuch as the sympathetic vasomotor arm of the reflex, which is paramount in carotid sinus hypotension, has a response time that is much slower than the time permitted between imposed pressure changes, the results are difficult to interpret. Eckberg (1980) later overcame this limitation by directly recording muscle sympathetic nerve activity (see Chapter 3).

The Importance of Arterial Baroreflexes in Upright Posture. When humans stand, both central venous and aortic *pulse pressures* fall suddenly (pulse pressure falls because of the decline in stroke volume) so that both these pressure signals contribute to the neural and humoral adjustments. In addition, carotid sinus pressure falls below aortic pressure because of the difference in hydrostatic pressure (see Figure 1-2).

Figure 2-8 shows a threshold, at -20 mmHg, for responses to lower body suction at which aortic pulse pressure began to fall and heart rate started to rise as arterial baroreflexes came into play. The progressive decline in aortic pulse pressure was closely paralleled by (and highly correlated with $[r = 0.94]$) the rising heart rate and also by a more pronounced decline in splanchnic blood flow. The findings suggest that arterial baroreceptors initiated the rise in heart rate and most of the splanchnic vasoconstriction, whereas forearm (skin and muscle) vasoconstriction was elicited mainly by the cardiopulmonary baroreflexes. That is, most of the forearm vasoconstriction had occurred before aortic pulse pressure fell

(Figure 2-8). This scheme was tested by suddenly raising carotid sinus transmural pressure while at the same time firing of both cardiopulmonary and arterial baroreceptors was reduced by lower body suction at −40 mmHg. The splanchnic vasoconstriction accompanying lower body suction appeared to be reversed by neck suction, but forearm vasoconstriction was maintained as long as central venous pressure was reduced (Abboud et al., 1979). In subsequent experiments, neck suction (−40 mmHg) was rapidly applied on the electrocardiogram R wave preceding each heartbeat and released a few milliseconds before the next heartbeat. The forearm remained vasoconstricted as long as body suction at −40 mmHg continued, but so did the splanchnic vasoconstriction (Escourrou et al., 1991). (Indicator dye can accumulate in neck veins during sustained neck suction, making splanchnic blood flow appear to rise.) The findings of Escourrou and associates (1991) seem more consistent with findings concerning humoral control of splanchnic blood flow, discussed in Chapter 3. Thus, the cardiopulmonary and possibly aortic baroreceptors appear to maintain the splanchnic vasoconstriction despite opposition by the carotid sinus receptors.

Further details related to the relative magnitude and time course of vasomotor responses to orthostasis were obtained when lower body suction was applied in a step and maintained for 13 to 25 min (Rowell et al., 1972) (Figure 2-12). The changes in cardiac output, heart rate, stroke volume, central blood volume, regional blood flow, and vascular resistance shown in Figure 2-12 were very rapid and similar in magnitude to the changes observed during upright posture. Only the rise in splanchnic vascular resistance occurred more slowly.

Interaction Between Cardiopulmonary and Arterial Baroreflexes. The potential for interaction between two mechanoreflexes—cardiopulmonary and arterial baroreflexes—has special importance in humans because of their simultaneous inhibition during orthostasis. A depletion of thoracic blood volume by gravity or lower body suction appears to increase the sensitivity of the arterial baroreflex, and the converse applies when thoracic blood volume and central venous pressure are elevated. Ample evidence exists for this interaction in animals (for reviews see Abboud and Thames, 1983; Bishop et al., 1983; Mancia and Mark, 1983; and Mark and Mancia, 1983).

The basic idea is that heart rate and vasomotor outflow would be increased in upright posture by much smaller changes in arterial pressure than are needed for the same changes while supine. This idea has been tested by observing the changes in systemic arterial pressure caused by neck suction both with and without lower body suction at −40 mmHg (to simulate upright posture). The changes in systemic arterial pressure in response to a given increase in carotid sinus transmural pressure by neck suction were greatest when central venous pressure was reduced by lower body suction (Bevegård et al., 1977). Note, however, that the level of

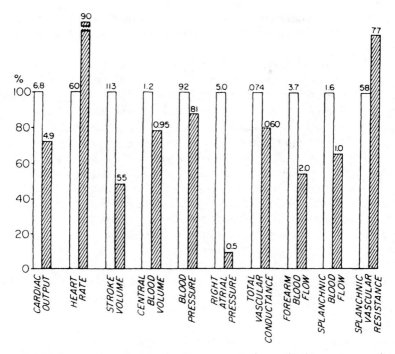

Figure 2-12 Average cardiovascular responses to lower body suction applied at −50 mmHg below the iliac crests and sustained for 8 to 21 minutes (until aortic mean pressure began to fall rapidly). Averages refer to stable periods. Control values (open bars) (100%) with resting values (in conventional units) above each bar. Hatched bars show percent changes (height of bar) during negative pressure with values above each bar (Rowell et al., 1972). (From Rowell, 1986, with permission of Oxford University Press.)

lower body suction (−40 mmHg) is sufficient to lower aortic pulse pressure (Figure 2-8) and this could explain the augmentation of the response. This concern was put to rest by showing that forearm vasoconstriction in response to positive pressure (+20 to +30 mmHg) at the neck (decreased carotid sinus transmural pressure) was greatly augmented by a mild lower body suction of only −10 mmHg. The augmentation far exceeded the sum of the responses to lower body suction alone plus that to neck pressure alone (Victor and Mark, 1985).

The Importance of Regional Vasoconstriction. The relative importance of each vascular bed in maintaining arterial mean pressure was calculated from the changes in total and regional vascular conductance (Rowell et al., 1972). The decrements in splanchnic vascular conductance accounted for one-third of the total peripheral vascular adjustment. Together, skin and muscle could account for about 40 percent if their responses over the entire body correspond with those in the forearm. Most of the remaining

28 percent of the fall in total vascular conductance must have occurred in the kidneys; this is in accordance with changes in renal perfusion measured by others.

In addition to its effects on arterial pressure, vasoconstriction also has the important effect of lowering the high capillary pressures that are especially prevalent in the legs. The effects on fluid transfer are by far the largest and most rapid in skeletal muscle (Lundvall and Länne, 1989). Figure 1-11 shows that, without vasoconstriction, net filtration pressure would be 86 to 91 mmHg in human ankles during upright rest. The dashed line in Figure 1-11 shows the combined effects of vasoconstriction, which markedly reduces pressure on the arterial end of the capillaries, and of the muscle pump, which reduces pressure on their venous end.

Recently, Essandoh and colleagues (1986) and Rusch and colleagues (1981) reported relatively smaller vasomotor changes in a leg than were observed in a forearm when suction was applied to only one leg. This has created a puzzle because the measured sympathetic neural responses, discussed in Chapter 3, were the same in both limbs. Nevertheless, the importance of vasoconstriction in the dependent legs during upright posture is undisputed. Without it, blood pressure cannot be maintained (see Chapter 4).

Is There Rapid Resetting of Arterial Baroreceptors? In 1956, J.W. McCubbin and his colleagues found that arterial baroreceptor firing rate was "reset" in chronically hypertensive dogs. Figure 2-13 schematically illustrates the phenomenon of "resetting." The frequency of baroreceptor firing seen at normal arterial pressure is observed at higher-than- (or lower-than-) normal arterial pressure after resetting has occurred. Traditionally baroreceptor resetting was thought to require from days to weeks.

We are discussing the *resetting at the receptor* and not resetting of the entire baroreflex; it is assumed that there is no change in how the central nervous system interprets a change in the firing rate from the receptor, whether it be due to a change in pressure or to an adaptation of the receptor to a constant pressure stimulus. That is, a change in receptor firing rate from *x* to *y* units will always be interpreted centrally as a change in pressure from 100 to 90 units, for example. Central "resetting" of the entire baroreflex is dealt with in Chapter 12. Technically, the term "resetting," borrowed from the field of engineering, describes a change in one definite preset control value for blood pressure called a *"set point"* or "operating point." For simplicity, a lateral shift in the operating point to a new baroreflex function curve (Figure 2-13) is called resetting.

Recently a rapid resetting of the arterial baroreceptors has been reported to occur within 5 to 10 minutes (see Mendelowitz and Scher, 1988; and Chapleau et al., 1989). This resetting of receptors resulted from brief exposures of isolated baroreceptors to high or low static conditioning pressures, and was observed as shifts in the relationship among baroreceptor pressure, systemic arterial pressure, renal sympathetic nerve activity,

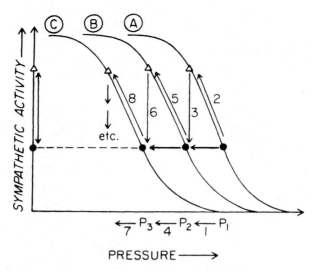

Figure 2-13 Consequence of rapid baroreceptor resetting if mean arterial pressure falls during orthostasis. If pressure at P_1 (normal) falls to P_2 (1), the reflex compensation to prevent further fall in pressure is to increase sympathetic activity at (2). Resetting of the baroreceptors to a new pressure at P_2 (new operating point) means that baroreceptor firing will fall to what it was at P_1 and sympathetic activity will return back to normal (3). The loss of vasoconstriction attributable to resetting will permit P_2 to fall to P_3 (4). As a result sympathetic activity will again rise (5) to restrict the fall in pressure. But again the rapid resetting of the baroreceptor to P_3 will mean that P_3 is now the "accepted pressure" (normal baroreceptor firing) so that again sympathetic activity is returned (6) to its normal level—again pressure can fall (7), sympathetic activity rise (8), and so on, until hypotension causes collapse.

or heart rate. Baroreceptors are mechanoreceptors that adapt rapidly to static pressures as partly illustrated in Figure 2-14. Two processes could explain the rapid adaptation: *First*, relaxation of a viscoelastic tissue could gradually restore wall tension and receptor activity in a distended vessel. *Second*, stretch of the receptor might activate the sodium-potassium (Na-K) pump causing hyperpolarization of the baroreceptor membrane and an increase in receptor threshold.

The consequence of rapid baroreceptor resetting in upright humans could be catastrophic. A decline in mean arterial pressure during orthostasis (a decline occurs immediately in some people) would lead to a continuous downward spiral in blood pressure, and eventual collapse. A hypothetical, stepwise sequence of events is schematically illustrated in Figure 2-13 and described in its legend. Briefly, as blood pressure declines, sympathetic activity increases to maintain pressure; were the baroreceptors to reset to (or to "accept") a new "set point" or operating point at a lower pressure, sympathetic activity would, as a consequence, be shut off at that point (no error exists) until blood pressure again fell below its new operating point. Once again, receptors would reset to the lower blood

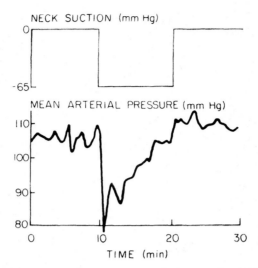

Figure 2-14   Rapid recovery of aortic pressure during sustained (10 minutes) application of neck suction at −65 mmHg. Recovery was due to adaptation of aortic
baroreceptors (mechanoreceptors adapt rapidly) and partly to reflex opposition of
aortic baroreceptors to hypotension. (From Rowell, Johnson, and Blackmon, unpublished.)

pressure, sympathetic activity would stop and pressure would fall again,
and so on. The stepwise description is only for illustration—the real
changes would be continuous.

Fortunately carotid baroreceptors do not adapt rapidly to pulsatile
pressures. Exposure of arterial baroreceptors to elevated or depressed
mean pressures with normal pulsations elicits sustained reflex responses
(Mendelowitz and Scher, 1988; Chapleau et al., 1989).

O'Leary and Scher (1989) examined baroreflex-induced responses in
peripheral vascular resistance and atrial rate during sustained (20-minute)
square-wave changes in mean arterial pressure (pulsatile) and cardiac
output (cardiac output and blood pressure were controlled by ventricular
pacing in dogs with atrioventricular block). If the baroreceptors reset
rapidly, the responses to these sudden changes should decrease rapidly as
the receptors reset to the prevailing pressure. This did not happen. Instead,
compensatory responses to the changes in blood pressure were sustained
and actually increased over the 20 minutes.

Sympathetic Venoarteriolar "Reflexes"

A local sympathetic axon "reflex," called a "venoarteriolar reflex"
(which, like any axon "reflex," is not a true reflex) may, as an adjunct to
central activation of vasomotor ouflow, modify vascular resistance in
dependent regions in upright humans (Henriksen, 1977). Relative changes
in rates of washout of locally injected ^{133}Xe revealed increments in local

arteriolar resistance when veins were distended by upright posture, external negative pressure, or local venostasis. The receptor sites appear to be in the small veins of skin, subcutaneous tissue, and skeletal muscle. The effector sites are in the corresponding arterioles (other tissues have not been studied in humans, but the "reflex" is present in the canine mesenteric circulation).

Figure 2-15 schematically illustrates the evidence that part of the vasoconstriction during orthostasis is *not* of central origin. In Figure 2-15A vasoconstriction persisted in dependent regions when central sympathetic ouflow was prevented by spinal anesthesia or by proximal sympathetic nerve blockade. Figure 2-15B shows a supine subject with no central sympathetic activation; vasoconstriction in the dependent limb is entirely local. This vasoconstriction could be reduced by local application of anesthetic, by an α-antagonist, or by external counterpressure to reduce venous transmural pressure. In general, the findings suggested that the myogenic reaction to vascular stretch is at least not a major factor in the response (Henriksen, 1977; Skagen, 1983). Although Henriksen (1977) observed no local vasoconstriction in chronically denervated upper limbs (after peripheral nerve fibers had degenerated), Zolte and associates (1989) found significant vasoconstriction in dependent microvessels of skin flaps that had long before been surgically transferred to the legs of trauma victims (no sympathetic nerves). These results show that a myogenic reaction can also elicit this local vasoconstriction.

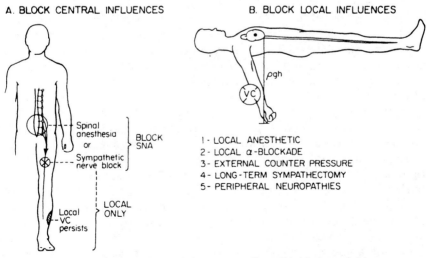

A. BLOCK CENTRAL INFLUENCES   B. BLOCK LOCAL INFLUENCES

Spinal anesthesia or Sympathetic nerve block } BLOCK SNA

Local -VC persists

LOCAL ONLY

ρgh

VC

1 - LOCAL ANESTHETIC
2 - LOCAL α-BLOCKADE
3 - EXTERNAL COUNTER PRESSURE
4 - LONG-TERM SYMPATHECTOMY
5 - PERIPHERAL NEUROPATHIES

Figure 2-15 Sympathetic venoarteriolar axon "reflexes" initiate part of the vasoconstriction in dependent limbs. **(A)** Demonstration that vasoconstriction (*VC*) is not of central origin. It persists after proximal blockade or spinal blockade of sympathetic nerve traffic. **(B)** Demonstration that vasoconstriction is of local origin. Local sympathetic vasoconstriction is prevented by counteracting venous distension and by local destruction or blockade of sympathetic fibers (Henriksen, 1977).

These local vasoconstrictor responses may help to explain why para-plegic and quadriplegic people with complete spinal cord transection can withstand upright tilting without syncope, whereas subjects with severe autonomic neuropathy cannot (see Chapter 4).

Is Neural Control of the Veins Important in Orthostasis?

This section asks whether reflexly induced, active changes in venous diameter and volume regulate right ventricular filling pressure. The discussion of active and passive control of the venous system is concentrated in this chapter to eliminate repetition later on; it provides the review necessary for further discussion of flow- and pressure-volume relationships in later chapters.

The magnitude and significance of venous capacitance was discussed in Chapter 1. The venous compartment is viewed as a reservoir for the cardiovascular system because large changes in volume can attend small changes in its transmural pressure, thereby buffering stresses such as upright posture and hemorrhage. Smooth muscle lines the walls of large parts of the venous system so that its volume can be *actively* reduced by *venoconstriction*. Such an event could minimize venous "pooling" in orthostasis and, by providing more blood for filling the heart, could raise cardiac output. Keep in mind that the magnitude of volume transferred out of dependent veins will be lessened by the added effects of gravity on their transmural pressure. *Vasoconstriction* will slow the time course of this rise in pressure and reduce its magnitude.

It seems logical that veins might be among the principal targets of the "orthostatic reflexes." On the other hand, one could argue that the volume of blood *passively* expelled from the veins by elastic recoil of their walls when their transmural pressure is reduced by *vasoconstriction* is as great as that expelled actively. The purely passive effects on venous volume are illustrated in Figure 1-5 and Figures 2-6 and 2-7.

Controversy over the significance of active versus passive mobilization of blood volume out of veins persists, partly because of the physical complexity of the system (Gow, 1980; Rothe, 1983a, 1983b). Consider, for example, the plight of some tiny imaginary observers positioned at the right atrium who must decide whether an increase in the return of blood to that chamber stems from its active expulsion back into the heart from peripheral veins. One observer could favor venoconstriction, whereas another could conclude that veins had not constricted—rather, cardiac output and peripheral blood flow had simply fallen. But another observer could still argue against venoconstriction, even if cardiac output had not fallen, by proposing that the distribution of cardiac output had shifted from compliant vascular beds to the less compliant ones.

There are four fundamental points to extract from this discussion:

1. Active vasoconstriction can in its effects mimic active venocon-striction.

2. The distribution of blood flow determines the distribution of blood volume.
3. Right atrial pressure reflects active changes in venous tone or capacitance only if cardiac output and its distribution are constant.
4. Reflex venoconstriction and vasoconstriction appear not to occur independently, or separately; venoconstriction would serve regulation if accompanied by powerful vasoconstriction.

Passive Effects of Changing Organ Blood Flow

The marked vasoconstriction and the fall in blood flow accompanying upright posture decreases the volume of blood that would otherwise be transferred by gravity into dependent veins as soon as one stands up. The importance of this response is emphasized by cases in which vasoconstriction is lost (Chapter 4). Again Figures 2-6 and 2-7 illustrate the importance of blood flow and vasoconstriction on venous volume.

Passive effects of blood flow on organ volume are greatest in the hepatic-splanchnic circulation, which is the largest and most compliant region and receives approximately 25 percent of resting cardiac output and contains approximately 20 percent of total blood volume. Because of its high compliance, the volume of this region is uniquely sensitive to changes in blood flow. For example, a mechanical reduction in inflow to the splanchnic region was observed by Brooksby and Donald (1971) to decrease downstream splanchnic venous pressure. When central venous pressure was normal or below, the volume of blood passively expelled from these organs was 65 percent of the maximum that could be expelled by reflexes. Raising or lowering central venous pressure would decrease or increase, respectively, the volume of blood returned to the heart by changing the pressure gradient between the veins and the atrium. Rothe (1983a) concluded that changing splanchnic blood flow with central venous pressure constant will reduce splanchnic blood volume (in dogs) by 0.2 ml ml^{-1} min^{-1} change in blood flow per kilogram of organ weight. Based on more recent numbers (see below), this number must be at least 0.3 ml ml^{-1} min^{-1} or higher (Rothe and Gaddis, 1990). If these numbers are applied to a 70-kg human, a 70 percent reduction in splanchnic blood flow would displace between 350 and 525 ml of blood or approximately 35 to 50 percent of total splanchnic blood volume with no venoconstriction. Therefore, the volume transferred by splanchnic vasoconstriction is highly dependent on the blood flow through the region and the pressures in the right atrium and hepatic veins. Volume transferred out of the region is maximum when central venous pressure is low.

Dependency of Central Venous Pressure on the Distribution of Cardiac Output

When humans increase or decrease cardiac output, they usually actively change the distribution of blood flow among different organs by sympathetic vasoconstriction (hypoxemia appears to be one exception [Rowell,

1986]). This vasoconstriction can determine the volume of blood available to fill the heart because some organs are much more compliant than others. Again, the splanchnic region is the largest and most compliant region in mammals. Also bear in mind that humans may be the only mammals with two large, highly compliant regions, the second being the skin.

In 1912, August Krogh offered a simple conceptual model of the circulation which he divided into two circuits, one compliant (C_1) and one noncompliant (C_2) (Figure 2-16). Krogh's idea was that the volume of blood available to the heart is determined by the distribution between such regions (the idea appears to have originated with DeJager in 1886; see Rothe, 1983a). Figure 2-17 provides another view of how flow through different circuits could affect the distribution of blood volume. Krogh saw the splanchnic circulation as the principal regulator of the supply of blood to the right atrium. Krogh's model would explain why Barcroft and Samaan (1935) saw that occlusion of the aorta above the mesenteric arteries caused a sudden increase in cardiac output, whereas occlusion below these arteries had the opposite effect. In the former maneuver, pressures (and volume) in the splanchnic region fell, meaning that blood moves centrally toward the heart, raising filling pressure. In the latter maneuver, the opposite changes occurred. Since that time, others have shown that large volumes can be passively transferred in and out of this organ system (see Skokland, 1983).

What Veins Are Innervated?

The only known neural control of veins in humans or other species is by adrenergic sympathetic nerves; the release of norepinephrine from these

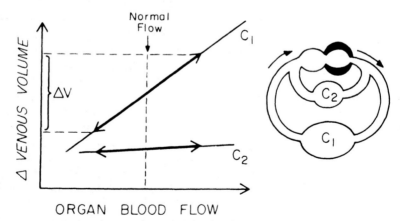

Figure 2-16 *Right*: The Krogh model divides the circulation into two circuits, one complaint (C_1) and one noncompliant (C_2). *Left*: The relationship between the change in organ venous volume and blood flow through a compliant organ (C_1) and a noncompliant organ (C_2). The volume of blood available to the heart is determined by the distribution of blood flow between such circuits. (From Rowell, 1986, with permission of Oxford University Press.)

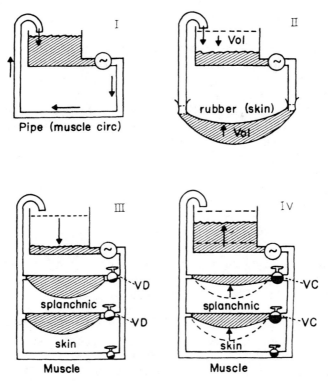

Figure 2-17 Hydraulic model contrasting effects of increasing blood flow through noncompliant **(I)** versus compliant circuits **(II, III, and IV)**. In **III**, vasodilation (*VD*) of compliant circuits depletes the volume (vol) of central reservoirs (blood volume of heart and pulmonary vessels). In **IV**, vasoconstriction (*VC*) of compliant circuits reduces their flows and passively displaces their volumes to partially restore central reservoir volume. (From Rowell, 1986, with permission of Oxford University Press.)

nerve terminals causes all veins containing α_1, α_2-adrenoreceptors to constrict (Shepherd and Vanhoutte, 1975; Hainsworth and Linden, 1978; Rothe, 1983a, 1983b; Hainsworth, 1986). It appears that postjunctional α_2 rather than the usual α_1 adrenoceptors are predominant in causing reflex constriction of cutaneous veins (Flavahan et al., 1985).

Donegan (1921) was the first to show that the responsiveness of veins to adrenergic stimulation varies among different regions. His conclusions, which still hold, were that mesenteric and superficial cutaneous veins were highly reactive to stimulation by either sympathetic nerves or catecholamines. Except for the mesenteric veins, Donegan found that in general, deep veins were unresponsive.

It is clear today that splanchnic and cutaneous veins are richly innervated by adrenergic nerve fibers, whereas veins of skeletal muscle contain sparse and possibly functionally insignificant innervation (Marshall, 1982; Hébert and Marshall, 1988). On the other hand, Faber (1988) found that the venules of rat skeletal muscle have both α_1 and α_2 adrenoceptors and can constrict in response to norepinephrine. Particular importance has been placed on the view that small venules (20 to 100 μm) are sparsely innervated and have little smooth muscle. In general, these venous microvessels are the most distensible portion of the vascular system (Gaehtgens and Uekermann, 1971; Fung, 1978) and are estimated to contain as much as 25 percent of the total blood volume. Therefore their ability or inability to constrict in certain regions is an important and unresolved issue. For example, when the pressure of *intestinal* venous microvessels (diameters ranging from 22 to 148 μm) was raised from 0 to 30 mmHg, their volume increased about 360 percent. Keep in mind that if venoconstriction were restricted to larger veins upstream, their rise in resistance should cause venular pressure and volume to increase as a consequence *if blood flow did not fall markedly at the same time.* That is, sustained venoconstriction could actually have a deleterious effect on filling pressure (see below).

Available evidence suggests that the splanchnic and cutaneous venous beds are the only ones that are richly innervated in humans; they are also the most capacious volume reservoirs in the human cardiovascular system.

Does the Venous System Actively Regulate Thoracic Blood Volume?

Many investigators argue that veins *actively* regulate ventricular filling pressure, whereas others argue that they do so passively. The dispute stems from serious methodological problems, which have been ably reviewed by Hainsworth and Linden (1978), Rothe (1983c), and Hainsworth (1986).

How Can We Measure Venoconstriction? In humans, measurements of venous capacitance have been confined to the limbs. Recently, a nuclide imaging technique (technetium-labeled red blood cells) called "quantitative equilibrium blood-pool scintigraphy" has been used to determine changes in blood volume within a specified region of the splanchnic bed in humans (Robinson et al., 1990). This technique, coupled with the ability to measure blood flow to some major vessels within the splanchnic region by Doppler techniques (Altobelli et al., 1985) opens the way to demonstrating noninvasively the relative magnitude of changes in splanchnic blood volume. However, separation of changes in volume owing to active venoconstriction, as opposed to passive effects of falling flow, requires the invasive measurement of splanchnic venous pressures at the proper sites. That is, the hepatic venous (or outflow) pressure will not reflect the pressures distending the most compliant veins where volume will change most in relation to flow, as shown in Figure 2-7.

Changes in venous volume are considered active if they occur while venous transmural pressure is constant. A valid measurement requires vascular isolation of the region and perfusion at constant flow with constant venous pressure. Volume changes due to filtration (equivalent to a delayed compliance at the capillaries) can still complicate the measurement. Alternatively, one can totally arrest blood flow to a region so that a purely qualitative index of venoconstriction is derived from the rise in pressure within the isovolumic veins as they contract. The latter has been used to show unambiguous changes in cutaneous venous tone in human limbs when they respond to changes in temperature; they do not respond to either arterial or cardiopulmonary baroreflexes (nor do veins of skeletal muscle).

Some have attempted to measure the compliance of the entire systemic vascular bed (determined primarily by venous compliance) by measuring the change in right atrial pressure associated with a known change in blood volume. The total systemic vascular compliance was calculated to be 2.3 ml mmHg^{-1} kg^{-1} of body weight, which is similar to estimates made in other animals. This procedure was repeated in humans during a constant infusion of norepinephrine at a rate sufficient to constrict resistance vessels and veins; the calculated total systemic compliance fell by 25 percent—from 2.3 to 1.73 ml mmHg^{-1} kg^{-1} (Echt et al., 1974). This would mean that 130 ml rather than 173 ml would be required to raise central venous pressure by 1 mmHg in a 75-kg human *were cardiac output constant*. The fundamental problem with this approach, however, is that in the intact circulation *the change in blood volume required to elicit a unit change in right atrial pressure reflects total compliance or capacitance only if cardiac output and its distribution are constant* (e.g., Hill and Barnard, 1897).

A preparation similar to that illustrated schematically in Figure 2-18 has been used to quantify active changes in venous tone. The circulation is broken at the junction of the vena cavae and right atrium with a mechanical pump interposed between them. Cardiac output is kept constant by this pump as long as the return of blood is adequate. Venous return, which can *transiently* differ from left ventricular outflow when vascular capacity changes, is fed into a reservoir. Any change in the reservoir volume, or pressure, means that venous return has changed with respect to cardiac output (i.e., the volume in the vascular system is assumed to be constant). Systemic venous pressure is changed by adjusting the height of the reservoir so as to regulate venous outflow pressure and back pressure. With cardiac output held constant, an increase in reservoir volume is taken as evidence that veins have constricted and forced blood centrally—but now into a reservoir instead of the right atrium (the distribution of cardiac output is assumed to stay constant).

How Important Is Active Venoconstriction? Inasmuch as richly innervated cutaneous veins do not respond to baroreflexes and (in dogs) splanchnic veins do respond (Donald, 1983), and, given the lack of significant venous innervation in other organs (including skeletal muscle, the largest organ), venoconstriction could be limited primarily to the splanchnic region in humans (Rowell, 1986). The bulk of evidence in support of

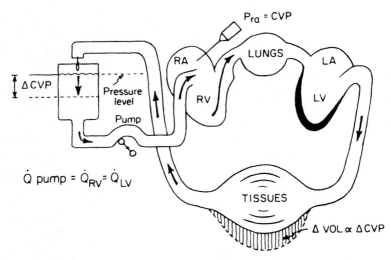

Figure 2-18   Schematic illustration of a constant cardiac output technique for estimating systemic vascular compliance from changes in total vascular volume. The rate
of outflow from the pump to the right atrium determines cardiac output. Compliance is
calculated from changes in central venous pressure (CVP) or height of the reservoir
and the volume that moves into and out of the reservoir when its level is changed or
when the level is adjusted to keep CVP constant. Because flow is constant the pressure
gradients across the venous bed are also assumed to be constant. Note that the
distribution of cardiac output can change even though total flow stays constant. (From
Rowell, 1986, with permission of Oxford University Press.)

significant reflex venoconstriction in response to changes in arterial pressure comes from investigations of the hepatic-splanchnic circulation in
cats and dogs (Donald, 1983; Greenway, 1983). In general, the volume of
blood actively transferred from the splanchnic region is not much less than
that transferred from the total systemic vasculature in response to large
reductions in isolated carotid sinus pressure (Shoukas and Sagawa, 1973;
Rothe, 1983a; Hainsworth, 1986). In dogs, active mobilization from the
entire vascular system is approximately 4.5 ml kg^{-1} with an additional 3
ml kg^{-1} (or 40 percent of the total) coming from the spleen. Inasmuch as
humans do not have large contractile spleens, the maximal transfer of
blood volume out of constricted veins should be about 340 ml in a 75-kg
man if the maximal capacitance response for man is also 4.5 ml kg^{-1}. This
would be entirely consistent with the view that the *splanchnic region could
be the only significant site of active volume transfer* (Hainsworth, 1986;
Rowell, 1986).
   Rothe and Gaddis (1990) used a preparation similar to that illustrated
in Figure 2-18 to quantify the magnitude of blood volume transferred out
of or into the systemic vasculature as a consequence of a change in cardiac
output per se—and as a consequence of changes in both cardiac output
and vascular capacitance. All venous return was pumped into the reser-

voir, central venous pressure was held constant, and cardiac output was maintained at various levels by pumping blood from the reservoir into the right atrium. When reflexes were intact, 9.2 ml kg^{-1} of blood were transferred to the reservoir by a 27 percent reduction in cardiac output. The same reduction in cardiac output caused a 6.8-ml kg^{-1} transfer of blood when reflexes were blocked by hexamethonium. Referred to a 75-kg human, a 27 percent decrease in cardiac output would shift 690 ml and 510 ml of blood centrally with and without reflexes intact, respectively. Thus, the constriction of veins would transfer only 180 ml or about 25 percent of the total 690 ml if these changes per kilogram of dog can be extrapolated to man. Recall that a 70 percent reduction in splanchnic blood flow could transfer between 350 and over 500 ml of blood out of this region in humans. The authors' conclusion is noteworthy: ''Passive blood volume redistribution between the peripheral vasculature and the heart after changes in blood flow, ..., provides a more powerful compensatory mechanism to maintain the cardiac output than do active reflex changes in vascular capacitance'' (Rothe and Gaddis, 1990).

The Problem of Venous Resistance. If venoconstriction raises venous resistance, it could over time actually reduce venous return and raise venous pressure in capacious venules upstream from the site where venous resistance increased, as shown schematically in Figure 2-19. Note that a change in vessel radius (r) has a larger effect on resistance (proportional to $1/r^4$) than to volume (proportional to r^2). For example, if the radius of

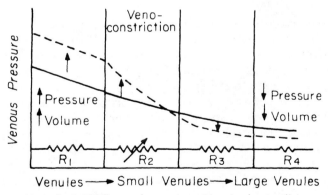

Figure 2-19 Hypothetical effects of venoconstrition in the small innervated veins with blood flow constant. Venoconstriction occurred at R_2 (most venules appear to lack innervation, and are highly compliant). Increased resistance at R_2 raised venous back pressure, increasing venule volume, and the increased pressure drop lowered downstream venous pressure so that ultimately venous outflow pressure or central venous pressure fell. In this scheme, the rise in venule pressure and volume would have to be counteracted by arteriolar constriction, which would reduce all venous pressures. (From Rowell, 1986, with permission of Oxford University Press.)

veins of 2-mm diameter decreased by 30 percent, volume would be reduced by 50 percent, but their resistance would increase by 420 percent.

Two occurrences could minimize the potentially deleterious effects of increased venous resistance on central venous pressure. The first is if venules of the splanchnic region constrict along with the other venous segments of the region so that volume transfer would be toward the heart and not back into the venules. Furness and Marshall (1974) were first to show that venules of the intestines are innervated. Shoukas and Bohlen (1990) found that small venules (20 to 100 μm) of rat intestine show significant decrements in their diameter at constant venular pressure when blood pressure is lowered by hemorrhage. These changes were blocked by denervation, indicating an active sympathetically mediated constriction occurred. The second occurrence that will counteract any effect of increased venous resistance is the constriction of the resistance vessels along with the veins. *We have no evidence that reflex venoconstriction and vasoconstriction ever occur independently* (Gow, 1980). The reduction in blood flow attending vasoconstriction will transfer much of the volume out of the venules and small veins. In effect, the splanchnic region could be viewed as having changed from a circuit with high flow, volume, and capacitance to one with low flow, volume, and capacitance. The passive effect of blood flow appears to be the dominant mechanism for transferring blood volume. Active venoconstriction of splanchnic veins may make an additional but smaller contribution.

SUMMARY

In summary, most of the blood transferred out of the peripheral vasculature (mainly veins) in response to hypotension is attributable to the purely passive effects of vasoconstriction and decreased blood flow. Reflex venoconstriction (except for thermoregulatory responses in the skin) appears to be largely confined to the splanchnic region. Vasoconstriction in this region mimics venoconstriction because of its high sensitivity to changes in blood flow. Although venoconstriction could transfer additional volume out of the region, the changes are probably relatively small. The argument that venoconstriction increases venous resistance upstream from the venules and thereby raises their transmural pressure and volume (Rowell, 1986) is counteracted by the finding that even the smallest splanchnic venules appear able to constrict actively. This effect on venous resistance would also be minimized by the vasoconstriction, which occurs simultaneously with venoconstriction, and causes most of the fall in venous volume.

When humans stand up, a large volume of blood shifts into the dependent veins of the legs and pelvic organs (approximately 600 to 900 ml), yet no venoconstriction has ever been observed in the legs. If most of the active transfer of blood by both vaso- and venoconstriction is from the splanchnic vessels, then all of our "capacitance reserve" would be used up when we stand. Although the capacitance response is small, loss of the ability to prevent a gravitationally caused rise in splanchnic blood volume in upright posture leads to severe postural hypotension (Chapter 4).

REFERENCES

Abboud, F.M., and M.D. Thames (1983). Interaction of cardiovascular reflexes in circulatory control. In J.T. Shepherd, F.M. Abboud, and S.R. Geiger, eds. *Handbook of Physiology. The Cardiovascular System: Peripheral Circulation and Organ Blood Flow*, sect. 2, vol. III, part 2, pp. 675–753. American Physiological Society, Bethesda, MD.

Abboud, F.M., D.L. Eckberg, U.J. Johannsen, and A.L. Mark (1979). Carotid and cardiopulmonary baroreceptor control of splanchnic and forearm vascular resistance during venous pooling in man. *J. Physiol. (Lond.) 286*, 173–184.

Ahmad, M., C.G. Blomqvist, C.B. Mullins, and J.T. Willerson (1977). Left ventricular function during lower body negative pressure. *Aviat. Space Environ. Med. 48*, 512–515.

Aksamit, T.R., J.S. Floras, R.G. Victor, and P.E. Aylward (1987). Paroxysmal hypertension due to sinoaortic baroreceptor denervation in humans. *Hypertension 9*, 309–314.

Altobelli, S.A., W.F. Volyes, and E.R. Greene (eds.) (1985). *Cardiovascular Ultrasonic Flowmetry*. Elsevier, New York.

Amberson, W.R. (1943). Physiologic adjustments to the standing posture. *Univ. Md. Sch. Med. Bull. 27*, 127–145.

Arieli, R., and L.E. Farhi (1987). Gravity-induced hyperventilation is caused by a reduced brain perfusion. *Respir. Physiol. 69*, 237–244.

Barcroft, H., and A. Samaan (1935). Explanation of the increase in systemic flow caused by occluding the descending thoracic aorta. *J. Physiol. (Lond.) 85*, 47–61.

Beaconsfield, P., and J. Ginsburg (1955). The effect of body posture on the hand blood flow. *J. Physiol. (Lond.) 130*, 467–473.

Bevegård, S., J. Castenfors, L.E. Lindblad, and J. Tranesjo (1977). Blood pressure and heart rate regulating capacity of the carotid sinus during changes in blood volume distribution in man. *Acta Physiol. Scand. 99*, 300–312.

Bevegård, S., B. Jonsson, I. Karlof, H. Lagergren, and E. Sowton (1967). Effect of changes in ventricular rate on cardiac output and central pressures at rest and during exercise in patients with artificial pacemakers. *Cardiovasc. Res. 1*, 21–33.

Bishop, V.S., A. Malliani, and P. Thoren (1983). Cardiac mechanoreceptors. In J.T. Shepherd, F.M. Abboud, and S.R. Geiger, eds. *Handbook of Physiology. The Cardiovascular System: Peripheral Circulation and Organ Blood Flow*, sect. 2, vol. III, part 2, pp. 497–555. American Physiological Society, Bethesda, MD.

Bridgen, W., S. Howarth, and E.P. Sharpey-Schafer (1950). Postural changes in the peripheral blood flow of normal subjects with observations of vasovagal fainting reactions, as a result of tilting, the lordotic posture, pregnancy and spinal anesthesia. *Clin. Sci. 9*, 79–91.

Brooksby, G.A., and D.E. Donald (1971). Dynamic changes in splanchnic blood flow and blood volume in dogs during activation of sympathetic nerves. *Circ. Res. 29*, 227–238.

Chapleau, M.W., G. Hajduczok, and F.M. Abboud (1989). Peripheral and central mechanisms of baroreflex resetting. *Clin. Exp. Pharmacol. Physiol. (Suppl. 15)*, 31–43.

Cornish, K.G., J.P. Gilmore, and T. McCulloch (1988). Central blood volume and blood pressure in conscious primates. *Am. J. Physiol. 254 (Heart Circ. Physiol. 23)*, H693–H701.

Culbertson, J.W., R.W. Wilkins, F.J. Ingelfinger, and S.E. Bradley (1951). The effect of the upright posture upon hepatic blood flow in normotensive and hypertensive subjects. *J. Clin. Invest. 30*, 305–311.

Donald, D.E. (1983). Splanchnic circulation. In J.T. Shepherd, F.M. Abboud, and S.R. Geiger, eds. *Handbook of Physiology. The Cardiovascular System: Peripheral Circulation and Organ Blood Flow.* sect. 2, vol. III, part 1, pp. 219–240. American Physiological Society, Bethesda, MD.

Donegan, J.F. (1921). The physiology of veins. *J. Physiol. (Lond.) 55*, 226–245.

Echt, M., J. Duweling, O.H. Gauer, and L. Lange (1974). Effective compliance of the total vascular bed and the intrathoracic compartment derived from changes in central venous pressure induced by volume changes in man. *Cir. Res. 34*, 61–68.

Eckberg, D.L. (1980). Parasympathetic cardiovascular control in human disease: a critical review of methods and results. *Am. J. Physiol. 239 (Heart Circ. Physiol. 8)*, H581–H593.

Escourrou, P., B. Raffestin, Y. Papelier, E. Pussard, and L.B. Rowell (1991). Splanchnic and forearm vasomotor responses to neck suction and lower body negative pressure. *FASEB J. 5*, 1414.

Essandoh, L.K., D.S. Houston, P.M. Vanhoutte, and J.T. Shepherd (1986). Differential effects of lower body negative pressure on forearm and calf blood flow. *J. Appl. Physiol. 61*, 994–998.

Faber, J.E. (1988). In situ analysis of α-adrenoceptors on arteriolar and venular smooth muscle in rat skeletal muscle microcirculation. *Circ. Res. 61*, 37–50.

Flavahan, N.A., L.-E. Lindblad, T.J. Verbeuren, J.T. Shepherd, and P.M. Vanhoutte (1985). Cooling and α_1- and α_2-adrenergic responses in cutaneous veins: role of receptor reserve. *Am. J. Physiol. 249 (Heart Circ. Physiol. 18)*, H950–H955.

Florkin, M., H.T. Edwards, and D.B. Dill (1930). Oxygen utilization in the legs of normal men. I. Effect of posture. *Am. J. Physiol. 94*, 459–463.

Franklin, D.L., R.L. Van Citters, and R.F. Rushmer (1962). Balance between right and left ventricular output. *Circ. Res. 10*, 17–26.

Fung, Y.B. (1978). Mechanical properties of blood vessels. In P.C. Johnson, ed. *Peripheral Circulation*, pp. 45–79. Wiley, New York.

Furness, J.B., and J.M. Marshall (1974). Correlation of the directly observed responses of mesenteric vessels of the rat to nerve stimulation and noradrenaline with the distribution of adrenergic nerves. *J. Physiol. (Lond.) 239*, 75–88.

Gaehtgens, P., and U. Uekermann (1971). The distensibility of mesenteric venous microvessels. *Pflugers Arch. 330*, 206–216.

Gow, B.S. (1980). Circulatory correlates: vascular impedance, resistance, and capacity. In D.F. Bohr, A.P. Somlyo, and H.V. Sparks Jr., eds. *Handbook of Physiology. The Cardiovascular System: Vascular Smooth Muscle*, sect. 2, vol. II, pp. 353–408. American Physiological Society, Bethesda, MD.

Greenway, C.V. (1983). Role of splanchnic venous system in overall cardiovascular homeostasis. *Fed. Proc. 42*, 1678–1684.

Guyton, A.C., C.E. Jones, and T.G. Coleman (1973). *Circulatory Physiology: Cardiac Output and Its Regulation*, 2nd ed. W.B. Saunders, Philadelphia.

Guz, A., J.A. Innes, and K. Murphy (1987). Respiratory modulation of left ventricular stroke volume in man measured using pulsed Doppler ultrasound. *J. Physiol. (Lond.) 393*, 499–512.

Hainsworth, R. (1986). Vascular capacitance: its control and importance. *Rev. Physiol. Biochem. Pharmacol. 105*, 101–173.

Hainsworth, R., and R.J. Linden (1978). Reflex control of vascular capacitance. *Int. Rev. Physiol. (Cardiovascular Physiology III* [A.C. Guyton and D. Young, eds.]) *18*, 67–124.

Hèbert, M.T., and J.M. Marshall (1988). Direct observations of the effects of baroreceptor stimulation on skeletal muscle circulation of the rat. *J. Physiol. (Lond.) 400*, 45–59.

Heistad, D.D., and H.A. Kontos (1983). Cerebral circulation. In J.T. Shepherd, F.M. Abboud, and S.R. Geiger, eds. *Handbook of Physiology. The Cardiovascular System: Peripheral Circulation and Organ Blood Flow*, sect. 2, vol. III, part 1, pp. 137–182. American Physiological Society, Bethesda, MD.

Henriksen, O. (1977). Local sympathetic reflex mechanism in regulation of blood flow in human subcutaneous adipose tissue. *Acta Physiol. Scand. 101 (Suppl. 450)*, 7–48.

Henry, J.P., and O.H. Gauer (1950). The influence of temperature upon venous pressure in the foot. *J. Clin. Invest. 29*, 855–861.

Hesse, B., H. Ring-Larsen, I. Nielsen, and N.J. Christensen (1978). Renin stimulation by passive tilting: the influence of an anti-gravity suit on postural changes in plasma renin activity, plasma noradrenaline concentration and kidney function in normal man. *Scand. J. Clin. Lab. Invest. 38*, 163–169.

Heymans, C. (1929). *Le Sinus Carotidien*. H. K. Lewis, London.

Hill, L. (1895). The influence of the force of gravity on the circulation of the blood. *J. Physiol. (Lond.) 18*, 15–53.

Hill, L., and H. Barnard (1897). The influence of the force of gravity on the circulation. *J. Physiol. (Lond.) 21*, 323–352.

Hoffman, J.I.E., A. Guz, A.A. Charlier, and D.E.L. Wilcken (1965). Stroke volume in conscious dogs: effect of respiration, posture, and vascular occlusion. *J. Appl. Physiol. 20*, 865–877.

Johnson, J.M. (1986). Nonthermoregulatory control of human skin blood flow. *J. Appl. Physiol. 61*, 1613–1622.

Johnson, J.M., L.B. Rowell, and G.L. Brengelmann (1974a). Modification of the skin blood flow-body temperature relationship by upright exercise. *J. Appl. Physiol. 37*, 880–886.

Johnson, J.M., L.B. Rowell, M. Niederberger, and M.M. Eisman (1974b). Human splanchnic and forearm vasoconstrictor responses to reductions of right atrial and aortic pressure. *Circ. Res. 34*, 515–524.

Kirchheim, H.R. (1976). Systemic arterial baroreceptor reflexes. *Physiol. Rev. 56*, 100–176.

Krogh, A. (1912). Regulation of the supply of blood to the right heart (with a description of a new circulation model). *Skand. Arch. Physiol. 27*, 227–248.

Levy, M.N. (1979). The cardiac and vascular factors that determine systemic blood flow. *Circ. Res. 44*, 739–746.

Lundvall, J., and T. Länne (1989). Large capacity in man for effective plasma volume control in hypovolaemia via fluid transfer from tissue to blood. *Acta Physiol. Scand. 137*, 513–520.

Mancia, G., and A.L. Mark (1983). Arterial baroreflexes in humans. In J.T. Shepherd, F.M. Abboud, and S.R. Geiger, eds. *Handbook of Physiology. The Cardiovascular System: Peripheral Circulation and Organ Blood Flow*, sect. 2, vol. III, part 2, pp. 755–793. American Physiological Society, Bethesda, MD.

Mark, A.L., and G. Mancia (1983). Cardiopulmonary baroreflexes in humans. In J.T. Shepherd, F.M. Abboud, and S.R. Geiger, eds. *Handbook of Physiology. The Cardiovascular System: Peripheral Circulation and Organ Blood Flow*. sect. 2, vol. III, part 2, pp. 795–813.

Marshall, J.M. (1982). The influence of the sympathetic nervous system on individual vessels of the microcirculation of skeletal muscle of the rat. *J. Physiol. (Lond.) 332*, 169–186.

McDowall, R.J.S. (1924). A vago-pressor reflex. *J. Physiol. (Lond.) 59*, 41–47.

McDowall, R.J.S. (1956). *The Control of the Circulation of the Blood*. Dawson, London.

Mendelowitz, D.D., and A.M. Scher (1988). Pulsatile sinus pressure changes evoke sustained baroreflex responses in awake dogs. *Am. J. Physiol. 255 (Heart Circ. Physiol. 24)*, H673–H678.

Mohanty, P.K., M.D. Thames, J.A. Arrowood, J.R. Sowers, C. McNamara, and S. Szentpetery (1987). Impairment of cardiopulmonary baroreflex after cardiac transplantation in humans. *Circulation 75*, 914–921.

O'Leary, D.S., A.M. Scher, and J.E. Bassett (1989). Effects of steps in cardiac output and arterial pressure in awake dogs with AV block. *Am. J. Physiol. 256 (Heart Circ. Physiol. 25)*, H361–H367.

Poliner, L.R., G.J. Dehmer, S.E. Lewis, R.W. Parkey, C.G. Blomqvist, and J.T. Willerson (1980). Left ventricular performance in normal subjects: a comparison of the responses to exercise in the upright and supine positions. *Circulation 62*, 528–534.

Ring-Larsen, H., B. Hesse, J.H. Henriksen, and N.J. Christensen (1982). Sympathetic nervous activity and renal and systemic hemodynamics in cirrhosis: plasma norepinephrine concentration, hepatic extraction, and renal disease. *Hepatology 2*, 304–310.

Robinson, B.F., S.E. Epstein, G.D. Beiser, and E. Braunwald (1966). Control of heart rate by the autonomic nervous system: studies in man on the interrelation between baroreceptor mechanisms and exercise. *Circ. Res. 19*, 400–411.

Robinson, V.J.B., O.A. Smiseth, N.W. Scott-Douglas, E.R. Smith, J.V. Tyberg, and D.E. Manyari (1990). Assessment of the splanchnic vascular capacity and capacitance using quantitative equilibrium blood pool scintigraphy. *J. Nucl. Med. 31*, 154–159.

Rothe, C.F. (1983a). Reflex control of veins and vascular capacitance. *Physiol. Rev. 63*, 1281–1342.

Rothe, C.F. (1983b). Venous system: physiology of the capacitance vessels. In

J.T. Shepherd, F.M. Abboud, and S.R. Geiger, eds. *Handbook of Physiology. The Cardiovascular System: Peripheral Circulation and Organ Blood Flow* sect. 2, vol. III, part 1, pp. 397–452. American Physiological Society, Bethesda, MD.

Rothe, C.F. (1983c). Measurement of circulatory capacitance and resistance. In R.J. Linden, ed. *Techniques in the Life Sciences*, vol. P3/1, pp. P306/1–P306/28. Elsevier, New York.

Rothe, C.F., and M.L. Gaddis (1990). Autoregulation of cardiac output by passive elastic characteristics of the vascular capacitance system. *Circulation 81*, 360–368.

Rowell, L.B. (1977). Reflex control of the cutaneous vasculature. *J. Invest. Dermatol. 69*, 154–166.

Rowell, L.B. (1986). *Human Circulation: Regulation During Physical Stress.* Oxford University Press, New York.

Rowell, L.B., J.-M.R. Detry, J.R. Blackmon, and C. Wyss (1972). Importance of the splanchnic vascular bed in human blood pressure regulation. *J. Appl. Physiol. 32*, 213–220.

Rusch, N.J., J.T. Shepherd, R.C. Webb, and P.M. Vanhoutte (1981). Different behavior of the resistance vessels of the human calf and forearm during contralateral isometric exercise, mental stress, and abnormal respiratory movements. *Circ. Res. 48*, 111–1130.

Shepherd, J.T. (1963). *Physiology of the Circulation in Human Limbs in Health and Disease.* W.B. Saunders, Philadelphia.

Shepherd, J.T., and P.M. Vanhoutte (1975). *Veins and Their Control.* W.B. Saunders, Philadelphia.

Shoukas, A.A., and H.G. Bohlen (1990). Rat venular pressure-diameter relationships are regulated by sympathetic activity. *Am. J. Physiol. 259 (Heart Circ. Physiol. 28)*, H674–H680.

Shoukas, A.A., and K. Sagawa (1973). Control of systemic vascular capacity by the carotid sinus baroreceptor reflex. *Circ. Res. 33*, 22–33.

Skagen, K. (1983). Sympathetic reflex control of blood flow in human subcutaneous tissue during orthostatic maneuvres. *Dan. Med. Bull. 30*, 229–241.

Skokland, O. (1983). Factors contributing to acute blood pressure elevation. *J. Oslo City Hosp. 33*, 81–95.

Sprangers, R.L.H., K.H. Wesseling, A.L.T. Imholz, B.P.M. Imholz, and W. Wieling (1991). Initial blood pressure fall on stand up and exercise explained by changes in total peripheral resistance. *J. Appl. Physiol. 70*, 523–530.

Tyden, G. (1977). Aspects of cardiovascular reflex control in man. *Acta Physiol. Scand. Suppl. 448*, 1–62.

Tyden, G., H. Samnegard, and L. Thulin (1979). The effects of changes in the carotid sinus baroreceptor activity on splanchnic blood flow in anesthetized man. *Acta Physiol. Scand. 106*, 187–189.

Vatner, S.F., and M. Zimpfer (1981). Bainbridge reflex in conscious, unrestrained, and tranquilized baboons. *Am. J. Physiol. 240 (Heart Circ. Physiol. 9)*, H164–H167.

Victor, R.G., and A.L. Mark (1985). Interaction of cardiopulmonary and carotid baroreflex control of vascular resistance in humans. *J. Clin. Invest. 76*, 1592–1598.

Wilkins, R.W., J.W. Culbertson, and F.J. Ingelfinger (1951). The effect of splanchnic sympathectomy in hypertensive patients upon estimated hepatic blood

flow in the upright as contrasted with the horizontal position. *J. Clin. Invest.*
    31, 312–317.
Youmans, J.B., J.H. Akeroyd, Jr., and H. Frank (1935). Changes in the blood and
    circulation with changes in posture: the effect of exercise and vasodilatation.
    J. Clin. Invest. 14, 739–753.
Zolte, N., C. Young, I. Faris, and E. Tan (1989). The veno-arteriolar reflex in free
    skin flaps. *Clin. Physiol. 9,* 183–188.

3

Neural-Humoral Adjustments to Orthostasis and Long-Term Control

Without rapid constriction of resistance vessels, upright posture would not be possible without severe arterial hypotension in any animal whose heart lies considerable distance above the remainder of the circulation. The most rapid vasoconstriction is initiated by sympathetic vasomotor fibers. If the stress is prolonged, blood pressure is supported by circulating hormones that modify renal salt and water excretion and, in higher concentrations, are also vasoactive. Both neural and humoral effectors can act as efferent arms of the cardiopulmonary and arterial baroreflexes.

The primary objective of this chapter is to show when and how neural and humoral factors play their key roles in maintaining blood pressure during orthostasis. In Chapter 2 the term *reflex vasoconstriction* was used repeatedly without coming to grips with the evidence. Was the vasoconstriction actually mediated by increasing the firing rate of sympathetic adrenergic nerves? Perhaps the vasoconstriction was initiated by sympathetic nerves and maintained by circulating hormones. How could we know? This chapter outlines first the information that underlies our basic understanding of how sympathetic vasomotor nerves control vascular conductance. It explains the techniques we use to measure sympathetic nervous activity and shows how the measures of this activity change during orthostasis. The discussion will also reveal the problems of quantitatively relating the vasomotor response to this activity. Another objective is to show that time-dependent changes in the circulation during orthostasis require that adjustments go beyond neurogenic vasoconstriction in order to minimize progressive central hypovolemia. The volume of blood sequestered in dependent veins increases slowly at a given transmural pressure because their viscoelastic properties lead to a phenomenon called "creep" or "delayed compliance." Despite vasoconstriction, continued capillary filtration increases interstitial fluid volume (edema), so that eventually the rise in interstitial pressure limits further loss of intravascular volume. These gradual changes are accompanied by a slow and continuous decline in central venous pressure, arterial pulse pressure, and plasma volume. The progressive hypovolemia must be counteracted by circulating hormones that act slowly as both salt- and water-retaining hormones. Some of these hormones also act rapidly and directly as vasoconstrictor agents, thus serving in parallel with neurally mediated vasoconstriction.

One of the most important ideas put forward in this chapter is that we are protected by multiple, redundant feedback loops, most of which have rather high gain. This redundancy means that the removal of one feedback control mechanism can be almost fully compensated for (depending on its gain) by the action of additional (redundant) controllers, which may or may not have been tonically active. Although this improves our chances of survival, it creates a nightmare for the investigator who seeks to establish the relative importance of one of these feedback mechanisms.

NEURAL CONTROL

Sympathetic Adrenergic Innervation: The Efferent Neural Arm of Homeostatic Reflexes

The sympathetic or thoracolumbar division of the autonomic nervous system innervates the entire arterial tree down to the smallest arterioles before metarterioles and capillaries are reached. It also innervates veins of the splanchnic organs down to small venules. Adrenergic innervation of skeletal muscle veins and venules is still questioned (Marshall 1991). The neural transmitter is norepinephrine, which is often released with a cotransmitter, neuropeptide Y (Pernow et al., 1987; Eckberg et al., 1988). This cotransmitter is released at higher rates of nerve firing than trigger norepinephrine release alone, and the neuropeptide's powerful constriction of vascular smooth muscle persists longer.

Liberation of norepinephrine from nerve varicosities is modulated by a number of substances, some of which can, in effect, amplify the action of norepinephrine on α_1-adrenoceptors by decreasing reuptake and increasing release. Other substances, such as locally released metabolites, can interfere with the actions of norepinephrine on the postjunctional α-adrenoceptors or inhibit its release from the nerve varicosities (prejunctional inhibition). The last point is especially important for later discussion, for it is the basis for the notion that activation of sympathetic vasoconstriction is severely blunted in metabolically active organs (see also discussion of hypoxemia in Chapter 4).

Three important generalizations about sympathetic vasoconstrictor innervation to bear in mind are as follows:

1. Only the adrenergic or noradrenergic fibers are ubiquitously distributed throughout the entire cardiovascular system.
2. Only the adrenergic fibers are tonically active and contribute to resting vascular tone.
3. Only the adrenergic fibers compromise the efferent arm of the major homeostatic reflexes, such as baroreflexes, chemoreflexes, and reflexes associated with exercise.

The only known exception to 2 and 3 above is the putative neurogenic vasodilator transmitter (probably peptidergic) released by sympathetic nerves in human skin (Hökfelt et al., 1980), which serves, along with sweating (mediated by sympathetic cholinergic nerve fibers), as a primary effector of temperature regulation.

In contrast, the known sympathetic "vasodilator" fibers (excluding those just referred to in human skin) have the following characteristics:

1. A relatively sparse distribution to particular organs or to specialized tissues within an organ
2. Not tonically active and thus do not contribute to resting vascular conductance
3. Appear to play no active role in baroreflexes and other homeostatic reflexes
4. Appear not to open more capillaries, indicating that neurogenic vasodilation does not increase exchange of materials across the microcirculation

Sympathetic nerve fibers may contain several cotransmitters, which include peptides, purines (e.g., adenosine triphosphate, dopamine, vasoactive intestinal polypeptide, and so on (Hökfelt et al., 1980; Burnstock, 1986; Pernow et al., 1987).

There are also cholinergic nerve fibers originating in the craniosacral, parasympathetic outflow that are known to supply arterioles in the brain, heart, erectile tissue of the genitalia, and various glands in the gastrointestinal tract. For the most part the role played by these vasodilator fibers is unknown. Their importance in contributing to hyperemia in certain glands and permitting the engorgement of erectile tissue of the genitalia is well established. The vasomotor portion of the parasympathetic nervous system appears not to participate in any quantitatively significant way in the major homeostatic reflexes (Rowell 1986).

Neural Influences in Differential Vasomotor Control

Various organs may respond differently to a given magnitude of sympathetic vasoconstrictor nerve activity. This stems from regional variations in the responsiveness of resistance vessels to sympathetic activity and to humoral influences as well. Bevan (1979) reviewed this topic, and only some of the more important influences are reviewed here. First, the density of α-adrenergic innervation varies among organs. Arterioles supplying skin, skeletal muscle, splanchnic organs, kidneys, and adipose tissue are richly innervated. Innervation is particularly variable in veins, being least in the deep veins of a limb and greatest in the splanchnic and cutaneous veins. Second, sensitivity of vascular smooth muscle to norepinephrine varies from region to region. The density of α-adrenoceptors can contribute to this variation. Third, there is some heterogeneity of α-adrenergic receptors; for example, in the brain they are different from those in other regions (Bevan, 1979; Vanhoutte et al., 1981). Fourth, modes of norepinephrine removal differ from region to region, depending partly on the density of innervation and also on the width of the junctional cleft. In some regions, neuronal reuptake predominates, whereas in others, norepinephrine is removed extraneurally after it spills over into the bloodstream (Esler et al., 1990).

Intrinsic and Local Influences in Differential Vasomotor Control

In addition to neural influences, there are intrinsic and local influences as well that cause regional differences in vasomotor control. The level of intrinsic vascular tone or basal tone varies among different organs and influences the responses to sympathetic stimulation (Bevan, 1979). For example, basal tone is commonly found to be low in the kidneys and appears to be greatest in the heart, brain, and skeletal muscle. An important generalization is that *tissues with the greatest range of metabolism have the greatest range of basal tone*. It is this basal tone that is modulated by neural and humoral influences.

Vascular size and structure vary and contribute to the heterogeneity of responses to adrenergic stimulation. The smaller the vessel, the smaller the junctional cleft, the more localized the action of released norepinephrine, and the more the rate of neuronal reuptake of the transmiter will affect the overall response (this also has important bearing on the amount of norepinephrine that leaks from nerve terminals into circulating blood [Esler et al., 1990]).

Release of endogenous vasoactive substances (autacoids) such as the prostaglandins, adenine nucleotides, histamine, and 5-hydroxytryptamine can compete with adrenergic effects. Also, locally produced vasoactive metabolites can attenuate vasoconstriction when rates of sympathetic activation are low (Vanhoutte et al., 1981). Circulating humoral agents can impede or potentiate the response to neurogenic vasoconstriction (e.g., angiotensin II potentiates effects of norepinephrine). Vasomotor influences can be augmented by cooling or attenuated by heating as in cutaneous vessels, or can cause the opposite effects in other vessels such as in deep veins of the limbs (Vanhoutte, 1980; Vanhoutte et al., 1981). Cold-induced cutaneous vasomotion is mediated by α_2-adrenoreceptors rather than α_1-adrenoceptors (Flavahan, 1985). Finally, the interaction among neurotransmitters, circulating humoral agents, and potent substances released by vascular endothelium may prove to be the most potent local influences (Vanhoutte, 1988).

Summary. In summary, the factors that account for regional differences in response to sympathetic vasoconstrictor discharge include differences in density and distribution of α_1- and α_2-adrenoceptors, affinity of the receptors for norepinephrine, and modes of norepinephrine removal from the junctional cleft (release of the cotransmitters probably varies from region to region). Regional differences in basal tone, densities of sympathetic innervation and neurotransmitter receptor sites, quantity of smooth muscle, competing action of local metabolites, and different receptor types can all be factors.

Diffuse Versus Punctate Activation of Sympathetic Nerves

An old but recurrent question regarding the mode of activation of the sympathetic nervous system is whether it is "turned on" more or less en masse with different regional responses being determined by variations in competing local influences. Alternatively, sympathetic activity could be directed from higher centers of the central nervous system to more or less specific target sites. In one view, activation of the sympathetic nervous system is equivalent to throwing the master switch that turns on all the lights in the house at once, whereas the counterview is that each light could be turned on separately.

Scher and associates (1991) summarized the findings from retrograde labeling of sympathetic preganglionic neurons in the hypothalamus, pons, and medulla. The observation that each neuron appeared to project from a central area to only a single spinal segment could suggest a specificity for the sympathetic connections from each central neuron pool. Conversely, one could argue for a lack of specificity because the neurons projecting to different spinal segments were intermixed at their central origins so as to reveal no topographical organization. Neither observation offers conclusive evidence.

Could a principal source of regional variation in sympathetically mediated vasomotor responses be found in discrete patterns of sympathetic outflow to different organs? Or, conversely, could differences in responsiveness to a fixed rate of sympathetic nerve stimulation be the major cause of this variation? The concept once put forward by Walter B. Cannon, that the entire sympathetic nervous system is activated en masse so as to produce a uniform outflow, must be modified. More recent studies on humans and other species put to rest any notion that sympathetic nervous outflow is always diffuse and that its differential effects are due only to local modulation at specific receptor and vascular sites (Simon and Riedel, 1975; Wennergren, 1975; Vallbo et al., 1979). We will find examples suggesting that either pattern of activation might occur. Scher and colleagues (1991) suggest that the specificity found in some situations (e.g., temperature regulation) may not be evident in the baroreflexes (or possibly during exercise, as discussed later).

Direct Assessments of Sympathetic Nerve Activity

The proof that regional vasoconstriction is directly mediated by release of norepinephrine from sympathetic nerve varicosities comes from two main sources; (1) measurement of plasma concentration and spillover of norepinephrine, and (2) direct intraneural measurements of muscle sympathetic nerve activity (MSNA) by the microneurographic technique (Vallbo et al., 1979).

Spillover of Norepinephrine to the Circulation

This topic was reviewed by Esler and coworkers (1990). In humans only a small fraction of the norepinephrine in plasma is derived from adrenal medullary secretions; the rest is released from sympathetic nerve varicosities, along with neuropeptides and other putative neurotransmitters (Burnstock, 1986; Pernow et al., 1987). Only 10 to 20 percent of the norepinephrine released from the varicosities escapes from the synaptic cleft into the interstitial spaces and spills into plasma where it is degraded by monoamine oxidases, largely in the liver and kidneys. The remaining 80 to 90 percent of this neurotransmitter is either taken up by the sympathetic neurons (neuronal reuptake) where it is reincorporated into vesicular stores or taken up by smooth muscle cells and methylated. Despite the relatively small fraction of the total neuronal release, the rate of norepinephrine spillover into venous drainage of individual organs is usually (but not always) proportional to the rate of firing of their sympathetic nerve supply (local inhibition of neuronal release or extreme changes in neuronal reuptake can alter this relationship).

Regional Norepinephrine Spillover. Organ spillover is determined not only by local sympathetic firing rate and neuronal reuptake, but also by organ mass, organ blood flow, the width of the synaptic or junctional clefts, and diffusion-concentration gradients and capillary permeability of norepinephrine. Nevertheless, the use of regional measures of norepinephrine spillover into plasma as a measure of sympathetic nervous activity is justified if the rate at which norepinephrine spills from sympathetic varicosities into venous drainage of an organ is *proportional* to the rate of sympathetic nerve firing to that organ. Electrical stimulation of sympathetic nerves supplying the heart, kidneys, liver, skeletal muscle, spleen, and pancreas reveals that this proportionality exists, but the quantitative relationships vary substantially from organ to organ, depending on perfusion, mass, and so on (Esler et al., 1990). Also, for a given organ these relationships can vary greatly among different individuals (e.g., Oliver et al., 1980).

Organ spillover of norepinephrine is greatest in skeletal muscle and kidneys. The lungs were thought to have high spillover rates as well (Esler et al., 1990), but this has been challenged experimentally (Hjemdahl et al., 1989). Skeletal muscle contributes somewhere between 20 and 50 percent, the kidneys approximately 25 percent, the splanchnic region approximately 10 percent, skin about 5 percent, and the heart only 2 to 3 percent of the total norepinephrine spillover in resting humans (Esler et al., 1990).

Total Norepinephrine Spillover. Esler and colleagues (1990) pointed to the hope that whole-body norepinephrine spillover rate would prove to be a reliable method for measuring overall sympathetic nerve activity or integrated nerve firing rate. They carefully outlined the pitfalls, including cases in which spillover and firing rate can change in opposite directions. A major problem is that determination of spillover rates depends on the sampling site. For example, if a substantial fraction of the total norepinephrine spillover were to occur in the pulmonary circulation or outside of the systemic circuit or mixing chamber into which radiolabeled norepinephrine is infused, errors would occur.

Determination of Norepinephrine Spillover. Measurement of norepinephrine spillover is based on traditional metabolic clearance rate methods. Dilution of tritiated norepinephrine ($[^3H]NE$) in plasma is used to measure its rate of spillover into plasma. The $[^3H]NE$ is infused so that in a steady state (which must exist for the technique to be valid):

$$\text{Total NE spillover rate (ng min}^{-1}) = \frac{[^3H]NE \text{ infusion rate}}{\text{plasma NE specific activity}} \quad (3\text{-}1)$$

To calculate net overflow from an organ by the Fick principle, both the arteriovenous concentration difference for norepinephrine and the plasma flow are needed. Because norepinephrine is being both released as well as taken up, net spillover is underestimated without the simultaneous measurement of $[^3H]NE$ extraction by the organ. In at steady state:

$$\text{Organ NE spillover (ng min}^{-1}) = [(C_{VNE} - C_{ANE}) + C_{ANE} (NE_{Extr})] \cdot Q \quad (3\text{-}2)$$

where C_{ANE} and C_{VNE} are arterial and venous plasma concentrations of norepinephrine, NE_{Extr} is the fraction of $[^3H]NE$ extracted, and Q is organ plasma flow (Esler et al., 1990).

Others have substituted the extraction of unlabeled epinephrine by an organ for $[^3H]NE$ extraction to estimate that organ's norepinephrine extraction. This is feasible because there is normally no neuronal release of epinephrine, routes of uptake are the same for both catecholamines, and the extraction of epinephrine is consistently 70 percent of the norepinephrine extraction.

Despite the limitations in using the plasma concentration of norepinephrine as an index of total or regional sympathetic activity, norepinephrine levels in arterial and forearm venous blood (locally biased mainly by release and reuptake within forearm muscle) nevertheless closely parallel sympathetically mediated increases in heart rate and vascular resistance measured either as regional vasoconstriction or directly determined by neural recordings (see Figure 3-1). The norepinephrine concentration often provides a crude but valid qualitative index of overall sympathetic nerve activity in normal humans under a wide variety of stressful conditions (Christensen, 1979; Goldstein et al., 1983; Hjemdahl et al., 1989). The measurement of concentration provides important clues about disturbances in sympathetic control as well (see Chapter 4). The close relationships among plasma norepinephrine concentration, sympathetically medi-

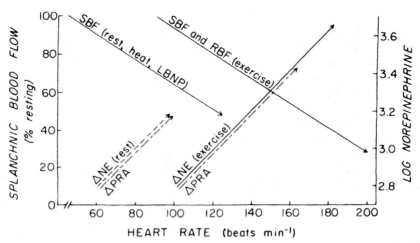

Figure 3-1   Schematic summary of relationship among splanchnic (*SBF*) and renal blood flows (*RBF*) and changes in plasma norepinephrine concentration (*NE*) and renin activity (*PRA*) in relation to heart rate. Subjects were physically stressed during rest and exercise. In exercise, sympathetic activity did not increase until heart rate approached 100 beats min^{-1}. Rightward shift of slopes with exercise is important (see Chapter 6) (for references, see Rowell, 1983, 1984). Real slopes for PRA are not available because of variation in published units, but intercepts with heart rate during stresses applied at rest or during exercise were similar to those for NE. Figure emphasizes predictability of regional vasoconstriction and plasma NE concentration relative to heart rate during stresses that increase sympathetic nervous activity. (From Rowell, 1986, with permission of Oxford University Press.)

ated regional vasoconstriction, and heart rate are referred to frequently in this book and are illustrated in Figure 3-1.

Norepinephrine Spillover During Orthostasis

When humans stand up, both plasma concentration and spillover of norepinephrine increases (Davis et al., 1987), but the total rate of spillover will be lessened in relation to the rise in sympathetic activity, owing to the reduction in blood flow to major organs by vasoconstriction. For example, during a 60° head-up tilt, plasma norepinephrine concentration rose from 242 to 570 pg ml^{-1}, total spillover increased from 2 to 3.4 nM min^{-1} per m^2 of body surface, and plasma clearance of norepinephrine fell from 1.43 to 1.0 L min^{-1} per m^2. The fall in clearance must stem mainly from the fall in splanchnic blood flow, inasmuch as most of the norepinephrine is normally cleared by the liver.

Directly Measured Sympathetic Nerve Activity by Microneurography

Our understanding of sympathetic control has grown with the development of microneurographic techniques that permit continuous registration of firing from the sympathetic axons within a fascicle containing fibers that innervate either the skin or skeletal muscle of an extremity (Vallbo et al., 1979; Wallin and Fagius, 1988). This technique permits a close look at the timing of sympathetic activation (or inactivation) unimpeded by the much slower events at the effector sites of a target organ. Also, sympathetic effects can sometimes be separated from those attributable to hormonal or other actions.

Multiunit nerve recordings are made via tungsten microelectrodes with tip diameters of a few micrometers. The electrode is percutaneously inserted into a nerve fascicle of a large peripheral nerve of an extremity, specifically the median, radial, or ulnar nerves in the arm, or, more commonly, the peroneal or tibial nerves in the leg are used (Wallin 1983). Sympathetic axons within these nerves supply mainly muscle and skin. The sympathetic origin of the impulses is assured by showing that changes in burst frequency and/or amplitude accompany events known to be sympathetically mediated; examples are changes in arterial pressure (e.g., during a Valsalva maneuver), changes in vascular resistance, or specifically for skin, changes in skin electrical resistance or plethysmograph pulse amplitude (Wallin and Fagius, 1988). The efferent nature of the impulses was shown by effects of injecting local anesthetic proximal or distal to the recording electrode and by demonstrating that activity was reversibly abolished by intravenous administration of a ganglion-blocking drug. Also, impulses were found to be conducted at about 1 m sec^{-1}, which matches conduction velocity of a sympathetic axon. Sympathetic bursts picked up by the electrode are amplified, filtered, rectified, and integrated. Recorded sympathetic nerve activity is quantified by measuring the number of bursts and their average amplitude per unit time; this activity is reported either as *burst frequency* (burst min^{-1}) or as a dimensionless *total activity*. The latter is the product of burst frequency and average amplitude. Amplitude is a function of the number of axons firing near the electrode at a given instant. Figure 3-2 shows a recording of muscle sympathetic nerve activity (MSNA).

Distinction between sympathetic axons supplying the skin and those supplying skeletal muscle is straightforward. In contrast to the sympathetic axons supplying the muscle, those supplying skin are characterized by an irregular burst pattern, the magnitude of which varies markedly with arousal or emotion and with environmental temperature (Wallin and Fagius, 1988). In contrast, MSNA shows a periodic bursting pattern that is synchronized with the cardiac cycle by the arterial baroreflex (Figure 3-2). This pulse synchrony is also modulated by respiratory rhythm through effects of breathing on arterial pressure and also through the lung inflation reflexes (Seals et al., 1990). This synchrony of MSNA with the heartbeat is lost when the arterial baroreflex is not functional (even if the cardiopulmonary baroreflex is intact (Aksamit et al., 1987).

An important feature of MSNA in *resting* individuals is that burst patterns measured from axons in the arms and legs have striking similarity (Sundlöf and Wallin, 1977). This has led to the important assumption

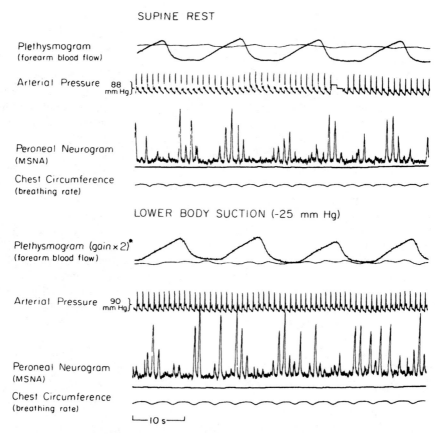

Figure 3-2 Direct measurement of muscle sympathetic nerve activity (MSNA) by microneurography in the peroneal nerve of a normal subject during supine rest (*top*) and lower body suction at −25 mmHg (*bottom*). Large spikes on neurogram are bursts of sympathetic activity. Lower body suction increased amplitude and burst frequency of MSNA (see averaged results in Figure 3-5). Forearm blood flow (slope of plethysmograph curve) fell by approximately one-half during stress (actual slope is doubled by gain increase). Arterial pressure was unchanged and heart rate increased slightly. (From Rowell and Seals, 1990.)

(discussed in later chapters) that the MSNA recorded in one limb in an individual undergoing stress is probably the same as the activity in another limb from which MSNA cannot be recorded for one reason or another. This is known *not* to be true during mental stress (Anderson et al., 1987), but similar levels of MSNA in different limbs have been seen during static exercise (Wallin et al., 1989), and lower body suction (Rea and Wallin, 1989). A second important feature of MSNA is that its strength at rest differs markedly between individuals, and it can vary greatly in a given individual with very slight changes in the recording site (e.g., Rowell and Seals, 1990).

Muscle Sympathetic Nervous Activity and Its Relation to Plasma Norepinephrine Levels and Vasomotor Responses

Microneurography records impulses from a small fraction of the potentially active sympathetic fibers within a nerve fascicle. Thus, a consistent and close relationship between MSNA and the concentration of norepinephrine in the venous blood draining the site of both measurements might not be expected. Commonly MSNA is determined in the leg and norepinephrine concentration is measured in forearm venous blood. A close relationship between nerve activity and norepinephrine concentration would surely not be expected under any circumstances in which changes in MSNA in the arm differed substantially from changes in the leg.

Significant correlations between MSNA determined in a leg and forearm venous norepinephrine concentration have been observed in subjects undergoing dynamic exercise (Seals et al., 1988), a cold pressor test (Victor et al., 1987), and in subjects in whom blood pressure was altered by vasopressor or vasodilator drugs (Eckberg et al., 1988). One reason for the good correlations may be that most of the norepinephrine appearing in forearm venous blood is derived from sympathetic varicosities within the forearm muscles (Esler et al., 1990), which presumably receive the same levels of MSNA as the leg muscles. Wallin and Fagius (1988) and Hjemdahl et al., (1989) observed a significant positive correlation between MSNA in the peroneal nerve and spillover of [3H]NE into femoral venous blood.

The next question to be answered about direct measurement of sympathetic activity is whether it can be quantitatively related to the effector response, namely, to increased vascular resistance in the target organ. Again, this is asking a lot from a sampling of activity from an unknown fraction of the local axon population. Wennergren (1975) pointed out four drawbacks in the neurophysiological approach to analyzing quantitatively the reflex involvement of the effectors. *First,* small changes in discharge frequency are difficult to determine in multifiber preparations; small changes in frequency can have major functional significance. *Second,* even if one knows that a recording is from a vasomotor fiber, it is often not possible to know which vascular bed or vascular section is innervated (the problem of separating muscle versus skin in the limbs has been dealt with satisfactorily in humans). *Third,* there appears to be a pool of preganglionic sympathetic neurons, which are averaged in with others and are not influenced by superspinal structures and therefore do not participate in baroreflexes, thus the meaning of an average discharge is questioned. *Fourth,* the relationship between vasomotor fiber discharge frequency and vasomotor response is not linear and tends to be more sensitive at low discharge frequencies. The alternative to nerve recording is measurement of blood flow, blood pressure, and vascular resistance. It is quantitative—but again responses are slow and cannot always inform us about the effector mechanism for the response, that is, it could be humorally mediated.

Seals (1989) related the sympathetic neural discharge to muscles of one lower leg (peroneal nerve) with vascular resistance in the contralateral lower leg before, during and after isometric handgrip exercise. Figure 3-3 shows the similar time course of the changes in calf vascular resistance and MSNA. Rowell and Seals (1990) found close correlations between changes in forearm vascular resistance and MSNA in individual subjects undergoing lower body suction (see below), but the slopes relating the two variables varied by orders of magnitude among different subjects, making correlation coefficients for pooled data statistically insignificant. Thus, it has not been possible to predict, froma given relative or absolute change in MSNA, what will happen, in either relative or absolute terms, at the effector site (see Figure 3-4).

The findings of Oliver and coworkers (1980) amplify this point. They measured renal blood flow, renal vascular resistance, and release of norepinephrine into the renal vein in dogs while renal sympathetic activity was controlled by direct electrical stimulation. Correlations among renal sympathetic activity, renal venous norepinephrine concentration and renal vascular resistance among individual dogs were very high; but, as in Figure 3-4, the slopes relating these variables among the different dogs varied so greatly that there were no significant correlations when data for all dogs were pooled. Incidentally, these findings on the kidney suggest that rela-

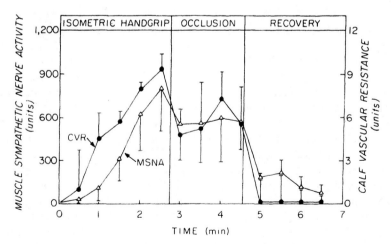

Figure 3-3 Examples of close parallel between direct measurements of sympathetic activity in the peroneal nerve of one leg and the increase in vascular resistance in contralateral leg. Sympathetic activity was increased by isometric forearm exercise, followed by vascular occlusion (see Chapter 11). (Adapted from Seals, 1989.)

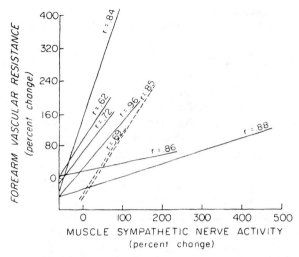

Figure 3-4 Correlation between changes in forearm vascular resistance and muscle sympathetic nerve activity in the leg is mostly high in individuals (stress was lower body suction via protocol in Figure 3-5). However, slopes vary greatly among different individuals, causing low and insignificant correlations for pooled data. (From Rowell and Seals, 1990.)

tionships between MSNA and vascular resistance (or norepinephrine) among different human subjcts do not differ simply because the nerve activity is recorded from different limbs.

So far, no experiments have been carried out to show the relationships among simultaneously measured MSNA, vascular resistance, and norepinephrine concentration or norepinephrine spillover in two different groups of muscles. Possibly one should not expect the changes in arm and leg norepinephrine concentration and spillover to equal or even parallel one another because organ masses, blood flows, and the proportions of skin, muscle, and bone releasing and taking up the transmitter are markedly different in the two limbs.

Summary. In summary, there are two main points:

1. Among individuals there is often a close temporal relationship between MSNA and plasma norepinephrine concentration as well as with muscle vascular resistance at moderate to high levels of sympathetic activity.
2. Among different individuals the absolute changes in MSNA for a given absolute change in plasma, norepinephrine concentration or in vascular resistance will vary greatly.

Nevertheless, the close relationship among these variables in individuals provides good evidence that the sympathetic nervous system is participating importantly in the responses.

Muscle Sympathetic Nerve Activity During Orthostasis and Central Hypovolemia

MSNA increases markedly when humans are upright (Wallin and Fagius, 1988). Although it is clear that the cutaneous vessels are also constricted (see Chapter 2), direct evidence of a sympathetically mediated vasoconstriction is still lacking (Wallin and Fagius, 1988).

Most experiments have used different magnitudes of lower body suction (Chapter 2) to simulate different levels of orthostasis. For example, lower body suction of -45 to -50 mmHg appears to simulate a 90° head-up tilt.

Figure 3-5 shows the progressive rise in MSNA of one leg during very mild lower body suction imposed in 5-mmHg steps up to -25 mmHg. Heart rate and aortic pulse pressure change significantly at a pressure of -20 mmHg; prior to that level, only central venous pressure is decreased (see Figure 2-8). As shown in Figure 3-5, MSNA rises significantly with time throughout lower body suction (Victor and Leimbach, 1987; Rowell and Seals, 1990), although the increments were very small at the lower levels of body suction. Note in Figure 3-5 that there was no significant rise in norepinephrine during lower body suction after -5 mmHg and up through -20 mmHg. The relative increase in MSNA exceeded 100 percent only at -25 mmHg. Based on earlier findings (Victor et al., 1987; Seals et al., 1988), only small, if any, increments in forearm venous norepinephrine concentration would be expected with these increments in MSNA. Nevertheless, the average rise in forearm vascular resistance roughly paralleled the rise in MSNA highlighting, as expected, the greater sensitivity of vascular resistance over norepinephrine concentration as an index of sympathetic activity.

The finding that neural (Rea and Wallin, 1989) and vasomotor responses (Vissing et al., 1989) to lower body suction were similar in the forearm and leg is at odds with the quantitatively different effects of lower body suction on forearm and calf blood flow found by Essandoh and associates (1986). The cause of the discrepancy may stem from the marked differences that can exist in the relationship between recorded nerve activity and degree of vasoconstriction (Figure 3-4) (Wennergren, 1975; Oliver et al., 1980).

Presumably the sympathetic responses to lower body suction up to -20 mmHg in Figure 3-5 are in response to the inhibition of cardiopulmonary baroreceptors and not arterial baroreceptors. As discussed in Chapter 2, any "interaction" between these two reflexes has special importance to humans because of their simultaneous engagement during orthostasis. Presumably, the marked augmentation of forearm vasoconstriction by application of neck suction during mild lower body suction is due to augmented MSNA (see Chapter 2).

Microneurography during higher levels of lower body suction that simulate 90° head-up tilt has not been feasible because the position of

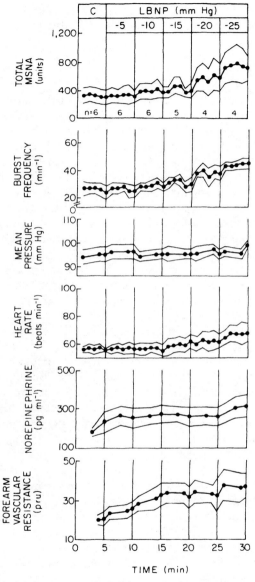

Figure 3-5 Graded increments in muscle sympathetic nerve activity (MSNA) in humans undergoing graded levels of orthostatic stress imposed as mild to moderate lower body suction. Average MSNA and forearm vascular resistance rose together, but not in the same proportions (see Figure 3-4). In contrast, MSNA (peroneal nerve) and forearm venous norepinephrine concentration were often unrelated at such low levels of stress (note relationship improved when stress was increased; see Figure 4-16). (From Rowell and Seals, 1990.)

sympathetic nerve recording electrodes can be significantly altered by the slightest motion attending higher levels of suction.

HUMORAL CONTROL

The main objective of this section is to discuss the importance of humoral control in prolonged orthostasis, during which a significant fraction of the plasma volume leaks out of the capillaries into the interstitial spaces. The focus is on a second line of defense of arterial (and central venous?) pressure via "cardiac" or "atriorenal" reflexes that act on the kidney and the renin-angiotensin-aldosterone axis and also on the pituitary gland to activate secretion of arginine vasopressin. The primary target of these reflexes is the kidney, where they act to regulate plasma volume through the hormonal and neural control of renal water and sodium loss of retention. Another objective here is to weigh evidence about the importance of the cardiorenal reflexes (Henry-Gauer reflex) against growing evidence that arterial baroreflexes may dominate this humoral control in bipeds.

The most important hormones released during orthostasis are angiotensin II, arginine vasopressin, aldosterone, and epinephrine. Atrial peptides have not yet secured a strong place in this scheme for reasons mentioned later (Goetz, 1988). In humans, norepinephrine is not released as a circulating hormone in significant quantities from the adrenal medulla along with epinephrine. Rather, norepinephrine is a neurotransmitter that leaks from sympathetic nerve terminals into plasma. Only during highly stressful conditions does neuronal leakage of norepinephrine become so great that its plasma concentration reaches vasoactive levels. This occurs above concentrations of 1 to 1.5 ng ml^{-1} (three to four times normal resting levels) (Silverberg et al., 1978). Norepinephrine can also directly stimulate renin release despite reflex effects that oppose it (see below) (Licht and Izzo, 1989).

The importance of some circulating hormones to human cardiovascular function in orthostasis remains unclear, for example, the atrial peptides (Goetz, 1988). Their pharmacological effects may be well established but pharmacological doses often far exceed those accompanying natural endogenous release. Primary emphasis here is on angiotensin II and arginine vasopressin; their actions are not only important to the regulation of plasma volume but they are also thought to represent important adjuncts to sympathetic neural control as well. The release of epinephrine from the adrenal medulla is not discussed until Chapter 4, where the focus is on its potentially disruptive effects on regulation during prolonged orthostasis.

The Renin-Angiotensin-Aldosterone System

Figure 3-6 schematically summarizes the causes of, and effects of, activation of the renin-angiotensin system during a prolonged head-up tilt. The

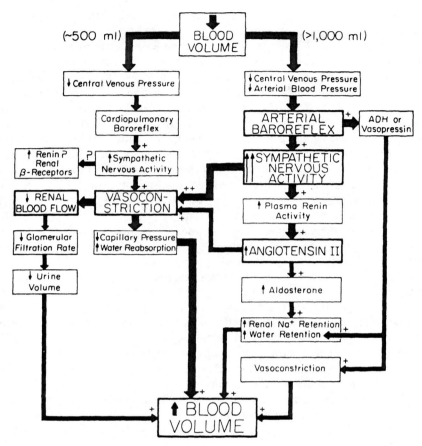

Figure 3-6 Two standard schemes for role of renin-angiotensin-aldosterone axis in maintaining blood volume. Small volume loss (*left*) reduces only central venous pressure. Cardiopulmonary baroreflex mediates increase in sympathetic activity, but renin release is not observed in humans (unless stress is prolonged; see text). Large volume loss (*right*) activates arterial baroreflex which activates renin-angiotensin-aldosterone system. Marked fall in aortic pulse pressure and especially a fall in mean pressure causes antidiuretic hormone (*ADH*) or vasopressin release.

most controversial part of this summary concerns the events that initiate the first significant stimulation of renin release from the kidney. The commonly held view that the inhibition of the cardiopulmonary baroreceptors is the most important initial step (i.e., via the Henry-Gauer reflex) has been challenged because it may apply mainly to quadrupeds and not to bipeds. The challenge is logical if we consider that humans change body position frequently with consequent large fluctuations in central venous pressure that would cause activation and inhibition of the renin release to fluctuate frequently and erratically. Quadrupeds do not experience such erratic shifts in central venous pressure. This issue is discussed in more depth at the end of this chapter.

The scheme in Figure 3-6 highlights two major actions of angiotensin II; namely, it is a vasoconstrictor and it stimulates the release of aldosterone. As a vasoconstrictor, angiotensin II has about 40 times the potency of norepinephrine on a mole-for-mole basis, that is, when the effects are derived from circulating concentrations of both the hormone and the neurotransmitter. Bear in mind, however, that angiotensin II is carried to its target organs by the circulation in which it is diluted before it exerts its vasomotor effects. In contrast, we must consider the concentration of norepinephrine released directly into the junctional cleft of the vascular effector site of its target organ, where its concentration vastly exceeds that reached after it has leaked out into the circulation. In short, such comparisons of potency can be misleading. A better comparison of the relative strengths of the systems outlined in Figure 3-6 is the ability of each to counteract a given reduction in arterial pressure (i.e., the feedback gain) (see Cowley and Liard, 1987).

Angiotensin II is formed in plasma through the action of a proteolytic enzyme, *renin,* contained within the secretory granules of endothelial cells, called juxtaglomerular cells, located near the glomerular end of the renal afferent arteriole. When juxtaglomerular cells are stimulated, renin is released into plasma where it acts on an α_2-globulin called angiotensinogen, from which it cleaves off a decapeptide fragment to form the inactive *angiotensin I.* In its passage from the renal vein through the microcirculation of the lungs, angiotensin I is converted to its active form, *angiotensin II,* by a converting enzyme bound to the vascular endothelium. Any conversion to angiotensin II not completed in the lungs will take place in other organs, all of which contain converting enzyme bound to their vascular endothelium.

The stimuli for the release of renin from kidney are as follows:

1. *Increased activity of the sympathetic nerve fibers that innervate afferent and efferent arterioles of the renal glomerulus.* This neurally induced release of renin is mediated via β_1-adrenergic receptors on juxtaglomerular cells and can be blocked by β-adrenergic antagonists, such as propranolol.
2. *A reduction of the pressure distending afferent arterioles.* The afferent arteriole behaves as a "baroreceptor" so that when renal perfusion pressure is reduced, renin secretion is stimulated. This mechanism of release is not blocked by β-antagonists.
3. *A reduction of the sodium concentration in the early distal tubule.* It is thought that the macula densa, a group of cells in the distal tubules and adjacent to the juxtaglomerular cells, somehow monitors the ionic concentration of the tubular fluid and relays to the juxtaglomerular cells the stimulus for renin secretion.

Also, norepinephrine directly stimulates release of renin in proportion to the circulating concentration of the neurotransmitter (Licht and Izzo, 1989). The effect was shown by norepinephrine infusion (which suppressed sympathetic activity and endogenous norepinephrine release) to be a direct one.

Angiotensin II constricts arterioles by its direct effects on their smooth muscle. This action is not modified by blockade of α- or β-adrenoreceptors. Angiotensin II also raises vascular resistance and stimulates the heart indirectly through its potentiating actions on the sympathetic nervous system. It stimulates sympathetic ganglia; it facilitates responses to sympathetic activity and vasoconstrictor drugs; it accelerates the synthesis of norepinephrine; it increases norepinephrine release in response to impulse traffic; and it delays the neuronal reuptake of the transmitter. Thus, angiotensin II appears to amplify the effects of sympathetic nervous activity by increasing the availability of norepinephrine at the effector sites. If so, angiotensin II might have important effects on peripheral vascular resistance even when its plasma concentration is too low to exert direct effects on vascular smooth muscle. The greatest direct vascular effects of angiotensin in dogs are on renal, hepatic, gastrointestinal, and cutaneous vascular resistances. Equivalent information from humans is not available.

A more gradual and long-term effect of angiotensin II, lasting over hours and days, is its stimulation of aldosterone synthesis and secretion by the adrenal cortex. Because of the importance of this latter function, the system is often referred to as the ''renin-angiotensin-aldosterone system.'' Aldosterone is a mineralocortacoid hormone that increases the reabsorption of sodium by the collecting duct in Henle's loop in the kidney, and it also reduces sodium excretion. As a consequence, water is retained by the kidney, and plasma volume expands. This is an important facet of cardiovascular regulation under conditions in which cardiac filling pressure, cardiac output, and arterial pulse or mean pressures are reduced by inadequate blood volume. It may *not* be important under other conditions that cause reductions only in cardiac filling pressure (see below).

An additional effect of angiotensin II is its action on the central nervous system to provoke water ingestion, secretion of the water-saving hormone vasopressin, or antidiuretic hormone (ADH), and increased sodium ingestion. The diverse peripheral and central effects of the renin-angiotensin-aldosterone system are viewed as having in common a defense of the extracellular fluid volume in the hypovolemic, hypotensive animal.

How Important Is the Renin-Angiotensin System in Orthostasis?

Shepherd (1963) reviewed studies showing that vasoconstriction of the forearm during head-up tilt is sympathetically mediated. Patients with cervical sympathectomies or normal subjects with acute anesthetic blockade of sympathetic nerves supplying the arm were unable to vasoconstrict the limb. Also, any effects of circulating humoral agents were not observable during 10 minutes of maintained full 90°, head-up tilt. Evidence favors a neurally mediated vasoconstriction during the first few minutes of upright posture. Patients without kidneys (no renin) and maintained on dialysis regulate blood pressure normally during a 20-minute head-up tilt at 80° (Oparil et al., 1970).

It is now clear that in normally hydrated, salt-replete humans, release of renin plays no significant role in the immediate hemodynamic responses to orthostasis or lower body suction. Blockade of renin release (or lack of release in anephric patients) or blockade of angiotensin I-converting enzyme does not interfere with hemodynamic adjustment to posture. In contrast, salt-deprived hypovolemic humans require the renin-angiotensin system to maintain arterial pressure during orthostasis; when this system is blocked there is postural hypotension (Oparil and Haber, 1974). In normal subjects salt-depleted by diuretics to increase plasma renin activity, 10 to 15 minutes of lower body suction (severe enough to lower mean arterial pressure by 10 mmHg) caused a marked rise in splanchnic vascular resistance. Pretreatment of the same individuals with angiotensin-converting enzyme inhibitor abolished the splanchnic vasoconstriction, reduced the rise in peripheral vascular resistance and caused a more pronounced fall in arterial pressure (Stadeager et al., 1989). This enzyme inhibitor also reduced plasma norepinephrine levels. Apparently the main constrictor effects of angiotensin II are on the splanchnic and renal circulations; blockade of angiotensin had no effect on forearm vasoconstriction in a later study (Stadeager et al., 1990).

Levels of lower body suction known to lower only central venous pressure without changing arterial pulse pressure cause marked vasoconstriction but do not raise plasma renin activity unless suction is sustained for longer than 10 or 20 minutes (cf. Fasola and Martz, 1972; Bevegård et al., 1977; Mark et al., 1978; Mohanty et al., 1985, 1988). As soon as lower body suction is applied at a level that will *lower aortic pulse pressure* (i.e., at levels exceeding −20 mmHg; see Figure 2-8), renin levels start to rise but still may not reach the levels needed to cause hemodynamic changes (Bevegård et al., 1977; Mark et al., 1978; Mohanty et al., 1988). The important point here is that when lower body suction is applied at low levels sufficient to lower only central venous pressure, the stress must be prolonged in order to stimulate renin secretion.

As shown in Figure 2-1, aortic pulse pressure falls immediately when humans stand up. In upright posture, release of renin parallels the increases in renal vascular resistance and plasma norepinephrine concentration (Hesse et al., 1978; Ring-Larson et al., 1982). Finally, the importance of the renin-angiotensin system appears to depend mainly on how long an orthostatic stress is applied and how much volume leaves the vascular space (see Chapter 4 for further discussion).

Renal retention of salt and water through the actions of aldosterone could constitute an effective long-term adjustment to upright posture by opposing to some degree the gravitational effects on plasma volume. Further, vasoconstrictor actions of angiotensin II (and vasopressin) could serve as important adjuncts to sympathetic vasoconstriction in the maintenance of blood pressure. This could be particularly important during protracted periods of orthostatic stress during which sympathetic nerve activity gradually becomes unable to maintain adequate peripheral vascular resistance.

What Reflexes Initiate Renin Secretion?

Baroreflexes. Debate has centered on what the primary cause of renin release might be. Is it the fall in central venous pressure or the fall in arterial pulse pressure? In dogs, cardiopulmonary vagal afferents appear to exert tonic restraint on renin release; a fall in central venous pressure raises plasma renin activity (Mancia et al., 1975; Thames, 1977). In contrast, Fisher and Malvin (1980) observed no effect of cardiopulmonary baroreceptor denervation on suppression of renin release in volume-expanded dogs. Nevertheless, arterial baroreceptors in dogs can also play a major role as well (Cunningham et al., 1978).

Attempts to separate cardiopulmonary and arterial baroreflex influences on renin release in humans have produced conflicting results, referred to above. Again, the findings shown in Figure 2-8 reveal why this may be true, namely, that levels of lower body suction exceeding −20 mmHg will significantly reduce aortic pulse pressure and inhibit arterial baroreceptors. It may be that renin release in humans, in contrast to dogs, requires inhibition of arterial baroreflexes as appears to be the case for secretion of vasopressin (see below)—or, as some conclude, possibly both ventricular and arterial baroreceptors must be inhibited (Bishop et al., 1983).

Humans, monkeys, and dogs show a decline in plasma renin levels when cardiac chambers are *stretched* by water immersion. Incidentally, the suppression of renin and aldosterone secretion could contribute to the natriuresis accompanying thoracic engorgement (see below) (Krasney et al., 1989).

Cardiorenal Reflexes. Henry and Gauer were the first to propose an important functional link between receptors in the atria and the kidney after they observed that left atrial distension in dogs caused increased urine flow (see Gauer and Henry, 1976). The "reflex" is called the *Henry-Gauer reflex,* or atrio- or cardiorenal reflex. Their logic was, first, that the most distensible regions of the circulation (e.g., the atria) would be best suited to "monitor" small changes in intrathoracic blood volume. Second, all conditions eliciting a change in intrathoracic volume should produce the expected effect on the excretory function of the kidney. For example, stress, such as orthostasis, lower body suction, and venous tourniquets, which lower thoracic blood volume, should cause salt and water retention. Water immersion (at neutral temperature), lower body positive pressure, blood volume expansion, bed rest, and weightlessness should cause natriuresis and diuresis. By and large the findings were consistent with the hypothesis. Eventually volume control by atrial reflexes was considered to be mediated mainly by regulation of renal water clearance through reflex changes in *vasopressin* (antidiuretic hormone) secretion.

Arginine Vasopressin or Antidiuretic Hormone

The neurohormone arginine vasopressin, or simply vasopressin (in some species the arginine is replaced by lysine), is synthesized in cells of the hypothalamus and is stored and released from axon terminals located in the neurohypophysis of the pituitary gland. It is called vasopressin because its powerful vasoconstrictor action was discovered first. In some species (e.g., the rat) this action can exceed that caused by angiotensin II by 30-fold on a mole-for-mole basis. The sensitivity of vascular smooth muscle is less in dogs than in rats, whereas human resistance vessels have only one-tenth the sensitivity to vasopressin seen in dogs. Its vasoconstrictor effects are, like those of other hormones, nonuniform among different organs. Regional differences are not well quantified for humans; in dogs vasoconstriction is greatest in skeletal muscle and some splanchnic organs, but renal blood flow was unchanged. The effects are not purely local effects on vascular smooth muscle; vasopressin can centrally reduce sympathetic vasomotor activity and increase cardiac vagal activity (Cowley and Liard, 1987; Cowley et al., 1988).

Vasopressin later became known as *antidiuretic hormone* ([ADH] or water-retaining hormone) when its potent faciliation of water reabsorption at the distal and collecting tubules of the kidney was recognized. A rise in plasma vasopressin levels reduces free-water clearance by the kidney and has little or no effect on osmotic water clearance, owing to increased sodium clearance (natriuresis). A fall in plasma vasopressin levels has the opposite effect on free-water clearance. In humans, the dose of vasopressin required to raise arterial pressure by 5 mmHg (a poor index of vasoconstriction owing to reflex buffering) is about two times greater than the dose needed for its maximal antidiuretic effect. This may suggest that vasopressin exerts its major physiological effects on renal water reabsorption and plasma volume rather than on vascular resistance in humans—except possibly during severe hemorrhage. During severe hemorrhage, it is clear that vasopressin can become an important factor in preserving blood pressure. Infusion of a competitive inhibitor of vasopressin can reverse the restoration of blood pressure in severely hemorrhaged dogs (Cowley and Liard, 1987). A rise in plasma vasopressin levels can become an important adjunct to sympathetic vasoconstriction when prolonged gravitational stress significantly reduces plasma volume. Further reductions with time are minimized when vasopressin reduces renal water clearance.

What Reflexes Control Vasopressin Secretion in Orthostasis and Volume Expansion?

We come now to the central issue of whether a cardiorenal reflex (the Henry-Gauer reflex) is the dominant controller of the renal water clearance, which serves the maintenance of plasma volume. Conversely, might arterial baroreflexes be more important and might any effect on plasma volume be mediated by altered control of renal sodium clearance as well as water clearance?

Goetz and colleagues (1975) objected to the indirect nature of the evidence for an atriorenal reflex, and argued that the changes required to elicit renal responses were not necessarily confined to the atria and that a necessary link was never established between cardiac "volume" receptors and sodium balance. That is, their point was that extracellular fluid volume is governed largely by renal sodium retention or excretion whereas adjustments in renal free-water clearance are regulated primarily by *vasopressin* secretion, which is dominantly controlled by osmoreceptors (see below). Today the question of what reflexes might govern salt and water management by the kidney presents a complex issue.

Experimental tests on humans to determine how secretion of vasopressin might be controlled have relied heavily on the technique of water immersion to the neck in a thermoneutral bath to raise intrathoracic volume. Water immersion engorges thoracic vessels with blood (Figure 1-9) and raises cardiac output and mean pressure by a marked increase in stroke volume (via Frank-Starling), *which in turn raises aortic pulse pressure;* heart rate does not change. This contrasts with what was seen in dogs; because of their Bainbridge reflex heart rate increases so that neither stroke volume or aortic pulse pressure rise. It will be seen that this species difference helps to unravel a puzzle; changes in aortic pulse pressure could have primary importance in initiating reflex-induced diuresis in humans.

Osmoreceptors. Alternative controllers of vasopressin release are the specialized cells within the hypothalamus called osmoreceptors. If the large fluid translocations within the body during water immersion should reduce plasma osmolarity, vasopressin release would be suppressed. Up to a point, osmolarity is far better guarded than is "volume," which is detected as pressure by baroreceptors. Osmoreceptors detect 1 or 2 percent changes in plasma osmolarity and change vasopressin secretion appropriately (Bie, 1980). In contrast an iso-osmotic change in plasma volume in the order of 5 to 10 percent is required to alter vasopressin by measurable degrees (Cowley and Liard, 1987). To date, the evidence indicates that plasma osmolarity is not significantly altered by orthostasis or water immersion (Norsk and Epstein, 1988).

Cardiopulmonary and Arterial Baroreceptors. If baroreceptors provide the stimulus, is the effect a change in the stretch exerted on mechanoreceptors in the atria and great pulmonary vessels (Gauer and Henry, 1976), or do the baroreceptors in the carotid sinus and aortic arch dominate the control of vasopressin secretion? Many have supported the growing view that dogs or quadrupeds rely predominantly upon an atrio- or cardiorenal-reflex, whereas primates rely mainly on inhibition or activation of arterial baroreceptors to control vasopressin secretion (e.g., Gilmore, 1983). Tele-ologically such a difference in control in quadrupeds versus bipeds would make sense because of the large and frequent excursion in intrathoracic volume and pressure experienced by bipeds. The reviews of Goetz et al., (1975), Gauer and Henry (1976), Gilmore (1983), Norsk and Epstein (1988), and Krasney et al., (1989) provide excellent background.

Central Hypovolemia, Humans. Selective inhibition of cardiac barorecep-tors by lower body suction has no effect on vasopressin levels. Conversely, when the level of suction was increased so as to raise heart rate and lower arterial pulse pressure, without changing mean pressure, vasopressin lev-els rose slightly (Goldsmith et al., 1982). Again, the change in arterial pulse pressure is viewed as being essential to the response.

Responses to upright posture vary among studies. In both young and old subjects vasopressin rose along with angiotensin II and aldosterone during 70 minutes of 70° head-up tilt (Vargas et al., 1986). Although the rise in arterial vasopressin level in well-hydrated subjects during 30 minutes of quiet standing was not significant, venous vasopressin levels rose a significant 31 percent, presumably due to reduced peripheral clearance of the hormone (Os et al., 1984) (recall that standing and head-up tilt are not the same stress).

Central Hypervolemia, Humans. In general, most have found that en-gorgement of thoracic vessels by water immersion to the neck in a ther-moneutral bath (34.5°C) causes a significant fall in plasma renin activity and in vasopressin levels (Norsk and Epstein, 1988). Hydration of subjects tends to suppress this response; nevertheless, their vasopressin levels do decrease and free-water clearance increases (but much less). Prior dehydration of subjects is required to reveal a significant depression in vasopressin levels, partly because low resolution of the assay requires larger changes. Paradoxically, in the dehydrated subjects, the diuresis was attributable to *natriuresis,* which is not an effect of lowered vasopressin levels. Apparently the fall in vasopressin is not sufficient to change signifi-cantly free-water clearance.

Reduction in angiotensin II and aldosterone could contribute to the natriuresis as could a decrease in renal sympathetic nerve activity (dis-cussed below), or the marked increase in plasma atriopeptin levels (dis-cussed later) observed by Norsk and Epstein (1988). The argument against a contribution of aldosterone is that it takes about 40 minutes for its levels to change. Norsk and Epstein (1988) and Norsk (1989) emphasize the poor correlation as well as discrepancies in the time course of the changes in central venous pressure and vasopressin levels. They concluded that in dehydrated subjects suppression of vasopressin levels is not a likely mediator of immersion-induced diuresis.

Elevation in central venous pressure by inflating antishock trousers, by isotonic volume loading, or by 30° head-down tilt failed to reduce plasma vasopressin levels (Goldsmith et al., 1984). The conclusion was that plasma vasopressin levels do not respond to *moderate* iso-osmotic loading of both cardiopulmonary baroreceptors (central venous pressure rose 4 mmHg) *and* arterial baroreceptors (mean arterial pressure rose 7 mmHg). The implication argued by Norsk (1989) is that an elevation in arterial pulse pressure is needed.

Responses to Water Immersion in Primates. The existence of a cardiorenal reflex in primates was questioned in a series of studies by Gilmore and his colleagues (reviewed by Gilmore, 1983; Krasney et al., 1989). This reflex was never demonstrated in monkeys under the same experimental conditions used to show its existence in dogs. Peterson and colleagues (1987) showed that cardiopulmonary afferent neural pathways are not required in anesthetized monkeys to elicit the diuresis and natriuresis in response to water immersion, confirming earlier findings that neither cervical vagotomy nor thoracic sympathectomy altered the renal responses in primates (Gilmore, 1983). However, renal responses to thoracic hypervolemia are markedly changed by anesthesia (Peterson et al., 1987; Krasney et al., 1989). Vatner and coworkers (1986) showed a significant vagal control of renal function in unanesthetized monkeys with chronic sinoaortic denervation to eliminate the (dominant?) influence of these receptors. This suggests that the entire diuresis cannot be explained by stimulation of arterial baroreceptors.

A pivotal finding in this complicated story is that stimulation of *cardiac mechanoreceptors—or arterial baroreceptors—or both could elicit natriuresis and diuresis by reflex inhibition of renal sympathetic activity.* A direct inhibitory effect of renal nerve activity on renal sodium clearance is now viewed as an essential effector mechanism for diuresis in dogs (DiBona, 1985). Adrenergic nerve terminals make direct contact with basement membranes of the proximal and distal renal tubules; in dogs, maneuvers that raise renal sympathetic nerve activity reduce sodium excretion even when renal blood flow does not change (DiBona, 1985). Originally this direct neural effect on natriuresis was not found in anesthetized primates, but in more recent studies on conscious primates renal denervation was found to augment diuresis and natriuresis (see Peterson et al., 1987). (NOTE: Anesthesia apparently blunts natriuretic responses to atrial volume expansion [Krasney et al., 1989].)

Is Renal Regulation of Salt and Water Secretion Transferred From Cardiac Receptors in Dogs to Arterial Baroreceptors in Humans and Primates?

Evidence From Water Immersion: Thoracic Hypervolemia. The engorgement of cardiac chambers in humans and monkeys is not accompanied by any change in heart rate. Humans and other primates, in contrast to dogs, have no *Bainbridge reflex.* As a consequence, *stroke volume and aortic pulse pressure rise* so that arterial baroreceptors are stimulated by increases in both mean and pulse pressure. In animals having a Bainbridge reflex, *a change in central venous pressure is accompanied by a parallel change in heart rate and cardiac output. The Bainbridge reflex minimizes the effect of filling pressure on stroke volume and on arterial pulse pressure* (Hajduczok et al., 1987). Note the exception here to the usual case in which the rise in cardiac output would reduce central venous pressure. Here water immersion opposes the increase in peripheral vascular volume normally attending a rise in cardiac output. Therefore the signals fed back to the central nervous system from cardiac and arterial baroreceptors are different in dogs and primates during immersion and volume loading. This has greatly complicated the interpretation of experimental results, but now recognition of this difference can help us to understand some of the apparent discrepancies.

Despite the species differences in the hemodynamic effects of volume expansion and water immersion on arterial pulse pressure, the diuresis is uniformly dominated by the *natriuretic component.* This is consistent with the idea that the natriuresis is induced by a reflex inhibition of renal sympathetic nerve activity (DiBona, 1985). In dogs, cardiac denervation does not diminish the diuresis (Hajduczok et al., 1987); rather, it changes its character so that free-water clearance is increased, presumably via vasopressin. Accordingly, cardiac receptors are needed for full expression of the natriuretic response, presumably via reflex modulation of the sympathetic nerves supplying the renal tubules (DiBona, 1985). Cardiac denervation abolishes the Bainbridge reflex so that the same rise in cardiac output in response to volume loading is achieved by a rise in stroke volume rather than in heart rate. The rise in stroke volume increases aortic pulse pressure and stimulates arterial baroreceptors, which in turn inhibits vasopressin release and increases free-water clearance.

Figure 3-7 summarizes what has been presented so far. It highlights the importance of the Bainbridge reflex in explaining species differences. In conscious dogs, cardiac afferent nerves appear to be primarily responsible for the natriuretic response mediated mainly by renal sympathetic nerves. If cardiac receptors are denervated the diuresis in response to water immersion and iso-osmotic volume loading persists, but the diuresis originates mainly from increased renal free-water clearance rather than from sodium clearance. In both dogs and hydrated humans, and other primates, the arterial baroreceptors can dominate the control of vasopres-

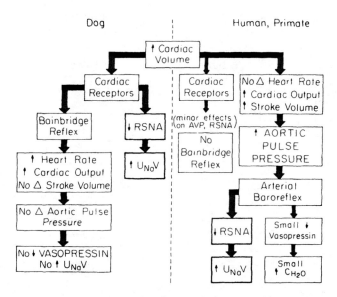

Figure 3-7 Schematic summary of *reflexes* governing renal excretion of salt and water following increased thoracic blood volume. The scheme emphasizes the importance of the Bainbridge reflex in determining renal response to increased cardiac volume. In dogs, stimulation of cardiac receptors reduces renal sympathetic nerve activity (RSNA), which explains the natriuresis ($\uparrow U_{Na}V$). Without the Bainbridge reflex the increments in aortic pulse pressure further activate the arterial baroreflex, which reduces RNSA and increases $U_{Na}V$ and also (small effect) lowers vasopressin.

sin secretion and renal free-water clearance. This supports the thinking of Gilmore (1983) and his coworkers, Peterson and coworkers (1987), Norsk and Epstein (1988), Krasney and coworkers (1989), and Norsk (1989). The most confusing point is that, in contrast to cardiac-denervated dogs, the diuresis in mildly dehydrated humans is not caused by the decrease in vasopressin; free-water clearance does not increase very much. Rather, the diuresis is associated with natriuresis and appears to be caused by the inhibition of renal sympathetic nerve activity caused by stimulation of arterial baroreceptors.

Physical (Nonreflex) Factors Governing Renal Excretion. Cowley and Skelton (1991) pointed out the importance of distinguishing between compensatory mechanisms attending acute thoracic hypervolemia induced by isotonic saline loading (400 ml) and those induced by equivalent loading of the thorax with whole blood (100 ml). They showed in dogs that the dominant mechanism controlling renal excretion of salt and water acutely (within the first 5 to 6 hours in which 85 percent of the load was excreted) was the fall in plasma colloid osmotic pressure caused by hemodilution. The reduction in plasma oncotic pressure would increase glomerular filtra-

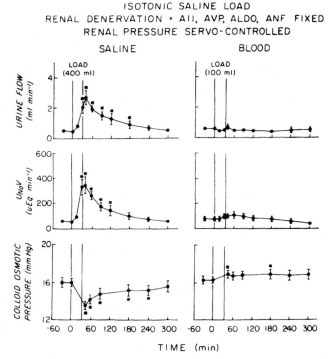

Figure 3-8 Experimental results demonstrating the dominance of a physical (nonre-flex) effect of volume expansion with isotonic saline (400 ml) in dogs with renal denervation, renal perfusion pressure servocontrolled, and endocrine levels (angio-tensin II, arginine vasopressin, aldosterone, and atrial natriuretic factor) fixed by constant infusion. The increases in urine flow and $U_{Na}V$ with saline loading (400 ml) were caused by a fall in plasma colloid osmotic pressure (increased glomerular filtration and decreased reabsorption). An equivalent volume load with 100 ml of whole blood had no effect on renal excretion. (Adapted from Cowley and Skelton, 1991.)

tion across the entire glomerulus (the rise in protein concentration initially not being large enough to stop filtration—and reabsorption force would be diminished along the peritubular capillaries as well). Renal salt and water excretion was maximally affected when Cowley and Skelton (1991) either fixed or eliminated endocrine controllers. The kidneys were dener-vated and renal perfusion pressure was servocontrolled. The results shown in Figure 3-8 contrast the diuretic effects of isotonic saline loading with the lack of effects of an equivalent loading with whole blood. The latter changed neither plasma oncotic pressure nor renal salt and water ex-cretion.

The preceding description reveals still another redundancy in the con-trol of renal salt and water excretion, but this time it involves only one

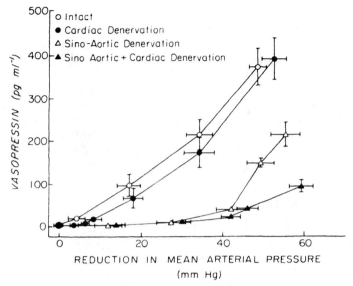

Figure 3-9   Effect of stepwise denervation of the heart, the carotid sinus and aortic arch (sinoaortic denervation), baroreceptors, and, finally, both the heart and sinoaortic receptors in three groups of splenectomized dogs. Cardiac denervation alone did not alter vasopressin secretion, whereas sinoaortic denervation virtually abolished it until hypotension was severe. Vasopressin rise with severe hypotension in sinoaortic denervated dogs was markedly reduced by cardiac denervation, revealing that a small role for cardiac receptors had been hidden by dominance of arterial baroreceptors. (From Shen et al., 1991.)

simple physical change—plasma oncotic pressure. As Cowley and Skelton (1991) point out, their findings do not negate the importance of the endocrine controllers which act over longer periods—and which correct volumes when loading is with isotonic, iso-oncotic fluids.

Thoracic Hypovolemia.   Although the evidence is still indirect, the findings from humans exposed to decrements in intrathoracic volume *that do not alter arterial pulse pressure* (e.g., lower body suction) reveal no effect of the stimulus on plasma vasopressin levels; plasma renin activity rises only if the stress is prolonged. If the imposed reduction in intrathoracic volume incurs changes in arterial pulse pressure such as occur in upright posture, then almost immediate increments in vasopressin and renin release are seen. An important indicator that pulse pressure has fallen is a rise in heart rate (e.g., see Figure 2-8).

Despite the growing evidence suggesting a dominant role for arterial baroreceptors in the control of vasopressin secretion, conflicting reports continue to appear (see Goetz and Wang in Cowley et al., 1988). However the results in Figure 3-9 reinforce the main thread of this discussion. Shen et al. (1991) found that neither acute cardiac denervation (intrapericardial lidocaine) nor chronic surgical cardiac denervation blunted the augmented release of vasopressin during progressive hemorrhage in conscious, splenectomized dogs (Figure 3-9). However, denervation of sinoaortic baroreceptors significantly reduced the rise in vasopressin levels. A major role was seen for arterial baroreceptors in mediating vasopressin secretion, wheres no significant role could be assigned to cardiac receptors. But the combined denervation of both cardiac and arterial baroreceptors caused further blunting of vasopressin release. This meant that a modest role for cardiac receptors was hidden by the dominance of arterial baroreceptors in controlling vasopressin secretion during hypovolemia.

Atriopeptin (Atrial Natriuretic Factor)

The atrial peptides might also contribute to human plasma volume regulation in orthostasis and hypervolemia. It is clear that intravenous infusions of atriopeptin in pharmacological doses rapidly elicit a natriuresis in humans and other species (Goetz, 1988; Brenner et al., 1990). However, this does not inform us about the effects of the peptide levels that attend a physiological stimulus. Some doubts about the role of atrial peptides in eliciting natriuresis in response to atrial distension have been ably expressed by Goetz (1988). These doubts stem from several key observations, not the least of which is that elevations in atriopeptin associated with blood volume expansion or water immersion in human subjects or experimental animals are far too small to initiate or sustain the degree of natriuresis that is observed. Water immersion in humans increases atriopeptin levels only twofold. However, when atriopeptin is infused into humans at rates that raise its plasma levels to exceed basal levels by about 10- to 25-fold, there is only two- to threefold rise in renal sodium clearance. Normally, these levels of natriuresis can occur at far lower circulating levels of atriopeptin.

Other points are that when plasma atriopeptin levels rise promptly in response to water immersion, the rise in renal sodium clearance lags about a hour or more behind, making the two events appear unrelated. Finally, cardiac denervation (dogs) does not affect the magnitude of increase in circulating atriopeptin levels attending atrial distension; nevertheless, this denervation markedly diminishes and can even abolish the natriuretic response. Thus, in humans and dogs, the small fluctuation in circulating atriopeptin levels that occur under normal conditions appear to have little or no effect on renal sodium excretion. Although the peptide appears not to play any primary causal role in eliciting natriuresis, it is clearly premature to conclude that it plays no role—or that its role might not become far greater after sustained loss of other feedback mechanisms in plasma volume control. Goetz (1988) also reviewed evidence that renal responses to volume expansion may be far more dependent on atriopeptin in other species (i.e., the rat) than is currently apparent in humans or dogs.

The Henry-Gauer Reflex Revisited: Summary

It is now clear that the simple link between left atrial distension and vasopressin secretion originally proposed by Henry and Gauer cannot account for the diuresis in response to volume loading or for the water retention in response to central hypovolemia. Nevertheless, there is little doubt that a cardiorenal reflex modifies renal function when intracardiac pressures are altered. In tribute to those who planted the seed, it might be called a "modified Henry-Gauer reflex"; the reflex is simply not quite what its original proposers had in mind (and surely that is not new).

Perhaps we will find no better example of the complications and complexity caused by the existence of multiple, redundant feedback loops in a control system than in the hormonal systems of the baroreflex-renal axis. In systems with redundant feedback controllers, the removal of one feedback mechanism may be almost fully compensated for by the expression of another controller, which may or may not normally be active. The unfolding story of the reflex control of plasma volume is far from complete, and the role of atriopeptin appears destined to add still another complex chapter.

A general summary of the factors that are currently felt to dominate the control of total blood volume in response to thoracic engorgement with blood are schematized in Figure 3-10. Figure 3-10 can also be adapted to summarize the effects of reduced cardiac pressures, such as occur in orthostasis, but with less confidence because of fewer data. The figure has an epicenter, namely, increased *thoracic volume* (stretch), which is one functional link to the kidney but not the only one. The cardiac receptors, particularly in quadrupeds, are considered to be the dominant controllers of renal sodium clearance effected by their reflex modulation of sympathetic nerve traffic to the kidney. This nerve traffic directly affects tubular clearance of sodium and is thought to be an important regulator of natriuresis.

Denervation of the dog's heart eliminates the tachycardia (via the Bainbridge reflex) that normally raises cardiac output without changing stroke volume or aortic pulse pressure. Diuresis persists after cardiac denervation, but it appears to be initiated reflexly by arterial baroreflexes activated by the rise in aortic pulse pressure (due to the increased stroke volume accompanying unchanged heart rate). Diuresis after cardiac denervation is due mainly to increased renal free-water clearance now apparently regulated by vasopressin.

Humans and other primates have no Bainbridge reflex. The cardiac response to volume loading parallels that of the cardiac-denervated dog: heart rate does not change but cardiac output, stroke volume, and aortic pulse pressure all rise. The latter initiates an arterial baroreflex, which is thought to cause the fall in vasopressin levels, but this diuresis is not associated with significantly increased free-water clearance. Rather, natriuresis dominates the renal response in previously dehydrated humans

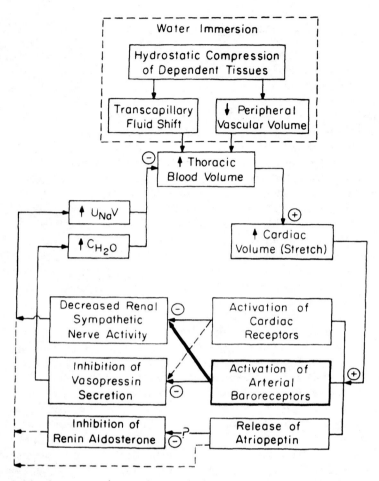

Figure 3-10 Summary of normal control of renal excretion of sodium ($U_{Na}V$) and water (C_{H_2O}) in response to water immersion. Physical effects of water immersion (in broken line box at the top) do not alter plasma osmotic pressure. Increased cardiac volume decreases renal sympathetic nerve activity, which causes natriuresis (increased $U_{Na}V$). In humans the increased cardiac volume activates arterial baroreceptors, which also cause natriuresis—presumably via reduction of renal sympathetic nerve activity. Vasopressin release is also inhibited, but increased C_{H_2O} is minor (in cardiac-denervated dogs with no Bainbridge reflex, increased cardiac volume raises aortic pulse pressure, reduces vasopressin, and increases C_{H_2O}). Arial stretch increases atriopeptin secretion, but resultant concentrations exert small effects on $U_{Na}V$. (Modified scheme of Krasney et al., 1989.)

and other primates during cardiac distension. The natriuresis persists in primates with surgically denervated cardiopulmonary receptors, suggesting that arterial baroreceptors stimulate natriuresis, possibly by activating renal sympathetic nerves.

In humans, the correlations between central venous pressure and plasma vasopressin levels are poor. Available evidence suggests that the primary *reflex controllers of the renin-angiotensin-aldosterone system and of vasopressin are the arterial baroreceptors* because the changes in thoracic volume required to alter their secretion must be large enough to alter arterial pulse pressure (or otherwise stresses must be applied for long periods of time, for reasons still unknown). This generalization appears to be valid for both expansion and contraction of thoracic blood volume.

REFERENCES

Aksamit, T.R., J.S. Floras, R.G. Victor, and P.E. Aylward (1987). Paroxysmal hypertension due to sinoaortic baroreceptor denervation in humans. *Hypertension 9*, 309–314.

Anderson, E.A., B.G. Wallin, and A.L. Mark (1987). Dissociation of sympathetic nerve activity in arm and leg muscle during mental stress. *Hypertension 9* (*Suppl. III*), III-114–III-119.

Bevan, J.A.(1979). Some bases of differences in vascular response to sympathetic activity. *Circ. Res. 45*, 161–171.

Bevegård, S., J. Castenfors, and L.E. Lindblad (1977). Effect of changes in blood volume distribution on circulatory variables and plasma renin activity in man. *Acta Physiol. Scand. 99*, 237–245.

Bie, P. (1980). Osmoreceptors, vasopressin, and control of renal water excretion. *Physiol. Rev. 60*, 961–1048.

Bishop, V.S., A. Malliani, and P. Thoren (1983). Cardiac mechanoreceptors. In J.T. Shepherd, F.M. Abboud, and S.R. Geiger, eds. *Handbook of Physiology. The Cardiovascular System: Peripheral Circulation and Organ Blood Flow*, sect. 2, vol. III, part 2, pp. 497–555. American Physiological Society, Bethesda, MD.

Brenner, B.M., B.J. Ballermann, M.E. Gunning, and M.L. Zeidel (1990). Diverse biological actions of atrial natriuretic peptide. *Physiol. Rev. 70*, 665–699.

Burnstock G. (1986). The changing face of autonomic neurotransmission. *Acta Physiol. Scand. 126*, 67–91.

Christensen, N.J. (1979). Plasma noradrenaline and adrenaline measured by isotope-derivative assay. *Dan. Med. Bull. 26*, 17–56.

Cowley, A.W. Jr., and J.-F. Liard (1987). Cardiovascular actions of vasopressin. In D.M. Gask and G.J. Boer, eds. *Vasopressin: Principles and Properties*, pp. 389–433. Plenum Press, New York.

Cowley, A.W. Jr., J.-F. Liard, and D.A. Ausiello (eds.) (1988). *Vasopressin: Cellular and Integrative Functions*. Raven Press, New York.

Cowley, A.W. Jr., and M.M. Skelton (1991). Dominance of colloid osmotic pressure in renal excretion after isotonic volume expansion. *Am. J. Physiol. 261* (*Heart Circ. Physiol 30*) H1214–H1225.

Cunningham, S.G., E.O. Feigl, and A.M. Scher (1978). Carotid sinus reflex influence on plasma renin activity. *Am. J. Physiol. 234 (Heart Circ. Physiol. 3)*, H670–H678.

Davis, D., L.I. Sinoway, J. Robison, J.R. Minotti, F.P. Day, R. Baily, and R. Zelis (1987). Norepinephrine kinetics during orthostatic stress in congestive heart failure. *Circ. Res. 61 (Suppl. 1)*, I-87–I-90.

DiBona, G.F. (1985). Neural regulation of renal tubular sodium reabsorption and renin secretion. *Fed. Proc. 44*, 2816–2822.

Eckberg, D.L., R.F. Rea, O.K. Andersson, T. Hedner, J. Pernow, J.M. Lundberg, and B.G. Wallin (1988). Baroreflex modulation of sympathetic activity and sympathetic neurotransmitters in humans. *Acta Physiol. Scand. 133*, 221–231.

Esler, M., G. Jennings, G. Lambert, I. Meredith, M. Horne,and G. Eisenhofer (1990). Overflow of catecholamine neurotransmitters to the circulation: source, fate, and functions. *Physiol. Rev. 70*, 963–985.

Essandoh, L.K., D.S. Houston, P.M. Vanhoutte, and J.T. Shepherd (1986). Differential effects of lower body negative pressure on forearm and calf blood flow. *J. Appl. Physiol. 61*, 994–998.

Fasola, A.F., and B.L. Martz (1972). Peripheral venous renin activity during 70° tilt and lower body negative pressure. *Aerospace Med. 43*, 713–715.

Fisher, S.J., and R.L. Malvin (1980). Role of neural pathways in renin response to intravascular volume expansion. *Am. J. Physiol. 238 (Heart Circ. Physiol. 7)*, H611–H617.

Flavahan, N.A., L.-E. Lindblad, T.J. Verbeuren, J.T. Shepherd, and P.M. Vanhoutte (1985). Cooling and α_1- and α_2-adrenergic responses in cutaneous veins: role of receptor reserve. *Am. J. Physiol. 249 (Heart Circ. Physiol. 18)*, H950–H955.

Gauer, O.H., and J.P. Henry (1976). Neurohormonal control of plasma volume. *Int. Rev. Physiol. 9*, 145–190. (*Cardiovascular Physiology II* [A.C. Guyton and A.W. Cowley, eds.]).

Gilmore, J.P. (1983). Neural control of extracellular volume in the human and nonhuman primate. In J.T. Shepherd, F.M. Abboud, and S.R. Geiger, eds. *Handbook of Physiology. The Cardiovascular System: Peripheral Circulation and Organ Blood flow*, sect. 2, vol. III, part 2, pp. 885–915. American Physiological Society, Bethesda, MD.

Goetz, K.L. (1988). Physiology and pathophysiology of atrial peptides. *Am. J. Physiol. 254 (Endocrinol. Metab. Gastrointest. Physiol. 17)*, E1–E15.

Goetz, K.L., G.C. Bond, and D.D. Bloxham (1975). Atrial receptors and renal function. *Physiol. Rev. 55*, 157–205.

Goldsmith, S.R., A.W. Cowley, Jr., G.S. Francis, and J.N. Cohn (1984). Effect of increased intracardiac and arterial pressure on plasma vasopressin in humans. *Am. J. Physiol. 246 (Heart Circ. Physiol. 15)*, H647–H651.

Goldsmith, S.R., G.S. Francis, A.W. Cowley, and J.N. Cohn (1982). Response of vasopressin and norepinephrine to lower body negative pressure in humans. *Am. J. Physiol. 243 (Heart Circ. Physiol. 12)*, H970–H973.

Goldstein, D.S., R. McCarty, R.J. Polinsky, and I.J. Kopin (1983). Relationship between plasma norepinephrine and sympathetic neural activity. *Hypertension 5*, 552–559.

Hajduczok, G., K. Miki, S.K. Hong, J.R. Claybaugh, and J.A. Krasney (1987). Role of cardiac nerves in response to head-out water immersion in conscious dogs. *Am. J. Physiol. 253 (Regulatory Integrative Comp. Physiol. 22)*, R242–R253.

Hesse, B., H. Ring-Larsen, I. Nielsen, and N.J. Christensen (1978). Renin stimulation by passive tilting: the influence of an anti-gravity suit on postural changes in plasma renin activity, plasma noradrenaline concentration and kidney function in normal man. *Scand. J. Clin. Lab. Invest. 38*, 163–169.

Hjemdahl, P., J. Fagius, U. Freyschuss, B.G. Wallin, M. Daleskog, G. Bohlin, and A. Perski (1989). Muscle sympathetic activity and norepinephrine release during mental challenge in humans. *Am. J. Physiol. 257 (Endocrinol. Metab. Gastrointest. Physiol. 20)*, E654–E664.

Hökfelt T., O. Johansson, A. Ljungdahl, J.M. Lundberg, and M. Schultzberg (1980). Peptidergic neurones. *Nature 284,* 515–521.

Krasney, J.A., G. Hajduczok, K. Miki, J.R. Claybaugh, J.L. Sondeen, D.R. Pendergast, and S.K. Hong (1989). Head-out water immersion: a critical evaluation of the Gauer-Henry hypothesis. In J.R. Claybaugh and C.E. Wade, eds. *Hormonal Regulation of Fluid and Electrolytes,* pp.147–185. Plenum, New York.

Licht, M.R., and J.L. Izzo Jr. (1989). Humoral effect of norepinephrine on renin release in humans. *Am. J. Hypertension 2,* 788–791.

Mancia, G., J.C. Romero, and J.T. Shepherd (1975). Continuous inhibition of renin release in dogs by vagally innervated receptors in the cardiopulmonary region. *Circ. Res. 36,* 529–535.

Mark, A.L., F.M. Abboud, and A.E. Fitz (1978). Influence of low- and high-pressure baroreceptors on plasma renin activity in humans. *Am. J. Physiol. 235 (Heart Circ. Physiol. 4)*, H29–H33.

Marshall, J.M. (1991). The venous vessels within skeletal muscle. *News Physiol. Sci. 6,* 11–15.

Mohanty, P.K., J.R. Sowers, F.W.J. Beck, M.F. Godschalk, J. Schmitt, M. Newton, C. McNamara, J.G. Verbalis, and M. McClanahan (1985). Catecholamine, renin, aldosterone, and arginine vasopressin responses to lower body negative pressure and tilt in normal humans: effects of bromocriptine. *J. Cardiovasc. Pharmacol. 7,* 1040–1047.

Mohanty, P.K., J.R. Sowers, C. McNamara, and M.D. Thames (1988). Reflex effects of prolonged cardiopulmonary baroreceptor unloading in humans. *Am. J. Physiol. 254 (Regulatory Integrative Comp. Physiol. 23)*, R320–R324.

Norsk, P. (1989). Influence of low- and high-pressure baroreflexes on vasopressin release in humans. *Acta Endocrinol. 121 (Suppl. 1)*, 1–32.

Norsk, P., and M. Epstein (1988). Effects of water immersion on arginine vasopressin release in humans. *J. Appl. Physiol. 64,* 1–10.

Oliver, J.A., J. Pinto, R.R. Sciacca, and P.J. Cannon (1980). Basal norepinephrine overflow into the renal vein: effect of renal nerve stimulation. *Am. J. Physiol. 239 (Renal Fluid Electrolyte Physiol. 8)*, F371–F377.

Oparil, S., and E. Haber (1974). The renin-angiotensin system. *N. Engl. J. Med. 291,* 389–401.

Oparil, S., C. Vassaux, C.A. Sanders, and E. Haber (1970). Role of renin in acute postural homeostasis. *Circulation 41,* 89–95.

Os, I., S.E. Kjeldsen, I. Aakesson, J. Skjoto, A. Westheim, I. Eide, and P. Leren (1984). Arteriovenous difference of plasma vasopressin in normal man and effect of posture. *Acta Physiol. Scand. 122,* 49–53.

Pernow, J., A. Ohlen, T. Hökfelt, O. Nilsson, and J.M. Lundberg (1987). Neuropeptide Y: presence in perivascular noradrenergic neurons and vasoconstrictor effects on skeletal muscle blood vessels in experimental animals and man. *Regulatory Peptides 19,* 313–324.

Peterson, T.V., B.A. Benjamin, and N.L. Hurst (1987). Effect of vagotomy and thoracic sympathectomy on responses of the monkey to water immersion. *J. Appl. Physiol. 63*, 2467–2481.

Rea, R.F., and B.G. Wallin (1989). Sympathetic nerve activity in arm and leg muscles during lower body negative pressure in humans. *J. Appl. Physiol. 66*, 2778–2781.

Ring-Larsen, H., B. Hesse, J.H. Henriksen, and N.J. Christensen (1982). Sympathetic nervous activity and renal and systemic hemodynamics in cirrhosis: plasma norepinephrine concentration, hepatic extraction, and renal release. *Hepatology 2*, 304–310.

Rowell, L.B. (1983). Cardiovascular adjustments to thermal stress. In J.T. Shepherd, F.M. Abboud, and S.R. Geiger, eds. *Handbook of Physiology. The Cardiovascular System: Peripheral Circulation and Organ Blood Flow*, sect. 2, vol. III, part 2, pp. 967–1023. American Physiological Society, Bethesda, MD.

Rowell, L.B. (1984). Reflex control of regional circulations in man. *J. Auton. Nerv. Syst. 11*, 101–114.

Rowell, L.B., and D.R. Seals (1990). Sympathetic activity during graded central hypovolemia in hypoxemic humans. *Am. J. Physiol. 259 (Heart Circ. Physiol. 28)*, H1197–H1206.

Scher, A.M., D.S. O'Leary, and D.D. Sheriff (1991). Arterial baroreceptor regulation of peripheral resistance and of cardiac performance. In P. Persson and H. Kirchheim, eds. *Baroreceptor Reflexes*. Springer-Verlag, Heidelberg.

Seals, D.R. (1989). Sympathetic neural discharge and vascular resistance during exercise in humans. *J. Appl. Physiol. 66*, 2472–2478.

Seals, D.R., N.O. Suwarno, and J.A. Dempsey (1990). Influence of lung volume on sympathetic nerve discharge in normal humans. *Circ. Res. 67*, 130–141.

Seals, D.R., R.G. Victor, and A.L. Mark (1988). Plasma norepinephrine and muscle sympathetic discharge during rhythmic exercise in humans. *J. Appl. Physiol. 65*, 940–944.

Shen, Y.-T., A.W. Cowley, and S.F. Vatner (1991). Relative roles of cardiac and arterial baroreceptors in vasopressin regulation during hemorrhage in conscious dogs. *Circ. Res. 68*, 1422–1436.

Shepherd, J.T. (1963). *Physiology of the Circulation in Human Limbs in Health and Disease*. W.B. Saunders, Philadelphia.

Silverberg, A.B., S.D. Shah, M.W. Haymond, and P.E. Cryer (1978). Norepinephrine: hormone and neurotransmitter in man. *Am. J. Physiol. 234 (Endocrinol. Metab. Gasrointest. Physiol. 3)*, E252–E256.

Simon, E., and W. Riedel (1975). Diversity of regional sympathetic outflow in integrative cardiovascular control: patterns and mechanisms. *Brain Res. 87*, 323–333.

Stadeager, C., B. Hesse, O. Henriksen, F. Bonde-Petersen, J. Mehlsen, and S. Rasmussen (1990). Influence of the renin-angiotensin system on human forearm blood flow. *J. Appl. Physiol. 68*, 527–532.

Stadeager, C., B. Hesse, O. Henriksen, N.J. Christensen, F. Bonde-Petersen, J. Mehlsen, and J. Giese (1989). Effects of angiotensin blockade on the splanchnic circulation in normotensive humans. *J. Appl. Physiol. 67*, 786–791.

Sundlöf, G., and B.G. Wallin (1977). The variability of muscle nerve sympathetic activity in resting recumbent man. *J. Physiol (Lond.) 272*, 383–397.

Thames, M.D. (1977). Reflex suppression of renin release by ventricular receptors with vagal afferents. *Am. J. Physiol. 233 (Heart Circ. Physiol. 2)*, H181–H184.

Vallbo, A.B., K.-E. Hagbarth, H.E. Torebjork, and B.G. Wallin (1979). Somatosensory, proprioceptive,and sympathetic activity in human peripheral nerves. *Physiol. Rev. 59*, 919–957.

Vanhoutte, P.M. (1980). Physical factors of regulation. In (D.F. Bohr, A.P. Somlyo, and H.V. Sparks Jr., eds. *Handbook of Physiology. The Cardiovascular System: Vascular Smooth Muscle*, sect. 2, vol. II, pp. 443–474. American Physiological Society, Bethesda, MD.

Vanhoutte, P.M. (ed.) (1988). *Vasodilatation*. Raven Press, New York.

Vanhoutte, P.M., T.J. Verbeuren, and R.C. Webb (1981). Local modulation of adrenergic neuroeffector interaction in the blood vessel wall. *Physiol. Rev. 61*, 151–247.

Vargas, E., M. Lye, E.B. Faragher, C. Goddard, B. Moser, and I. Davies (1986). Cardiovascular haemodynamics and the response of vasopressin, aldosterone, plasma renin activity and plasma catecholamines to head-up tilt in young and old healthy subjects. *Age Ageing 15*, 17–28.

Vatner, S.F., W.T. Manders, and D.R. Knight (1986). Vagally mediated regulation of renal function in conscious primates. *Am. J. Physiol. 250 (Heart Circ. Physiol. 19)*, H546–H549.

Victor, R.G., and W.N. Leimbach Jr. (1987). Effects of lower body negative pressure on sympathetic discharge to leg muscles in humans. *J. Appl. Physiol. 63*, 2558–2562.

Victor, R.G., W.N. Leimbach Jr., D.R. Seals, B.G. Wallin, and A.L. Mark (1987). Effects of the cold pressor test on muscle sympathetic nerve activity in humans. *Hypertension 9*, 429–436.

Vissing, S.F., U. Scherrer, and R.G. Victor (1989). Relationship between sympathetic outflow and vascular resistance in the calf during perturbations in central venous pressure: evidence for cardiopulmonary afferent regulation of calf vascular resistance in humans. *Circ. Res. 65*, 1710–1717.

Wallin, B.G. (1983). Intraneural recording and autonomic function in man. In R. Bannister, ed. *Autonomic Failure* pp. 36–51. Oxford University Press, Oxford.

Wallin, B.G., and J. Fagius (1988). Peripheral sympathetic neural activity in conscious humans. *Annu. Rev. Physiol. 50*, 565–576.

Wallin, B.G., R.G. Victor, and A.L. Mark (1989). Sympathetic outflow to resting muscles during static handgrip and postcontraction muscle ischemia. *Am. J. Physiol. 256 (Heart Circ. Physiol. 25)*, H105–H110.

Wennergren, G. (1975). Aspects of central integrative and efferent mechanisms in cardiovascular reflex control. *Acta Physiol. Scand. [Suppl. 428]*, 5–53.

4

Orthostatic Intolerance

A goal of the previous chapters was to explain how neural and humoral mechanisms of vascular and cardiac control keep blood pressure from falling during orthostasis. The goal of this chapter is to amplify the discussion of essential adjustments to orthostasis by showing what happens when a particular part of the control system is either lost or malfunctioning. The cartoons in Figure 4-1 summarize both initial and long-term adjustments to orthostasis; they emphasize a time-dependent progression of centrifugal shifts in blood volume accompanied by falling central venous and arterial pressures. Despite the progressive neurally and humorally mediated corrections, they culminate in a failure of regulation called syncope. Normally, this sequence of adjustments occurs over many minutes during passive head-up tilt when muscles are relaxed. It takes longer during quiet standing because the tonically contracted postural muscles press against dependent veins, lessening their transmural pressure and, consequently, the volume they contain (Figure 1-14). In contrast, syncope may occur within seconds after patients with autonomic dysfunction stand up. Regardless of what the precipitating causes of syncope might have been, loss of consciousness due to inadequate cerebral perfusion is the end point.

The course of events leading to syncope is not always as illustrated in Figure 4-1. This chapter is about some weak links that can fail and disrupt this chain of regulatory events. The disruption can occur in normal individuals when some other (nongravitational) cardiovascular stress is added to that of orthostasis and causes a maldistribution of blood flow and blood volume. Or normal individuals may make appropriate adaptations to hypogravitational states (e.g., supine posture or zero gravity), but these adaptations work against adequate regulation during upright posture at 1 g. In other cases, a relatively common hormonal response to stress can precipitate syncope and collapse. Paradoxically, orthostatic tolerance appears to be embarrassed by either the improved cardiovascular function associated with physical conditioning, or by the diminished function associated with prolonged bed rest.

Patients with certain cardiovascular and neurologic diseases provide a means to dissect out some key elements of blood pressure control during orthostasis. The importance of these elements is punctuated by the failure of control that attends their absence. As will be seen below, there are

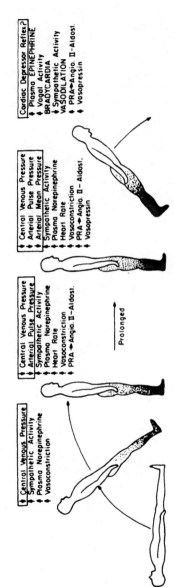

Figure 4-1 Summary of neural and humoral responses to increasing angle of head-up tilt (held for several minutes) and prolongation of tilt at 90° (for 20 to 30 minutes) until regulation of blood pressure fails and syncope occurs. Variables in boxes show stimuli at each stage until the last (syncope). Cause of putative cardiac depressor reflex in this setting is unknown. Note effect of changes in arterial pulse and mean pressure on hormonal responses. (Adapted from Rowell, 1986.)

cases in which severe cardiac dysfunction is paradoxically corrected by orthostasis and even aided further by a paradoxical vasodilation during the stress. Conversely, patients who have lost vital elements of autonomic control through spinal cord injury, surgical intervention, localized neuropathies, or widespread autonomic dysfunction provide a window for viewing the vital elements in a spectrum of controls. As pointed out in Chapter 3, there are multiple, redundant feedback controls of blood pressure and blood volume so that effects of removing one control mechanism may not be disabling, or may not even be evident. For example, individuals with complete transection of the spinal cord can tolerate a head-up tilt without syncope despite their lack of any reflex connections between the arterial baroreceptors and all parts of the body below the lesion. Conversely, patients with peripheral neuropathies may never be able to withstand even a mild orthostatic stress without syncope despite the multiple controllers of blood pressure; a vital link in the control of pressure is missing. In short, the site of the lesion is often critical to the outcome.

No pretense is made to offer in this book a thorough treatment of how certain diseases can alter cardiovascular and autonomic function. For this the reader must look elsewhere (e.g., Johnson and Spalding, 1974; Johnson et al., 1984; Bannister, 1988). The goal here is to offer illustrative examples of how defects in the control of the human vascular system impact on our ability to withstand orthostatic stress. It is hoped that the discussion offers a modest testimony to the value of heeding lessons from nature's experiments, as well as a personal recognition of the great value of working with clinical scientists.

NORMAL INDIVIDUALS: MALDISTRIBUTION OF BLOOD FLOW AND BLOOD VOLUME

If left upright and dependent for long periods of time, humans will succumb to hypotension, cerebral ischemia, syncope, and ultimately death if blood pressure is not restored (usually return to horizontal posture suffices). This chain of events can be accelerated in healthy individuals who are positioned upright after severe exercise (Bjurstedt et al., 1983) and/or when body temperature is elevated (Rowell, 1983).

To begin, Figures 2-3 through 2-6 are essential to this discussion because they make the point that an elevation in cardiac output in a resting individual (supine or upright) will cause central venous pressure and stroke volume to fall. Inasmuch as atrial pressure is already close to zero, Chapter 2 and these figures explain why cardiac output cannot be increased further because of the sensitive relationship between peripheral blood flow and vascular volume. Thus the consequence of an elevation in vascular conductance or "maldistribution" of cardiac output in upright posture will be immediate hypotension.

Postexercise Orthostatic Intolerance

The tendency for "orthostatic collapse" or syncope among runners who stand still after an exhaustive race is well known. The primary event is stoppage of the muscle pump so that an initially high cardiac output must be driven back up to the right ventricle by the left ventricle while the transmural pressure and volume of the leg vasculature increases. The other precipitating elements are a temporary mismatch between cardiac output and total vascular conductance with cardiac output falling faster than conductance so that arterial pressure falls. The slow abatement of muscle vasodilation coupled with a persistent elevation in cardiac output and muscle blood flow—*with no muscle pump*—will lower central venous pressure and stroke volume for reasons pointed out above and in Figure 2-5. Also, the vasoconstriction of visceral organs and the skin probably abates during the initial phase of recovery (before arterial pressure falls), and their contribution to total vascular conductance increases as cardiac output becomes smaller (i.e., they constitute a greater fraction of the total conductance).

Why does blood pressure continue to fall? A rise in heart rate will not help. Once central venous pressure approaches zero, nothing can be done to raise cardiac output (see Chapter 2) unless central venous pressure is restored by activation of the muscle pump or by repositioning the subject horizontally. Bjurstedt and colleagues (1983) suggested that maintained muscle acidosis and high internal temperature probably prevent the full expression of the vasoconstrictor response in skeletal muscle and skin, respectively. That is, it is not the degree of vasoconstriction that is affected, but rather it is that the magnitude of the blood flow during that vasoconstriction will still be much higher; for example, a 50 percent fall in blood flow from 100 to 50 units as opposed to a 50 percent fall from 10 to 5 units (Mosley, 1969; Johnson et al., 1973). The skin circulation may be the principal culprit, and this is discussed in the next section.

Heat-Induced Orthostatic Intolerance

The distribution of blood flow among organs during heat stress provides the best example in normal people of a cardiac output that is maldistributed to withstand orthostasis (or anything else for that matter). Blood flow is, however, optimally distributed for increasing heat loss to the environment (Rowell, 1983, 1986).

Figure 4-2 contrasts the distribution of blood flow and blood volume in a normothermic human with that in a hyperthermic individual. Assume the view is looking down on two supine people. The heat-induced increment in cardiac output drives central venous pressure down close to zero (Rowell et al., 1969, 1970), as shown in Figure 4-3 and in accordance with the schematic illustrations in Figures 2-5 through 2-7. All the energy

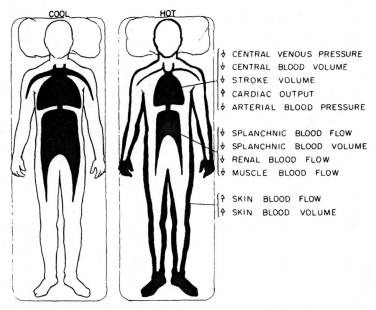

Figure 4-2   Altered distribution of blood volume caused by cutaneous vasodilation and visceral organ vasoconstriction in hyperthermic human (postures are supine). Heat stress reduces orthostatic tolerance because of redistribution of blood flow and blood volume away from heart into compliant cutaneous vasculature. (Adapted from Rowell, 1986.)

required to drive blood through the compliant microcirculation and the small veins was provided by the left ventricle (i.e., no "second heart" on the return side). The fall in right atrial mean pressure reflects the rise in peripheral venous volume, which in this case is out of proportion to the fraction of cardiac output directed to the skin where all of the vasodilation occurs. The cutaneous circulation has a specific compliance second only to the splanchnic circulation in humans (Chapter 1 in this book; Rowell, 1986). The point is that with cardiac output distributed in this manner, tolerance to orthostasis would be lost.

The only way to prevent a catastrophic fall in ventricular filling pressure in this setting is to constrict both the cutaneous and splanchnic vasculatures. Both regions are normally vasoconstricted in upright posture (Figure 2-1) and this is also true during heat stress, as shown for the skin in Figure 4-4. However, even after a marked cutaneous vasoconstriction, its blood flow remains elevated well above normal levels. Cardiac output cannot rise enough to match vascular conductance and blood pressure falls on standing up. With greater heat stress and higher skin blood flow, the symptoms of orthostatic intolerance will appear rapidly (Lind et al., 1968). Even activation of the muscle pump may not solve the problem because of the high percentage of leg blood flow that does not pass through the

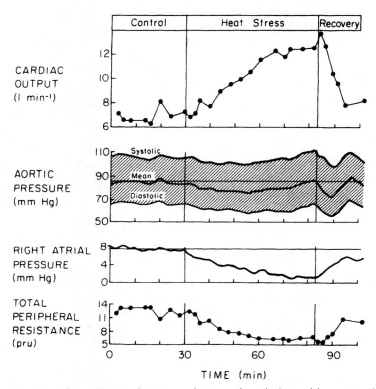

Figure 4-3 Data from a normal person who was directly heated by raising body skin temperature between 30 and 83 minutes (body temperature rose to 38.7°C). Vasodilation and increased cardiac output reduced right atrial pressure from 8 to 1.5 mmHg (in accordance with predictions in Figures 2-5 and 2-6). Flow-dependent increase in peripheral vascular volume decreases thoracic volume and causes orthostatic hypotension. (From Rowell et al., 1969.)

pump. An important reminder is that, normally, it is not possible in resting humans to raise cardiac output as much as shown in Figure 4-3 by either cardiac pacing or infusion of vasodilators (or by both). The consequent fall in ventricular filling pressure and stroke volume limit the increase to only 2 to 3 L min^{-1}. The higher cardiac output during heat stress stems from the powerful inotropic stimulation of the heart, marked hyperventilation (respiratory pump), and a passive shift of blood volume away from vasoconstricted splanchnic vessels to the heart (Rowell, 1983, 1986).

Prolonged Weightlessness, Simulated and Real

Prolonged exposure to zero gravity, sustained periods of bed rest, and periods of intense physical conditioning for activities requiring endurance have all been associated with reduced orthostatic tolerance or, in the case of weightlessness, frank orthostatic intolerance. The deficits in regulation

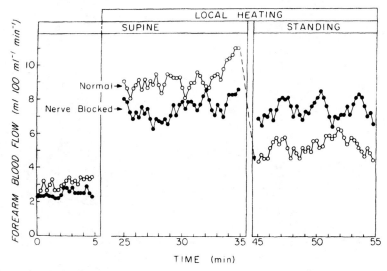

Figure 4-4   Effect of a change from supine to upright posture on forearm skin blood flow in a normal arm (*open circles*) and an arm that had received an intra-arterial infusion of bretylium tosylate to block sympathetic vasoconstriction (*closed circles*). At 5 minutes both arms were locally heated at 42°C. (Adapted from Mosely, 1969; reproduced from Rowell, 1986, with permission of Oxford University Press.)

have been extremely difficult to identify, especially in the endurance-trained individuals.

Normal subjects exposed to hypogravic states such as space flight (commonly simulated in part by prolonged bed rest or water immersion), develop orthostatic intolerance (Gauer and Thron, 1965; Blomqvist and Stone, 1983). Gauer and Henry (1976) and their colleagues emphasized the need for chronic orthostatic stress in order to maintain a blood volume that is adequate for optimal ventricular filling pressure. In their view, the adaptation to reduced gravitational stress simply returns overall hemodynamic function to what would normally exist in upright posture, that is, lower intrathoracic and cardiac blood volumes. However, the consequence of this adaptation is a reduction in the ability of the circulation to readjust when normal gravitational force is reintroduced. A salient feature of hypogravic states is that there is no longer a gravitationally dependent distribution of venous and arterial pressures and of blood volume in peripheral vessels. Thus, without gravity, blood volume is redistributed throughout the vascular system in accordance with specific regional compliances. The volume translocation engorges thoracic vessels with blood.

The increased thoracic blood volume associated with weightlessness and prolonged bed rest is accompanied by only a brief transient shift in volume from the extravascular to the intravascular space. Thereafter

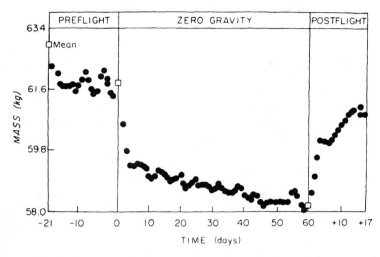

Figure 4-5 Determinations of body mass in a human before, during, and after a 60-day space flight (0 g). Mass was proportional to frequency of oscillation of a spring-loaded oscillator system. (Adapted from Blomqvist and Stone, 1983.)

plasma volume and body weight decline. Figure 4-5 shows the change in body mass of an astronaut during a 60-day space flight (mass was determined from the frequency of oscillation in a spring-loaded oscillating system). Approximately one-third of the early weight loss was caused by the loss of plasma volume (Blomqvist and Stone, 1983). Blomqvist and Stone (1983) reviewed the magnitudes and time courses of plasma volume losses during weightlessness, bed rest, and $-4°$ to $-6°$ head-down tilt. Commonly, losses are 10 to 12 percent (approximately 350 ml), and they begin within hours and plateau after a few days (for unknown reasons there is also a significant loss of red blood cells during space flight, so that total blood volume loss is much greater than for bed rest, for example).

The causes of orthostatic intolerance following hypogravic states appear to be far more complex than simply a response to hypovolemia. A loss of 10 to 12 percent of plasma volume is not likely to reduce orthostatic tolerance to the levels seen after space flight. Acute expansions of plasma volume did not restore orthostatic tolerance to normal. Nor did exercise in supine posture during prolonged bed rest ameliorate subsequent development of intolerance. A few hours of sitting or standing each day or short daily exposures to lower body suction were effective as countermeasures (Blomqvist, 1990). Large discrepancies beween the reported magnitudes of blood volume loss and the deficiency in orthostatic adjustments reviewed by Blomqvist and Stone (1983) led them and others to postulate some of the following additional factors that might contribute to orthostatic intolerance.

Increased Venous Capacitance

Although increased venous capacitance would exaggerate gravitational pooling, and both positive and negative results have been published, the strongest evidence appears to be against this hypothesis (Blomqvist and Stone, 1983). Nevertheless, Echt and coworkers (1974) observed a significant increase in forearm blood volume at a given venous transmural pressure after water immersion. This could contribute to the orthostatic intolerance reported to follow this particular stress.

Depressed Autonomic Function

Depressed autonomic function could blunt not only the rise in heart rate (this is not a problem) but also, and more seriously, the sympathetically mediated vasoconstriction that is so critical to accommodating a change to upright posture. Limited data on autonomic function after prolonged bed rest suggest that both cardiac acceleration and regional vasoconstriction are intact; pressor responses to norepinephrine and angiotensin infusions are normal; the turnover rate of norepinephrine is normal (Blomqvist and Stone, 1983). Although evaluation of autonomic function may reveal no obvious dysfunction, it clearly is not what it needs to be to prevent orthostatic intolerance. Small changes in a number of important autonomic effectors, possibly changes within errors of measurement, may somehow add together and exaggerate the effects of reduced plasma volume, smaller cardiac dimensions, and reduced efficiency of the muscle pump (see below). Or there may be changes for which the autonomic nervous system cannot compensate. Attention will be directed later to the "hyperadrenergic" state in the face of smaller cardiac dimensions.

Depressed Cardiac Function

Saltin and colleagues (1968) observed an 11 percent decrease in heart volume during 20 days of complete bed rest. They concluded that intrinsic myocardial function must be depressed by bed rest because stroke volume was also reduced during exercise. More recent studies employing nuclide imaging techniques suggest that ventricular filling (end-diastolic volume) is reduced in both upright and supine postures after bed rest together with an increase in left ventricular ejection fraction. The suggestion is that the increased ejection fraction combines with tachycardia to compensate for the reduction in end-diastolic volume so that cardiac function is not depressed (Blomqvist and Stone, 1983). Nevertheless, even if cardiac function were depressed, it should not alter orthostatic tolerance (unless it were extreme) because peripheral vascular rather than cardiac adjustments are the essential ones. This was revealed by the lack of effects of total autonomic blockade of the heart on the adjustments to orthostasis (see Tyden, 1977, and Chapter 2).

Reduced Cardiopulmonary and Arterial Baroreceptor Sensitivity

Reduced cardiopulmonary and arterial baroreceptor sensitivity would have the same effect as depressed autonomic function, that is, larger-than-normal changes in pressure would be required to elicit any given autonomic responses (Chapter 12 contains more detailed discussion of this concept and of baroreceptor "resetting"; see also Figure 2-13). Alternatively, one could argue that rather than depressed sensitivity, the operating point of the arterial baroreflex has been shifted ("reset") to operate most effectively (maximum "gain") at a lower blood pressure. If this were the case, autonomic functions comprising the efferent arm of the baroreflexes would appear normal, but they would simply be defending a lower arterial pressure, leaving less margin for any further decline during orthostasis. This still tempts the question: if the baroreflexes are intact and vasoconstrictor responses are normal, why does blood pressure fall so low as to cause syncope? What fails and why?

Reduced Skeletal Muscle Tone

Of the five possible factors (including the four preceding subsections) that might contribute to orthostatic intolerance, reduced muscle tone appears not only to be the simplest, but also may be the most feasible. Figure 1-13 stresses the importance of muscle tone and intramuscular pressures as determinants of venous transmural pressure and venous volume in dependent legs. In Chapter 1 it is pointed out that in patients exposed to prolonged bed rest, fainting occurred on standing when intramuscular pressure was only 80 to 120 mmH$_2$O, whereas fainting was not seen if intramuscular pressures rose to 200 to 300 mmH$_2$O. Unfortunately, the time course of this loss of tonic contraction in postural muscles is not established. If the time course proves to be out of phase with the defects in blood pressure control, it is not likely to be the major cause. Today, the primary cause (if there were only one) of orthostatic intolerance following hypogravic states and bed rest is still unknown. A potentially important clue is that many individuals suffering from orthostatic intolerance have what is called a "*hypovolemic hyperadrenergic* postural hypotension" (Blomqvist and Stone, 1983; Bannister, 1988). The importance of *epinephrine* in this intolerance is discussed in subsequent sections.

Physical Activity

Traditionally, the astronauts have been highly conditioned physically, but the reports of their postural hypotension after return from zero to normal gravity left doubts about the efficacy of conditioning. Some reports implied that less well-conditioned individuals experienced far less difficulty. Others pointed to a plethora of anecdotes concerning the orthostatic intolerance of highly conditioned endurance athletes. The literature became replete with studies that found either no beneficial effects, or a significant deleterious effect, of physical conditioning on orthostatic tolerance.

In an extensive investigation, Levine and coworkers (1991) appeared to have put the issue to rest—at least for people with a more or less normal range of maximal oxygen uptakes ($\dot{V}o_2$max). They investigated three groups of men: one group with higher-than-normal $\dot{V}o_2$max of 60 ml kg^{-1}; one group with normal $\dot{V}o_2$max of 48.9 ml kg^{-1} min^{-1}; and one group with a lower-than-normal value of 35.7 ml O_2 kg^{-1} min^{-1}. $\dot{V}o_2$max was a poor predictor of orthostatic tolerance determined by progressive lower body suction to an end point of presyncope. Also, the maximum sensitivity (or "open-loop gain") of the carotid sinus baroreflex was the same for the three groups. The study was strengthened by their analysis of three components of the baroreflex. They determined changes in heart rate, stroke volume, and peripheral vascular resistance in response to stepwise changes in carotid sinus transmural pressure (positive and negative neck pressure) applied over 2-minute periods. In previous studies, in which only the changes in heart (R-R) interval were used to evaluate the reflex, subjects with large stroke volumes (e.g., "athletes") had less change in R-R interval in response to a given change in neck pressure, that is, baroreflex sensitivity appeared to be subnormal. However, its sensitivity was not subnormal; the athletes simply required a smaller change in heart rate (owing to larger stroke volumes) to effect any given change in cardiac output and in arterial pressure.

There is an important lesson here concerning appropriate ways to assess the sensitivity of the arterial baroreflex. Unfortunately, investigators continue to use the change in heart interval in response to a change in blood pressure as an index of baroreflex sensitivity. Figure 4-6A shows the constant relationship between a given change in arterial pressure and the change in heart rate during rest and during some stress that raises heart rate. Figure 4-6B shows, in contrast, the effect of changing arterial pressure on heart interval. Arterial pressure was raised by a bolus injection of phenylephrine—a potent sympathomimetic and vasoconstrictor. The often false conclusion is that the greater slope of this relationship during rest (Figure 4-6B) as compared to the lower slope during a stress indicates that baroreflex sensitivity was reduced by the stress. Conversely, the lower slope during the stress could simply indicate that the rise in blood pressure was counteracted by a smaller fall in heart rate (or rise in heart interval) owing to a greater stroke volume during the stress. A more common explanation for a false conclusion about baroreflex sensitivity is shown in Figure 4-6C—namely for any given change in heart rate, the change in interval becomes smaller as baseline heart rate becomes higher. Therefore, the lower slope for stress in Figure 4-6B often means simply that baseline heart rate was higher when blood pressure was raised by the drug during the stress. We will return to this problem in Chapter 12.

Interindividual variations in tolerance to lower body suction were

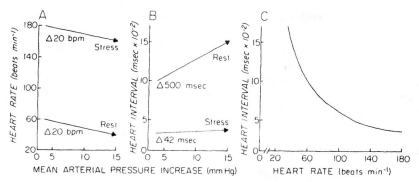

Figure 4-6 **(A)** The pitfall in using slopes relating interval between heartbeats (RR interval) to determine sensitivity of arterial baroreflex. **(B)** Despite constant relationship between Δ heart rate and mean arterial pressure increase (panel A) (by injection of a pressor drug), stress reduced the slope of heart interval by nearly eightfold. **(C)** The pitfall in equating the reduced slope with reduced baroreflex sensitivity is that for any change in *heart rate*, corresponding change in *heart interval* becomes less as initial heart rate becomes higher with stress.

found by Levine and colleagues (1991) to be best related to, first, the peak value for vascular conductance of the calf (i.e., conductance at the peak of reactive hyperemia produced by ischemic exercise) and, second, to the maximal steady-state gain of the carotid sinus baroreflex. Of particular interest is the fact that the subjects with the highest stroke volumes tended to have the largest decrements in stroke volume during lower body suction and also the poorest tolerance to this stress. Although the tolerance of the "athletes" to lower body suction tended to be slightly lower than that of the others, no simple relationship between $\dot{V}o_2$max (one index of physical conditioning) and orthostatic tolerance was found.

One is tempted to conclude that if functionally important deficits in orthostatic tolerance normally attend physical conditioning, they would have been far more obvious. The comprehensive study by Levine and colleagues (1991) makes that point. The siren call from outer space seems to invite us to "come as we are."

In fairness, a final comment should be added about those exceptional endurance athletes around whom stories and observations of orthostatic intolerance gravitate. Systematic laboratory studies rarely, if ever, include individuals with values for $\dot{V}o_2$max that reach 80 to 85 ml kg^{-1} min^{-1}; their maximal cardiac outputs exceed 40 L min^{-1} and their stroke volumes exceed 200 ml (Ekblom and Hermansen, 1968). They are difficult to find and difficult to study; personal experience has cautioned many of us about their propensity for fainting when a needle appears. Blomqvist (1990) offers a hypothetical explanation for this phenomenon. It rests on the suggestion that athletes with large diastolic volumes normally operate on the steep portion of the curve describing the relationship between left ventricular end-diastolic volume and end-diastolic pressure. Conversely, sedentary individuals operate at near maximal volume (when supine) mostly over a flatter region of the curve. The idea is, therefore, that it takes less of a fall in central venous pressure to drop left ventricular volume to very low levels in an athlete. The unstated notion is that "*a cardiac depressor reflex*" (described below) may be activated more easily in the athlete.

Fainting: Vasovagal Syncope

Orthostatic intolerance commonly ends in syncope. Fainting or syncope refers to a sudden loss of consciousness stemming from a precipitous decline in blood pressure and cerebral blood flow.

In 1876, "Salathe suggested that patients who have lain long in bed lose the power of adapting themselves to change of position and become like quadrupeds and hence the faintness, dizziness, and danger of syncope ... when the patient first rises from bed." (Hill, 1895).

Piorry in 1826 distinguished between emotional "cerebral" syncope and "cardiac" syncope. He stated: "In cerebral syncope, the heart continues to beat, but the beats have not force enough to overcome the resistance which is given by gravity." (cited by Hill, 1895). Hill states: "It therefore seems legitimate to suggest that ordinary emotional syncope is produced by sudden and temporary inhibition of the vasomotor center ...."

In Quain's *Dictionary of Medicine,* 1894, it states that: "Syncope consists essentially in sudden failure of the action of the heart." Hill (1895) added: "Now, no nerve is known which can produce such an effect except the vagus nerve ...."

The complex and poorly understood phenomenon of fainting can occur in response to a variety of stresses (e.g., Johnson and Spalding, 1974; Hainsworth, 1988; Van Lieshout, 1989). By whatever cause, once arterial pressure falls below 50 to 60 mmHg, autoregulatory corrections in cerebral vascular resistance fail and cerebral blood flow falls. When arterial pressure falls below 40 mmHg, consciousness is lost. The predisposing event is a reduction in venous return to the heart. This can be caused by vasodilation or by a gravitational (e.g., orthostasis) or mechanical impedance (e.g., straining maneuvers) to venous blood flow. Syncope takes two main forms. The first was called "vasovagal syncope" by Sir Thomas Lewis in 1932, because of the vasodilation (vaso) and profound bradycardia of vagal origin. The bradycardia could be blocked by atropine, but *not* the vasodilation and hypotension. The second form of syncope is sometimes called "vasodepressor syncope," with the hypotension caused simply by a fall in vascular resistance; heart rate responses vary (Van Lieshout, 1989). Without an active muscle pump, central venous pressure and then cardiac output, and then blood pressure fall. Any tachycardia attending the vasodilation does not ameliorate the hypotension.

Is the Vasodilation During Syncope Active or Passive?

In one view the rise in peripheral vascular conductance is due to a loss of the vasoconstriction needed to maintain blood pressure and minimize the sequestration of blood in dependent vasculature. The opposing view is that sympathetic vasodilator nerves contribute to the vasodilation, making it an active process as well. Some species (e.g., cats and dogs) appear to have sympathetic cholinergic vasodilator fibers supplying skeletal muscle. Although these fibers are not found in primates, some indirect evidence suggests their presence in humans (keep in mind Sir Thomas Lewis' observation that atropine does not prevent the hypotension of vasovagal syncope).

A brief review of the evidence concerning cholinergic vasodilation in human limbs unearthed little to support its existence (Rowell, 1981; Hainsworth, 1988). It is established that strong emotional stress (fright and revolting suggestions), reduce tonic vasoconstriction, and even the mild stress of mental arithmetic can lead to vasodilation in the forearm (see Rowell, 1981; Hainsworth, 1988). Some evidence suggests that the rise in forearm blood flow under these conditions can far exceed that which would attend withdrawal of tonic sympathetic vasoconstriction. The question is whether this vasodilation is neural or humoral in origin.

Arguments for a neural component cite the rapidity of the response and its reduction by sympathetic nerve blockade or local atropine administration. Arguments for a dominant humoral component cite the long latency of the response and the maintained response after sympathectomy, stellate ganglion blockade, and local atropine infusion. An obvious conclusion is that responses to emotional stress are as variable as the stress itself.

An early suggestion of neurogenic vasodilation came from a study by Barcroft and Edholm (1945) in which syncope was induced by venous congestion in the subjects' legs. They prevented the transient rise in forearm blood flow accompanying vasovagal syncope by local sympathetic nerve blockade. However, quantitative comparison of forearm blood flows in these two conditions (with or without blockade) was extremely difficult. Baseline flow values differed markedly and blood pressure fell precipitiously. Inasmuch as blood flows during this stress were similar, and because vascular conductances could not be estimated, it is difficult to ascertain that active vasodilation had occurred.

Support for the existence of cholinergic vasodilation in human skeletal muscle comes from the following observations, each of which is prefaced by *sometimes*:

1. Acute sympathetic nerve blockade reduced emotionally induced vasodilation.
2. Forearm blood flow peaked at levels unattainable by release of vasoconstrictor tone.

3. Intra-arterial infusion of atropine reduced the vasodilation.
4. Anesthetic blockade of cutaneous nerves in the forearm appeared
   not to reduce the response.

The existence of cholinergic vasodilation in human skeletal muscle is
not supported by the following observations obtained during emotional
stress (usually mental arithmetic):

1. Acute sympathetic nerve blockade did not abolish the response to
   stressful mental arithmetic.
2. Suppression of the skin circulation in an arm by epinephrine iontophoresis reduced the vasodilator responses in that arm.
3. The vasodilation is reduced in patients after adrenalectomy and can
   be mimicked by epinephrine infusion.
4. Vasoconstriction is commonly observed in the hand which is mainly
   skin; epinephrine vasoconstricts skin and vasodilates muscle.

It is a long leap from the stress of mental arithmetic to the strong
emotional stress imposed by Blair and colleagues (1959), or to the stress
preceding vasovagal syncope. Figure 4-7 shows blood flow to a normal

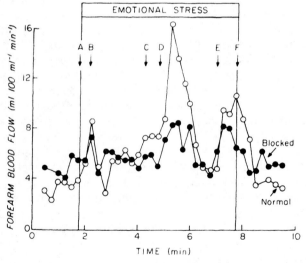

Figure 4-7   Evidence that putative sympathetic vasodilator system exists in human
forearm. A normal subject was exposed to revolting suggestions. **(A)** A dead and
dissected (postmortem) rabbit was produced. **(B)** The rabbit was held to the subject's
face and he was asked to smell it. **(C)** The rabbit's heart was opened and the blood
poured into a glass. **(D)** The subject was asked to drink the blood; he agreed, but the
request was withdrawn. **(E)** The rabbit's stomach was opened and its contents were
offered to the subject to eat, and then the offer was withdrawn. **(F)** He was told to
"relax" (perhaps the greatest challenge). Blood flow rose more in the normal arm
(*open circle*) than in the nerve-blocked arm (*closed circle*). (Adapted from Blair et
al., 1959, p. 639.)

forearm and one with its deep nerves blocked (blood pressure is unknown) during *severe* emotional stress. In most of the experiments in this report, the onset of forearm vasodilation was slow, suggesting a humoral component.

Experiments of this type, although technically well executed, are difficult to interpret for two reasons. First, the sites or origins of the response must often be identified in separate experiments. Second, the stress is neither constant nor repeatable, and, as a consequence, conclusions depend on a statistical approach in which variations in responses to unknown variations in input must be determined.

Transient neurogenic vasodilator responses to emotion do appear in facial skin and are called "blushing." The response is not, however, confined to skin. Holling (1964) described a "rectal blush" in a male subject who became embarrassed by the sudden presence of a female nurse at the subject's sigmoidoscopic examination. The observations were not unlike those made by Alexis St. Martin at the other end of the alimentary canal, and suggest that an emotion-triggered vasodilation may exist in the human gastrointestinal tract. The functional significance of these well-hidden "blushes" is unknown (Rowell, 1981).

Release of Tonic Vasoconstriction

The early investigations of Hill (1895) clearly revealed the essentiality of vasoconstrictor control in quadrupeds placed in head-up position. It has been clear since then that loss of tonic vasoconstriction can by itself explain the sudden hypotension attending syncope. The clinical examples in subsequent sections provide additional evidence. Wallin and Sundlof (1982) observed an abrupt fall in directly recorded sympathetic nervous activity in skeletal muscle (MSNA; see Chapter 3) during vasovagal fainting. Figure 4-8 shows another example of near-syncope during lower body suction (Rowell and Seals, 1990). Heart rate and blood pressure declined, and there was a virtual cessation of muscle sympathetic nervous activity (MSNA) (peroneal nerve). As yet, no one has observed an increase in the activity of nerve fascicles supplying skeletal muscle, suggestive of activation of sympathetic vasodilator fibers during syncope.

Hormonal Factors in Syncope

The discussion of hormonal control in Chapter 3 directs attention to the evidence that arterial blood pressure during orthostasis is initially well maintained by arterial and cardiopulmonary baroreflexes. The renin-angiotensin-aldosterone system is not summoned until enough blood has been translocated away from the heart into deep veins so as to lower aortic pulse pressure (Figure 4-1). Vasopressin secretion is initially activated by decrements in aortic pulse pressure; secretion is augmented by falling arterial mean pressure.

Experience with human subjects exposed to severe (-50 to -70 mmHg) lower body suction maintained to presyncopal levels points to a

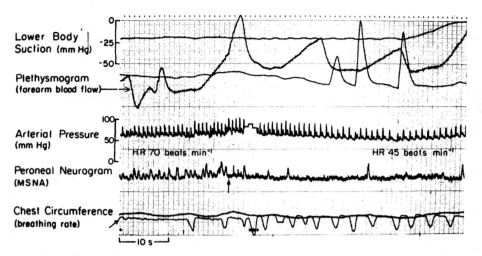

Figure 4-8 Onset of vasovagal syncope in normal subject during lower body suction. At arrow muscle sympathetic nerve activity (MSNA) virtually stopped, heart rate slowed and blood pressure fell, while forearm blood flow became unstable, and at the last plethysmograph curve on right, flow rose markedly (all of this subject's responses are summarized in Figure 4-13B). Note also hyperventilation (breathing rate). (From Rowell and Seals, 1990.)

powerful defense of mean pressure as pulse pressure gradually declines (for example, see Figure 4-9). However, as soon as mean arterial pressure begins to fall, its regulation deteriorates rapidly and the only route to recovery is cessation of suction as illustrated in Figure 4-9 (Rowell et al., 1972).

Figure 4-10 shows a progressive decline in arterial pulse pressure while little else changes over 19 minutes (average) of 60° head-up tilt. During the final minute of tilt, mean pressure fell precipitously from 94 to 50 mmHg and was accompanied by a sudden bradycardia. The sudden elevation in circulating hormones is expected (Chapter 3), except for the marked rise in *epinephrine* from 130 to 270 pg ml^{-1} (comparisons could only be made between the final 10 minutes of tilt and the onset of syncope) (Sander-Jensen et al., 1986a). The rise in pancreatic polypeptide, an indicator for vagal cholinergic activity, parallels the rise in cardiac vagal activity. As expected, norepinephrine rose (along with sympathetic activity) but did not rise further at the point of syncope when sympathetic nerve traffic stops (Figure 4-8). The rise in vasopressin from 4 to 126 pg ml^{-1} occurred without change in plasma osmolarity. Its elevation may contribute to the nausea during syncope (Cowley et al., 1988).

The most important feature in Figure 4-10 may be the sudden and marked increase in epinephrine prior to syncope. Within the range of 200 to 500 pg ml^{-1}, epinephrine will raise peripheral vascular conductance by 40 to 50 percent, reduce left ventricular end-diastolic volume by 30 per-

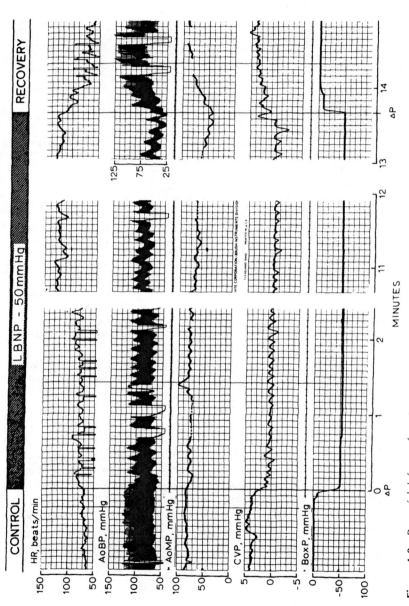

Figure 4-9 Powerful defense of aortic mean pressure (*AoMP*) during severe lower body suction for 13 minutes despite marked diminution of aortic pulse pressure (*AoBP*) and maintained zero right atrial pressure (*CVP*). Note the sudden decline in mean pressure from 80 to 40 mmHg after 13 minutes. (From Rowell et al., 1972, with permission of the American Physiological Society.)

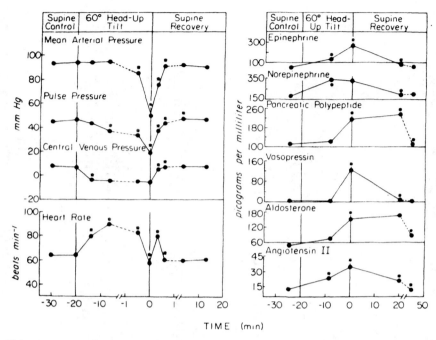

TIME (min)

Figure 4-10 (*Left*): Average circulatory responses to prolonged (average 19 minutes) head-up tilt at 60° until onset of syncopal symptoms in seven normal subjects. Time is normalized from time = 0, marking onset of syncopal symptoms. Asterisks mark significant differences ($p < 0.05$) from the preceding value. (*Right*): Average hormonal responses during the same head-up tilt (same seven subjects) shown on right. Note rise in epinephrine and no change in norepinephrine in response to near-syncope. Pancreatic polypeptide is a marker for increased vagal activity. (Adapted from Sander-Jensen et al., 1986a.)

cent, and raise stroke volume by 30 to 40 percent (i.e., in supine subjects), primarily by increasing left ventricular ejection fraction (to above 80 percent) (Stratton et al., 1985). The beneficial effects of epinephrine on cardiac performance cannot be realized during orthostasis, particularly if reduced vasoconstriction further compromises ventricular filling.

Consistent observations of a close parallel between rising plasma epinephrine levels and presyncopal symptoms appear in the latter 1980s (Sander-Jensen et al., 1986a; Tatar et al,. 1986; Robinson and Johnson, 1988; Rowell and Blackmon, 1989; Rowell and Seals, 1990). The rise in epinephrine can occur very suddenly (see below) and its β_2-adrenergic vasodilator effects on skeletal muscle could well explain the forearm vaso-dilation observed in earlier studies of syncope. Most important, perhaps, are its β-adrenergic effects on the splanchnic circulation. As Hill and Barnard pointed out in 1897 (Chapter 2), anything that diminishes the compensation stemming from splanchnic vasoconstriction in head-up position causes "pressure to fall enormously through the blood passing into the veins of the splanchnic area .... The splanchnic flood gates are thrown open."

Could the rise in vascular conductance and hypotension during syncope be explained entirely by the β-adrenergic effects of epinephrine? Probably not. A more sinister possibility focuses on the inotropic effects of epinephrine on a volume-depleted left ventricle. This effect is called the *cardiac depressor reflex*.

Cardiac Depressor Reflexes

An old idea is that strong inotropic stimulation of a left ventricle, nearing emptiness as a consequence of hemorrhage, leads to a powerful depressor reflex that originates from the heart itself. The partially hypothetical sequence of events leading up to cardiac or ventricularly induced syncope is summarized in Figure 4-11.

In 1867, Albert von Bezold observed that injection of veratrum alkaloids into the heart caused a sudden, vagally mediated decrease in heart rate and blood pressure. The responses could be prevented by cutting the vagal nerves. Von Bezold attributed the vasodepression to direct stimulation of sensory nerve endings in the heart by the alkaloids (Thoren, 1987). Since then, cardiac "receptors" or afferent fibers have been investigated extensively (Bishop et al., 1983, Thoren, 1987).

In 1949, Adolf Jarisch was apparently the first to suggest a depressor reflex from the heart might be the mechanism behind vasovagal syncope (the reflex became known as the Bezold-Jarisch reflex).

Oberg and White (1970) showed in cats that the vasovagal bradycardia in severe hemorrhage was due to activation of cardiac receptors. In fact, Oberg and Thoren (1972), directly recorded the increased activity in left ventricular C fibers. So far, evidence that the cardiac depressor reflex triggers vasovagal syncope in humans is indirect. The bradycardia (rather than the expected tachycardia) and the concomitant release of pancreatic polypeptide in humans suffering severe hemorhage is suggestive. Sander-Jensen and colleagues (1986b) pointed out that treatment of these patients with atropine or adrenergic agonists could prove fatal.

Additional indirect support for ventricular-induced syncope came from normal subjects who experienced bradycardia and hypotension when the β-agonist isoproterenol was infused during head-up tilt. Syncope could also be induced in this way in patients (with normal electrocardiograms) who suffered from recurrent episodes of neurally mediated syncope. Also, the spontaneous neural syncope could be prevented by blockade of β_1-adrenoreceptors in the heart (Almquist et al., 1989). Rowell and Blackmon (1989) observed a marked and sudden reduction in left ventricular end-systolic volume in a presyncopal subject during lower body suction (-30 mmHg) (Figure 4-12). At the same time plasma epinephrine concentration rose sharply while heart rate and blood pressure fell. Another clue linking syncope to epinephrine release is that acute hemorrhagic

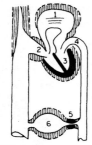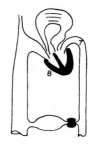

STAGE I   STAGE II

1. ↓ Central Blood Volume   1.-6.
2. ↓ Central Venous Pressure   7. ↓ Aortic Pulse Pressure
3. ↓ Stroke Volume   8. ↑ Heart Rate
4. ↓ Cardiac Output   9. ↑ Plasma Renin Activity
5. ↑ Sympathetic Activity (↑NE, MSNA)
6 ↓ Blood Flow (Splanchnic, Renal,
      Skin, Muscle)

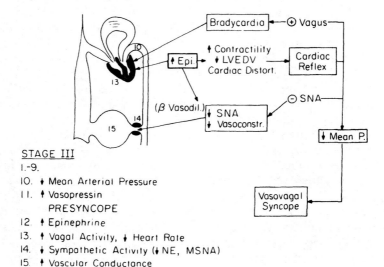

STAGE III

1.-9.
10. ↓ Mean Arterial Pressure
11. ↑ Vasopressin
       PRESYNCOPE
12. ↑ Epinephrine
13. ↑ Vagal Activity, ↓ Heart Rate
14. ↓ Sympathetic Activity (↓NE, MSNA)
15 ↑ Vascular Conductance
       SYNCOPE

Figure 4-11   Stages of orthostatic adjustment to central (thoracic) hypovolemia. *Stage I* is primarily response to cardiopulmonary baroreflex inhibition. *Stage II* is response to reduced aortic pulse pressure; increments in heart rate and plasma renin activity are added to responses 1–6 from Stage I. *Stage III* is falling mean pressure in severe hypovolemia adding to responses 1–9 a rise in vasopressin and epinephrine along with bradycardia and passive vasodilation that mark the onset of putative cardiac depressor reflex.

Figure 4-12 Echocardiographic estimation of left ventricular end-diastolic volume (LVEDV) (*closed circles*) and end-systolic volume (LVESV) (*open triangles*) in a normal subject undergoing lower body negative pressure (LBNP) (or suction) during normoxia and moderate hypoxemia (10 percent oxygen). Syncopal symptoms in hypoxemia were accompanied by a marked increase in plasma epinephrine concentration from <100 pg ml^{-1} to >600 pg ml^{-1}, bradycardia, hypotension, and marked shrinkage in ventricular volume (cardiac depressor reflex?). $\dot{Q}$ represents calculated cardiac outputs (heart rate × Δ ventricular volume) before and during suction; low $\dot{Q}$ values on bottom panel coincide (in time) with low ventricular volumes. (See Rowell and Blackmon, 1989.)

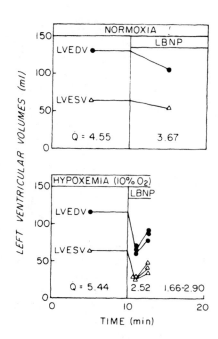

hypotension in rats was accompanied by reduced renal sympathetic nerve traffic, and *increased* traffic to the adrenal gland (this increases epinephrine release) (Victor et al., 1989). Again the evidence that epinephrine, acting via a cardiac depressor reflex, is a key link to human vasovagal syncope is suggestive but not conclusive.

CARDIOVASCULAR DYSFUNCTION

This section singles out some examples of orthostatic intolerance caused by a defective cardiovascular response to orthostatic stress. In one case, however, the function of dysfunctional hearts is actually improved by orthostatic stress and a paradoxical vasomotor response. The challenge has been to identify the site of the primary defect leading to intolerance—or, in one case, to its improvement. Hypoxemia is presented here as a more detailed example of a search for sometimes subtle causes of subnormal orthostatic adjustment. It is easy to look in the "wrong" places.

Hypoxemia
Background

Hypoxemia is commonly listed as a cause of syncope during orthostasis that is unassociated with cardiovascular disease (Hurst et al., 1990). Any orthostatic intolerance appears not to be associated with a maldistribution of blood flow or blood volume through excessive vasodilation. There is little vasodilation (except coronary and cerebral) in humans until arterial Po_2 falls to 30 or 35 mmHg (see Rowell, 1986). With such severe hypoxemia most of the vasodilation appears to be in skeletal muscle, a noncompliant region [Rowell and Blackmon (1987)].

On the one hand, there are findings that point to either a *central* or *peripheral* blunting (or possibly both) of sympathetic effector mechanisms in hypoxemia. On the other hand, there is clear evidence of powerful and sustained vasoconstriction during extreme hypoxemia ($Pao_2 < 20$ mmHg) as shown in the diving mammals. They maintain an intense α-adrenergic vasoconstriction that virtually stops blood flow to most organs except for the heart and brain (see chapter 12 in Rowell, 1986). Then there is the image of the climber (acclimatized to hypoxemia of course) who struggles to the summit of Mt. Everest (8,848 m) without supplemental oxygen and stands there quietly (without syncope) holding up a flag while his or her arterial Pao_2 is at approximately 28 mmHg.

In some cases, hypoxemia appears to impede vasoconstriction in response to sympathetic stimulation. For example, Heistad and Wheeler (1970) reported a larger fall in blood pressure and a subnormal forearm vasoconstriction during lower body suction when some (not all) of their normal subjects breathed 10 percent oxygen. Furthermore, they observed that hypoxemia lessened somewhat the forearm vasoconstriction in response to intra-arterial infusions of angiotensin II and norepinephrine. This suggests that hypoxemia depressed vascular contractile responses or somehow blunted receptor affinity for the hormones. In a study of hypoxemic patients with chronic lung disease ($Pao_2 = 27$ to 60 mmHg), several had significant impairment of their forearm vasomotor responses to lower body suction at -20 to -40 mmHg. Conversely, some of these patients, including several who were the most hypoxemic, showed no significant impairment in their responses. Nevertheless, when vasoconstriction was impaired, it could be restored by raising inspired oxygen up to 40 and 100 percent (Heistad et al., 1972). Figure 4-13 shows two more recent examples of a sudden onset of arterial hypotension during low levels of lower body suction.

Another body of evidence from humans points to maintained effectiveness of neural and vascular effector mechanisms in hypoxemia. For example, Heistad and Wheeler (1970) saw in approximately one-half of their subjects that hypoxemia (10 percent oxygen) had no effect on the rise in blood pressure or in leg vascular resistance in response to *intravenously* infused norepinephrine. Further, the pressor response to ice on the forehead was unaltered. Rowell and Blackmon (1986) observed the same pressor responses to intravenous norepinephrine infusion in normoxia and severe hypoxemia ($Pao_2 = 34.8$ mmHg), and there was no obvious blunting by hypoxemia of the splanchnic vasoconstriction in response to norepinephrine infusion. Finally, Henriksen and Rowell (1986) could detect no effect of hypoxemia (10 to 11 percent oxygen) on the washout rates of xenon 133 from skeletal muscle during 40° to 60° head-up tilt. Washouts of xenon, an index of blood flow, were measured in both an arm at venostatic level (i.e., to eliminate the local venoarteriolar reflex) and also in a dependent leg where both local and central reflex controls were operative. These findings are not consistent with an hypoxemia-induced orthostatic intolerance.

Central Versus Peripheral Defects in Autonomic Function

The inability of some individuals to maintain blood pressure during upright posture combined with hypoxemia could stem from a central effect of hypoxemia that reduces sympathetic nervous activity. Alternatively, it could result from a peripheral alteration in sympathetic action stemming from a reduced ability of sympathetic varicosities to release norepinephrine, that is, *prejunctional inhibition.*

Prejunctional Inhibition of Norepinephrine Release. Vanhoutte and colleagues (1981) listed several factors that depress neurally mediated vasoconstriction at a time when responses to exogenously administered norepinephrine exist. This effect characterizes a prejunctional inhibition of norepinephrine release from the sympathetic nerve varicosities. *Any inhibition from local metabolites occurs when their concentrations are below those that directly relax vascular smooth muscle—and such inhibition is most prominent at low levels of sympathetic activity* (keep in mind for later chapters: it would not be expected during severe stresses).

In isolated organs, both potassium and adenosine prejunctionally inhibit norepinephrine release (Vanhoutte et al., 1981). In some organs both substances may be increased by hypoxemia. However, Burcher and Garlick (1975) found no reduction in vasoconstrictor responses to either circulating or to neuronally released norepinephrine in dog skeletal muscle perfused with blood at $Po_2 = 17$ mmHg. When they added potassium to the deoxygenated blood, neurogenic vasoconstriction was abolished at high plasma concentrations, but vasoconstriction in response to circulating norepinephrine persisted. Possibly the marked vasoconstriction in diving mammals (mentioned earlier) is maintained by circulating norepinephrine release from the adrenal medulla (Gooden and Elsner, 1985) (this would not occur in humans, since norepinephrine release is almost entirely neuronal).

Despite what has just been said about inhibition of transmitter release, a puzzle exists. When normal young people are made acutely hypoxemic ($Pao_2 = 35$ to 27 mmHg) plasma norepinephrine concentration does not rise significantly (Rowell and Blackmon, 1986; Rowell et al., 1989) (note that $Pao_2 = 27$ mmHg was never maintained longer than 10 minutes; a rise in norepinephrine might well have accompanied a more prolonged exposure). This finding raised the obvious question: do central effects of hypoxemia inhibit sympathetic activity, or is neuronal release of norepinephrine inhibited?

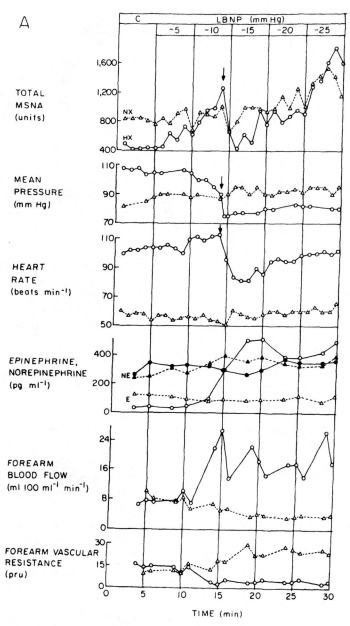

Figure 4-13 Sudden development of syncopal symptoms in two normal young men during graded lower body suction (−5 to −25 mmHg) while breathing 10 percent oxygen (HX = hypoxemia, open circles; NX = normoxia, open triangles). **(A)** Arrow marks sudden presyncope. Note marked rise in epinephrine and forearm blood flow. Note sudden drop in muscle sympathetic nerve activity followed by spontaneous recovery. **(B)** Sudden onset of presyncope with severe hypotension requiring stoppage

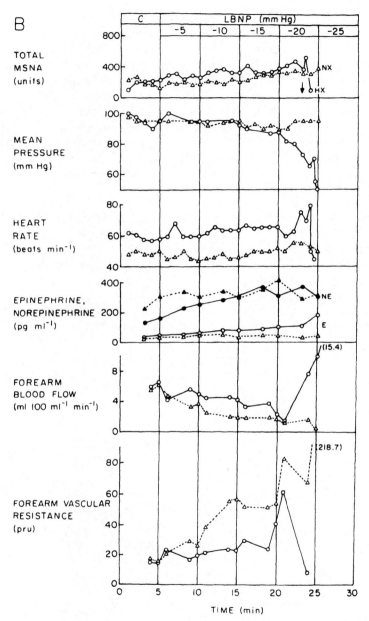

of lower body suction at 25 minutes. Recovery (not shown) was rapid. (From Rowell and Seals, 1990, with permission of the American Physiological Society.)

Rowell and Blackmon (1988) used the rise in pressure within isovolumic cutaneous veins to test whether or not sympathetic α-adrenergic constrictor mechanisms are intact in humans during both moderate and severe hypoxemia (Pao_2 = 35 to 28 mmHg). Veins are especially sensitive to small changes in sympathetic constrictor activity (Vanhoutte et al., 1981), and although veins and arteries are normally exposed to different chemical environments, neurotransmission in cutaneous veins is still subject to prejunctional inhibition by metabolites (Verhaeghe et al., 1978). Even the most severe local or central hypoxemia failed to impair venoconstriction, as illustrated in Figure 4-14. This strongly suggests that prejunctional inhibition of norepinephrine release does not explain the failure of plasma norepinephrine levels to rise during hypoxemia.

Central Influence on Sympathetic Nervous Activity. Could the failure to increase neuronal release of norepinephrine during hypoxemia stem from a central depression of sympathetic activity?

A direct approach to this problem was to measure by microneurography the effect of moderate to severe hypoxemia on MSNA (see Chapter 3) (Figure 4-15). The surprising result was that, in contrast to some other sympathoexcitatory stimuli such as exercise or cold stress (see Chapter 3), moderate (10 percent oxygen) to severe hypoxemia (8 percent oxygen)

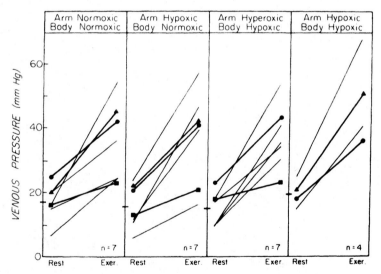

Figure 4-14 Pressure rise in occluded isovolumic forearm veins caused by reflex, sympathetic venoconstriction in response to exercise in seven (and four) normal young men. Arm versus body oxygen tensions were separated by occluding arm as one gas mixture breathed, then switching subject to another gas mixture as arm remained occluded. Neither central nor local hypoxemia, nor both, blunted venoconstriction. (From Rowell and Blackmon, 1988, with permission of the American Physiological Society.)

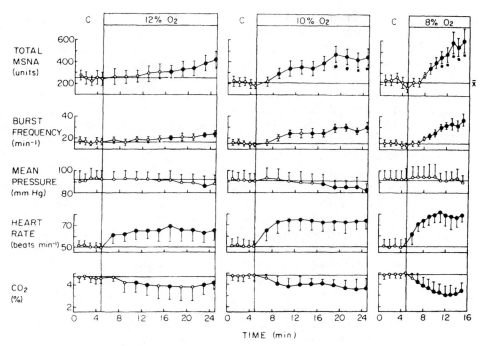

Figure 4-15 Moderate to severe hypoxemia increases muscle sympathetic nerve activity (MSNA) without increasing plasma norepinephrine concentration. Increases in MSNA were not correlated with changes in heart rate, end-tidal CO_2, or mean arterial pressure. MSNA did not increase in four of nine subjects breathing 12 percent oxygen; the small (83 percent) increase in five subjects was delayed 15 minutes. MSNA did not increase in three subjects breathing 10 percent oxygen; it rose (300 percent) in all breathing 8 percent oxygen. (From Rowell et al., 1989, with permission of the American Physiological Society.)

increased MSNA in the peroneal nerve by 260 and 300 percent, respectively, without raising plasma norepinephrine levels in resting humans. Based on the previous studies relating MSNA to plasma norepinephrine levels during exercise and cold stress, no significant rise in norepinephrine concentration would be expected during exposure to 12 percent oxygen because the rise in MSNA (83 percent) was too small to cause significant release.

Orthostatic Tolerance in Hypoxemia. At this point one might conclude that any propensity for orthostatic intolerance in hypoxemia could stem from a failure of sympathetic nerves to release norepinephrine. At least the amount released might not be sufficient to cause the degree of vasoconstriction needed to maintain arterial pressure. Parenthetically, one might conclude at this juncture that investigations sometimes proceed like the search for a coin beneath a street light; it was not where the coin was lost, but rather the only spot that provided light.

Rowell and Seals (1990) asked whether any inhibitory effects of hypoxemia on autonomic or cardiovascular function would be unmasked by a very mild orthostatic stress applied as small, −5-mmHg increments of lower body suction. Recall that Figure 2-8 shows that very low levels of lower body suction elicit significant vasoconstriction in normoxic subjects. Figure 4-16 compares the responses of six subjects to two exposures to this graded stress. They breathed air during one sequence of suction and 10 percent oxygen (two breathed 12 percent oxygen) during a second identical sequence. Two of the subjects failed to finish the test, as shown in Figure 4-13.

Hypoxemia significantly augmented both the absolute and percentage *changes* in total MSNA (amplitude × burst frequency) and in burst frequency. Forearm venous norepinephrine concentration was significantly increased by lower body suction in both normoxia and hypoxemia, but was increased additionally by hypoxemia only at the highest levels of suction (−20 and −25 mmHg). Arterial pressure was well maintained and unaffected by hypoxemia, unless presyncopal symptoms occurred (e.g., Figure 4-13). Figure 4-16 shows smaller absolute increments in forearm vascular resistance when subjects were hypoxemic, but the percentage increments were the same in both conditions; forearm resistance was lower (and blood flow higher) in the control period during hypoxemia. One could either argue that vasoconstriction was blunted by hypoxemia, or that it was not, but this matter is not easily resolved (see Rowell and Seals, 1990). Even if the percent changes in vessel diameter were the same in both situations, different values for absolute increments in resistance would be obtained for normoxic and hypoxemic vasodilated states owing to the different initial resistance values. In any case, release of norepinephrine was not blunted by hypoxemia once a small stress was added. Therefore no defect in sympathetic control could be found during mild, gradually applied orthostatic stress as long as plasma *epinephrine* levels did not rise.

An important clue (which seems to have been missed) comes from a study in which 3 of 13 normal subjects exposed to 7 to 10 percent oxygen during 45° head-up tilt experienced a vasovagal reaction (no one fainted when tilted while normoxic) (Anderson et al., 1946). Their precipitous bradycardia and hypotension were accompanied by a sudden and marked vasodilation in the forearm. The response was much like that seen by Barcroft and Edholm (1945) in severe hemorrhage (Anderson and colleagues thought this vasodilation was caused by some muscle twitching during hypoxemia). In the nonfainters, vasovagal symptoms did not appear even when inspired oxygen was decreased to 7 percent and subjects actually became unconscious (Anderson et al., 1946). Rowell and Blackmon (1989) made similar observations in eight subjects exposed to lower body suction while breathing air and then 10 percent oxygen. Heart rate and blood pressure fell suddenly in four subjects during suction only while low

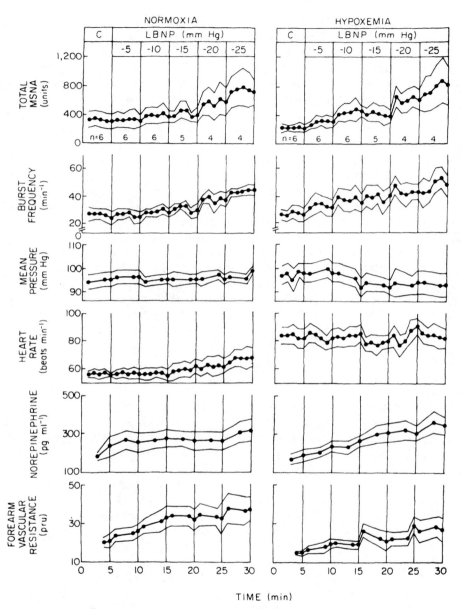

Figure 4-16 Graded increments in muscle sympathetic nerve activity (MSNA) in normoxic versus hypoxemic humans during mild to moderate lower body suction. Hypoxemia significantly increased the changes in total MSNA and burst frequency and in forearm venous norepinephrine concentration. Absolute increases in forearm vascular resistance were lower in hypoxemia but relative (percent) increments were the same in both conditions. Arterial pressure was not significantly affected by hypoxemia. (From Rowell and Seals, 1990, with permission of the American Physiological Society.)

oxygen was breathed (see Figure 4-12). Two courses of events very much like those described by Anderson and collagues are shown in Figure 4-13 (note the rapid decline in muscle sympathetic nerve firing and the rise in epinephrine). Note also in Figure 4-13A that the subject nearly fainted, but then showed spontaneous recovery; this unexplained phenomenon was also observed by Anderson and collagues (1946).

Figures 4-13 and 4-17 provide additional clues pertaining to reduced orthostatic tolerance in hypoxemia. The rise in MSNA in this individual was normal throughout lower body suction and unaffected by hypoxemia, whereas arterial blood pressure and forearm vascular resistance fell throughout the stress. These changes all paralleled a progressive rise in plasma *epinephrine* concentration that was never seen when these subjects were stressed during normoxia. The concentrations of epinephrine were sufficient to vasodilate skeletal muscle and splanchnic organs, thereby lessening their contribution to increased vascular resistance. It was this observation that prompted this discussion of orthostatic intolerance associated with hypoxemia as an example of cardiovascular rather than autonomic dysfunction. Epinephrine release could be a primary factor in any of the orthostatic intolerance associated with hypoxemia. One objective of this discussion is to reveal how difficult it can be to uncover causes of orthostatic intolerance. It pays tribute to those who discover the defects in patients with multiple disorders.

Valvular Heart Disease

In the nineteenth century, Adams and Stokes described (in separate publications) the occurrence of syncope associated with permanent slowing of heart rate in calcific aortic valve disease. They established the coexistence of cardiac arrhythmias and ventricular obstruction as causes for "cardiac syncope" (see Hurst et al., 1990).

Another example of recurrent orthostatic intolerance is seen in patients with mitral valve prolapse (Blomqvist, 1990). This syndrome is commonly characterized by a small left ventricle that is poorly matched anatomically to a large mitral valve. These patients may have a variety of symptoms, which include marked orthostatic hypotension. Relative to their orthostatic intolerance, the most important aspects of mitral valve prolapse appear to be the reduced blood volume, low ventricular volumes, and low stroke volume in upright posture. Many experience excessive sympathetic activity along with the inordinately large decreases in left ventricular end-diastolic volume. Exaggerated sympathetic vasoconstriction is required to maintain arterial blood pressure and in some patients the vasoconstriction is so exaggerated that blood pressure is above normal despite low cardiac output. They are said to exist in an "hyperadrenergic state" (Blomqvist, 1990). Hearts with low ventricular volumes are susceptible to adrenergic stimulation (see below).

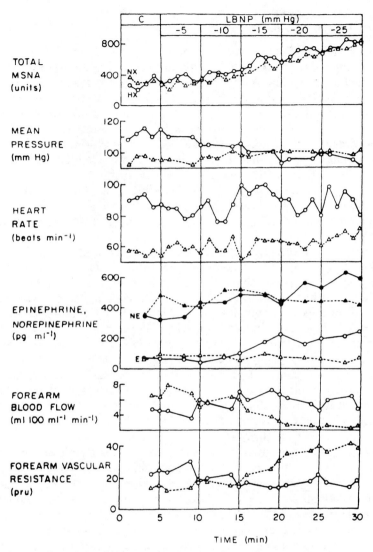

Figure 4-17 Borderline orthostatic intolerance during hypoxemia (10 percent oxygen) in one subject during graded lower body suction. A progressive rise in plasma epinephrine concentration was accompanied by a gradual fall in mean pressure and forearm vascular resistance while forearm blood flow remained above control (C). Total muscle sympathetic nerve activity rose normally and was unaffected by hypoxemia. (From Rowell and Seals, 1991, with permission of the American Physiological Society.)

Congestive Heart Failure

Congestive heart failure is most commonly associated with chronic cardiac dilatation secondary to ischemic heart disease, chronic mitral regurgitation, or congestive cardiomyopathy. The disease is characterized by low resting cardiac output and chronically increased cardiac filling pressures and systolic volumes. Vascular resistance is increased so that the primary determinant of left ventricular output is the left ventricular *afterload* or outflow resistance. Unlike the normal heart, the performance of the chronically failing heart is virtually independent of preload; thus one might expect the output of the failing heart during orthostasis to be dependent on a steep relationship to afterload (Zelis et al., 1981; Kassis, 1989). As pointed out in Chapter 2, performance of the normal heart is highly dependent on changes in filling pressure or preload (Frank-Starling relationship).

Bridgen and Sharpey-Schafer (1950) observed that patients with congestive heart failure responded abnormally to a head-up tilt. Instead of vasoconstriction, a paradoxical vasodilation was observed in the forearm. Further, plasma concentration of norepinephrine does not rise and may even fall in these patients during a tilt. Rather than the normal doubling of [³H]NE spillover, a marked reduction is observed (Davis et al., 1987). One hypothesis offered to explain these paradoxical findings has been that baroreflex function is blunted in this disease. Abboud and coworkers (1981) proposed that the sudden reduction in the size of an overdistended heart during a tilt might alter the firing of ventricular afferents so as to prevent normal inhibition of the cardiopulmonary reflex. A different explanation was offered by Kassis (1989), whose experimental findings are summarized in Figure 4-18.

Kassis (1989) confirmed previous findings that systemic vascular resistance falls markedly in patients with congestive heart failure during a 45° head-up tilt. The contrast in Figure 4-18 is with a control group of patients under examination for possible ischemic heart disease, but whose left ventricular function and orthostatic responses were basically normal. This fall in resistance in the congested patients is accompanied by large decrements in mean arterial pressure. Although their heart rates failed to increase, their cardiac outputs *rose* during the tilt as a consequence of the *increase in stroke volume*. The fall in left ventricular afterload led to marked improvement of left ventricular function in these patients. The improvement in stroke volume occurred despite equivalent orthostatic pooling of blood in the patients and controls, that is, right atrial pressure fell by approximately 5 mmHg in both groups. Neglecting for now the hypothesis of Abboud and colleagues (1981), cardiopulmonary baroreceptors could have been inhibited to the same degree in both groups. If true (and it may not be) why did vasoconstriction occur in one group (the control) and vasodilation in the other? Kassis (1989) suggested that the

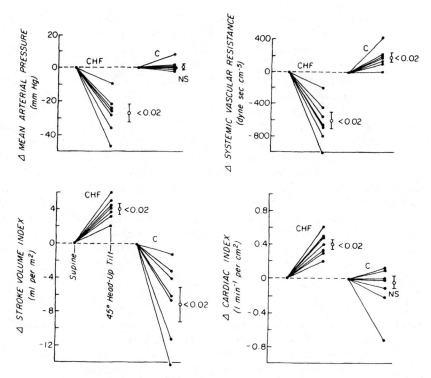

Figure 4-18 Orthostasis improves cardiac function in patients with congestive heart failure (CHF). The fall in arterial pressure and vascular resistance with head-up tilt reduces ventricular afterload (preload remains high) and favors increased cardiac output and stroke volume. Aortic baroreceptors may be stimulated by increased pulse pressure (higher stroke volume) causing reflex withdrawal of vasoconstrictor tone. (Adapted from Kassis, 1989.)

increase in aortic pulsatile stretch owing to the increase in stroke volume *stimulated* aortic baroreceptors and reflexly released vasoconstriction. For this to occur, however, the rise in stroke volume would need to precede the fall in arterial pressure that presumably permits the rise in stroke volume. Normally, aortic receptors are inhibited in orthostasis by reduced pulse pressure, so this situation would be the opposite of that shown in Figure 2-8 (which shows high baroreflex sensitivity to decreased aortic pulse pressure). Although the rise in aortic pulse pressure may contribute to the paradoxical vasodilation, it would appear not to have initiated it.

Tests in the patients with heart failure for autoregulatory responsiveness of resistance vessels to changes in transmural pressure revealed normal vascular function. The same was true for their local sympathetic venoarteriolar "axon" reflexes (see Chapter 2). In contrast, there was vasodilation and increased blood flow to forearm skin and muscle in response to a 45° head-up tilt. A key finding was that the heart-failure patients *increased plasma epinephrine* concentration during head-up tilt, and the control subjects did not. The paradoxical vasodilation during the tilt could be prevented by β-adrenergic blockade (Kassis, 1989).

Although there is no vasoconstriction in the forearm of patients in congestive heart failure, significant nonneurally induced vasoconstriction may occur in splanchnic organs and kidneys. During 1 hour of lower body suction at − 10 and at −40 mmHg, Creager and colleagues (1990) observed vasoconstriction in visceral organs but not in the forearm. Could this mean that, despite the inhibition of sympathetically mediated vasoconstriction, plasma levels of renin and angiotensin II nevertheless increase, making angiotensin II the primary controller of visceral vascular resistance (see Stadeager et al., 1989). Arterial pulse pressure in these patients did not change, so the hypothesis of Abboud and colleagues (1981) warrants consideration.

Cardiac Transplants

For the most part, transplanted hearts function well, so it is not entirely appropriate to reintroduce this topic in a section on dysfunction. However, as pointed out in Chapter 2, transplantation causes the loss of ventricular mechanosensitive afferents. The blunted forearm vasoconstriction and the small increase in plasma norepinephrine levels during lower body suction in transplant patients emphasizes the role of *ventricular receptors* in the responses (Chapter 2). A note of caution is needed here: although the dorsal portion of the atria including neural pathways from left atrial receptors are intact, mechanical uncoupling of atrial receptors and atrial muscle could attend chronic atrial distension, so that receptor function is abnormal. This impairment of the vasomotor response was not caused by the patient's treatment with immunosuppressive agents. Other patients who had received renal transplants and who underwent similar immunosuppressive treatment did not have depressed vasoconstrictor responses (they were actually greater than normal).

Figure 2-9 shows that baseline levels of forearm vascular resistance were much higher in the transplant patients (blood pressure was also 10 to 15 mmHg higher as well, yet plasma norepinephrine levels were low). Increments in forearm vascular resistance and plasma norepinephrine concentration during a cold-pressor test were the same in both groups; this reveals that there was no significant defect in vasoconstrictor effector mechanisms. That is, despite the higher baseline vascular resistance in the transplant patients, there was still ample latitude for further vasoconstriction and thus no reason to invoke any peripheral impairment in vasoconstriction.

AUTONOMIC DYSFUNCTION

The points here are made from a few enlightening examples. These examples give us some end points by revealing what it takes to cause complete orthostatic intolerance. It is an incapacitating disease.

Damage to the Sympathetic Chain and the Spinal Cord

Van Lieshout (1989) outlined a unique case of disabling orthostatic hypotension caused by surgical sympathectomies performed to prevent severe hyperhydrosis (excessive sweating). The piecemeal surgical destruction of the sympathetic ganglia (as outlined in Figure 4-19) in a physically active 38-year-old woman took place over 2 years. The surgeons began with bilateral thoracic ganglionectomies; subsequent procedures extended to

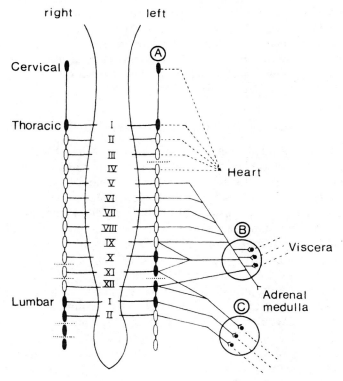

Figure 4-19 Schematic illustration of surgical ganglionectomies to prevent hyperhydrosis in 38-year-old woman. Black denotes intact sympathetic ganglia, and white denotes ganglionectomy. (A) Cervical ganglia. (B) Celiac and superior mesenteric ganglia. (C) Lower abdominal sympathetic ganglia. Disabling orthostatic intolerance was precipitated by removal of celiac and superior mesenteric ganglia. (From Van Lieshout, 1989, with permission of the author and Elsevier, Holland.)

lumbar levels with right and left sides operated separately. Despite the thoracolumbar sympathectomies (note that sympathetic control of one leg remained intact) this woman continued to compete in field hockey at a high level. She did not complain of orthostatic problems until after her final surgery.

The final surgery produced almost complete denervation of the splanchnic region, and thereafter she was disabled by severe orthostatic intolerance (reports from the 1950s had shown that splanchnic sympathectomy by itself led to postural hypotension in humans). Parasympathetic control of heart rate was normal, and its sympathetic control was only partly affected. Upright posture did not increase plasma levels of either norepinephrine or epinephrine. The latter reflected the loss of sympathetic control of the adrenal medulla.

We are reminded of the dictum of Hill (1895) who first pointed out the critical importance of the splanchnic region in maintaining blood pressure in orthostasis (Chapter 2). Its singular importance in this case is emphasized by the fact that all of the damage to the sympathetic nervous system that preceded splanchnic denervation appeared not to have had much apparent effect. Parenthetically, these findings also argue against the concept of an "abdominal water jacket" that counteracts hydrostatic pooling in abdominal organs (see Chapter 2).

Injury to the Spinal Cord: Spinal Man (Tetraplegia)

Cardiovascular control in humans with high spinal cord lesions (tetra- or quadriplegia) is dissociated from any cerebral or medullary regulatory component. "... they form a human physiological model in whom the afferent, central, and vagal efferent components of the baroreflex arc are intact, but where the spinal and peripheral sympathetic nervous system is isolated" (Mathias and Frankel, 1988). Supine tetraplegics have low tonic sympathetic activity and low plasma levels of norepinephrine and epinephrine. Plasma renin activity tends to be above normal.

Their responses to a 45° head-up tilt differ markedly from those patients with autonomic neuropathy. The two responses are contrasted in Figure 4-20. In the tetraplegic patient, blood pressure falls immediately and markedly with rapid partial recovery, and thereafter it tends to settle at a lower-than-normal level. The fall in blood pressure is ameliorated by some "secondary mechanism" if postural changes are made frequently, that is, there is some sort of gradual adaptation. This "maintenance" of arterial pressure above presyncopal levels is coupled with an apparent extension of effective cerebral autoregulation to lower arterial pressures. Adequate cerebral perfusion appears to be maintained even when arterial pressure is below the normal lower limit (approximately 60 mmHg for autoregulation) (Bannister, 1988; Mathias and Frankel, 1988). Plasma norepinephrine and epinephrine levels do not increase during head-up tilt unless sympathetic nerves are activated by local spinal sympathetic reflexes caused by skeletal

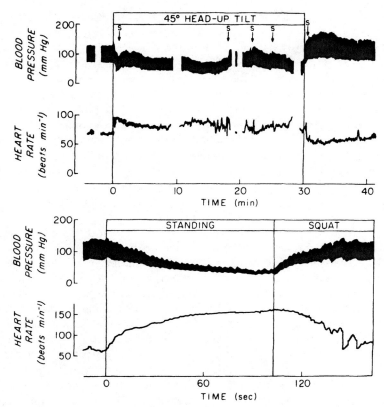

Figure 4-20 Remarkable orthostatic tolerance in a quadriplegic man during 45°
head-up tilt (*top*). With tilt pressure falls with prompt partial recovery caused by
muscle spasms (S) inducing spinal sympathetic activity. Plasma renin levels rose
markedly (measured where pressure record is interrupted). In latter phase of tilt
frequent spasms raised pressure. Venoarteriolar "reflexes" are also active (see Figure
2-15). (Adapted from Mathias and Frankel, 1988.) The contrast is with severe orthostatic hypotension (*bottom*) in a patient with autonomic neuropathy. Squatting at
the verge of syncope expresses volume out of splanchnic vessels, restoring cardiac
output and blood pressure. (Adapted from Van Lieshout, 1979.)

muscle spasms or urinary bladder contractions (see Figure 4-20). The rise
in heart rate is a vagally mediated response to hypotension. Rate does not
usually exceed 100 beats min^{-1}, the rate at which vagal withdrawal is
virtually complete in humans.

How does spinal man maintain blood pressure so well? In contrast to
patients with autonomic neuropathy, tetraplegics limit the fall in blood
pressure by vasoconstriction. This vasoconstriction could be caused by
the renin-angiotensin system (Chapter 3), by local sympathetic venoarteriolar "reflexes" (see Chapter 2), or by local spinal sympathetic reflexes.

The rise in plasma renin activity during head-up tilt is greater than normal in tetraplegic patients (Mathias and Frankel, 1988). The renin release cannot be elicited by sympathetic nerves and therefore must be initiated nonneurally by the fall in pressure distending the afferent arterioles (the renal "baroreflex," Chapter 3). The importance of angiotensin II as a vasoconstrictor of the human splanchnic region (see Chapter 3 in this book, and Stadeager et al., 1989) and the renal circulation (Creager et al., 1990) during orthostatic stress in normal, salt-depleted subjects and in patients with congestive heart failure suggest that angiotensin II may play an especially important role in patients with spinal cord injury. Mathias and Frankel (1988) comment that administration of captopril, which inhibits the enzyme that converts angiotensin I to angiotensin II, exacerbates postural hypotension in these patients. In addition to angiotensin II, the marked rise in vasopressin seen in tetraplegics may also play a role (Mathias and Frankel, 1988).

The sustained vasoconstriction in the legs of upward-tilted tetraplegics contributes significantly to the maintenance of arterial pressure (Skagen, 1983). Simply lowering one leg of a supine patient caused a 47 percent decrease in subcutaneous blood flow in that limb. During head-up tilt, a similar reduction in blood flow occurred and could not be abolished by proximal blockade of sympathetic nerves. This finding is consistent with the vasoconstriction being caused by a local sympathetic venoarteriolar "reflex" and/or a local myogenic reaction. Vasoconstriction was also observed in an arm positioned at venostatic level (no venoarteriolar "reflex") in a tilted tetraplegic patient. Anesthetic blockade of the proximal sympathetic nerve supply of the arm prevented the vasoconstriction. This vasoconstriction was therefore throught to be elicited by spinal sympathetic reflexes (Skagen, 1983).

Autonomic Neuropathy

The highly complex topic of autonomic neuropathy, reviewed by Johnson and Spalding (1974), Johnson and coworkers (1984), and Bannister (1988), can only be touched on briefly. There is a striking contrast between patients with severe autonomic deficiency who have virtually no orthostatic tolerance and tetraplegic patients who develop a surprising degree of tolerance. Considering the complexity as well as the redundancy in the physiological mechanisms that defend blood pressure during orthostasis, why is it that patients with autonomic neuropathies do so poorly in upright posture (see Figure 4-20)? The example of patients with diabetic autonomic neuropathy will suffice to make the point.

Long-term diabetes mellitus causes degeneration of both somatic and autonomic nerves. Irrespective of its etiology, orthostatic hypotension can be the result of (1) an abnormally low blood volume, (2) excessively low cardiac output, or (3) inadequate vasoconstriction. In diabetes any or all of these factors may be involved. Figure 4-21 summarizes some findings from seven diabetic patients (age 40 years) with autonomic neuropathy

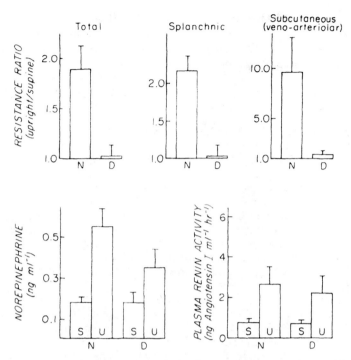

Figure 4-21 Causes of severe orthostatic intolerance in seven patients with diabetic neuropathy (D) during quiet standing. Comparison is with seven normal control subjects (N). Note increased vascular resistance ratio (ratio of resistances in upright versus supine posture) in group N and virtual absence of vasoconstriction in group D (top). In contrast, increments in plasma norepinephrine concentration and plasma renin activity going from supine (S) to upright (U) (bottom) in group N did not differ significantly from those in group D. (Adapted from Hilsted et al., 1981.)

and orthostatic hypotension (systolic blood pressure fell 50 mmHg within 1 minute after standing up). Their decrements in cardiac output and plasma volume and their increments in heart rate were no different from the changes observed in seven normal control subjects (age 30 years). The defect that underlay their orthostatic intolerance was an inability to increase vascular resistance, as shown in Figure 4-21.

Plasma renin activity rose normally (but not greater than normal, as in tetraplegics). This rise is presumably mediated by the "renal baroreflex." A reduction in renin responses is seen when nephropathy affects the juxtaglomerular apparatus. The inability to constrict resistance vessels in dependent regions, including the splanchnic circulation is the critical and consistent defect. Splanchnic vascular resistance does not change. In addition, the local venoarteriolar reflex is also lost as a consequence of sympathetic nerve dysfunction. There was no significant increase in plasma norepinephrine concentration nor in peripheral vascular resistance in upright posture. Therefore, blood moves without restriction into dependent veins, causing a rapid loss of ventricular filling pressure and a sudden onset of syncope. A normal rise in plasma renin activity would not be expected to supplant sympathetic vasomotor control.

REFERENCES

Abboud, F.M., M.D. Thames, and A.L. Mark (1981). Role of cardiac afferent nerves in regulation of circulation during coronary occlusion and heart failure. In F.M. Abboud, H.A. Fozzard, J.P. Gilmore, and D.J. Reis, eds. *Disturbances in Neurogenic Control of the Circulation*, pp. 65–86. American Physiological Society, Bethesda, MD.

Almquist, A., I.F. Goldenberg, S. Milstein, M.-Y. Chen, X. Chen, R. Hansen, C.C. Gornick, and D.G. Benditt (1989). Provocation of bradycardia and hypotension by isoproterenol and upright posture in patients with unexplained syncope. *N Engl. J. Med. 320*, 346–351.

Anderson, D.P., W.J. Allen, H. Barcroft, O.G. Edholm, and G.W. Manning (1946). Circulatory changes during fainting and coma caused by oxygen lack. *J. Physiol. (Lond.) 104*, 426–433.

Bannister, R. (ed.) (1988). *Autonomic Failure: A Textbook of Clinical Disorders of the Autonomic Nervous System*. Oxford University Press, Oxford, UK.

Barcroft, H., and O.G. Edholm (1945). On the vasodilatation in human skeletal muscle during post-haemorrhagic fainting. *J. Physiol. (Lond.) 104*, 161–175.

Bishop, V.S., A. Malliani, and P. Thoren (1983). Cardiac mechanoreceptors. In J.T. Shepherd, F.M. Abboud, and S.R. Geiger, eds. *Handbook of Physiology. The Cardiovascular System: Peripheral Circulation and Organ Blood Flow*, sect. 2, vol. III, part 2, pp. 497–555. American Physiological Society, Bethesda, MD.

Bjurstedt, H., G. Rosenhamer, U. Balldin, and V. Katkov (1983). Orthostatic reactions during recovery from exhaustive exercise of short duration. *Acta Physiol. Scand. 119*, 25–31.

Blair, D.A., W.E. Glover, A.D.M. Greenfield, and I.C. Roddie (1959). Excitation of cholinergic vasodilator nerves to human skeletal muscles during emotional stress. *J. Physiol. (Lond.) 148*, 633–647.

Blomqvist, C.G. (1990). Orthostatic hypotension. In W.W. Parmley, and K. Chatterjee eds. *Cardiology*, vol. 1, pp. 1–20. Lippincott, Philadelphia.

Blomqvist, C.G., and H.L. Stone (1983). Cardiovascular adjustments to gravitational stress. In J.T. Shepherd, F.M. Abboud, and S.R. Geiger, eds. *Handbook of Physiology. The Cardiovascular System: Peripheral Circulation and Organ Blood Flow*, sect. 2, vol. III, part 2, pp. 1025–1063. American Physiological Society, Bethesda, MD.

Bridgen, W., and E.P. Sharpey-Schafer (1950). Postural change in peripheral blood flow in cases with left heart failure. *Clin. Sci. 9*, 93–100.

Burcher, E., and D. Garlick (1975). Effects of exercise metabolites on adrenergic vasoconstriction in the gracilis muscle of the dog. *J. Pharmacol. Exp. Ther. 192*, 149–156.

Cowley, A.W. Jr., J.-F. Liard, and D.A. Ausiello (eds.). (1988). *Vasopressin: Cellular and Integrative Functions*. Raven Press, New York.

Creager, M.A., A.T. Hirsch, V.J. Dzau, E.G. Nabel, S.S. Cutler, and W.S. Colucci (1990). Baroreflex regulation of regional blood flow in congestive heart failure. *Am. J. Physiol. 258 (Heart Circ. Physiol. 27),* H1409–H1414.

Davis, D., L.I. Sinoway, J. Robison, J.R. Minotti, F.P. Day, R. Baily, and R. Zelis (1987). Norepinephrine kinetics during orthostatic stress in congestive heart failure. *Circ. Res. 61 (Suppl. I),* I87–I90.

Echt, M., L. Lange, and O.H. Gauer (1974). Changes of peripheral venous tone and central transmural pressure during immersion in a thermoneutral bath. *Pfluegers Arch. 352,* 211–217.

Ekblom B., and L. Hermansen (1968). Cardiac output in athletes. *J. Appl. Physiol. 25,* 619–625.

Gauer, O.H., and J.P. Henry (1976). Neurohormonal control of plasma volume. *Int. Rev. Physiol. 9,* 145–190.

Gauer, O.H., and H.L. Thron (1965). Postural changes in the circulation. In W.F. Hamilton and D. Dow, eds. *Handbook of Physiology. Circulation,* sect. 2, vol. III, pp. 2409–2439. American Physiological Society, Washington, D.C.

Gooden, B., and R. Elsner (1985). What diving animals might tell us about blood flow regulation. *Perspect. Biol. Med. 38,* 465–474.

Hainsworth, R. (1988). Fainting. In R. Bannister, ed. *Autonomic Failure: A Textbook of Clinical Disorders of the Autonomic Nervous System,* 2nd ed., part I, pp. 142–156. Oxford University Press, Oxford, UK.

Heistad, D.D., F.M. Abboud, A.L. Mark, and P.G. Schmid (1972). Impaired reflex vasoconstriction in chronically hypoxemic patients. *J. Clin. Invest. 51,* 331–337.

Heistad, D.D., and R.C. Wheeler (1970). Effect of acute hypoxia on vascular responsiveness in man. *J. Clin. Invest. 49,* 1252–1265.

Henriksen, O., and L.B. Rowell (1986). Lack of effect of moderate hypoxemia on human postural reflexes to skeletal muscle. *Acta Physiol. Scand., 127,* 171–175.

Hill, L. (1895). The influence of the force of gravity on the circulation of the blood. *J. Physiol. (Lond.) 18,* 15–53.

Hilsted, J., H.-H. Parving, N.J. Christensen, J. Benn, and H. Galbo (1981). Hemodynamics in diabetic orthostatic hypotension. *J. Clin. Invest. 68,* 1427–1434.

Holling, H.E. (1964). Effect of embarrassment on blood flow to skeletal muscle. *Trans. Am. Clin. Climatol. Assoc. 76,* 49–57.

Hurst, J.W., R.C. Schlant, C.E. Rackley, E.H. Sonnenblick, and N.K. Wenger (eds.) (1990). *The Heart,* 7th ed. McGraw-Hill, New York.

Johnson, J.M., M. Niederberger, L.B. Rowell, M.M. Eisman, and G.L. Brengelmann (1973). Competition between cutaneous vasodilator and vasoconstrictor reflexes in man. *J. Appl. Physiol. 35,* 798–803.

Johnson, R.H., D.G. Lambie, and J.M.K. Spalding (1984). *Neurocardiology.* W.B. Saunders, London.

Johnson, R.H., and J.M.K. Spalding (1974). *Disorders of the Autonomic Nervous System.* F.A. Davis, Philadelphia.

Kassis, E. (1989). Baroreflex control of the circulation in patients with congestive heart failure. *Dan. Med. Bull. 36,* 195–211.

Levine, B.D., J.C. Buckley, J.M. Fritsch, C.W. Yancy, Jr., D.E. Watenpaugh, P.G. Snell, L.D. Lane, D.L. Eckberg, and C.G. Blomqvist (1991). Physical

fitness and cardiovascular regulation: mechanisms of orthostatic intolerance. *J. Appl. Physiol. 70,* 112–122.

Lind, A.R., C.S. Leithead, and G.W. McNicol (1968). Cardiovascular changes
during syncope induced by tilting men in the heat. *J. Appl. Physiol. 25,*
268–276.

Mathias, C.J., and H.L. Frankel (1988). Cardiovascular control in spinal man.
Annu. Rev. Physiol. 50, 577–592.

Mosley, J.G. (1969). A reduction in some vasodilator responses in freestanding
man. *Cardiovasc. Res. 3,* 14–21.

Oberg, B., and P. Thoren (1972). Increased activity in left ventricular receptors
during hemorrhage or occlusion of caval veins in the cat: a possible cause
of the vaso-vagal reaction. *Acta Physiol. Scand. 85,* 164–173.

Oberg, B., and S. White (1970). The role of vagal cardiac nerves and arterial
baroreceptors in the circulatory adjustments to hemorrhage in the cat. *Acta
Physiol. Scand. 80,* 395–403.

Robinson, B.J., and R.H. Johnson (1988). Why does vasodilatation occur during
syncope? *Clin. Sci. 74,* 347–350.

Rowell, L.B. (1981). Active neurogenic vasodilatation in man. In P.M. Vanhoutte
and I. Leusen, eds. *Vasodilatation,* pp. 1–17. Raven Press, New York.

Rowell, L.B. (1983). Cardiovascular adjustments to thermal stress. In J.T. Shepherd, F.M. Abboud, and S.R. Geiger, eds. *Handbook of Physiology. The
Cardiovascular System: Peripheral Circulation and Organ Blood Flow,*
sect. 2, vol. III, part 2, pp. 967–1023. American Physiological Society,
Bethesda, MD.

Rowell, L.B. (1986). *Human Circulation. Regulation During Physical Stress.*
Oxford University Press, New York.

Rowell, L.B., and J.R. Blackmon (1986). Lack of sympathetic vasoconstriction in
hypoxemic humans at rest. *Am. J. Physiol. 251 (Heart Circ. Physiol. 20),*
H562–H570.

Rowell, L.B., and J.R. Blackmon (1987). Human cardiovascular adjustments to
acute hypoxaemia. *Clin. Physiol. 7,* 349–376.

Rowell, L.B., and J.R. Blackmon (1988). Venomotor responses during central and
local hypoxia. *Am. J. Physiol. 255 (Heart Circ. Physiol. 24),* H760–H764.

Rowell, L.B., and J.R. Blackmon (1989). Hypotension induced by central hypovolaemia and hypoxaemia. *Clin. Physiol. 9,* 269–277.

Rowell, L.B., G.L. Brengelmann, J.R. Blackmon, and J.A. Murray (1970). Redistribution of blood flow during sustained high skin temperature in resting
man. *J. Appl. Physiol. 28,* 415–420.

Rowell, L.B., G.L. Brengelmann, and J.A. Murray (1969). Cardiovascular responses to sustained high skin temperature in resting man. *J. Appl. Physiol.
27,* 673–680.

Rowell, L.B., J.-M.R. Detry, J.R. Blackmon, and C. Wyss (1972). Importance of
the splanchnic vascular bed in human blood pressure regulation. *J. Appl.
Physiol. 32,* 213–220.

Rowell, L.B., D.G. Johnson, P.B. Chase, K.A. Comess, and D.R. Seals (1989).
Hypoxemia raises muscle sympathetic activity but not norepinephrine in
resting humans. *J. Appl. Physiol. 66,* 1736–1743.

Rowell, L.B., and D.R. Seals (1990). Sympathetic activity during graded central hypovolemia in hypoxemic humans. *Am. J. Physiol. 259* (*Heart Circ. Physiol. 28*), H1197–H1206.

Sander-Jensen, K., N.H. Secher, A. Astrup, N.J. Christensen, J. Giese, T.W. Schwartz, J. Warberg, and P. Bie (1986a). Hypotension induced by passive head-up tilt: endocrine and circulatory mechanisms. *Am. J. Physiol. 251* (*Regulatory Integrative Comp. Physiol. 20*), R742–R748.

Sander-Jensen, K., N.H. Secher, P. Bie, J. Warberg, and T.W. Schwartz (1986b). Vagal slowing of the heart during haemorrhage: observations from 20 consecutive hypotensive patients. *Br. Med. J. 292,* 364–366.

Saltin, B., G. Blomqvist, J.H. Mitchell, R.L. Johnson, Jr., K. Wildenthal, and C.B. Chapman (1968). Response to exercise after bed rest and after training. *Circulation 38* (*Suppl. 7*), 1–78.

Skagen, K. (1983). Sympathetic reflex control of blood flow in human subcutaneous tissue during orthostatic maneuvres. *Dan. Med. Bull. 30,* 229–241.

Stadeager, C., B. Hesse, O. Henriksen, N.J. Christensen, F. Bonde-Petersen, J. Mehlsen, and J. Giese (1989). Effects of angiotensin blockade on the splanchnic circulation in normotensive humans. *J. Appl. Physiol. 67,* 786–791.

Stratton, J.R., M.A. Pfeifer, J.L. Ritchie, and J.B. Halter (1985). Hemodynamic effects of epinephrine: concentration-effect study in humans. *J. Appl. Physiol. 58,* 1199–1206.

Tatar, P., J. Bulas, R. Kvetnansky, and V. Strec (1986). Venous plasma adrenaline response to orthostatic syncope during tilting in healthy men. *Clin. Physiol. 6,* 303–309.

Thoren, P. (1987). Depressor reflexes from the heart during severe haemorrhage. In R. Hainsworth, P.N. McWilliam, and D.A.S.G. Mary, eds. *Cardiogenic Reflexes,* sect. 5, pp. 389–401. Oxford University Press, Oxford, UK.

Tyden, G. (1977). Aspects of cardiovascular reflex control in man. *Acta Physiol. Scand* (*Suppl. 448*), 1–62.

Vanhoutte, P.M., T.J. Verbeuren, and R.C. Webb (1981). Local modulation of adrenergic neuroeffector interaction in the blood vessel wall. *Physiol. Rev. 61,* 151–247.

Van Lieshout, J.J. (1989). *Cardiovascular Reflexes in Orthostatic Disorders.* Rodopi, Amsterdam.

Verhaeghe, R.H., R.R. Lorenz, M.A. McGrath, J.T. Shepherd, and P.M. Vanhoutte (1978). Metabolic modulation of neurotransmitter release: adenosine, adenine nucleotides, potassium, hyperosmolarity, and hydrogen ion. *Fed. Proc. 37,* 208–211.

Victor, R.G., P. Thoren, D.A. Morgan, and A.L. Mark (1989). Differential control of adrenal and renal sympathetic nerve activity during hemorrhagic hypotension in rats. *Circ. Res. 64,* 686–694.

Wallin, B.G., and G. Sundlöf (1982). Sympathetic outflow to muscles during vasovagal syncope. *J. Auton. Nerv. Syst. 6,* 287–291.

Zelis, R., S.F. Flaim, A.J. Liedtke, and S.H. Nellis (1981). Cardiocirculatory dynamics in the normal and failing heart. *Annu. Rev. Physiol. 43,* 455–476.

5

Central Circulatory Adjustments to Dynamic Exercise

This chapter describes the basic hemodynamic adjustments to mild to severe dynamic exercise and, in particular, the basic mechanisms underlying them. Cardiac adjustments to chronic high loads (physical conditioning) are discussed also. These adjustments occur over a range that can be precisely defined by objectively determined maximal values. The concept of a maximum for cardiovascular function is developed in some detail. The primary focus is on how heart rate, stroke volume, and oxygen extraction increase and also on how ventricular and vascular pressures are maintained by physical or hemodynamic means. This includes a treatment of those nonreflex mechanical adjustments that counteract the flow-dependent fall in cardiac filling pressures seen when cardiac output rises during rest. Except for the role of cardiac vagus and sympathetic nerves, neural and reflex control are covered in subsequent chapters. In addition to providing a summary and some basic background for the chapters that follow, new material is presented.

CARDIOVASCULAR FUNCTIONAL CAPACITY: THE CONCEPT

Exercise provides a precise and powerful tool that permits the study of the regulation of the cardiovascular system under rigorously controlled and highly reproducible conditions, which include the full range of its "functional capacity." Exercise more than any other stress taxes the regulatory ability of the cardiovascular system. The obvious advantage to the investigator is that more is learned about how a system operates when it is forced to perform than when it is idle.

The chapter is organized mainly around the Fick principle, which is expressed in Equation 5-1:

$$\dot{V}o_2 = HR \times SV \times AVo_2\text{diff}, \qquad (5\text{-}1)$$

where $\dot{V}o_2$ is oxygen uptake, HR is heart rate, SV is stroke volume, and $AVo_2\text{diff}$ is arterial-mixed venous oxygen difference (or total systemic arteriovenous oxygen difference). The degree to which each of these variables can increase determines the upper limit for whole-body oxygen consumption. This limit is called the *maximal oxygen uptake* ($\dot{V}O_2$max).

The fact that there is a truly maximal value for oxygen uptake called $\dot{V}O_2$max and that this value can be accurately measured experimentally is of fundamental importance. A more complete understanding of cardiovascular control during exercise developed when physiologists found a means of quantifying the *functional capacity* of the entire cardiovascular system. This means that cardiovascular responses to exercise—or to any other stress—can be scaled in relation to an objectively defined "full-scale" response. The functional capacity of the cardiovascular system is expressed as its maximal ability to transport oxygen to the working muscle during severe exercise, that is, at the limit of the system's regulatory ability.

The ability to define the functional limits of an entire system has provided a strong scientific base from which to investigate its regulation. It is essential, however, that this *maximum* be a reproducible characteristic of the individual and that it not be a "pseudomaximum," which depends on factors such as skill or motivation of the subject or on other confounding variables (see below).

By definition, the limit of circulatory function is reached at the highest attainable oxygen uptake, that is, the $\dot{V}O_2$max. *The $\dot{V}O_2$max has an exact physiological definition, which is*

$$\dot{V}O_2\text{max} = HR_{max} \times SV_{max} \times AVO_2\text{diff}_{max}. \qquad (5\text{-}2)$$

Equation 5-2 restates the Fick principle in Equation 5-1 and is modified simply to show that the highest attainable oxygen uptake is achieved at the maximum values for each variable in the equation. Unfortunately, it is usually not technically feasible to satisfy this unambiguous physiological definition. The alternative is to measure directly the $\dot{V}O_2$max by the procedure illustrated schematically in Figure 5-1. An intensity of exercise is established, beyond which further increments in rate of work raise oxygen uptake no further—a plateau or maximal value has been reached. If this is done correctly, then by definition we have reached the unique value for oxygen uptake defined in Equation 5-2. The experimental evidence indicates that each variable in this equation has reached a maximum for a particular individual.

The Classical Concept of $\dot{V}O_2$max

Why is it not better simply to measure oxygen uptake at rest and express values in exercise as multiples of rest? Barcroft (1934) explored this question in a chapter entitled "The Principle of Maximal Activity." Scaling from measurements at rest suffers from the marked random variation characterizing that loosely defined state. Barcroft asked: "In what terms are we to describe organs of the body, in terms of rest, regarding exercise

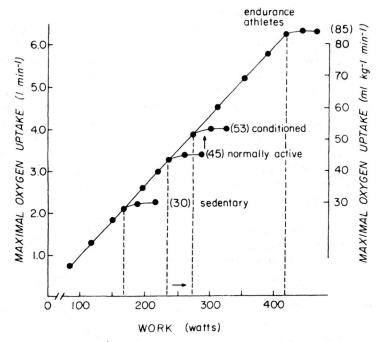

Figure 5-1   Values for $\dot{V}O_2$max in normal young people range from 30 ml kg^{-1} min^{-1} (or even lower in the most sedentary individuals) up to 85 ml kg^{-1} min^{-1} in elite endurance athletes. By comparison, the range over which $\dot{V}O_2$max increases in normal individuals (e.g., from 45 to 53 ml kg^{-1} min^{-1}) with 2 to 3 months of physical conditioning is small. Also illustrated is the linear relationship between oxygen uptake and workload up to the $\dot{V}O_2$max. Thereafter, oxygen uptake reaches a plateau as work rate increases. This plateau is the basis for an objective determination of the maximal value. (From Rowell, 1986, with permission of Oxford University Press.)

as a variant or in terms of its [sic] capacity to do work?'' Barcroft (1934) applied his ideas to the investigation of metabolism of single organs and glands. He stated ''... the impression which I have carried away from these researches is that it is much more easy to obtain uniform values for active than for resting organs .... It seems that the most uniform measure of an organ is in terms of the maximum which it can accomplish.''

Hill and Lupton (1923) showed that oxygen uptake does not continuously increase with increasing work intensity until intolerable levels of effort are reached. Rather, a *plateau* of oxygen upake is eventually reached well before the effort becomes intolerable. Hill and colleagues went on to show that individuals could exercise for brief periods at levels exceeding those required to elicit this plateau, that is, beyond $\dot{V}O_2$max. This is an important point because it showed that $\dot{V}O_2$max occurred at submaximal rates of power output, that is, submaximal for whatever rate of work muscles could perform. Beyond $\dot{V}O_2$max muscles are partly supported metabolically by anaerobic processes. Hill and Lupton (1923) argued that oxygen uptake cannot exceed this plateau level or upper limit because of limitations of the cardiovascular and respiratory systems. This view became known as the *classical concept of* $\dot{V}O_2$max.

Before and well after Hill's work, investigators showed that exercise with small muscle mass elicited low peak values for oxygen uptake, whereas peak values were much higher when large masses of muscle were active. Liljestrand and Stenstrom (1920) observed a plateau of oxygen uptake in a subject who ran at successively increasing speeds. When the arms were added to running in cross-country skiing, oxygen uptake increased further, but the increase was only 150 to 200 ml min^{-1} despite the fact that added metabolic costs of arm work were much greater than the increment in oxygen uptake. These authors concluded that the failure of this subject to raise oxygen uptake further was due to increased mechanical efficiency (i.e., rather than to the cardiovascular-respiratory limitation proposed later by Hill and colleagues).

The physiologist's concept of a $\dot{V}O_2$max requires the establishment of a plateau of oxygen uptake with increasing work rate or an equivalent *objective* measure showing that a true maximum is attained. For example, a blood lactate concentration exceeding 90 mg 100 ml^{-1} is taken as another criterion (Åstrand, 1952). Once this upper limit for oxygen uptake has been objectively established, it has been shown to be insensitive to a variety of acute stresses that do not directly affect its determinants (Taylor et al., 1963). It is a reproducible characteristic of the individual and it has a day-to-day variability of only 2 to 4 percent, or similar to that for body height and weight and is less variable than the basal metabolic rate.

Muscle Mass as a Determinant of $\dot{V}O_2$max

A pivotal aspect of the concept of $\dot{V}O_2$max is that attainment of a true maximum requires that a certain fraction of the total muscle mass be engaged. Unfortunately, this fraction has not been established. As already mentioned, it is assumed to be about 50 percent of the total (Rowell, 1974; Åstrand and Rodahl, 1977). It is clear that peak values for oxygen uptake can be attained when muscle groups of any size are taxed to their inherent contractile limits (or to subjective limits of fatigue) over brief periods of time. There is no unique "peak value" because it is directly related to the mass of active muscle, and to the motivation to exert it to an extreme (e.g., Figure 7-13). In short, no upper limit that fits the definition of $\dot{V}O_2$max can be defined. The term $\dot{V}O_2$max applies strictly to the highest value attainable for the whole body.

It is therefore meaningless to speak of a $\dot{V}O_2$max for small muscle groups. The *peak* $\dot{V}O_2$, or the highest attainable oxygen uptake for small muscle groups, depends on limitations that vary with conditions, and not on fixed physiological end points expressed in Equation 5-2 and illustrated in Figure 5-2. This distinction between a unique oxygen uptake that is

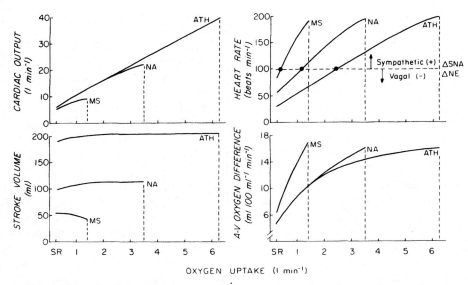

Figure 5-2 The four determinants of $\dot{V}O_2$max. Representative cardiovascular responses to graded dynamic exercise in three groups of individuals whose levels of $\dot{V}O_2$max are (a) very low (patients with "pure" mitral stenosis [MS]), (b) normal (normally active subjects [NA]), or (c) very high (elite endurance athletes [ATH]). Vertical dashed lines at the end of each curve identify $\dot{V}O_2$max of each group. Note marked differences in maximal cardiac outputs and stroke volumes and the similarity in maximal heart rates and systemic arteriovenous oxygen differences. In the heart rate panel dashed horizontal line at heart rate = 100 and solid circles on heart rate curves show points at which sympathetic nerve activity (ΔSNA) and plasma norepinephrine (ΔNE) increase. Above the dashed line, heart rate is increased slowly by elevated (+) sympathetic activity (see Figure 5-5). Below this dashed line heart rate is increased rapidly by vagal withdrawal (−) (see Figure 5-5). (Adapted from Rowell, 1986.)

truly maximal and a peak value is a vital one. *It is essential to differentiate between limitations that are simply brought on by some local factors as opposed to those that are brought forth by a well-defined functional limit.* It is impossible to identify what factors limit oxygen uptake unless we properly define its limit (Chapter 9).

Although the fraction of the total muscle mass that must be active to elicit a $\dot{V}O_2$max is commonly estimated to be about 50 percent, the accuracy of this estimate is unknown. We still lack ways to quantify the total mass of active muscle. Some have assumed that all muscles must be active; however, the concept of a $\dot{V}O_2$max would be meaningless if its value were attained in an asymptotic approach to a limiting value in some task, ultimately requiring the contraction of every muscle in the body at a level eliciting a peak oxygen uptake for each individual muscle. This would mean that cardiac output and systemic arteriovenous oxygen difference would be functions of the percentage of the total muscle mass utilized.

Available evidence argues strongly against this idea (but it is a fundamental aspect of other schemes; see Weibel, 1984).

A practical problem is raised whenever the task used to determine $\dot{V}O_2$max fails to elicit a true maximum. For example, many individuals cannot reach $\dot{V}O_2$max by leg exercise alone on a cycle ergometer but they do commonly reach 90 to 95 percent of the true maximum (e.g., Bergh et al., 1965). This has been demonstrated by combining arm plus leg exercise (cycling). The peak value in the latter equals the highest value and presumably the true maximum observed during treadmill running at a grade (Bergh et al., 1976). Parenthetically, Taylor and colleagues (1955) were unable to establish a true plateau of oxygen uptake simply by increasing treadmill speed; oxygen uptake asymptotically approaches some upper limit such as seen during exercise with small muscle groups (see Figure 7-13).

In a number of studies combined arm and leg exercise has been used to show independence of $\dot{V}O_2$max on muscle mass once a critical mass is active (see Rowell, 1974; Bergh et al., 1976; Clausen, 1977). In contrast, others have found that, even during treadmill exercise (on a grade), a slightly higher value for oxygen uptake can be achieved when arms are exercised during running (in all such experiments, however, the cost of arm exercise far exceeds the small rise in oxygen uptake) (Hermansen, 1973). The problem may be that well-conditioned individuals often have cardiovascular systems adapted to supply abnormally large fractions of total muscle mass (e.g., as in cross-country skiers). As a consequence, these individuals may have to exert a larger percentage of their total muscle mass to attain a $\dot{V}O_2$max than sedentary individuals.

These discrepancies can be important because normalization of responses to values that are not truly maximal can create artificial differences between individuals. For example, so-called "maximal" cardiac output and arteriovenous oxygen difference would be lower than normal. Another example is if the assumed $\dot{V}O_2$max were actually a submaximal peak value, then addition of more muscle will increase oxygen uptake, leading in this case to a false conclusion that $\dot{V}O_2$max was limited by the metabolic capacity of muscle rather than by the cardiovascular system.

DETERMINANTS OF OXYGEN UPTAKE: A BRIEF REVIEW

The four parts of Figure 5-2 summarize the relationship of each determinant of oxygen uptake to the rate of total oxygen consumption during graded levels of exercise up to and including the level required to elicit a $\dot{V}O_2$max (the abbreviated term used to describe this particular intensity of exercise is "maximal exercise," even though this intensity is submaximal for work rate and only maximal for oxygen uptake). The line for each group ends at their average value for $\dot{V}O_2$max.

The comparisons are between three groups whose values for $\dot{V}O_2$max average 1.4, 3.5, and 6.2 L min^{-1}. The lowest values are from a selected group of patients with "pure" mitral stenosis (MS) ("pure" meaning no cardiac failure, no pulmonary hypertension, or congestion) who had approximately normal cardiac output and blood gases at rest (Blackmon et al., 1967). They were chosen as a model for low maximal cardiac output. The highest values of $\dot{V}o_2$max are extreme values from some elite endurance athletes (ATH) studied by Ekblom and Hermansen (1968) and Ekblom (1969). The values for normally active (NA) subjects were derived from sources reviewed by Rowell (1974) and Clausen (1977). The values apply to dynamic upright exercise, predominantly with the legs, in a neutral thermal environment at sea level in well-hydrated, postprandial subjects who were appropriately familiarized with the exercise test and their laboratory surroundings (i.e., well-standardized conditions).

Cardiac Output

Cardiac output rises nearly linearly with oxygen uptake with a slope of approximately 6 L min^{-1} of cardiac output per L min^{-1} increase in oxygen uptake in normally active subjects and endurance athletes. Some (e.g., Åstrand et al., 1964) have observed a tendency for the slope to decrease as $\dot{V}o_2$max is approached. Values of cardiac output as high as 42 L min^{-1} have been observed in elite endurance athletes (Ekblom and Hermansen, 1968). The low cardiac outputs of the mitral stenosis patients are attributable to the mechanical filling defect caused by a stenotic mitral valve (Blackmon et al., 1967).

Cardiac Index Versus Cardiac Output: Criticism of a Tradition. The use of indices based on body surface area in studies of cardiovascular function in exercise is unfortunate. It is recognized that long tradition has made it useful for comparing patients in clinical medicine even though the surface area index is based on assumptions that have been thoroughly refuted (see Tanner, 1949; Kleiber, 1975). The original idea that led to the surface area index was that metabolic rate is a function of the rate of heat loss to the environment, which is in turn proportional to body surface area. However, this assumption is not even correct for resting snakes, which are poikilotherms and have, unlike humans, an easily quantifiable body surface area (Galvao et al., 1965).

During weight-bearing exercise, body mass and not surface area determines oxygen uptake, whereas on a cycle ergometer, the resistance to movement determines power output and total oxygen uptake. Thus, comparison of values based on body weight is valid for weight-bearing exercise. On the ergometer, we compare absolute oxygen uptakes. Both have the advantage that oxygen uptake is related to the variable that determines its magnitude.

Heart Rate

Under properly standardized conditions the relationship between heart rate and oxygen uptake is quite reproducible in any individual (see Taylor et al., 1963). "Maximal" heart rate or the heart rate at which $\dot{V}O_2$max is achieved tends to be fixed at 190 to 195 beats min^{-1} in normal young subjects (such rates were observed in several of the mitral stenosis patients as well [Blackmon et al., 1967]). Parenthetically, heart rate can reach slightly higher values under highly stressful conditions such as hyperthermia or dehydration. Figure 5-2 shows that the *range* of heart rate response is mainly a function of the resting heart rate, which can be as low as 30 beats min^{-1} in the athletes and up to 80 or 90 beats min^{-1} in the mitral stenosis patients.

The slope of the relationship between heart rate and oxygen uptake is a function of the $\dot{V}O_2$max. When heart rate is plotted against the percent of $\dot{V}O_2$max required (*relative oxygen uptake*), the slopes become virtually identical and almost superimposed down to the respective resting heart rates for each group. Viewed in this relative manner, the three groups are separated by the range over which heart rate can increase. Figure 5-2 reveals that, at any given submaximal oxygen uptake, heart rate and stroke volume are functions of $\dot{V}O_2$max, whereas cardiac output is not.

Arteriovenous Oxygen Difference

The difference for oxygen concentration in arterial and the mixed venous or pulmonary arterial blood widens with increasing oxygen consumption (Figure 5-2). At rest arteriovenous oxygen difference is normally 4.5 ml 100 ml^{-1} (approximately 23 percent extraction) and at $\dot{V}O_2$max this difference is commonly close to 16 ml 100 ml^{-1}. Usually 80 to 85 percent of the available oxygen is extracted from the total blood volume at $\dot{V}O_2$max. Arteriovenous oxygen difference at $\dot{V}O_2$max reached 17 ml 100 ml^{-1} in the mitral stenosis patients as it often does in well-conditioned individuals. Absolute differences were somewhat lower in the athletes with very high maximal cardiac outputs because their hemoglobin concentrations and arterial oxygen contents were below normal (see Ekblom, 1969). Also, in some athletes the saturation of arterial blood with oxygen may decline as $\dot{V}O_2$max is approached and this will further reduce the arteriovenous oxygen difference (see Chapter 9). Nevertheless, the athletes still extract 85 percent or more of the available oxygen from blood. To some extent the lower resting hemoglobin concentration and arterial desaturation are compensated for by the hemoconcentration associated with loss of plasma water into muscle during severe exercise.

The Physiological Basis for Differences in $\dot{V}O_2$max

The three groups in Figure 5-2 were chosen to make two points. First, inasmuch as maximal heart rate and maximal arteriovenous oxygen difference are usually so similar, the factor most commonly accounting for the different values of $\dot{V}O_2$max in different individuals is stroke volume. The numbers in Table 5-1 express values for each variable of the Fick equation

Table 5-1 Physiologic Basis for Differences in $\dot{V}O_2$max in Three Subject Groups

Subjects	$\dot{V}O_2$max (ml min^{-1})	=	Heart Rate (beats min^{-1})	×	Stroke Volume (ml)	×	Arteriovenous Oxygen Difference (ml 100 ml^{-1})
ATH	6,250	=	190	×	205	×	16
NA	3,500	=	195	×	112	×	16
MS	1,400	=	190	×	43	×	17

ATH, elite endurance athletes; NA, normally active subjects; MS, subjects with pure mitral stenosis.

and illustrate the basis for the differences in $\dot{V}O_2$max in the three sample groups. Each oxygen uptake on the left equals the product of the three variables on its right. Table 5-2 shows the range of adjustment for each determinant of $\dot{V}O_2$max and emphasizes again that stroke volume determines the range over which cardiac output and heart rate can increase, whereas the increase in arteriovenous oxygen difference is similar among different groups.

The second point is that, if heart rate and arteriovenous oxygen difference are normalized or scaled by expressing them in relation to the relative oxygen uptake (i.e., percent of $\dot{V}O_2$max), then diverse groups such as those in Figures 5-1 and 5-2 appear to respond in virtually identical fashion (Åstrand et al., 1964; Rowell et al., 1964; Blackmon et al., 1967). That is, these cardiovascular responses are more closely related to the *relative* metabolic demands than to the absolute demands (note that expressing cardiac output in relation to relative oxygen uptake often increases the difference between individuals and can be misleading).

Bear in mind that there are many exceptions to the generalizations made in Figure 5-2 and in Tables 5-1 and 5-2. For example, the range over which heart rate can increae can be greatly reduced in cardiac patients as a consequence of their disease. Anemia, hypoxemia, and pulmonary disease will reduce arteriovenous oxygen difference by lowering arterial oxygen

Table 5-2 Magnitudes of Increase in the Determinants of $\dot{V}O_2$max in Three Subject Groups Characterized by Different Stroke Volumes

Subjects	$\dot{V}O_2$max (ml min^{-1})*	Heart Rate (beats min^{-1})	Stroke Volume (ml)	Arteriovenous Oxygen Difference (ml 100 ml^{-1})
ATH	25 × (250–6,250)*	6.4 × (30–190)	1.1 × (190–205)	3.56 × (4.5–16)
NA	14 × (250–3,500)	3.6 × (55–195)	1.1 × (100–112)	3.56 × (4.5–16)
MS	5.6 × (250–1,400)	2.3 × (83–190)	0.8 × (53–43)	3.1 × (5.48–17)

ATH, elite endurance athletes; NA, normally active subjects; MS, subjects with pure mitral stenosis.
* Range of absolute values in parentheses.

content. One example will suffice to show the sensitivity of $\dot{V}O_2$max to a change in arterial oxygen content. Figure 5-3 shows how simulated high altitude (4,000 m) reduces $\dot{V}O_2$max. $\dot{V}O_2$max falls in direct proportion to the fall in arterial oxygen content and arteriovenous oxygen difference; the ability to reduce mixed venous oxygen content was not significantly affected. Maximal heart rate and cardiac output were unaffected by acute hypoxemia. Maldistribution of blood flow between muscle and inactive regions will also reduce arteriovenous oxygen difference by raising mixed venous oxygen content (Chapter 6).

Summary. In summary, heart rate, cardiac output, and oxygen uptake increase over a range that is normally determined by the size of the stroke volume. Maximal extraction of oxygen tends to be similar among athletes, sedentary individuals, and some cardiac patients. This means that the $\dot{V}O_2$max is limited by whatever determines the capacity of these variables to increase.

The following sections examine the regulation of each of these variables discussed above and in addition, analyzes the variables that determine ventricular performance, acutely and over prolonged periods of repeated stress.

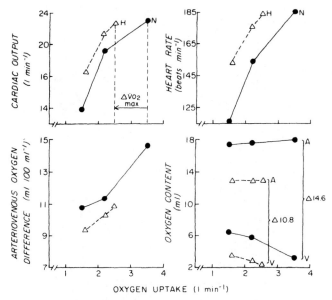

Figure 5-3   Effects of simulated high altitude (4,000 m) on cardiovascular responses to graded exercise up to $\dot{V}O_2$max in both conditions. Triangles and H denote values at simulated altitude. Comparison is with values at sea level (*solid circles*). Dashed lines in upper left panel show hypoxemia-induced reduction in $\dot{V}O_2$max. Moderate hypoxemia had no effect on maximal heart rate or cardiac output. (Adapted from Stenberg et al., 1966.)

REGULATION OF THE CENTRAL CIRCULATION

Heart Rate

Heart rate is under the control of both the parasympathetic and the sympathetic branches of the autonomic nervous system as illustrated in Figure 5-4. Blockade of parasympathetic control of heart rate with atropine reveals that most of the initial heart rate response to exercise, up to a heart rate of approximately 100 beats min^{-1}, is mainly attributable to the withdrawal of tonic vagal activity. Two points of major importance to subsequent discussion of reflex control are first that *vagal withdrawal provides very rapid changes in heart rate and cardiac output.* Figure 5-5 compares the rate of responses of the heart to vagal and sympathetic stimulation. The second important point is that the range over which heart rate and cardiac output can be *rapidly* increased varies greatly among the three groups because of large differences in their resting heart rates and stroke volumes. Table 5-3 shows how much of a rise in cardiac output is possible by rapidly raising heart rate to 100 beats min^{-1}.

Above a heart rate of 100 beats min^{-1} the slower sympathetic activation of the heart becomes the dominant factor in increasing rate. This was demonstrated (as with vagal effects) by pharmacological blockade of cardiac receptors; in this case β_1-adrenoceptors were blocked with propranolol. *The response of heart rate and cardiac output to sympathetic activa-*

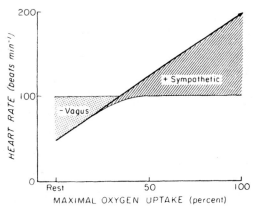

Figure 5-4 Relative contribution of sympathetic and parasympathetic nervous systems to the rise in heart rate during exercise. Stippled region (Vagus) shows most of heart rate increase up to 100 beats min^{-1} is caused by vagal withdrawal (also shown in Figure 5-2). Above heart rate of 100 beats min^{-1}, heart rate is increased by sympathetic activation of cardiac β_1-adrenoceptors by norepinephrine. Schematically illustrated from experiments with parasympathetic cholinergic blockade (atropine) and sympathetic β-adrenergic blockade (propranolol). (Adapted from Robinson et al., 1966, and Rowell, 1986.)

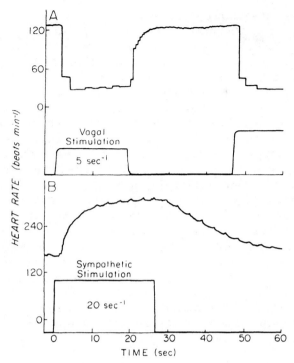

Figure 5-5 **(A)** Speed and magnitude of heart rate responses to vagal stimulation. Vagal response required less than 1 second (on) and about 2 seconds for "off" response. **(B)** Sympathetic stimulation changes heart rate much more slowly; the response is not fully complete for 10 to 20 seconds ("off" response is even slower). (Adapted from Warner and Cox, 1962.)

Table 5-3 Magnitudes of Increase in Cardiac Output* Attributable to Vagal Withdrawal and Increase in Heart Rate from Resting Value to 100 Beats per Minute

Subjects	Resting Heart Rate (beats min^{-1})	Δ Heart Rate to 100 (beats min^{-1})	Stroke Volume (ml)	ΔCardiac Output (L min^{-1}) to HR = 100	ΔCardiac Output (% of maximal output)
ATH	30	70	200	14	35
NA	55	45	100	4.5	21
MS	83	17	50	0.85	10

ATH, elite endurance athletes; NA, normally active subjects; MS, subjects with pure mitral stenosis; HR, heart rate.

Values for resting heart rate and for stroke volume based on basal measurements, supine rest. Resting heart rate and stroke volume determine how much the change in heart rate to 100 beats min^{-1} will raise cardiac output.

*Absolute in liters per minute and relative as percent of the maximal cardiac output.

tion is several times slower than the response to vagal withdrawal at the onset of exercise. This means that below approximately 40 percent of $\dot{V}o_2$max, the relative oxygen uptake at which heart rate reaches 100 beats min^{-1}, the rate of rise of cardiac output at the onset of exercise is rapid, whereas above 40 percent of $\dot{V}o_2$max, the response takes much longer. Therefore, when resting heart rate is close to 100 beats min^{-1}, as in the mitral stenosis patients, most of the increase in heart rate and cardic output occurs slowly because most of the tonic vagal outflow is already withdrawn. The contrast is with athletes in whom almost half of the rise in cardiac output occurs very rapidly owing to vagal withdrawal. This analysis is consistent with the findings of Jones and coworkers (1970), who derived aortic blood flow velocity by applying the Navier-Stokes equation to pressure recordings from the ascending aortas of 10 normal men varying widely in physical conditioning. Response times for heart rate and cardiac output at mild to heavy exercise are also shown in Figure 5-6. Response times were shortest in mild exercise and longest in heavy exercise. As would be expected from Figure 5-2, response times in moderate exercise were shortest in the best conditioned subjects (this point is not illustrated in Figure 5-6). Eriksen and colleagues (1990) used the Doppler ultrasound technique to show that in response to mild (supine) leg exercise, heart rate, cardiac output and femoral arterial blood flow all rose together, with

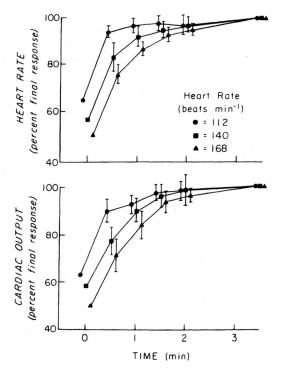

Figure 5-6 Time course of heart rate and cardiac output responses to three levels of supine exercise in 10 normal young men. Severity of exercise is indicated by the three average heart rates. Cardiac output was calculated from the aortic pressure pulse wave and Navier-Stokes equation. Time courses of heart rate and cardiac output were the same and both responded most rapidly at the lowest work rate and most slowly at the highest work rate. (Adapted from Jones et al., 1970.)

their increments being virtually complete in 10 to 15 seconds (see Figure 7-11).

It is also important to remember that as heart rate reaches 100 beats min^{-1}, the first significant leakage of norepinephrine from sympathetic nerve endings into circulating plasma occurs. This leakage reflects generalized sympathetic outflow to the heart and blood vessels of many organs (even active muscle) (Chapter 3).

Summary. In summary, parasympathetic blockade with atropine reveals the importance of the vagus nerve in controlling heart rate at low levels of exercise. β-Adrenergic blockade with propranolol reveals the importance of augmented sympathetic nervous activity to raising heart rate at higher levels of exercise; also, sympathetic nerve activity to the blood vessels of many organ systems increases as well.

Stroke Volume

Despite the decrease in ventricular filling time from 0.55 seconds at rest (heart rate 70 beats min^{-1}) to 0.12 seconds at a heart rate of 195 beats min^{-1}, adjustments in cardiac performance permit stroke volume to be maintained or even increased somewhat over values measured at supine rest (see Åstrand et al., 1964; Wang et al., 1960). An apparent exception to this finding came from a detailed study of 24 normal men in whom cardiac output was measured both by direct Fick method and by thermal dilution with stroke volume being computed from heart rate as is customary (Higginbotham et al., 1986). In agreement with others, stroke volume during supine rest and peak oxygen uptake ($\dot{V}O_2$max was not determined) were the same, but nevertheless stroke volume tended to decline slightly from values at 70 percent of peak oxygen uptake (this tendency appears to be statistically insignificant).

Although a treatment of cardiac mechanics is not within the purview of this book, the major determinants of stroke volume warrant discussion here and will be used in subsequent chapters. Adjustments associated with exercise increase the performance of the heart. The improvement is brought about by extrinsic influences on the heart that affect the stroke volume. These include ventricular filling pressure. In addition, cardiac performance is dependent on intrinsic properties of the myocardial cells, which affect their inherent contractile properties. The distinction between extrinsic and intrinsic influences on the heart is an important one (for concise reviews, see Huntsman and Feigl, 1990; Katz, 1992).

Extrinsic Factors

In accordance with the Frank-Starling or length-tension relationship, stroke volume is determined by ventricular filling pressure or *preload*. Contractile force increases with increasing myocardial fiber length, an observation referred to sometimes as *Starling's law of the heart*. Stroke volume is also influenced by the aortic pressure or *afterload* against which left ventricular stroke volume is driven outward. With all else constant, stroke volume increases with decreased afterload and vice versa. Afterload is determined by the peripheral vascular adjustments described in Chapter 6, and it exerts its influence by affecting the velocity of ventricular contraction in what is called the *force-velocity* relationship.

Intrinsic Factors

The vigor of cardiac contractions can be increased (or decreased) by factors that are independent of myocardial fiber length or the ventricular afterload. The force of a *skeletal* muscle contraction is increased by recruiting more motor units and by activation of more muscle fibers; but in the heart all muscle fibers are activated during each beat. Thus, each cardiac fiber must respond to those alterations in its chemical environment that change the force of each contraction. This intrinsic myocardial cell property is called *contractility*.

Three factors that increase the intrinsic myocardial contractile state, or inotropic state, during exercise are increased heart rate per se, increased activity of cardiac sympathetic nerves, and an increase in circulating epinephrine concentration. The interval between heart beats is a determinant of intrinsic contractile force because of its influence on the quantity of calcium available to the cell. The heart rate–related increase in contractility is referred to as the *interval-strength* relationship. Both norepinephrine, which is released from cardiac sympathetic nerves, and circulating epinephrine released from the adrenal medulla, have powerful positive inotropic effects on the heart mediated by β_1-adrenoreceptors. Again, these agents affect the availability of calcium to the myocardial cell by increasing calcium influx across the sarcolemma (e.g., Huntsman and Feigl, 1990; Katz, 1992).

Over the years considerable controversy has revolved around the relative importance of extrinsic factors versus the intrinsic contractile properties of the heart during exercise. Up to the mid-1950s the emphasis was on the Frank-Starling (length-tension) relationship. Those who related stroke volume determined during exercise to determinations made during upright rest when end-diastolic volume and stroke volume are reduced markedly (as in Figures 5-7 and 2-1) could make a strong case for the importance of the length-tension relationship in determining stroke volume during exercise. In upright posture, ventricular filling pressure, end-diastolic volume, and stroke volume increase as soon as muscle contraction begins (see Figure 2-1). Those who relate stroke volume in exercise with control measurements made during supine rest had a less convincing argument for the dominance of length-tension effects. In fact, Rushmer (1960) made observations suggesting *reductions* in end-diastolic volume and thus in myocardial fiber length in exercising dogs. This prompted support for the primacy of inotropic effects in maintaining stroke volume

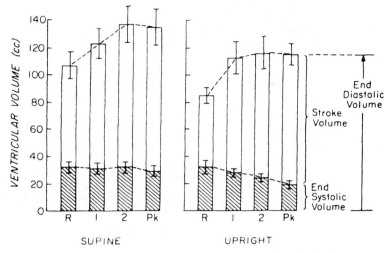

Figure 5-7 Left ventricular volumes (means with standard errors) at rest and at three levels of supine and upright exercise in normal young subjects. Exercise was mild (*1*), moderate (*2*), and at "peak" levels (*Pk*). End-diastolic volumes increased significantly during exercise in both postures. In upright posture 85 percent of the ventricular volume was ejected at peak exercise. (Adapted from Poliner et al., 1980, and reproduced from Rowell, 1986, with permission of Oxford University Press.)

during exercise. Clearly the initial cardiac response to exercise in an upright biped is fundamentally different from that in a quadruped.

Ventricular Performance During Exercise

The techniques of radionuclide angiography or ventriculography have made it possible to evaluate human cardiac performance in terms of changes in *end-diastolic volume, end-systolic volume,* and *ejection fraction* of the left ventricle in response to changes in *preload* (right atrial and pulmonary wedge pressures) and *afterload* (aortic blood pressure). Of the techniques utilizing radionuclide scintigraphy, measurement of left ventricular ejection fraction is the most accurate and reproducible (Gould, 1982). The potential errors in the measurement of ventricular volumes and also in measurement of pressures reflecting preload are substantial.

Figure 5-8 shows results of attempts to quantify right and left ventricular filling pressures. Ekelund and Holmgren (1967) observed that right and left ventricular filling pressures (pulmonary wedge pressure) appeared to change in opposite directions with increasing cardiac output during *supine* exercise in which cardiac output reached nearly 25 L min^{-1}. On the same figure are pressures at the same sites measured during *upright* exercise in the 24 subjects of Higginbotham and colleagues (1986). One problem is that these pressures had to be referenced to atmospheric pressure and

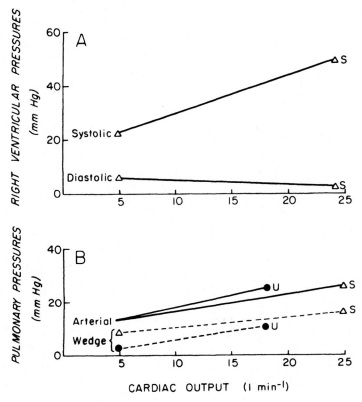

Figure 5-8 **(A)** Relationship between right ventricular systolic and diastolic pressures at rest (supine) and during supine exercise (S) in normal subjects. Note the fall in diastolic pressure. **(B)** Relationship between pulmonary arterial mean pressure and wedge pressure during rest and supine (S) exercise. Same subjects as in Figure A (Ekelund and Holmgren, 1967). Note the rise in wedge pressure. Solid line (U) and dashed line (U) show pulmonary arterial (solid) and wedge pressures (dashed) from different subjects during upright exercise up to peak cardiac output; averages are from 24 normal men aged 20 to 50 years (Higginbotham et al., 1986). (Adapted from Rowell, 1986.)

thus do not provide measures of transmural pressure or (effective) filling pressure. At a constant or even decreasing atrial or ventricular pressure (referred to atmospheric pressure), effective filling pressure can increase because intrapleural pressure or the pressure outside the atria and ventricles becomes increasingly negative as the rate and depth of breathing increases. However, Holmgren (1956) concluded from his attempts to determine right atrial transmural pressure from simultaneous measurements of right atrial and intraesophageal pressures (via esophageal balloon) that right ventricular filling pressure did not increase (and intraesophageal pressure did not fall) with increasing severity of exercise. The adequacy of intraesophageal pressure as a measure of intrapleural pressure during exercise has been repeatedly questioned (see Holmgren, 1956).

Although pulmonary wedge pressure does increase, as anticipated by those who emphasized the length-tension relationship, these pressure measurements must also be viewed with caution. Presumably pulmonary wedge pressure is a measure of left ventricular filling pressure. This pressure, which is measured from a catheter wedged into a small pulmonary vessel, is determined by differences between alveolar pressure, intrapleural pressure, and the pressures in the small collateral vessels that link the wedge site to upstream and downstream arteries and veins. Also, the phase and amplitude of the pulsations are more important to left atrial filling than the damped "mean" pressure that is measured. The same applies to the right atrium.

In conclusion, because of the problems in assessing transmural pressures within the thorax, the magnitude of the increase in ventricular filling pressures during moderate to heavy exercise must be treated cautiously. Small but functionally important increases are undoubtedly hidden by the unknown changes in intrapleural pressure that are exaggerated by hyperventilation during exercise.

Ventricular volume measurements provide indirect but important information about ventricular filling pressure. A rise in left ventricular end-diastolic volume indicates that an increase in effective ventricular filling pressure has occurred (i.e., a sudden increase in ventricular compliance is highly unlikely). Figure 5-7 shows the changes in left ventricular systolic volume and stroke volume and ejection fraction (stroke volume divided by end-diastolic volume) during supine and upright rest and exercise at three levels. The intensity of exercise was characterized as low (50 watts), intermediate (100 to 125 watts), and "peak" exercise ($\dot{V}o_2$max was not established). The increase in end-diastolic volume from 107 ml at supine rest to 135 ml at peak supine exercise means that filling pressure must have increased. When compared with values during upright rest, there is clearly a large increase in end-diastolic volume and filling pressure during upright exercise; however, comparison with supine resting values reveals an increase of only 9 percent (from 107 to 116 ml) up to peak exercise. Figure 5-7 reveals that an increase in end-diastolic volume contributes approximately two-thirds and a reduction in end-systolic volume contributes about one-third to the increase in stroke volume from seated rest to upright exercise.

The reduction in end-systolic volume and greater ejection fraction at a time when peak systolic pressure or afterload is rising is viewed as a manifestation of increased myocardial contractility. The data in Figure 5-7 support the conclusion that stroke volume is maintained through the effects of both increased myocardial fiber length and increased contractile state. This means that the muscle pump provides optimal filling pressure for the heart at all levels of exercise, even when heart rate reaches 195 beats min^{-1}. The results of Higginbotham and colleagues (1986) are not in full agreement with this view. As with stroke volume, left ventricular end-diastolic volume tended to decline slightly beyond 70 percent of the peak oxygen uptake; clearly it did not increase. End-systolic volume declined as in Figure 5-7, but ejection fraction rose only to 76 percent, starting from 59 percent at supine rest, and at 61 percent at upright rest, respectively. Ejection fraction rose from 65 to 85 percent in the study of Poliner and coworkers (1980), which is similar to the increments measured by others. Bear in mind that Higginbotham and colleagues' subjects were a nonhomogeneous group with respect to age, which ranged from 20 to 50 years, and more importantly, peak oxygen uptakes ranged from 2.0 to 3.8 L min^{-1}. In short, a wide range of cardiovascular capacities were mixed together.

Pericardial Constraints

As described in Chapter 2 (see Figure 2-2), left ventricular stroke volume decreases during inspiration rather than increasing along with right ventricular stroke volume because of limited space within the pericardium. In human cardiac patients, both right and left ventricular stroke volumes increase during inspiration after pericardectomy. If it is true that the muscle pump can provide ample filling pressure for the heart at all levels of exercise, then one might expect the elimination of any pericardial constraints on stroke volume to allow stroke volume and cardiac output to increase further. Figure 5-9 shows cardiac output and stroke volume during graded exercise up to the $\dot{V}o_2$max in a healthy and active man who had previously had cardiac surgery to destroy the bundle of His in order to abolish chronic tachycardia. The pericardium had been cut, and a pacemaker catheter was implanted and equipped with a programmable rate controller. When heart rate was held constant, for example, at 100 beats min^{-1}, during exercise by electrical pacing, cardiac output (thermal dilution) and oxygen uptake rose normally with increasing work intensity (Figure 5-9). The rise in cardiac output was achieved by marked increases in stroke volume; stroke volume rose primarily because of the increase in myocardial fiber length, as reflected in the increase in pulmonary wedge pressure shown in Figure 5-9. In addition, adrenergic effects on the heart are presumably responsible for the reduction in end-diastolic volume (radionuclide angiography) and increased ejection fraction (also shown in Figure 5-9). These changes reflect an augmentation of contractile force. Changing heart rate to a different constant value changed only the range over which cardiac output could increase. Stroke volume was not affected.

In dogs, even when heart rate is allowed to increase normally during exercise, stroke volume will still increase above normal after the pericardium is removed. Figure 5-10 shows average heart rate and stroke volume in dogs during graded exercise up to "maximal" levels (cardiac output and heart rate reached a plateau) before and after surgical removal of the pericardium. Both submaximal and "maximal" exercise intensities were the same before and after surgery, meaning that "maximal" stroke volume was less than it could have been at that particular level of exertion because

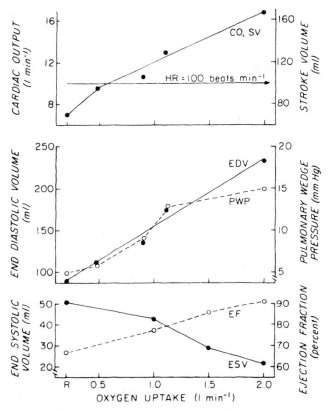

Figure 5-9 Cardiac responses to upright exercise (cycle ergometer) in one middle-aged healthy and physically active man who had previously had cardiac surgery (pericardium cut) and a cardiac pacemaker implanted. Cardiac output rose normally in relation to oxygen uptake up to 2.0 L min⁻¹ despite constant heart rate at 100 beats min⁻¹. Note the extreme increases in stroke volume (values superimpose with cardiac output × 10), left ventricular end-diastolic volume (radionuclide imaging) and pulmonary wedge pressure (PWP) (these pressure measurements were made in a separate diagnostic study as were those in bottom panel). Left ventricular ejection fraction (EF) and end-systolic volume responded normally. (From data that were kindly provided by the late Professor P.D. Gollnick.)

of the pericardial constraints. Clearly the muscle pump provides sufficient filling force for the ventricles so that stroke volume can be increased by length-tension effects when pericardial constraints are removed (Stray-Gundersen et al., 1986). This suggests that the skeletal muscle pump is as effective as the left ventricular pump in providing flow. Inasmuch as there are fewer contractions of the leg muscles than there are contractions of the left ventricle, the "stroke volume" of the muscle pump must exceed that of the ventricle; this assumes that at $\dot{V}o_2$max 85 percent of the cardiac output is passing through the muscle (see Chapter 7).

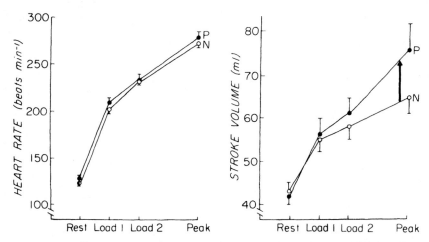

Figure 5-10 Effects of pericardectomy on stroke volume during submaximal and "maximal" (peak) exercise. Comparison is between 10 normal (N) dogs before pericardectomy and the same dogs after pericardectomy (P). Heart rate was the same before and after the surgery. Exercise loads were 6.4 km h⁻¹ with 8 and 16 percent grades (treadmill) and the highest speed and grade needed to identify a plateau of cardiac output. Peak exercise was at the same intensity before and after pericardectomy. (Adapted from Stray-Gundersen et al., 1986.)

Arterial Blood Pressure (Afterload) and Total Vascular Conductance

Figure 5-11 shows the increase in aortic mean and pulse pressures during upright rest and upright exercise at different fractions of $\dot{V}o_2$max (Rowell et al., 1968). The small rise in aortic mean pressure or ventricular afterload, which was only 25 mmHg from rest to "maximal" exercise, is striking. The rise in aortic pulse pressure was also small (from 112/68 to 154/70 mmHg) in comparison to the rise observed in the radial artery (from 133/66 to 236/58 mmHg) because of the peripheral amplification of the pulse wave (McDonald, 1974). Wave amplification by the peripheral vasculature prevents any meaningful evaluation from peripheral sites of the pulsatile strain on baroreceptors in central vessels (Rowell et al., 1968).

The small changes in aortic mean pressure from rest to "maximal" exercise reveal that rising total vascular conductance compensates well for the rise in cardiac output, which in the studies ranged from 6 L min⁻¹ at rest to over 30 L min⁻¹ at $\dot{V}o_2$max (Åstrand et al., 1964; Rowell et al., 1968).

The higher the maximal cardiac output, the higher the total vascular conductance, as shown in Figure 5-12. Vascular conductance is traditionally calculated from arterial minus central venous or right atrial pressures and from the cardiac output according to Ohm's law. This calculation assumes that the flow of blood from the left ventricle back to the right

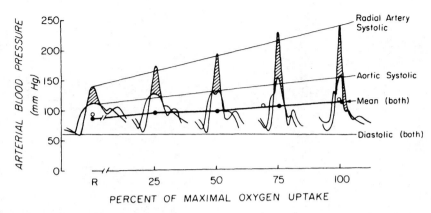

Figure 5-11 Simultaneously measured radial arterial and aortic pressures during rest (R) and upright exercise. Note the similarities in mean aortic pressures at a given percent of $\dot{V}O_2$max from two studies on subjects whose absolute values of $\dot{V}O_2$max varied widely (Åstrand et al., 1964, *open circles*; Rowell et al., 1968, *closed circles*). Peripheral wave amplification caused large increases in radial arterial pulse pressure. Pressure wave forms were traced from direct simultaneous recordings from a representative subject (Rowell et al., 1968). (Reproduced from Rowell et al., 1986, with permission of Oxford University Press.)

atrium is determined by the pressure difference between these two chambers, discounting the fact that the circuit is cyclically interrupted by a second (muscle) pump, which also delivers energy to drive blood flow.

Total Vascular Conductance and the Muscle Pump

We are warned not to compute, in a conventional manner, vascular conductance or resistance across the lung or across any circuit in which resistance to flow is also importantly affected by the external pressure surrounding the vessels. Such a circuit is sometimes called a "Starling resistor," an example of which is shown in Figure 1-4. Figure 5-13 shows that a more complex situation exists for exercise. The circuit is broken by a second pump, and a simple ohmic resistance does not exist across the contracting muscle. Virtually all of the energy needed to drive blood back to the heart from the active muscle is provided by the powerful driving force of the muscle pump. Computation of conductance across the muscle would require that we have a postcapillary pressure at a site that is protected by valves from the effects of the muscle pump on the veins. An extreme comparison would be the computation of the resistance between the pulmonary artery and the left ventricle from the blood flow and pulmonary arterial-left ventricular pressure difference (i.e., a negative resistance). Therefore we can speak only of a *virtual* total vascular conductance during exercise.

Figure 5-13 is a schematic representation of how the muscle pump might alter the pressure profile across the vascular system during exercise.

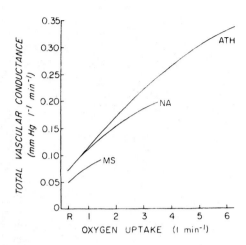

Figure 5-12 Total vascular conductance in relation to oxygen uptake from supine rest (R) up to $\dot{V}O_2$max (end of curves) in the same three groups described in Figure 5-2, Table 5-1, and text. Conductance was calculated from data of Åstrand et al., 1964; Blackmon et al., 1967; Rowell et al., 1968; and Clausen, 1977. Conductance based on cardiac output and arterial pressure is a *virtual* value because the circuit is broken at the muscle pump; see Figure 5-13 and text. (Adapted from Rowell, 1986.)

The features that make the muscle pump so effective are discussed in Chapter 1 and illustrated in Figure 1-14. The pump not only raises central venous volume and pressure, but it also improves muscle perfusion. Muscle perfusion pressure is increased by the pump because immediately after each contraction its veins are empty, venous valves prevent any back flow, and intravenous pressure is momentarily near zero, possibly negative. Thus in upright posture and immediately after a muscle contraction, when muscle venous pressure momentarily falls to zero, net arterial perfusion pressure is momentarily increased in proportion to the added hydrostatic effect on the arterial (but not the venous) side (Figure 1-14). The fact that the muscle pump can generate a high pressure of 90 mmHg (when veins are partially occluded) is not reflected in Figure 5-13 because the rise in muscle venous pressure in unobstructed small muscle veins is not known.

Laughlin (1987) took the preceding concepts a step further by suggesting that pressures within the smallest intramuscular veins could be negative following a contraction. This is the negative venous pressure shown under ''muscle pump'' in Figure 5-13. Muscle relaxes rapidly (in 50 to 100 msec) so that the sudden release of high compressive force could actually pull open—by elastic recoil—the empty collapsed veins, making their transmural pressure *negative*. Parenthetically, a similar argument is commonly offered to explain how the ventricles could suck blood during diastole. If the next muscle contraction were to precede both the refilling of the veins and the recovery of the precontraction pressure, then the repeated frequent contractions should maintain a low muscle venous pressure, a maintained increase in arterial venous driving pressure across the muscle, and a maintained central displacement of blood volume that raises ventricular filling pressure. In any event, venous valves mean that hydrosta.ic forces are not simply added equally onto the venous and arterial sides of a continuous vascular loop.

The action of the muscle pump has been suggested as one of the reasons why the peak blood flows and oxygen uptakes of voluntarily contracting muscles is so much greater than values observed in muscles made to contract by electrical stimulation of their motor nerves (Laughlin, 1987). Some serious problems with the latter approach, as far as the muscle itself is concerned, stem from the abnormal patterns of motor unit recruitment and force development. This appears to make the pump much less effective; it disturbs the distribution of blood flow causing pockets of ischemia and lactate release, and local increases in H^+ concentration reduce force development and diminish the effectiveness of the pump (this also explains why peak muscle blood flow is highest during voluntary contractions).

Figure 5-13 shows that after the venous blood leaves the muscle pump, it is exposed to another less powerful pump—the respiratory pump—which could exert a small but significant additional effect on ventricular filling. As mentioned previously, it is the effects of this respiratory pump on atrial and ventricular transmural pressures that make the measurement of effective cardiac filling pressures so difficult.

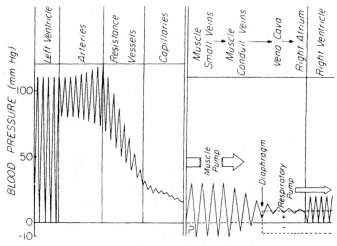

Figure 5-13   Schematic illustration of the pressure profile across the vascular system. Up to the capillaries pressure oscillations characterize only the changing magnitudes of pulse pressure and not cardiac frequency. The *circuit is broken in the muscle by the muscle pump* and pressure oscillations show *external* effects of muscle pumping and then respiratory pumping—four pumps in series. Blood flow from the left ventricle to the muscle is determined by the pressure difference between the heart and some unknown point in the muscle, whereas blood flow from active muscle to the right ventricle is determined by the force provided by the muscle pump.

Flow Dependency of Peripheral Vascular Volume and Ventricular Filling Pressure

A theme threaded throughout Chapters 1 through 4 is that peripheral vasculature volume is highly sensitive to changes in blood flow. It is possible to increase cardiac output only slightly in supine resting humans by increasing heart rate and/or administering vasodilators, before a fall in central venous pressure and stroke volume imposes a self-limiting constraint. The underlying cause is the high compliance of the peripheral vasculature and its high sensitivity to small changes in transmural pressure attending changes in blood flow. Cardiac preload, ventricular function, and thus the overall performance of the heart are importantly coupled to the control of the peripheral circulation. This control involves the mechanical effects of muscle contraction as well as the autonomic neural effects on vascular resistance. Guyton and colleagues (1962) saw the problem and stated that

> the normal [i.e., at rest] circulatory system operates near this limit [i.e., collapse of central venous pressure owing to increased cardiac output] so that an increase in efficacy of the heart as a pump cannot by itself increase the cardiac output more than a few percent, unless some simultaneous effect takes place in the peripheral circulatory system at the same time to translocate blood from the peripheral vessels to the heart.

The question to be answered here is what permits the maintenance of adequate (or more than adequate) ventricular preload during mild to severe dynamic exercise. How is it possible to increase cardiac output by four- to sevenfold and produce a 25- to 40-fold increase in muscle blood flow without depletion of thoracic blood volume and reduction in ventricular preload? Clearly a second pump (or "second heart") is needed to keep any flow-dependent rise in peripheral vascular volume from occurring during exercise. The task of the muscle pump is therefore to maintain the filling pressure of the heart. On the other hand, the task of the autonomic nervous system (covered in Chapter 6) is to assure that too large a fraction of the cardiac output is not directed through compliant regions that are unaffected by the muscle pump. *Therefore the maintenance of stroke volume and cardiac output during exercise requires a balance between the purely mechanical effects of the muscle pump and the sympathetic control of the blood vessels.*

Congenital Absence of Venous Valves and Varicose Veins

The importance of the muscle pump was revealed in the 1960s in several studies on patients with absence of valves in deep veins of the legs. These patients had a 35 percent reduction in stroke volume during exercise when body position was shifted from supine to sitting position (stroke volume may have been low to start with, even during exercise in supine posture). Cardiac output was maintained by a proportional increase in heart rate (Bevegård and Lodin, 1962). Others reported low stroke volumes in pa-

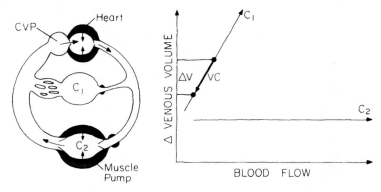

Figure 5-14 The volume of blood available to fill the heart depends on the distribution of blood flow between compliant (C_1) and noncompliant (C_2) circuits as in Figures 2-16 and 2-17. In exercise active muscle (noncompliant circuit $[C_2]$) becomes another pump actively returning blood to the heart. Cardiac filling pressures are determined by effectiveness of muscle pumping and sympathetic control of other circuits (e.g., C_1), that is, in effect the ratios of blood flows through C_1 and C_2.

tients with varicose veins (Grimby et al., 1964); stroke volume could be raised 30 percent during upright (seated) exercise by bandaging the legs.

Summary. In summary, Figure 5-14 shows that two things must happen to prevent the increase in peripheral blood flow from raising peripheral vascular volume and reducing ventricular filling pressure:

1. A large fraction of the cardiac output needs to pass through the noncompliant muscle that actively squeezes out its blood volume during contraction.
2. The flow of blood passing through circuits that are compliant (and whose volume increases with flow) must decrease.

Systemic Arteriovenous Oxygen Difference
Arterial Oxygen Content

Arterial oxygen content depends on the concentration of hemoglobin and its oxygen binding capacity, the alveolar Po_2, pulmonary diffusion capacity, and alveolar ventilation. It is commonly assumed that the arterial oxygen content and hemoglobin saturation are well maintained during exercise up to the level of $\dot{V}o_2$max in all normal individuals (Holmgren and Linderholm, 1958). Actually, arterial hemoglobin concentration and oxygen-carrying capacity rise approximately 10 percent above resting values during "maximal" exercise, because plasma water is lost into active muscle cells and interstitial fluid as the concentration of osmotically active particles in the muscles rises. Inasmuch as arterial oxygen-carrying capacity rises, whereas oxygen content remains nearly constant (in sedentary or

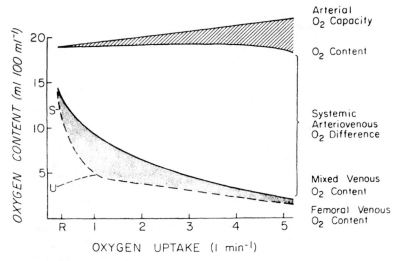

Figure 5-15 Oxygen contents in arterial, mixed venous (pulmonary artery), and femoral venous blood during rest (R) and exercise up to $\dot{V}_{O_2}$max (5.2 L min^{-1} in this illustration). Arterial oxygen-carrying capacity is increased by hemoconcentration, but content and saturation do not rise similarly. Femoral and mixed venous contents fall markedly and approach similar values near $\dot{V}_{O_2}$max because of the increased vasoconstriction and oxygen extraction in inactive regions (Chapter 6). The lowest femoral oxygen contents tend to occur in those with the highest $\dot{V}_{O_2}$max (Rowell, 1974) or in patients with very low maximal cardiac outputs (Wade and Bishop, 1962). (Adapted from Åstrand and Rodahl, 1977.)

normally active people), oxygen saturation falls slightly during "maximal" exercise, for example, from 96 to 93 percent (Rowell et al., 1964). This is illustrated in Figure 5-15. Some of this fall in saturation could be attributable to reduction in arterial pH and a rise in temperature, which lowers saturation at a given P_{O_2}. Figure 5-16 shows the rightward shift of the oxygen dissociation curve, called the Bohr shift, over the range of temperatures and pH values found in skeletal muscle during moderate to the most severe exercise. Substantial arterial desaturation by the Bohr effect when arterial P_{O_2} is close to 100 mmHg is only possible at extreme values of blood temperature and pH, whereas the unloading of oxygen in the muscle is significantly increased at a given venous P_{O_2}.

Mixed Venous Oxygen Content

The content of oxygen in pulmonary arterial or mixed venous blood falls with increasing oxygen uptake to values as low as 2 and 3 ml 100 ml^{-1} at $\dot{V}_{O_2}$max (Figure 5-15). The lowest values are observed in cardiac patients with low cardiac outputs (Wade and Bishop, 1962; Blackmon et al., 1967) and in physically conditioned subjects (Saltin et al., 1968; Ekblom, 1969). Total oxygen extraction is commonly estimated to be 85

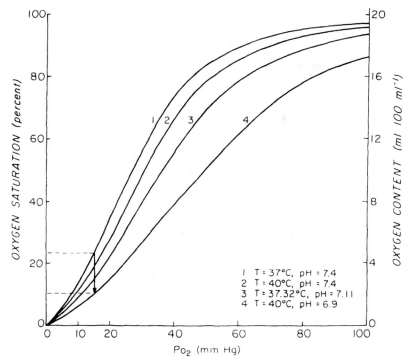

Figure 5-16 Effects of increased blood temperature and decreased pH on oxygen dissociation (Bohr shift). Curve 1 is normal resting curve. Curve 2 shows effect of hyperthermia only. Curve 3 shows effects of blood temperature and pH during brief exercise at $\dot{V}O_2$max. Curve 4 shows effects on oxygen dissociation of extreme values for muscle venous blood temperature and pH during exhaustive exercise. Only at such extremes could the Bohr shift account for the arterial desaturation observed in athletes (Chapter 7). (Curves calculated from data of Severinghaus, 1958.)

percent or more in conditioned athletes and between 80 and 85 percent in normally active and sedentary subjects (Rowell, 1974) (Figure 5-15). The oxygen content of femoral venous blood draining the exercising legs rarely falls below 2 ml 100 ml^{-1}, but reductions to 1.4 ml 100 ml^{-1} have been observed, for example, in physically conditioned individuals (Saltin et al., 1968) and in cardiac patients (Wade and Bishop, 1962).

Two factors account for the ability to extract 85 percent of the available oxygen from blood during exercise. The first is the increase in oxygen extraction by the muscle, and second is the regional vasoconstriction, which decreases resting organ blood flow so that their oxygen extraction increases (Chapter 6).

The widening extraction of oxygen in the active muscle is explained by several factors. Unlike cardiac muscle, in which most capillaries are open, only a small fraction of the total number of capillaries is perfused in resting muscle. As a result, diffusion distances between the capillaries and the muscle fibers are great. Also, the mean transit time of the red blood cells through so few capillaries must be short, that is, high blood flow per unit capillary blood volume and a short mean transit time. As a result of the large diffusion distances and short mean transit time, the gradient for oxygen between the capillaries and the muscle cells is large, explaining why intercellular Po_2 in resting muscle is only a few millimeters of mercury. Thus, blood leaves the capillaries unequilibrated with the muscle cells and with a relatively high Po_2 (approximately 35 mmHg) and a high oxygen content of approximately 14 ml 100 ml^{-1}. During exercise the enormous increase in the number of open capillaries greatly reduces diffusion distances and increases capillary blood volume so that capillary mean transit time does not become too brief to allow unloading of oxygen. Thus, each 100 ml of blood leaving the muscle may contain less than 2 ml of oxygen instead of 14 ml. As a consequence of the greater number of open capillaries, each muscle fiber is now supplied by more capillaries than it was at rest.

Therefore, in order to maintain a high extraction of oxygen across the muscle there must be a delicate balance between the optimal rates of blood flow, capillary blood volume, and the minimum mean transit time available for the exchange of oxygen across the skeletal muscle capillaries (see Duling, 1981). This balance is preserved at high rates of muscle blood flow; in fact, extraction of oxygen tends to increase with increasing $\dot{V}o_2$max and thus increasing blood flow. Capillary blood volume must be large enough and capillary mean transit time must be long enough to allow oxygen to be released from the hemoglobin and diffuse all the way from the capillaries to the mitochondria of the muscle cells.

Figure 5-16 shows how the rightward shift in the oxygen dissociation curve caused by the fall in muscle pH and the rise in muscle temperature (Bohr shift) will affect the unloading of oxygen in the muscle capillaries. When muscle is extremely active, its temperature may exceed 40°C, and its pH may fall below 7.0. If the Po_2 in the blood of venous capillaries drops to 15 mmHg, the Bohr shift would lower venous oxygen content from 4.2 to 2.0 ml 100 ml^{-1}. Were muscle blood flow 25 L min^{-1}, this shift would provide an added 625 ml min^{-1} of oxygen to the muscle. This effect decreases markedly when muscle capillary Po_2 falls to 10 mmHg or lower.

ADJUSTMENTS TO CHRONIC HIGH LOADS: PHYSICAL CONDITIONING

The cardiovascular system is changed by repeated exposure to high intensities of exercise over long periods. The process is called physical conditioning. $\dot{V}o_2$max is the measurement that has been most useful in quantifying the overall effects of physical conditioning on the cardiovascular system. The $\dot{V}o_2$max has *not* been as useful in assessing the effects of physical conditioning on endurance and/or work capacity which are primarily referable to metabolic changes within the skeletal muscle (Saltin and Rowell, 1980; Saltin and Gollnick, 1983).

Equation 5-2 tells where to look for the causes of any increase in $\dot{V}O_2$max; again, it does not tell us where to look for the cause of an improvement in work capacity. Work capacity (or endurance) is measured by *performance criteria* (power output times duration) rather than *functional criteria*. The following examples, as applied to automobiles, makes the distinction. Performance criteria show how far the vehicle will go on 20 liters of fuel. Functional criteria establish the maximal power that can be developed by the automobile's engine and say nothing about how far it can go. Returning to people, the increase in endurance or performance after physical conditioning usually exceeds by orders of magnitude the rise in $\dot{V}O_2$max or cardiovascular capacity. Commonly $\dot{V}O_2$max is increased by approximately 15 percent, but this improvement depends on the initial value (see below). In contrast, muscle endurance commonly increases by 200 to 300 percent during 2 to 3 months of intensive physical conditioning. This topic is the subject of reviews on skeletal muscle metabolism (Gollnick et al., 1985) (see Chapter 9).

How Much Does $\dot{V}O_2$max Increase?

The large range of $\dot{V}O_2$max in normal young adults is summarized in Figure 5-1. Values fall below 30 ml O_2 kg^{-1} min^{-1} in young sedentary individuals and reach 85 ml O_2 kg^{-1} min^{-1} in elite endurance athletes. Values of 45 to 50 ml O_2 kg^{-1} min^{-1} are commonly observed in normally active young adults (Taylor et al., 1963; Rowell, 1974; Åstrand and Rodahl, 1977; Clausen, 1977). In five different longitudinal studies on 39 young individuals, the rise in $\dot{V}O_2$max averaged 16 percent or from 44 to 51 ml O_2 kg^{-1} min^{-1} in response to 2 to 3 months of physical conditioning (see Rowell, 1974; Clausen, 1977). However, the farther the initial $\dot{V}O_2$max value is below 45 ml O_2 kg^{-1} min^{-1}, the greater the relative and absolute increase with conditioning. Increases exceeding 30 percent have been observed (e.g., Saltin et al., 1968). If the $\dot{V}O_2$max is relatively high, for example, between 50 and 60 ml O_2 kg^{-1} min^{-1}, then the increase with 2 to 3 months of physical conditioning will be only a few percent.

When physical conditioning is prolonged over years, additional adjustments in the cardiovascular system occur. Two previously sedentary subjects increased their $\dot{V}O_2$max by 44 percent (from 45 to 65 ml O_2 kg^{-1} min^{-1}) in response to 2 to 3 years of continuous physical conditioning (Ekblom, 1969). However, endurance athletes whose initial values for $\dot{V}O_2$max are very high may show little or no change after years of intensive conditioning (Rowell, 1974). It is not known if their extreme values for $\dot{V}O_2$max are genetically determined or if years of intensive physical conditioning, particularly during formative adolescent years, may have fostered their development (a possible role of the pericardium is discussed later in this chapter). Therefore the range of $\dot{V}o_2$max is large, but the range of adaptation may be smaller; values can be doubled when they are low at the beginning of conditioning, whereas those with high values may show little or no increase with years of conditioning. What changes in the cardiovascular system permit these increases?

How Does $\dot{V}o_2$max Increase?

Physical conditioning increases the functional capacity of the cardiovascular system in two ways: (1) it increases maximal cardiac output, and (2) it increases the fraction of oxygen extracted from the blood. Emphasis in this chapter is on how cardiac output is increased; oxygen extraction is covered in Chapter 7.

Physical conditioning of normal young sedentary individuals for 2 or 3 months increased $\dot{V}o_2$max by 16 percent as a consequence of 8 percent increases in maximal cardiac output and 8 percent increases in arteriovenous oxygen difference (Saltin et al., 1968; Rowell, 1974; Clausen, 1977). The increase in cardiac output was due entirely to increased stroke volume. Maximal heart rate is generally stable within any given age group and, if anything, may decrease slightly during the conditioning period.

The generalization that increased maximal cardiac output and arteriovenous oxygen difference contribute equally to the increase in $\dot{V}o_2$max is not uniformly applicable. In some individuals the rise in $\dot{V}o_2$max with physical conditioning is due almost completely to an increase in maximal stroke volume and cardiac output, whereas oxygen extraction is unaltered. This is observed in physically active individuals whose preconditioning levels of $\dot{V}o_2$max are high and it is also seen in middle-aged men (Hartley et al., 1969; Saltin et al., 1969) and middle-aged and elderly women (Kilbom, 1971). When conditioning was sustained over years and included significant anatomical changes, the 40 percent increase in $\dot{V}o_2$max was accompanied by a 32 percent increase in cardiac output and stroke volume and only an 8 percent increase in arteriovenous oxygen difference (Ekblom et al., 1968). Apparently the peripheral adjustments that determine oxygen extraction take place rapidly and the long-term circulatory changes, which may involve morphological adjustments in the heart, progress more slowly. Note that these adjustments occur when physical conditioning involves a large percentage of the total muscle mass.

Another departure from the generalization that changes in cardiac output and oxygen extraction contribute equally to the rise in $\dot{V}o_2$max was seen in the response of foxhounds to physical conditioning (Musch et al., 1985). This athletic animal responds like the physically active human with the entire 28 percent rise in $\dot{V}o_2$max (from 114 to 146 ml min^{-1} kg^{-1}) being attributable to the rise in maximal stroke volume and cardiac output. Despite the marked rise in cardiac output, arterial pressure at $\dot{V}o_2$max remained the same (mean: 140 mmHg), owing to a rise in total vascular conductance.

Summary. In summary, both central and peripheral circulatory adjustments to physical conditioning are a function of age, the initial level of $\dot{V}O_2$max, and the mass of muscle that is conditioned.

The remainder of this chapter focuses on possible mechanisms of cardiac adjustment to conditioning.

How Does Stroke Volume Increase?

Improvements in stroke volume have been explained by the effects of the Frank-Starling or length-tension relationship on the degree of shortening of myocardial fibers. If diastolic volume is increased, the associated lengthening of myocardial fibers will augment both the force and velocity of contraction. Conversely, others have assumed diastolic volume does not increase and have emphasized instead intrinsic changes in myocardial contractility, which are independent of ventricular volume and myofibril length and tension. For example, an upregulation of β_1-adrenoreceptors in the heart or augmented sympathoadrenal activity during exercise could increase the force of ventricular contraction and effect an increase in stroke volume by further reducing end-systolic volume (see Figure 5-7). The emphasis here is on (1) ventricular preload or filling pressure and the factors that might change it, and (2) geometrical or mechanical limits such as ventricular size or constraints of the pericardium; two other possibilities are (3) increases in the myocardial contractile state and (4) decreases in ventricular afterload. The last two possibilities are discussed first.

Myocardial Contractile State

Changes in myocardial contractility can be dispensed with quickly as an important mechanism for increased stroke volume. Although the findings of Poliner and colleagues (1980) (Figure 5-7) and Higginbotham and colleagues (1986) and others make it clear that contractile force increases with exercise intensity, any further effects caused by physical conditioning would be small and difficult to quantify. Left ventricular ejection fraction is already so high at 85 percent and end-systolic volume is so low at peak exercise in unconditioned subjects, that it would be difficult to see further improvements, given the limits in resolution (Gould, 1982); and further improvements would have only small effects on overall cardiac performance (Scheuer and Tipton, 1977; Blomqvist and Saltin, 1983).

Ventricular Afterload

The lack of significant effect of physical conditioning on ventricular *afterload* is important. Cross-sectional comparisons of sedentary individuals with highly conditioned athletes having extremely high maximal cardiac outputs reveal essentially the same mean arterial pressure at maximal cardiac outputs in both groups (Rowell, 1974, 1986; Clausen, 1977). If anything, mean arterial pressure tends to be a little lower in the athletes

(Ekblom, 1969). This means two things: (1) physical conditioning must be accompanied by some precise adjustment that matches total vascular conductance to maximal cardiac output, and (2) physical conditioning must be accompanied by an increase in muscle vascular conductance.

Ventricular Preload

A predominant notion has been that any increase in stroke volume during physical conditioning must originate from an increase in ventricular filling pressure. Does ventricular preload increase, and, if so, how does it happen?

Central venous pressure has not been measured before and after conditioning, but, even if it had been, we would be left with uncertainty about how well any changes might reflect effective filling pressure. That is, cardiac transmural pressures, as discussed previously in this chapter, are altered as intrapleural pressure becomes increasingly negative with rising ventilation. Even if right atrial pressure, referred to atmospheric pressure, did not increase with conditioning, the effective filling pressure could still be greater owing to the increase in maximal ventilation with higher oxygen uptake. Alternatively, the increase in cardiac volume means that less pressure is required to cause a given wall tension: the law of LaPlace. The heart functions on a steep portion of the curve relating stroke volume to end-diastolic pressure so that small changes in pressure could have large effects. It has therefore been more instructive to see if end-diastolic volume is greater during rest and exercise after conditioning. An increase could suggest that ventricular filling preload has risen.

Cross-sectional comparisons of end-diastolic volume in sedentary and well-conditioned individuals reveal the higher volumes as determined by radionuclide imaging techniques in the latter group (Morganroth et al., 1975; Roeske et al., 1975). In a longitudinal study Rerych (1980) reported substantial increases in end-diastolic volume in a group of 18 college athletes after 6 months of conditioning. End-diastolic volume rose from 133 to 167 ml at rest and from 166 to 204 ml during severe exercise after conditioning.

Some have argued that structural changes in the heart itself might contribute to the rise in stroke volume. Comparisons of cardiac dimensions among sedentary and well-conditioned individuals by radiographic, nuclide imaging and echocardiographic techniques, and even measurements at autopsy suggest that chronic physical exertion increases ventricular volume and ventricular wall thickness (see Grande and Taylor, 1965; Åstrand and Rodahl, 1977; Scheuer and Tipton, 1977; Blomqvist and Saltin, 1983). Significant correlations exist among heart size, Vo_2max, cardiac output and stroke volume. Saltin and coworkers (1968) reported parallel changes in heart volume and $\dot{V}o_2$max as both rose during physical conditioning, although the volume changes were quite small, averaging 9 percent.

In longitudinal investigations, cardiac dimensions do appear to increase with chronic activity as determined by echocardiographic techniques on active athletes (Morganroth et al., 1975). Endurance conditioning (running or swimming), which was viewed as "chronic volume loading," increased left ventricular end-diastolic volume without a change in left ventricular wall thickness (Morganroth et al., 1975). In contrast, frequent exposure to isometric exercise (e.g., wrestling), which raises arterial blood pressure and left ventricular afterload, increases left ventricular wall thickness but not left ventricular volume. Echocardiographic studies reviewed by Peronnet and colleagues (1981) support these conclusions (Morganroth et al., 1975).

Blood Volume. Despite numerous studies, it is still not clear whether physical conditioning invariably causes functionally significant increases in blood volume, and how much of an increase would suffice to augment preload over extended periods of time. Increases in blood volume with conditioning appear to be small; for example, the increase was only 100 to 200 ml in the study of Saltin and coworkers (1968). Could such increases in blood volume or even larger ones significantly raise ventricular preload or end-diastolic volume? If total systemic vascular compliance in humans is actually 2.5 ml mmHg^{-1} kg^{-1}, then a rise in blood volume of 200 ml in a 75-kg person would raise central venous pressure at rest by only 1 mmHg, that is, *if cardiac output and its distribution remain constant.* Convertino and coworkers (1991) reported in supine resting subjects (lateral decubitus position) that estimated "central venous pressure" (measured as antecubital venous pressure in the dependent arm) increased 1.8 mmHg or 19 percent along with a 380-ml (9 percent) rise in plasma volume attending 10 weeks of physical conditioning. The effect of the increase in blood volume on central venous pressure *during exercise* cannot be predicted, however, because exercise changes cardiac output and alters its distribution between various vascular beds; both affect central venous pressure at any given total blood volume (see Figure 5-17A,B).

Cross-sectional studies comparing athletes and sedentary individuals have also yielded inconsistent findings. The conclusions depend on whether volumes are expressed as milliliters per kilogram of total body weight, or as fat-free body weight (for references, see Moore and Buskirk, 1974). The conclusion from many studies is that any conditioning effect on blood volume is small and unlikely to be functionally significant. Nevertheless, there appears to be a consensus that physical conditioning does significantly increase blood volume and that the blood volumes of athletes exceed those of unconditioned individuals when expressed per kilogram of body weight (e.g., see Harrison, 1985).

Importance of the Pericardial Constraints

Whatever is finally decided about changes in blood volume and central venous pressure with physical conditioning, one fact stands out: *simply cutting the pericardium affords advantages to cardiovacular function via increased stroke volume and cardiac output that are similar to those afforded by months of physical conditioning* (Figure 5-10). Thus one could argue that, before physical conditioning, filling pressure is already higher than needed to improve stroke volume, but effects of this pressure on stroke volume are limited by the pericardium.

Central venous pressure has been increased acutely in sedentary and well-conditioned subjects and the conflicting results have caused confusion. For example, Robinson and coworkers (1966) raised central venous pressure by 7 mmHg in their *unconditioned subjects* by autotransfusion of whole blood, but stroke volume and cardiac output were not significantly increased during "maximal" exercise. Others have reported small but statistically significant increases in stroke volume during "maximal" exercise in unconditioned subjects and after acute expansion of plasma volume (Fortney et al., 1981). Furthermore, when Kanstrup and Ekblom (1982) expanded plasma volume by 700 ml in their *conditioned subjects,* they observed a 10 percent increase in maximal stroke volume and cardiac output (and no change in $\dot{V}o_2$max due to reduced hemoglobin concentration). In view of the dramatic effects of pericardectomy, it is surprising that any effect of raising filling pressure would be observed. That is, why would the pericardium be a constraint in one case and not another?

Could it be that hearts of conditioned subjects are more responsive to increases in plasma volume and presumably in preload than are the hearts of sedentary subjects? This suggestion prompted an interesting proposal by Blomqvist and Saltin (1983), who noted some relationship between maximal stroke volume before volume loading and the magnitude of increase in stroke volume after blood volume was increased. The higher the initial stroke volume, the greater the effect of volume loading on the subsequent stroke volume. They suggested that the constraint may lie in the pericardium and that physical conditioning might *alter apparent ventricular compliance by modifying right and left ventricular pericardial interactions.*Thus a greater diastolic reserve capacity could conceivably result from altered pericardial restrictions on stroke volume rather than alterations in myocardial function.

Could the effects of prolonged periods of heavy exercise on ventricular pressure have gradually stretched the pericardium so that the heart responds to a plasma volume and filling pressure that has been adequate all along? That is, no change in plasma volume was needed. The finding that acute volume loading raises stroke volume in some individuals argues against this idea, and supports the view that augmentation of filling pressure is a requirement for increased stroke volume (at least in these responsive individuals).

A question raised previously was if the rise in stroke volume during exercise after endurance training is merely the result of the chronic bradycardia (both at rest and submaximal exercise) that stretches the pericardium (Rowell, 1986). There is evidence suggesting that the bradycardia attending physical conditioning may initially reduce cardiac output slightly during submaximal exercise (Rowell, 1974; Clausen, 1977). Even a small reduction in cardiac output can markedly increase central venous pressure. Figure 5-17A shows this response in a dog which had atrioventricular conduction blocked so that cardiac output could be changed and held constant by servocontrol of a ventricular pacing catheter. Figure 5-17B shows the relationship between cardiac output in this dog (changed in the manner just described) and central venous pressure when the cardiac output is changed at rest and during exercise at 4 mph, 0 percent grade.

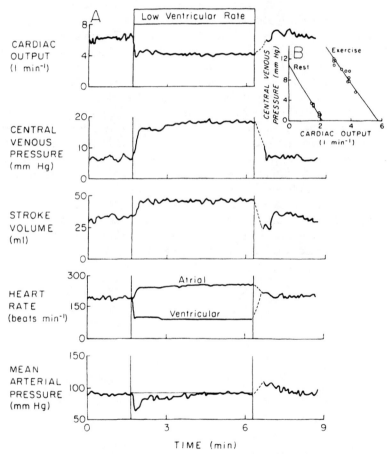

Figure 5-17 (A) Effect of reducing ventricular pacing rate during exercise in a dog with surgical atrioventricular block. Fall in cardiac output causes a marked increase in central venous pressure and stroke volume (pericardium was cut). Atrial rate rises in response to fall in blood pressure and reflexes from working muscle (Chapters 11 and 12). (B) Effects (on same dog) of changing cardiac output (by pacing) on central venous pressure at rest and during exercise after blockade of sympathetic nervous effects with hexamethonium to show effects on central venous pressure are not of reflex origin. (Data kindly provided by D. D. Sheriff et al., 1992.)

The rightward shift in the relationship between cardiac output and central venous pressure is attributable to the mechanical effect of the muscle pump on total vascular compliance and central vascular volume.

Studies of the mechanical properties of the pericardium in dogs reveal that pericardial volume increases markedly during chronic volume loading by arteriovenous fistula over a period of 21 to 107 days (Figure 5-18). Freeman and LeWinter (1984) concluded that the main effect on the pericardium was an increase in its unstressed volume due to its growth; that is, pericardial surface area and mass increased but its thickness did not change. The constant thickness meant that viscoelastic creep was not a primary cause of the increased pericardial volume. As a chamber, pericardial compliance increased, but, according to Freeman and LeWinter (1984), its intrinsic stiffness was unaltered, that is, the same material but different geometry. However, this latter conclusion was modified in a subsequent study, which found reduced stiffness as well (Lee et al., 1985).

The main points are that the pericardial constraints on stroke volume are greatly reduced by increasing cardiac filling pressure over time. Its greater compliance as a chamber constitutes a second form of adaptation that may explain why the volume loading of conditioned individuals increases their stroke volume (i.e., in contrast to the lack of effect in unconditioned individuals). Once the pericardium has hypertrophied (as, for example, by physical conditioning?) a much smaller rise in filling pressure is required to increase stroke volume. Also, the larger the heart to begin with, the smaller the rise in filling pressure required to increase pericardial volume and stroke volume during the conditioning (LaPlace's law). This reinforces the comment, made above, that a measurement of

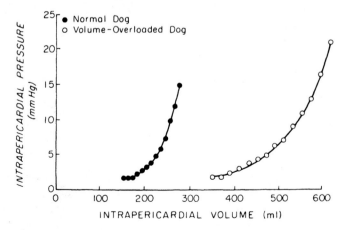

Figure 5-18 Chronic volume loading over several weeks by chronic arteriovenous (aorta to vena cava) fistula increases intrapericardial volume at any given intrapericardial pressure owing mainly to pericardial growth. (Adapted from Freeman and LeWinter, 1984.)

central venous pressure or filling pressure after conditioning may not reflect the change in effective filling pressure. Clearly, effects of a given change in plasma volume would have quite different effects on different individuals as well.

There are anecdotes about racing greyhounds with thoracotomy scars. The legend (which appears to be unconfirmed) is that many of these animals have had the pericardium cut to increase their maximal cardiac outputs, their racing performance, and their owners' profits. The procedure is said to be illegal, and is not known to have been applied to human athletes, along with blood transfusions and hormone supplements to improve performance.

REFERENCES

Åstrand, P.-O. (1952). *Experimental Studies of Physical Working Capacity in Relation to Sex and Age*. Munksgaard, Copenhagen.

Åstrand, P.-O., T.E. Cuddy, B. Saltin, and J. Stenberg (1964). Cardiac output during submaximal and maximal work. *J. Appl. Physiol. 19*, 268–274.

Åstrand, P.-O., and K. Rodahl (1977). *Textbook of Work Physiology*, 2nd ed. McGraw-Hill, New York.

Barcroft, H. (1934). *Features in the Architecture of Physiological Function*. Cambridge University Press, London.

Bergh, U., I.-L. Kanstrup, and B. Ekblom (1976). Maximal oxygen uptake during exercise with various combinations of arm and leg work. *J. Appl. Physiol. 41*, 191–196.

Bevegård, S., and A. Lodin (1962). Postural circulatory changes at rest and during exercise in five patients with congenital absence of valves in the deep veins of the legs. *Acta Med. Scand. 172*, 21–29.

Blackmon, J.R., L.B. Rowell, J.W. Kennedy, R.D. Twiss, and R.D. Conn (1967). Physiological significance of maximal oxygen intake in pure mitral stenosis. *Circulation 36*, 497–510.

Blomqvist, C.G., and B. Saltin (1983). Cardiovascular adaptations to physical training. *Annu. Rev. Physiol. 45*, 169–189.

Clausen, J.-P. (1977). Effect of physical training on cardiovascular adjustments to exercise in man. *Physiol. Rev. 57*, 779–815.

Convertino, V.A., G.W. Mack, and E.R. Nadel (1991). Elevated central venous pressure: a consequence of exercise training-induced hypervolemia? *Am. J. Physiol. 260 (Regulatory Integrative Comp. Physiol. 29)*, R273–R277.

Duling, B.R. (1981). Coordination of microcirculatory function with oxygen demand in skeletal muscle. In A.G.B. Kovach, J. Hamar, L. Szabo, eds. *Advances in Physiology, Cardiovascular Physiology: Microcirculation and Capillary Exchange*, vol. 7, pp. 1–16. Akademiai Kaido, Budapest.

Ekblom, B. (1969). Effect of physical training on oxygen transport system in man. *Acta Physiol. Scand. [Suppl. 328]*, 1045.

Ekblom, B., P.-O. Åstrand, B. Saltin, J. Stenberg, and B. Wallstrom (1968). Effect of training on circulatory response to exercise. *J. Appl. Physiol. 24*, 518–528.

Ekblom, B., and L. Hermansen (1968). Cardiac output in athletes. *J. Appl. Physiol.* *25*, 619–625.

Ekelund, L.-G., and A. Holmgren (1967). Central hemodynamics during exercise. *Circ. Res. 21 (Suppl. 1).* I-33–I-43.

Eriksen, M., B.A. Waaler, L. Walloe, and J. Wesche (1990). Dynamics and dimensions of cardiac output changes in humans at the onset and at the end of moderate rhythmic exercise. *J. Physiol. (Lond.) 426*, 423–437.

Fortney, S.M., E.R. Nadel, C.B. Wenger, and J.R. Bove (1981). Effect of acute alterations of blood volume on circulatory performance in humans. *J. Appl. Physiol. (Respir. Environ. Exercise Physiol.) 50*, 292–298.

Freeman, G.L., and M.M. LeWinter (1984). Pericardial adaptations during chronic cardiac dilation in dogs. *Circ. Res. 54*, 294–300.

Galvao, P.E., J. Tarasantchi, and P. Guertzenstein (1965). Heat production of tropic snakes in relation to body weight and body surface. *Am. J. Physiol. 209*, 501–506.

Gollnick, P.D., M. Riedy, J.J. Quintinskie, and L.A. Bertocci (1985). Differences in metabolic potential of skeletal muscle fibres and its significance for metabolic control. *J. Exp. Biol. 115*, 191–199.

Gould, K.L. (1982). Quantitative imaging in nuclear cardiology. *Circulation 66*, 1141–1146.

Grande, F., and H.L. Taylor (1965). Adaptive changes in the heart, vessels, and patterns of control under chronically high loads. In W.F. Hamilton and P. Dow, eds. *Handbook of Physiology. Circulation*, sect. 2, vol. III, pp. 2615–2678. American Physiological Society, Washington, D.C.

Grimby, G., N.J. Nilsson, and H. Sanne (1964). Cardiac output during exercise in patients with varicose veins. *Scand. J. Clin. Lab. Invest. 16*, 21–30.

Guyton, A.C., B.H. Douglas, J.B. Langston, and T.Q. Richardson (1962). Instantaneous increase in mean circulatory pressure and cardiac output at onset of muscular activity. *Circ. Res. 11*, 431–441

Harrison, M.H. (1985). Effects of thermal stress and exercise on blood volume in humans. *Physiol. Rev. 65*, 149–209.

Hartley, L.H., G. Grimby, A. Kilbom, N.J. Nilsson, I. Åstrand, J. Bjure, B. Ekblom, and B. Saltin (1969). Physical training in sedentary middle-aged and older men. *Scand. J. Clin. Lab. Invest. 24*, 335–344.

Hermansen, L. (1973). Oxygen transport during exercise in human subjects. *Acta Physiol. Scand. [Suppl. 299]*, 1–104.

Higginbotham, M.B., K.G. Morris, R.S. Williams, P.A. McHale, R.E. Coleman, and F.R. Cobb (1986). Regulation of stroke volume during submaximal and maximal upright exercise in normal man. *Circ. Res. 58*, 281–291.

Hill, A.V., and H. Lupton (1923). Muscular exercise, lactic acid, and the supply and utilization of oxygen. *Q. J. Med. 16*, 135–171.

Holmgren, A. (1956). Circulatory changes during muscular work in man: with special reference to arterial and central venous pressures in the systemic circulation. *Scand. J. Clin. Lab. Invest 8 (Suppl. 24)*, 1–97.

Holmgren, A., and H. Linderholm (1958). Oxygen and carbon dioxide tensions of arterial blood during heavy and exhaustive exercise. *Acta Physiol. Scand., 44*, 203–215.

Huntsman L.L., and E.O. Feigl (1989). Cardiac mechanics. In H.D. Patton, A.F. Fuchs, B. Hille, A.M. Scher, and R. Steiner, eds. *Textbook of Physiology*.

Circulation, Respiration, Body Fluids, Metabolism, and Endocrinology, 21st ed., vol. 2, sect. VIII, pp. 820–833. W.B. Saunders, Philadelphia.

Jones, W.B., R.N. Finchun, R.O. Russell Jr., and T.J. Reeves (1970). Transient cardiac output response to multiple levels of supine exercise. *J. Appl. Physiol. 28,* 183–189.

Kanstrup, I., and B. Ekblom (1982). Acute hypervolemia, cardiac performance, and aerobic power during exercise. *J. Appl. Physiol. (Respir. Environ. Exercise Physiol.) 52,* 1186–1191.

Katz, A.M. (1992). *Physiology of the Heart,* 2nd ed. Raven Press, New York.

Kilbom, A. (1971). Physical training in women. *Scand. J. Clin. Lab. Invest. 28 (Suppl. 119),* 7–34.

Kleiber, M. (1975). Body size and metabolic rate. In *The Fire of Life: An Introduction to Animal Energetics,* 2nd ed., pp. 179–222. Robert E. Drieger, Huntington, NY.

Laughlin, M.H. (1987). Skeletal muscle blood flow capacity: role of muscle pump in exercise hyperemia. *Am. J. Physiol. 253 (Heart Circ. Physiol. 22),* H993–H1004.

Lee, M.-C., M.M. LeWinter, G. Freeman, R. Shabetai, and Y.C. Fung (1985). Biaxial mechanical properties of the pericardium in normal and volume overload dogs. *Am. J. Physiol. 249 (Heart Circ. Physiol. 18),* H222–H230.

Liljestrand, G., and N. Stenstrom (1920). Respirationsversuche beim Gehen, Laufen, Ski- und Schlittschuhlaufen. *Skand. Arch. Physiol. 39,* 167–206.

McDonald, D.A. (1974). *Blood Flow in Arteries.* Williams & Wilkins, Baltimore.

Moore, R., and E.R. Buskirk (1974). Exercise and body fluids. In W.J. Johnson and E.R. Buskirk, eds. *Science and Medicine of Exercise and Sport,* 2nd ed., pp. 153–170. Harper & Row, New York.

Morganroth, J., B.J. Maron, W.L. Henry, and S.E. Epstein (1975). Comparative left ventricular dimensions in trained athletes. *Ann. Intern. Med. 82,* 521–524.

Musch, T.I., G.C. Haidet, G.A. Ordway, J.C. Longhurst, and J.H. Mitchell (1985). Dynamic exercise training in foxhounds. I. Oxygen consumption and hemodynamic responses. *J. Appl. Physiol. 59,* 183–189.

Peronnet, F., J. Cleroux, H. Perrault, D. Cousineau, J. DeChamplain, and R. Nadeau (1981). Plasma norepinephrine response to exercise before and after training in humans. *J. Appl. Physiol. (Respir. Environ. Exercise Physiol.) 51,* 812–815.

Poliner, L.R., G.J. Dehmer, S.E. Lewis, R.W. Parkey, C.G. Blomqvist, and J.T. Willerson (1980). Left ventricular performance in normal subjects: a comparison of the responses to exercise in the upright and supine positions. *Circulation 62,* 528–534.

Rerych, S.K., P.M. Scholz, D.C. Sabiston, and R.H. Jones (1980). Effects of exercise training on left ventricular function in normal subjects: a longitudinal study by radionuclide angiography. *Am. J. Cardiol. 45,* 244–252.

Robinson, B.F., S.E. Epstein, R.L. Kahler, and E. Braunwald (1966). Circulatory effects of acute expansion of blood volume: studies during maximal exercise and at rest. *Circ. Res. 19,* 26–32.

Roeske, W.R., R.A. O'Rourke, A. Klein, G. Leopold, and J.S. Karliner (1975). Noninvasive evaluation of ventricular hypertrophy in professional athletes. *Circulation 53,* 286–292.

Rowell, L.B. (1974). Human cardiovascular adjustments to exercise and thermal stress. *Physiol. Rev. 54*, 75–159.

Rowell, L.B. (1986). *Human Circulation: Regulation During Physical Stress.* Oxford University Press, New York.

Rowell, L.B., J.R. Blackmon, and R.A. Bruce (1964). Indocyanine green clearance and estimated hepatic blood flow during mild to maximal exercise in upright man. *J. Clin. Invest. 43*, 1677–1690.

Rowell, L.B., G.L. Brengelmann, J.R. Blackmon, R.A. Bruce, and J.A. Murray (1968). Disparities between aortic and peripheral pulse pressures induced by upright exercise and vasomotor changes in man. *Circulation 37*, 954–964.

Rushmer, R.F. (1960). Effects of nerve stimulation and hormones on the heart; the role of the heart in general circulatory regulation. In W.F. Hamilton and P. Dow, eds. *Handbook of Physiology. Circulation*, vol. I, sect. 2, pp. 533–550. American Physiological Society, Washington, D.C.

Saltin, B., G. Blomqvist, J.H. Mitchell, R.L. Johnson, Jr., K. Wildenthal, and C.B. Chapman (1968). Response to exercise after bed rest and after training, *Circulation 38 (Suppl. 7)*, 1–78.

Saltin, B., and P.D. Gollnick (1983). Skeletal muscle adaptability: significance for metabolism and performance. In L.D. Peachy, R.H. Adrian, and S.R. Geiger, eds. *Handbook of Physiology. Skeletal Muscle*, sect. 10, pp. 555–631. American Physiological Society, Bethesda, MD.

Saltin, B., L.H. Hartley, A. Kilbom, and I. Åstrand (1969). Physical training in sedentary middle-aged and older men. II. Oxygen uptake, heart rate, and blood lactate concentrations at submaximal and maximal exercise. *Scand. J. Clin. Lab. Invest. 24*, 323–334.

Saltin, B., and L.B. Rowell (1980). Functional adaptations to physical activity and inactivity. *Fed. Proc. 39*, 1506–1513.

Scheuer, J., and C.M. Tipton (1977). Cardiovascular adaptations to physical training. *Annu. Rev. Physiol. 39*, 221–251.

Severinghaus, J.W. (1958). Blood oxygen dissociation line charts: man. In D.S. Dittmer, and R.M. Grebe, eds. *Handbook of Respiration*, p. 72. W.B. Saunders, Philadelphia.

Sheriff, D.D., X. Zhou, A.M. Scher, and L.B. Rowell (1992). Peripheral vascular factors influencing cardiac output (CO) and central venous pressure (CVP) during dynamic exercise in conscious dogs. *FASEB J. 6*, A1470.

Stenberg, J., B. Ekblom, and R. Messin (1966). Hemodynamic response to work at simulated altitude, 4,000 m. *J. Appl. Physiol. 21*, 1589–1594.

Stray-Gundersen, J., T.I. Musch, G.C. Haidet, D.P. Swain, G.A. Ordway, and J.H. Mitchell (1986). The effect of pericardiectomy on maximal oxygen consumption and maximal cardiac output in untrained dogs. *Circ. Res. 58*, 523–530.

Tanner, J.M. (1949). The construction of normal standards for cardiac output in man. *J. Clin. Invest. 28*, 567–582.

Taylor, H.L., E. Buskirk, and A. Henschel (1955). Maximal oxygen intake as an objective measure of cardio-respiratory performance. *J. Appl. Physiol. 8*, 73–80.

Taylor, H.L., Y. Wang, L.B. Rowell, and G. Blomqvist (1963). The standardization and interpretation of submaximal and maximal tests of working capacity. *Pediatrics 32*, 703–722.

Weibel, E.R. (1984). *The Pathway for Oxygen: Structure and Function in the Mammalian Respiratory System*. Harvard University Press, Cambridge, MA.

Wade, O.L., and J.M. Bishop (1962). *Cardiac Output and Regional Blood Flow*. Blackwell, Oxford.

Wang, Y., R.J. Marshall, and J.T. Shepherd (1960). The effect of changes in posture and of graded exercise on stroke volume in man. *J. Clin. Invest.* *39*, 1051–1061.

Warner, H.R., and A. Cox (1962). A mathematical model of heart rate control by sympathetic and vagus efferent information. *J. Appl. Physiol.* *17*, 349–355.

Control of Regional Blood Flow During Dynamic Exercise

This chapter discusses the regulation of blood flow through nonmuscular or noncontracting organs (commonly called "inactive" or "resting" organs) during exercise. Those discussed are all major organs and none are involved directly with increasing oxygen transport nor do they contribute significantly to the rise in oxygen uptake during exercise. Two of these organs receive the largest fractions of cardiac output during rest (splanchnic and renal). The splanchnic circulation is one of the two most compliant vascular regions, the other being the cutaneous circulation.

Humans may be the only mammals having two major vascular beds that are highly compliant. A consequence of vasodilating both of these regions at the same time is the subject of the schematic drawing in Figure 2-17. As we will see, the consequence of not maintaining tight neural control of their vascular resistance during exercise is a diminution of cardiac performance

Finally, the regulation of cerebral blood flow is also discussed in the light of new evidence that its blood flow is not as constant as we once thought. The brain also provides an important example of a powerful blood pressure-raising reflex elicited by tissue ischemia. A similar reflex arises from ischemic muscle during exercise.

As in Chapter 5, the discussion here centers on the control of the cardiovascular system over a range in which blood flow is able to increase up to the limit of cardiac pumping capacity imposed by cardiac filling pressure and/or pericardial constraints on stroke volume, and by maximal heart rate. Chapter 5 emphasized that the effectiveness of the muscle pump is the factor that most importantly determines ventricular filling pressure. Another point was that the blood that does not flow through the muscle pump will, depending on how large a fraction of cardiac output it is, tend to diminish filling pressure and stroke volume. For example, at rest, without any muscle pumping, it is not possible to increase cardiac output more than 1 or 2 L min^{-1} or so because of the effect of blood flow on peripheral vascular volume (increased volume) and ventricular filling pressure (decreased pressure) (see Figures 2-5 and 2-6). Thus a final point of emphasis in Chapter 5, illustrated in Figure 5-14, is that two things must happen to preserve ventricular performance during exercise: (1) A large fraction of the cardiac output must pass through the muscles that pump blood back to the heart with each contraction, and (2) the blood flow through compliant circuits must decrease. Therefore the maintenance of stroke volume and cardiac output during exercise requires a balance between the mechanical effects of muscle contraction and the passive effects of sympathetic vasoconstriction to minimize peripheral vascular volume. This chapter is about the vasoconstriction.

The questions to be answered are as follows: *First,* what happens to the blood flow through "inactive or resting" organs during exercise, and how is it controlled? *Second,* what is the functional significance of regional blood flow to (a) the redistribution of blood volume, (b) the redistribution of oxygen, and (c) the maintenance of arterial pressure?

Table 6-1 shows the approximate blood flow, oxygen consumption, and oxygen extraction of the major vascular beds at rest. In contrast, Table 6-2 shows a combination of measured and estimated values for blood flow, oxygen consumption, and so on of the same vascular beds during maximal exercise (see Wade and Bishop, 1962).

SPLANCHNIC CIRCULATION

The splanchnic organs include the liver, gastrointestinal tract, pancreas, and spleen. Their vascular supply is exceedingly complex, but the most important features are (1) the gastrointestinal organs, spleen, and pancreas are supplied in parallel by separate arteries leaving the abdominal aorta, and (2) their venous drainages all converge and become confluent in the portal vein, which provides 70 percent of the total hepatic blood supply. The remaining 30 percent of the liver's blood supply is arterial and comes from the hepatic artery, which branches from the coeliac artery (Bradley, 1963). Accordingly, use of the Fick principle to determine liver blood flow by measuring the amount of an indicator extracted each minute by the

Table 6-1 Regional Blood Flow and Oxygen Consumption

Region	Blood Flow (ml min^{-1})	Cardiac Output (percent)	Oxygen Uptake (ml min^{-1})	Arteriovenous Oxygen Difference (ml 100 ml^{-1})
Splanchnic	1,500	27	60	4.0
Kidneys	1,200	22	14	1.2
Muscle	1,000(?)	18	60	6.0
Brain	750	14	60	8.0
Skin	500(?)	9	10	2.0
Coronary	250	5	35	14.0
Other	300(?)	5	11	3.7
Total	5,500	100	250	4.5

Table 6-2 Estimated Distribution of Cardiac Output in a Normal Human Subject During Exercise at the Level of $\dot{V}_{O_2}$max

Region	Blood Flow (ml min^{-1})	Cardiac Output (%)	Oxygen Uptake (ml min^{-1})	Arteriovenous Oxygen Difference (ml 100 ml^{-1})
Splanchnic	350	1.4	60	17.0
Kidneys	360	1.4	10	3.6
Muscle (active)	21,840	87.4	3,931	18.0
Muscle (inactive)	200	0.8	30	15.0
Brain	850	3.4	68	8.0
Coronary	1,000	4.0	140	14.0
Skin	300	1.2	10	3.3
Other	100	0.4	11	11.0
Total	25,000	100.0	4,260	17.0

Adapted from Wade and Bishop (1962) and Rowell (1974).

liver and the arterial hepatic-venous difference of the substance (e.g., indocyanine green) will also measure total splanchnic blood flow (Rowell, 1974b). This assumes there are no significant portacaval shunts (normally there are none). For methodological details, see Rowell (1974a).

Splanchnic Blood Flow and Blood Volume at Rest

Average splanchnic blood flow in adult humans at supine rest averages approximately 1,500 ml min^{-1}. Thus the region receives approximately 25 percent of the resting cardiac output, making it the largest regional circulation. This high blood flow passes through the liver, which weighs about 1.5 kg and is only approximately 2 percent of total body weight, making liver perfusion rate very high at approximately 100 ml 100 g^{-1} of liver each minute. Total splanchnic oxygen consumption at rest is only 50 to 60 ml min^{-1} and thus only 15 to 20 percent of the oxygen it receives each minute is extracted. Because of all the oxygen that is left over in the venous blood draining the organs, large reductions in splanchnic blood flow can occur without compromising the oxygen supply to the region. For example, a splanchnic blood flow of 350 ml min^{-1} can support the normal splanchnic oxygen uptake of 60 ml min^{-1} by increasing extraction from 4 ml 100 ml^{-1} to 17 ml 100 ml^{-1}.

Total splanchnic blood volume is estimated to be 1,200 to 1,500 ml of which 400 to 600 ml are in the intestinal circulation; the total constitutes approximately 20 to 25 percent of the total blood volume, making this by far the largest and most capacious region. Possibly the ability of the splanchnic region to rapidly transfer blood volume from its veins back to the heart is a more important hemodynamic function than its ability to divert to other organs major fractions of its high blood flow. Among the splanchnic organs, the liver has the greatest hemodynamic importance, not only because it receives all of the splanchnic blood flow, but also because its specific vascular compliance (ml kg^{-1} of tissue per mmHg) is 10 times greater than either intestinal or total systemic vascular compliance, both of which are approximately 2.5 ml mmHg^{-1} kg^{-1} (Rothe, 1983).

Measurements of splanchnic blood volume in anesthetized animals and available estimates from humans undergoing experimental hemorrhage reveal that the volume of the region can be reduced by as much as 40 percent or by 600 ml. These observations have spurred debate concerning the role of active splanchnic venoconstriction as opposed to the purely passive effects of arterial constriction and reduced blood flow on splanchnic venous volume (see Chapters 1 and 2). These observations lend credence to the old idea of Adolph Jarisch and Carl Ludwig (cited by Katz and Rodbard, 1939) that the splanchnic circulation is the "venesector and blood giver of the circulation." A number of the early physiologists such as Adolph Jarisch and Carl Ludwig, A.F. Dastre and J.P. Morat, Hermann Rein, O. Müller, and August Krogh thought there must be a reciprocal relationship between splanchnic blood flow and blood flow to other capacious regions, such as the skin. Dastre and Morat (1884) predicted that any increase in skin blood flow, for example, had to be compensated for by a reduction in splanchnic blood flow. The consequence of not vasoconstricting the splanchnic vasculature during exercise will be revealed later in this chapter.

Neural Control of Splanchnic Organs

Splanchnic organs are richly innervated by sympathetic noradrenergic fibers originating mainly from the splanchnic nerves. These nerves appear not to be tonically active because blood flow does not increase when they are blocked or surgically ablated (Lynn et al., 1952; Lautt, 1980) or when carotid sinus baroreceptor activity is increased (Tyden et al., 1979; Rowell et al., unpublished). Current evidence argues against the presence of significant cholinergic or other vasodilator innervation of human splanchnic blood vessels. Although glands of the gastrointestinal mucosa do receive sympathetic fibers that release cholinergic or peptidergic neurotransmitters and may also cause release of kinins which are potent local vasodilators, the effects of these neurotransmitters are probably confined to the glands and exert no significant control of the total splanchnic circulation.

Humoral Control

Epinephrine is probably the most important circulating "systemic" hormone acting on the splanchnic circulation. At the plasma concentrations observed during severe stress, epinephrine causes splanchnic vasodilation with blood flow reaching as high as 2.5 L min^{-1}, owing to the apparently dense distribution of β_2-adrenoceptors in the region. In high, pharmacological doses the effect of epinephrine on α-adrenoceptors dominates and the arterioles constrict (Greenway and Stark, 1971).

High circulating levels of angiotensin II and vasopressin can also vasoconstrict splanchnic vessels. Angiotensin II may exert its effects directly or by facilitating the responses to increased sympathetic nerve activity. Although vasopressin is a potent constrictor in some species, it appears to be far less so in humans and there is no evidence that it is released in vasoconstrictor quantities except under extreme conditions (see Chapter 3). The hypotension experienced by humans who have undergone splanchnic sympathectomy and cannot increase splanchnic vascular resistance, suggest a minor role or at least a slowly developing one for humoral control of splanchnic resistance in humans (van Lieshout, 1989).

Control of Splanchnic Veins

Inasmuch as approximately 20 percent of the total blood volume is contained within the splanchnic veins, their constriction could have a significant impact on right ventricular filling pressure. In fact, the liver can be viewed as a giant capacitor situated next to the right atrium. Again, the specific compliance of the liver (25 ml kg^{-1} mmHg^{-1}) is the highest of any region (Rothe, 1983).

Although most of the volume displaced from the splanchnic organs is attributable to the passive effects of reduced blood flow on their venous volume, active splanchnic venoconstriction has been demonstrated in anesthetized cats and dogs (see Chapter 2). Direct electrical stimulation of splanchnic nerves can dispel up to 50 percent of liver blood volume and up to 40 percent of intestinal volume. The fraction of splanchnic blood volume that is expelled by active venoconstriction depends on splanchnic blood flow, hepatic outflow resistance and central venous pressure, or the back pressure seen by the hepatic veins (Chapter 2). When central venous pressure is below normal, about 65 percent of the volume mobilized is the passive result of reduced flow on venous pressure and volume. When central venous pressure is greater than normal, the fraction of volume mobilized by venoconstriction increases. This is because the active component is greater when veins are distended and the venous pressure-volume curve is flatter so that changes in venous geometry do not influence the pressure-volume relationship (see Figure 1-5). Finally, the objection that venoconstriction would raise venous resistance so that pressure and volume would rise in the noninnervated venules upstream (Rowell, 1986) appears to be refuted by evidence that baroreflex constriction of small mesenteric venules has now been directly observed (Haase and Shoukas, 1991) (see Chapter 2).

Summary. In summary, the importance of any active splanchnic venocon- striction is highly dependent on the blood flow through the region and the pressures in the central and hepatic-splanchnic veins; venoconstriction without simultaneous vasoconstriction is highly unlikely so that passive effects of flow on volume should dominate at rest. However, if right atrial transmural pressure increases along with pulmonary wedge pressure during exercise, the increased back pressure on hepatic-splanchnic veins may necessitate a greater active venomotor contribution.

Control of the Splanchnic Circulation During Exercise
Blood Flow

The history of early efforts to study the splanchnic circulation during exercise was reviewed by Wade and Bishop (1962) and Rowell (1974c). The results varied because the methods of flow measurement, the physical condition of the subjects, and both the absolute and relative severity of exercise all varied, as well as the posture in which it was carried out. In some cases, marked reduction in clearance of indicators removed by the liver was observed and in other cases there were no changes.

Rowell and colleagues (1964) measured hepatic clearance and extrac- tion of indocyanine green in 10 normal subjects during rest and graded exercise at known fractions of their $\dot{V}o_2$max; $\dot{V}o_2$max varied widely among the subjects. At a given absolute oxygen uptake, the decrements in hepatic- splanchnic blood flow varied markedly among the subjects. At low abso- lute levels of oxygen uptake some showed no change from resting values, whereas others showed significant decreases. When blood flows were expressed in relation to the *relative oxygen uptake* (percent of $\dot{V}o_2$max) differences between individuals virtually disappeared, even when patients with abnormally low $\dot{V}o_2$max owing to their mitral stenosis were included, as shown in Figure 6-1 (Blackmon et al., 1967). The relationship between relative oxygen uptake and splanchnic blood flow was unaltered by physi- cal conditioning or by changing the mode of exercise to that with arms only or with legs only (Clausen, 1977).

Superimposition of heat stress on the stress of exercise caused the only exception seen so far in this relationship. At a given percent of $\dot{V}o_2$max, splanchnic blood flow was 20 percent lower during heat stress than at normal temperature (Rowell et al., 1965) (Figure 6-2). The cause of the leftward shift in the curve to a lower splanchnic blood flow at a given relative as well as absolute oxygen uptake was not ascertained at the time (see Chapter 12), but the obvious benefit to the subjects was a greater redistribution of a significant fraction of cardiac output to the skin (others noted earlier a similar effect of heat stress on renal blood flow at a given oxygen uptake; see below).

When several hundred observations (including those of Clausen [1977] and colleagues) were analyzed (Rowell, 1974c, 1983), it became obvious

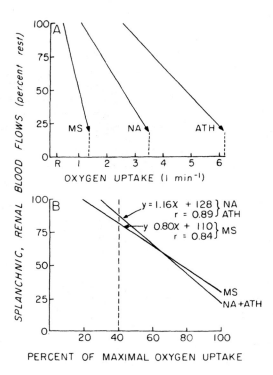

Figure 6-1 (**A**) Representative splanchnic and renal vascular responses to graded dynamic exercise up to $\dot{V}o_2$max (indicated by vertical dashed lines to x-axis) for the same three groups described in Figure 5-2. The three groups similarly decrease regional blood flow by 75 to 80 percent, but over very different ranges of total oxygen uptake. (**B**) Normalization of regional vasomotor responses shown in Figure A. Responses among the three groups are almost undistinguishable when oxygen uptake is expressed as percent of $\dot{V}o_2$max. (Data from Blackmon et al., 1967, and Rowell, 1974, 1986.)

that splanchnic blood flow most closely related to heart rate. *No matter what the stress during exercise, splanchnic blood flow did not start to fall until heart rate approached 100 beats min^{-1}* (Figure 6-3). For example, although splanchnic blood flow measured during exercise with heat stress was displaced to the left on the percent $\dot{V}o_2$max axis, all values for splanchnic blood flow became virtually superimposed on the heart rate axis irrespective of temperature.

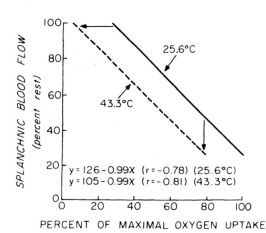

Figure 6-2 Leftward shift in relationship between splanchnic blood flow and percent of $\dot{V}o_2$max with environmental heat stress imposed during graded exercise. Despite the lower splanchnic blood flow at a given *relative* as well as absolute oxygen uptake; the relationship to heart rate (Figure 6-3) was unaltered (i.e., heat stress increased heart rate). (Adapted from Rowell et al., 1965.)

Figure 3-1 includes the data from Figure 6-3 and shows schematically the close relationship among splanchnic and renal blood flows, heart rate, plasma norepinephrine concentration and plasma renin activity once heart rate approaches approximately 100 beats min^{-1} during exercise (Rowell, 1984). In contrast, note that stresses applied to resting subjects increase all of these variables as soon as heart rate increases above a resting baseline. Although plasma norepinephrine concentration is only a rough index of sympathetic nervous activity, the consistency of its close relationship to heart rate during exercise is striking. Regional vasoconstrictor outflow is therefore proportional to heart rate and plasma norepinephrine concentration.

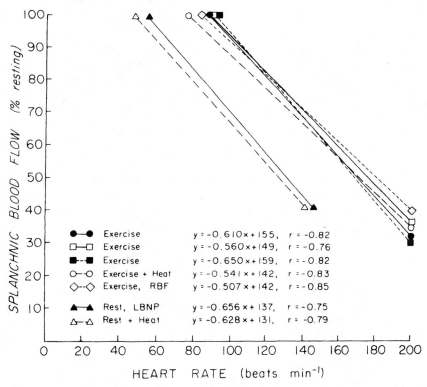

Figure 6-3 Relationship between splanchnic blood flow as percent of resting values and heart rate during exercise (five curves on the right). The two curves displaced to the left were derived from values measured in resting subjects exposed to other stresses. Exercise was carried out in neutral and hot environments, before and after physical conditioning, and with different muscle groups. Despite these differences and the various methodologies in the four different laboratories contributing these data, all regression lines were virtually the same (note the regression equations), including one study of renal blood flow (crosses and dashed lines) (for references see text and Rowell, 1983, 1984). (From Rowell, 1986, with permission of Oxford University Press.)

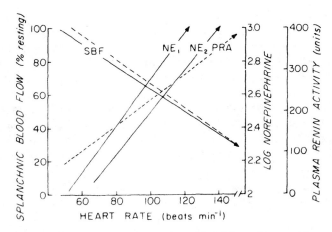

Figure 6-4   Relationship between splanchnic blood flow (*SBF*) and heart rate during heat stress and lower body negative pressure (*dashed line*). Also shown are relationships between plasma norepinephrine (*NE*) concentration and heart rate, and plasma renin activity (*PRA*) and heart rate. Units for PRA = ng angiotensin I 100 ml^{-1} NE = log pg ml^{-1}. Changes in each variable reflect relative increases in sympathetic nervous activity (see Rowell, 1984). (From Rowell, 1986, with permission of Oxford University Press.)

Figures 3-1, 6-3, and 6-4 all reveal an important difference between reflex control of the circulation during rest and exercise. For example, Robinson and colleagues (1966) showed that increased sympathetic activity caused most of the tachycardia in tilted (upright) resting subjects, whereas during exercise most of the rise in heart rate (up to approximately 100 beats min^{-1}) is attributable to withdrawal of vagal tone. Available data indicate, as shown in Figure 6-4, that norepinephrine increases as soon as heart rate rises and regional vasoconstriction begins during lower body suction and heat stress (applied at rest) (Rowell, 1983). These findings fit with directly measured increases in muscle sympathetic nerve activity (Victor and Leimbach 1987; Rowell and Seals, 1990) (see Chapters 2 and 3). Changes in plasma renin activity also fit the same scheme as for norepinephrine (Figure 6-4) (the actual slopes are not shown in Figure 3-1 because of variations in reported units of measurement).

As pointed out in Chapter 5, the increments in heart rate and cardiac output achieved by vagal withdrawal are rapid (1 to 2 seconds), whereas sympathetically mediated responses may require 15 to 20 seconds. Figures 3-1 and 6-3 reveal that *sympathetic vasoconstriction during exercise does not begin until the ability to increase heart rate and cardiac output rapidly by vagal withdrawal is exhausted.* This point is pivotal to the issue of what reflexes might govern sympathetic activity and thus control the circulation during exercise (Chapters 11 and 12).

Redistribution of Blood Volume

Figures 2-6 and 2-7 illustrate how *vaso*constriction could mimic *veno*constriction by changing the flow-dependent pressure gradient across the venous system of an organ and thereby reducing its blood volume. The splanchnic circulation is a prime example of how sensitive the volume of an organ can be to changes in blood flow (Rothe, 1983). Vasoconstriction reduces blood flow, and reduces the pressure gradient from arteries through veins causing pressure in the downstream veins to fall so that blood volume moves out of the organ (by elastic recoil) and back to the central circulation. This volume can be several hundred milliliters.

Measurements of splanchnic blood volume in exercising humans are rare and depend on the measurement of splanchnic blood flow and mean transit time of an indicator through a very complex venous network (Bradley et al., 1953; Wade et al., 1956; Clausen and Trap-Jensen, 1974). Reductions in splanchnic blood volume of 30 to 40 percent during relatively mild supine exercise in humans are a consistent finding with this technique. However, the decreases in splanchnic blood flow were small (350 ml min^{-1}) and prompted the suggestion that active *veno*constriction rather than vasoconstriction might explain such a large reduction in volume. At this time the occurrence of splanchnic venoconstriction in humans can neither be ruled in nor out.

Figure 6-5 is a sketch from a photograph of a scintigram taken from a

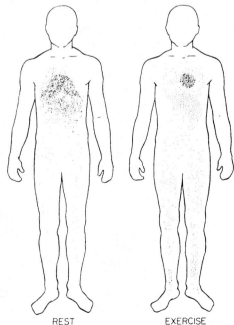

Figure 6-5 The distribution of technetium 99 in a human subject during rest and supine exercise. (Redrawn from a photograph kindly provided by Dr. F. Bonde-Petersen.) Note the marked shift of labeled red blood cells out of the splanchnic region. (From Rowell, 1986, with permission of Oxford University Press.)

REST   EXERCISE

human patient at rest and during exercise after the red blood cells had been labeled with technetium 99. A quantitatively large shift of labeled red blood cells out of the splanchnic region, however, has not been a consistent finding by those who have applied scintigraphic techniques. For example, two groups observed 40 to 50 percent decreases in splenic radioactivity (or volume), but only 14 percent decreases in liver and abdominal radioactivity (Sandler et al., 1984; Froelich et al., 1988). Reasons for the discrepancies are not known.

The intense splanchnic vasoconstriction seen in humans during severe exercise is not seen in dogs, even if the exercise is severe (Vatner, 1975). In accordance with these results is the finding that neuronal leakage of norepinephrine into plasma increases much less in dogs than in humans during exercise, indicating vasoconstrictor outflow is far less in dogs (Peronnet et al., 1981). These findings led to the view that regional vasoconstriction is not an important part of the exercise response in normal dogs. Contrary to this view, however, is the important fact that dogs raise splanchnic vascular resistance enough to maintain a nearly constant splanchnic blood flow when arterial pressure rises, even during severe exercise (Vatner, 1975; Fixler et al., 1976).

The significance of this splanchnic vasoconstriction first became obvious when Ashkar (1973) removed sympathetic innervation of splanchnic blood vessels and the adrenal medulla by thoracic sympathectomy. His chronically instrumented dogs could no longer maintain their normal cardiac output because of a marked fall in stroke volume during exercise, as shown in Figure 6-6. The interpretation of these findings was that after denervation of the splanchnic region, its blood flow rose passively during exercise along with arterial pressure. As a consequence, splanchnic blood volume increased markedly causing ventricular preload to fall. In short, the consequences of splanchnic denervation were the same as those observed in orthostatic intolerance (Chapter 4), during which increased gravitational force raises splanchnic vascular transmural pressure so that splanchnic blood volume increases markedly, if its blood flow is not curtailed by vasoconstriction (see Figure 4-20). Ventricular filling pressure falls so low that an adequate cardiac output can no longer be maintained. The patient who had orthostatic intolerance as a consequence of splanchnic denervation, like that shown in Figure 4-20, also had greatly reduced tolerance to exercise (van Lieshout, 1989). Up to a point, an adequate exercise response was permitted by a normal vagal control of heart rate, by the skeletal muscle and respiratory pumps, and by the abdominal compression associated with cycling, all of which contributed to a limited ability to raise cardiac output. Presumably because of the sequestration of blood in the splanchnic region, work capacity was severely impaired.

A more striking example from van Lieshout (1989) of the consequences of a maldistribution of cardiac output during exercise is seen in a patient with hypoadrenergic orthostatic hypotension. This defect was ameliorated to some degree by blood volume expansion (fludrocortisone) and clever

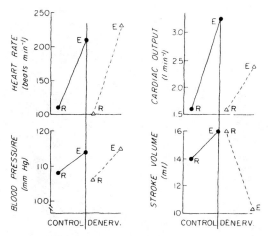

Figure 6-6   Circulatory responses to voluntary exercise in dogs with chronically implanted aortic flow meters. Variables measured during rest (R) and exercise (E) are compared before (control, *solid circles*) and after denervation (*open triangles, dashed lines*) of splanchnic organs and adrenal medulla by thoracic sympathectomy. Loss of adrenergic control of splanchnic flow and volume causes lower stroke volume and cardiac output during exercise. Maintenance of filling pressure and stroke volume requires control of flow through highly compliant regions, whether it be splanchnic or cutaneous (Ashkar, 1973). (From Rowell, 1986, with permission of Oxford University Press.)

maneuvers (by the patient) that relied on the muscle pump and abdominal compression to maintain ventricular filling pressure and thus arterial pressure. Figure 6-7 shows the inability of the muscle pump by itself to counteract the effects of volume sequestration in vascular beds that cannot constrict normally during exercise. This is revealed even during supine exercise (lower panel, Figure 6-7), which shows that arterial pressure progressively declined despite the fact that gravitational influences were virtually absent. Figure 6-7 reveals the problems experienced by this patient during daily cycling when she stopped at a traffic light. Arterial pressure fell precipitously and could only be restored when she pressed her thighs against her abdomen to express the blood sequestered in splanchnic vessels. In short, this patient had to use mechanical compression of splanchnic vessels in place of the compensatory vasoconstrictor responses illustrated in Figure 6-8. This figure schematically illustrates the balance that must exist among the blood flows through compliant skin and splanchnic regions and noncompliant muscle regions in order to maintain central venous pressure. Filling pressure in Figure 6-8A remains constant or increases when the fraction of total cardiac output going to muscle (Figure 6-8D) is high and splanchnic and cutaneous blood volumes shown in Figure 6-8B and C are passively reduced by vasoconstriction. Figure 6-8A (top) shows that filling pressure falls when one or both of these regions vasodilates (or does not vasoconstrict).

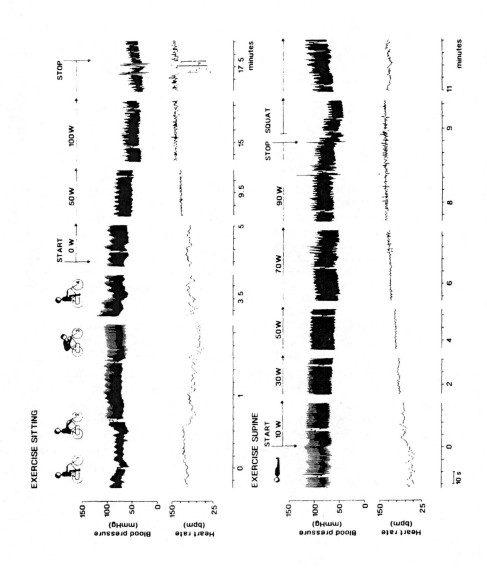

Redistribution of Oxygen by Splanchnic Vasoconstriction

The splanchnic circulation makes the largest contribution to the redistribution of oxygen delivery to working muscle during exercise when it vasoconstricts. This is made possible by its high blood flow of 1,500 ml min^{-1} and its small arteriovenous oxygen difference of 4 ml 100 ml^{-1}, that is, only 20 percent extraction. A reduction in splanchnic blood flow from 1,500 to 350 ml min^{-1}, such as seen at $\dot{V}o_2$max (Rowell et al., 1964), can redistribute 1,150 ml of blood flow and 230 ml of oxygen (1,150 ml min^{-1} × 20 ml 100 ml^{-1}) to active muscle each minute. The normal oxygen uptake of the splanchnic organs is preserved at 60 ml min^{-1} by expanding the arteriovenous oxygen difference of the region from 4 to 17 ml 100 ml^{-1} after vasoconstriction. Table 6-2 summarizes the additional oxygen and blood flow provided by regional vasoconstriction during "maximal" exercise.

Splanchnic Vasoconstriction and Blood Pressure Regulation

At rest the splanchnic circulation comprises 25 to 30 percent of total vascular conductance so that its changes in splanchnic vascular conductance have an important influence on blood pressure. For example, if splanchnic blood flow is decreased 80 percent from 1,500 to 300 ml min^{-1}, then arterial pressure would rise from 100 to 132 mmHg, a change of 32 mmHg (cardiac output was assumed to be 5 L min^{-1} and arterial pressure 100 mmHg, with total vascular conductance 0.05 L min^{-1}, and splanchnic vascular conductance fell from 0.015 to 0.003 L min^{-1} mmHg^{-1}). In severe exercise with cardiac output at 25 L min^{-1}, for example, and blood pressure at 115 mmHg, the same absolute decrease in splanchnic vascular conductance would raise blood pressure to 121 mmHg, or a change of 6 mmHg. Therefore, the effect of vasoconstriction on arterial pressure decreases in inverse proportion to the increase in cardiac output and total vascular conductance. The effects of all the regional vasoconstrictions on arterial pressure during severe exercise were summarized by Rowell (1974c).

Figure 6-7 Blood pressure tracing from a patient with acute dysautonomia and orthostatic hypotension. It shows the beneficial effects of maneuvers invented by the patient to counteract hypotension and fainting. Sitting on the bicycle without exercise caused hypotension (first cartoon). Placing feet on handle bars restored pressure (second cartoon), which was improved by bending forward (third cartoon). Note subsequent fall in pressure with sitting upright again. Pressure continued to fall throughout exercise despite increasing work rate from 0 to 100 watts. Lower panel shows progressive hypotension accompanying graded *supine* exercise showing the need for regional vasoconstriction despite the lack of orthostatic stress (note apparently normal heart rate response). (From van Lieshout, 1989, with permission of the author and Elsevier, Amsterdam.)

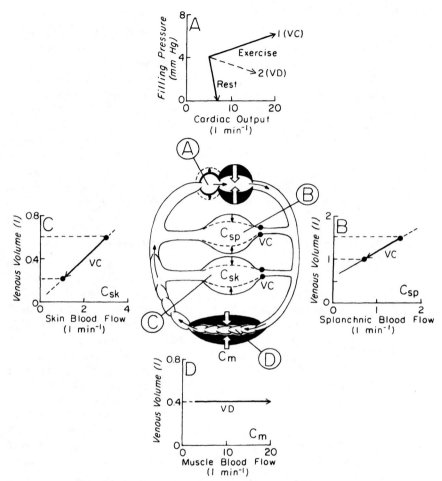

Figure 6-8 Schematic representation of the cardiovascular system as *compliant* splanchnic (C_{sp}) and cutaneous (C_{sk}) circuits and a *noncompliant* muscle pump (C_m). Cardiac filling pressure depends on ratio of flow through C_m to flow through C_{sp} and C_{sk}. The greater the fraction of total flow through C_{sp} and/or C_{sk} relative to the fraction through noncompliant muscle regions C_m, the lower the filling pressure Ⓐ at a given cardiac output. (**A**) Relationship between right atrial filling pressure and cardiac output at rest and during exercise (*arrow 1*) when C_{sp} and C_{sk} vasoconstrict (VC) so that most of the flow perfuses muscle (C_m), and (*arrow 2*) when C_{sp} and C_{sk} vasodilate (VD), causing a smaller fraction of cardiac output to perfuse muscle. With vasoconstriction (*arrow 1*), filling pressure may increase slightly along with cardiac output. With vasodilation of C_{sp} and C_{sk} (*arrow 2*), filling pressure decreases with increasing cardiac output, and maximal cardiac output is reduced. (**B and C**) Vasoconstriction and reduced splanchnic Ⓑ and skin Ⓒ blood flows (C_{sp} and C_{sk}) passively reduces their venous volumes, as shown by dashed lines in the schematic circuit (center). This vasoconstriction makes more volume available for cardiac filling as well as more flow for muscle Ⓓ. (**D**) shows no net effect of flow on volume of active muscle (C_m) because of its low compliance and pumping action.

CUTANEOUS CIRCULATION

The skin is a large organ, weighing as much as 2 kg in an average-size human with 1.8-m^2 surface area. It is our waterproof coating, vapor barrier, protection from mechanical injury, and our thermal insulation together with the underlying subcutaneous adipose tissue. Its role as a heat exchanger and insulator stems from its location on the body surface and its dense system of capillary loops that empty into a capacious subpapillary venous plexus. The low linear flow velocity of the large volume within this venous plexus and its close proximity to the body surface provides a means for rapid dissipation of heat. In effect, this plexus regulates the surface area from which heat can be conducted through the dermal layers.

Quantitative measurement of skin blood flow continues to be a problem. At present, we have no way of determining total skin blood flow. Measurements of flow, regardless of the organ, are indirect (except timed collection of volume in a calibrated container), being derived from variables that are related to flow. Some measurements provide estimates of absolute flow (e.g., Fick-based methods), whereas others can only provide information about relative changes in flow. None give quantitative measurements of skin blood flow in absolute units. Changes in regional skin blood flow have been assessed from changes in skin temperature (this is invalid), thermal conductivity, rates of heat loss by calorimetry, absorption of light by red cells and transilluminated skin, light-scattering techniques, and rates of isotope clearance. Laser-Doppler flowmetry has become especially useful because it appears to provide reasonable estimates of flow *changes* in any cutaneous region (Johnson et al., 1984). Although venous occlusion plethysmography permits quantitative estimates of changes in skin blood flow, the method is restricted to the arms and legs and the separate contributions of skeletal muscle, subcutaneous adipose, and skin to total limb blood flow must be determined. Changes in limb blood flow during heat stress do not include underlying muscle, to which blood flow may even decrease (Detry, et al., 1972; Johnson and Rowell, 1975).

Magnitudes of Cutaneous Blood Flow and Blood Volume

Total skin blood flow can be approximated from estimates of arteriovenous temperature difference across the skin and total heat exchange (Fick principle), but there are major assumptions. Such estimates place the value for total skin blood flow between 200 and 500 ml min^{-1} or 100 and 300 ml m^{-2} of body surface per minute. Skin "maximally" vasodilated by whole-body heating, or as near to maximal as the limits of thermal tolerance will allow, may receive as much as 7 to 8 L min^{-1} over the entire body surface or 3.5 to 4 L m^{-2} body surface per minute (Rowell, 1983). It is not known if vasodilation in subcutaneous fat contributes significantly to this high blood flow; other large organs do not (Rowell, 1983). The cutaneous circulation appears to be second only to skeletal muscle in its capacity to receive high blood flows at normal perfusion pressure, and can therefore compete seriously with skeletal muscle for cardiac output during exercise.

No quantitative estimates of cutaneous blood volume are available. Indirect evidence suggests that heated human skin comprises one of the largest venous "reservoirs" into which blood volume will accumulate when blood flow is high. Müller (1905) was possibly the first to show that temperature changes altered the distribution of blood volume in the human body. He measured shifts in the weights of various body segments in humans while they were supported horizontally on a series of weighing scales. Heating shifted body weight away from the center of the body (presumably away from visceral organs) to the limbs, whereas cooling did the opposite. Müller, like Dastre and Morat in 1884, concluded that an "antagonism" exists between superficial and visceral vessels so that when one region dilates, the other constricts. This "antagonism" has been demonstrated by measurements of regional blood flow and regional sympathetic nerve activity in nonhuman species (Schönung et al., 1971).

Neural Control

All cutaneous resistance vessels receive tonic outflow from sympathetic vasoconstrictor fibers. The first demonstration of this tonic vasoconstrictor activity was made in 1852 by Claude Bernard, who saw that cutting the nerves supplying a rabbit's ear caused an increase in its blood flow. The same result accompanies surgical section or pharmacological blockade of sympathetic nerves supplying human skin when ambient temperature is cool and tonic nerve activity is high; skin blood flow is approximately doubled when all vasoconstrictor tone is withdrawn (Shepherd, 1963). Tonic vasoconstrictor activity decreases with rising body temperature and skin temperature. Blood flow to nonacral skin (limbs and body trunk) is controlled by these fibers in cool environments, but tone is minimal in neutral environments. In contrast, when body temperature is normal and environmental temperature is neutral, tonic sympathetic vasoconstrictor outflow to acral regions is still so high that all vasodilation during heat stress is passively elicited by withdrawal of this tone.

The fundamental difference in the control of blood flow to acral as opposed to nonacral skin is that blood flow to acral skin is controlled by the frequency of impulse traffic over vasoconstrictor fibers, whereas nonacral skin possesses an *active* vasodilator system (Shepherd, 1963; Roddie, 1983). Humans are the only known species whose cutaneous vascular adjustment to heat stress depends almost entirely on active vasodilation and increased sweating; yet it is still not known whether the vasodilation is mediated neurally by specific vasodilator nerve fibers or by some neurohumoral effects accompanying sympathetic cholinergic activation of sweat glands. The proposal of Fox and Hilton (1958) that cutaneous vasodilation is caused by the formation of bradykinin in the cutaneous interstitium from an enzyme (kallikrein) released from sweat glands has not withstood close scrutiny (Rowell, 1977, 1981). Nevertheless, Brengelmann and colleagues (1981) observed that humans with congenital absence of sweat glands cannot vasodilate their skin; the two events appear to be functionally linked. These results are consistent with evidence from direct electrical stimulation of human cutaneous "vasodilator" (?) nerve fibers (Lundberg et al., 1989). The defect in vasodilation of the nonsweaters could not be related to any known deficiency in autonomic nervous function.

Hökfelt and coworkers (1980) postulated that cholinergic nerves release the vasodilator, vasoactive intestinal polypeptide (VIP), as a cotransmitter. In their scheme, illustrated in Figure 6-9, nerves containing these transmitters also supply cutaneous arterioles. Accordingly, blockade of acetylcholine with atropine would not affect release of VIP or the consequent vasodilation, but would abolish sweating because sweating is cholinergically mediated and VIP has no effect on it. This scheme fits the consistent observation that blockade of sympathetic cholinergic nerves by

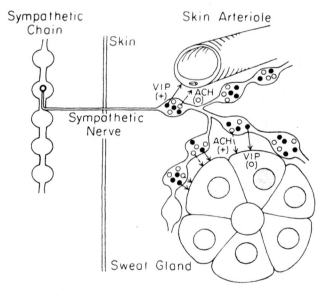

Figure 6-9 Hypothetical explanation for why cholinergic blockade (atropine) abolishes sweating but not active cutaneous vasodilation. Cutaneous sympathetic cholinergic nerves share acetylcholine (*ACH*) and vasoactive intestinal polypeptide (*VIP*) as cotransmitters. Despite blockade of ACH, VIP (+) is still released to vasodilate skin arterioles. ACH, whether released or blocked, has no effect on vasodilation (ACH O). The sweat gland, which is not affected by VIP (O) will respond only to ACH (+)—unless it, and sweating, are blocked. Final result is vasodilation and no sweating. (Adapted from Hökfelt et al., 1980.)

atropine prevents sweating, but *not* the cutaneous vasodilation (e.g., Roddie, 1983). Subsequently, VIP-like immunoreactivity was found in the nerves of human axillary sweat glands (see Savage et al., 1990). Savage and coworkers (1990) took advantage experimentally of the fact that patients with cystic fibrosis lack VIP fiber innervation of sweat glands. They proposed that a corresponding attenuation of active vasodilation in these patients would provide indirect evidence that VIP is involved as an effector mechanism in active cutaneous vasodilation. Despite confirmation of sparse VIP immunoreactive innervation in the cystic fibrosis patients, their cutaneous vasodilator responses to hyperthermia were normal. Savage and coworkers (1990) also found normal immunoreactivity for calcitonin gene-related peptide and for substance P in the cutaneous nerve fibers of these patients. They suggested that release of one or both of these peptides could provide a mechanism for the fully developed active cutaneous vasodilation. The mechanism of active cutaneous vasodilation is still an important unsolved mystery.

Other Factors Controlling Skin Blood Flow

Because of its lack of β_2-adrenoceptors and its high density of α-adrenoceptors, cutaneous vessels vasoconstrict at physiologically significant concentrations of epinephrine (Whelan, 1967). The effects of physiological levels of angiotensin II and vasopressin on the resistance vessels of human skin are not established.

Blood flow through the skin is also importantly influenced by its local temperature, which can vary over a much greater range than in other organs. Local cooling can reduce skin blood flow to zero, whereas elevations in skin temperature to 40°C or more will produce five- to ten-fold increases in flow. These are direct local effects of heat on vascular smooth muscle, which are fully expressed in denervated skin. The mechanisms of temperature-mediated vasomotor reactions have been investigated mainly in cutaneous veins (Keatinge and Harman, 1980; Vanhoutte, 1980), and are mentioned below.

Cutaneous Veins
Reflex Control

Cutaneous veins are richly innervated with sympathetic vasoconstrictor fibers. They constrict vigorously in response to local cold and are *reflexly* constricted in response to reductions in body skin or core temperatures. Together with splanchnic veins, cutaneous veins represent a potentially large volume reservoir that can be actively expelled when they constrict. When this venous reservoir is large during heat stress, a sudden venoconstriction in response to a rapid fall in skin temperatures causes large and immediate increases in central venous pressure, thoracic blood volume, and stroke volume (Rowell et al., 1969; Rowell et al., 1970) (see Figure

6-15). This venoconstriction also curtails heat loss by redirecting the high surface blood flow to deeper and better-insulated veins, providing in effect a "thermal short circuit."

Despite the potential importance of cutaneous veins in volume mobilization, their neural control by sympathetic nerves is dominated by thermoregulatory reflexes. Baroreflexes exert little influence on their tone despite the fact that they can contain enough blood to lower central venous pressure and thereby contribute significantly to orthostatic intolerance (Chapter 4). Cutaneous veins do, however, constrict reflexly in response to exercise (Rowell et al., 1971). They do not contain enough volume at neutral body temperatures to augment central venous pressure significantly when they constrict.

Local Temperature Effects

Cooling causes both arteries and veins of the skin to constrict even after sympathectomy (Keatinge and Harman, 1980; Vanhoutte, 1980). Cooling cutaneous vessels augments their response to sympathetic nerve stimulation and to catecholamines as a result of increased norepinephrine affinity of the α_2-adrenoceptors on vascular smooth muscle (Vanhoutte, 1980; Flavahan et al., 1985). In contrast, warming above normal temperatures reduces norepinephrine affinity and the vessels become less responsive to sympathetic activity.

Cutaneous veins are highly compliant, as revealed by the marked increases in limb blood volume that accompany elevated skin blood flow. It is commonly assumed that their compliance increases when venous wall temperature rises above normal. For example, an additional 250 ml of blood is displaced into cutaneous veins of the legs at a given transmural pressure during upright posture when leg skin temperature is elevated from 18°C to 44°C. The rise in "capacitance" with heating and the marked decrease with cooling has never been clearly distinguished from the purely passive effects of temperature-induced changes in blood flow on venous volume. The most important point is that locally induced *vaso*dilation and venous relaxation can only be partially overcome by sympathetic vasoconstriction.

Effect of Exercise on the Cutaneous Circulation

Is cutaneous blood flow during exercise determined by competing vasoconstrictor and vasodilator outflow or are both involved in moment-by-moment reflex modulation of flow? Despite the convenient location of cutaneous vessels on the body surface, this question has proven difficult to answer, not only for methodological reasons mentioned earlier, but also for reasons illustrated in Figure 6-10. This figure shows the complex competitive interaction between thermoregulatory and nonthermoregulatory reflexes in the control of skin blood flow. Thermoregulatory reflexes

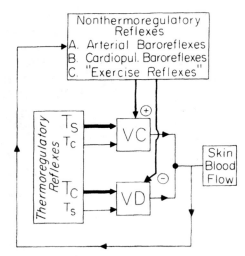

Figure 6-10 Schematic representation of control of skin blood flow via thermo- and nonthermoregulatory reflex control of vasoconstrictor (*VC*) and vasodilator (*VD*) outflow to skin. Thermoregulatory reflexes turn vasoconstriction and active vasodilation on (or off). Traditionally *nonthermoregulatory* reflexes were thought to modulate only vasoconstrictor tone, but current evidence also indicates inhibition $(-)$ of active vasodilation as well. (Revised from Rowell, 1986.)

are activated by the rise in body temperature during exercise. These reflexes inhibit vasoconstrictor outflow causing passive vasodilation, and at the same time they turn on the active (neurogenic?) vasodilator system. Also at the same time, reflexes associated with exercise (Chapters 11 and 12) activate the same sympathetic vasoconstrictor fibers whose tone would otherwise be withdrawn by rising body temperature. The net effects were reviewed by Rowell (1983) and by Johnson (1986).

The cutaneous vascular responses to exercise have been characterized as follows:

1. A transient vasoconstriction causes skin blood flow to fall below the resting, control level during the early moments of exercise before body temperature rises.
2. After reaching a nadir, skin blood flow increases to the pre-exercise control level and far beyond by a combination of withdrawal of vasoconstrictor outflow and by enlistment of active vasodilation as body temperature rises.
3. Relative to increments in even the most rapidly responding measures of central body temperature, the rise in skin blood flow is displaced to the right by exercise so that the *threshold* for vasodilation is reached at a higher body temperature than is so at rest.
4. Because of this elevated temperature threshold for vasodilation, skin blood flow is lower at any given internal temperature during exercise than it is at rest.

However, the rate of rise of skin blood flow in relation to rising internal temperature—the slope of the relationship—is usually unaffected by exercise (Johnson, 1986). Up to this point, there is currently agreement. The points are summarized in Figure 6-11.

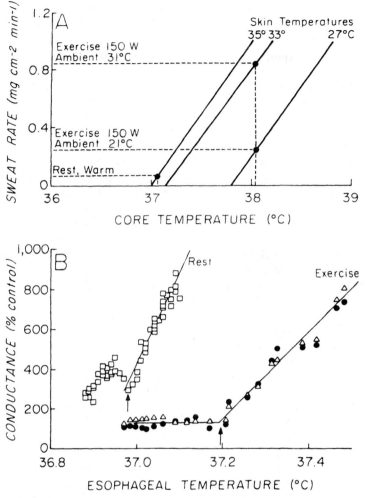

Figure 6-11   (A) Relationship between body core temperature and sweat rate at rest and exercise at two ambient temperatures. The rightmost slope (skin temperature 27°C) shows the rise in core temperature needed to cause the known sweating rate at that level of skin temperature and level of exercise. Less of a rise in core temperature is required to raise sweating to its observed level when skin temperature is elevated to 33°C by raising ambient temperature from 21 to 31°C. (Adapted from Brengelmann, 1989.) (B) Increase in vasodilator threshold (rise in skin vascular conductance at 37.2°C) caused by exercise. Open squares are normal skin at rest; solid circles are normal skin at exercise; open triangles are for skin with sympathetic adrenergic blockade by bretylium tosylate. (Adapted from Kellogg et al., 1991.)

The original interpretation of the preceding results was that exercise introduced an increase in sympathetic vasoconstrictor outflow that biased the relationship between skin blood flow and body temperature at all levels of exercise (Rowell, 1983). The rightward shift in skin blood flow relative to body temperature was seen as the consequence of the competition between vasoconstrictor outflow, which increases with severity of exercise, and vasodilator outflow, which also increases with severity of exercise because body temperature rises. It was assumed that vasodilator outflow was *not* influenced by nonthermoregulatory factors (based on the evidence that neurogenic vasodilators seem not to be effector mechanisms for major homeostatic reflexes) (e.g., Rowell, 1986).

The delayed increase in vasodilation (once believed due to competing vasoconstriction) *has the advantage of causing the rise in body temperature that is necessary to stimulate a sufficient increase in sweating* (see Figure 6-11) (Brengelmann, 1989). Inasmuch as skin temperature is little affected by an increase in work rate in a given environment, the increased heat production must be balanced by increased sweating. Sweating is driven upward mainly by a rise in core temperature. The increased sweat evaporation lowers skin temperature and widens the core temperature-skin temperature gradient so that more heat can be lost to the environment. This is crucially important to the prevention of hyperthermia during exercise.

Kellogg and coworkers (1990) have shown that baroreflexes can decrease skin blood flow by withdrawal of vasodilator outflow (this is in contrast to the widely held view that active vasodilator systems are not linked in any way with baroreflexes; that is, no one has seen activation of vasodilator mechanisms by baroreflexes other than transiently). Kellogg and coworkers (1990) used local iontophoresis of bretylium tosylate for selective blockade of sympathetic nerve fibers in local areas of skin. In another study, Kellogg and coworkers (1991a) compared the relative changes in laser-Doppler flowmetry signals in untreated areas of skin and showed that cutaneous vasoconstriction at the onset of exercise was actively mediated by sympathetic noradrenergic nerves and not passively mediated by withdrawal of vasodilator tone. They also showed that the elevated core temperature threshold for increased skin blood flow (i.e., the rightward shift in skin blood flow-core temperature curve in Figure 6-11) was caused by a delayed onset in vasodilator outflow to the skin (that is, bretylium blockade did not affect the response) (Kellogg et al., 1992) and *not* by increased vasoconstrictor outflow as proposed by Rowell (1983, 1986).

This discussion of neural control of skin blood flow is important because we are trying to understand how the cardiovascular system maintains a suitable balance between the fraction of cardiac output driven through the muscle pump and that supplied to the skin. As the fraction going through skin increases, the effect will be a decline in ventricular filling pressure and stroke volume (see Figure 6-15). The studies of Kellogg and colleagues (1991b) and Kenney and colleagues (1991) suggest that the control of skin blood flow during exercise, once skin blood flow has risen above control levels, is dominated by active vasodilation. Blockage of any sympathetic vasoconstriction by either bretylium tosylate or by α_1-adrenoceptor blockade (prazosin) did not affect the magnitude or rate of rise of forearm skin blood flow in relation to body temperature (these changes are confined to skin [Johnson and Rowell, 1975]).

Skin blood flow does not continue to rise without limit as body temperature increases during exercise. Several have shown that after a substantial rise in skin blood flow during exercise, there is a sudden decline in its rate of rise—a virtual plateau of skin blood flow in some cases. This occurs at or near a body temperature of approximately 38°C (Figure 6-12). The rate of rise of cardiac output has also been seen to decline similarly when external heat stress is imposed to raise skin blood flow and cardiac output (see Figure 6-15) (Rowell et al., 1969). This leveling off of skin blood flow and cardiac output was thought to be caused by arterial baroreflex activation of vasoconstrictor outflow to skin in order to prevent further decline in blood pressure (Brengelmann et al., 1977). This appears to be incorrect, because both Kenney and coworkers (1991) and Kellogg and coworkers (1991b) showed that adrenergic blockade did not alter this occurrence. Withdrawal of vasodilator outflow (or a marked [and improba-

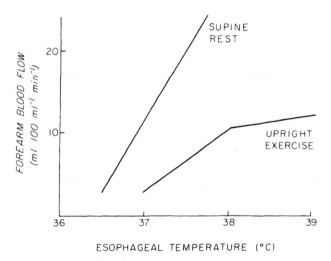

Figure 6-12   Forearm skin blood flow during direct whole-body heating at supine rest and moderate upright exercise. As in Figure 6-11B, exercise shifted the threshold for vasodilation to higher body temperature, causing skin blood flow to be lower at a given body temperature during rest than during exercise. When body temperature reached 39°C the rate of rise in skin blood flow decreased sharply (Brengelmann et al., 1977). Reduced vasodilator activity appears to account for this apparent upper limit for skin blood flow (Kellogg et al., 1991). (From Rowell, 1986, with permission of Oxford University Press.)

ble] rise in an unidentified circulating vasoconstrictor substance) appears to suppress the rate of rise in skin blood flow.

Is it still valid to postulate that the control of skin blood flow during exercise is mediated by baroreflexes as well as thermoregulatory reflexes? If it is valid, it would require that the baroreflex exert its control on skin blood flow by modulation of vasodilator activity. Although this would certainly be the most effective strategy, it is a unique one and clearly at odds with how we regard baroreflex control of sympathetic activity (e.g., Rowell, 1986).

Competing Demands for Cardiac Output: The Hemodynamic Consequences

The endogenous heat stress associated with prolonged high levels of exercise, with increased ambient temperature, or both, forces humans to deal with the two most powerful competing regulatory demands they ever face: the competition between skin and muscle for large fractions of cardiac output. Clearly at some level of exercise, cardiac output cannot rise enough to supply demands of both skin and muscle. We now know that cardiac output does not simply increase to supply both until the ability to raise cardiac output further is exhausted. This could occur at an oxygen uptake that is far below maximal because too large a fraction of cardiac output is going to skin where little oxygen is extracted (Rowell, 1974c, 1983).

This competition between skin and muscle for blood flow provides the best example of how the peripheral circulation determines the performance of the heart. Again, we return to Krogh's idea that the distribution of cardiac output determines the volume of blood available to the heart (Chapter 2). The shift in blood flow away from the muscle pump to a region of great capacitance (skin) means that the fraction of cardiac output perfusing the "second heart" is reduced. This causes a translocation of blood volume away from the heart and into peripheral veins along with a consequent decline in ventricular performance.

Figures 5-17 and 6-8 show the effects of raising and lowering cardiac output on right atrial pressure at a given rate of muscle blood flow. *The price we pay for pumping more blood through the skin or any "nonpumping" circuit during exercise, even if blood flow to active muscle stays constant, is a fall in ventricular filling pressure.* Even though movement helps to express some volume from cutaneous veins, which are well supplied with valves, Figure 6-13 schematically illustrates that the muscle pump does not work as well on cutaneous veins; ventricular filling pressure falls.

Central Hemodynamic Consequences of Cutaneous Vasodilation

Figure 6-14 shows the well-known phenomenon called "cardiovascular drift" associated with rising body temperature during prolonged exercise. Arterial and pulmonary pressures decline (central venous pressure also

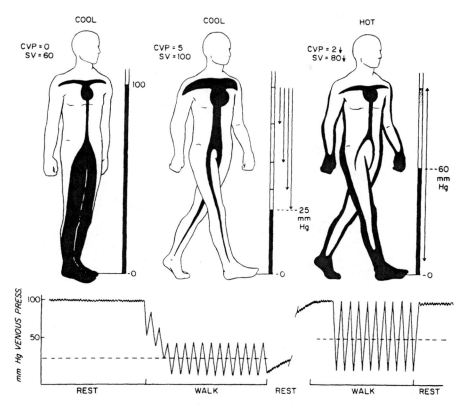

Figure 6-13   Heat stress alters the effectiveness of muscle pumping action on dependent cutaneous veins. Normally muscle contractions (cool) empty these veins and restore central venous pressure (*CVP*), stroke volume (*SV*), and central blood volume (darkened region extending from heart). Some rapid emptying of cutaneous veins in hot environments is counteracted by their rapid refilling, causing their average pressure and volume to be higher. As a consequence, central venous pressure, stroke volume, and central blood volume are lower in the heat. Note the rapid rise in venous pressure in the heat when exercise stops. (From Rowell, 1983, with permission of the American Physiological Society.)

declines) along with stroke volume (and thoracic blood volume) (Ekelund, 1967; Rowell, 1974c). This so-called drift is the consequence of progressive increase in the fraction of cardiac output directed to vasodilated skin as body temperature rises (Johnson and Rowell, 1975). Cardiac output may or may not increase with time despite the rise in skin blood flow; some see a progressive rise (Rowell, 1974c) and others do not (Saltin, 1964; Ekelund, 1967). Cooling the skin prevents cardiovascular drift during prolonged mild exercise (Rowell et al., 1969)

Figure 6-15 illustrates the points made so far about the effects of blood flow distribution on ventricular filling pressure and offers another

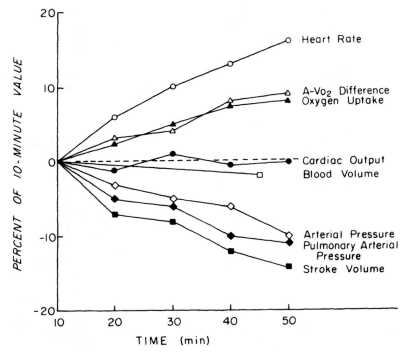

Figure 6-14 Circulatory responses to prolonged moderately heavy upright exercise in a neutral (20°C) environment. Values are expressed as the percentage change from values measured at the 10th minute of exercise. A gradual downward drift in systemic and pulmonary arterial pressures was accompanied by a fall in stroke volume. Cardiac output was maintained constant by increased heart rate. Most of the reduction in blood volume occurred before 10 minutes; little change occurred thereafter. Similar but less marked changes accompanied supine exercise (Ekelund, 1967). (From Rowell, 1986, with permission of Oxford University Press.)

experimental link to Figure 5-17. Figure 6-15 shows the "drift" during the first 30 minutes of exercise with body skin temperature held (by water-perfused suits) at neutral temperature. At 30 minutes, body skin temperature and skin blood flow were increased by rapidly raising skin temperature. Cardiac output rose and right atrial pressure and stroke volume fell in inverse proportion to the rise just as when cardiac output was changed by ventricular pacing in Figure 5-17.

A sudden drop in body skin temperature at 60 minutes in Figure 6-15 reflexly constricted cutaneous veins and that, along with the rapid fall in heart rate and cardiac output, promptly elevated right atrial pressure, stroke volume, and central blood volume.

The responses to heat stress (30 to 60 minutes in Figure 6-15) are analogous to those occurring in patients without control of the splanchnic circulation during exercise (Figure 6-7).

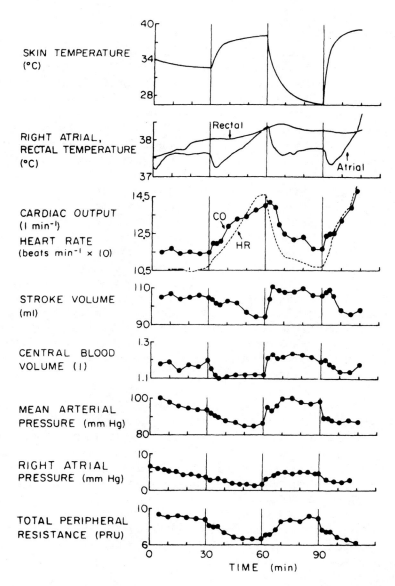

Figure 6-15   Cardiovascular responses to rapid changes in whole-body skin temperature (top panel) during upright exercise. Note rapid changes in right atrial blood temperature in contrast to rectal temperature (second panel). At 30 minutes and 90 minutes the rise in skin temperature caused reductions in stroke volume, central blood volume, and aortic and right atrial mean pressures. Cooling skin temperature at 60 minutes rapidly reversed these changes. Sustained cooling (60 to 90 minutes) abolished "cardiovascular drift." (From Rowell, 1986, with permission of Oxford University Press.)

Compensation for Cutaneous Vasodilation

Clearly we cannot sacrifice cutaneous blood flow for the sake of maintaining filling pressure; disabling hyperthermia would develop rapidly. The most striking regional vasomotor compensation observed during exercise in heat stress is the vasoconstriction in the splanchnic and renal circulations. Both have high blood flows that can be reduced markedly without compromising their oxygen supply. Rowell (1974c) estimated that the reduction in blood flow to these two regions during exercise and thermal stress could contribute an additional 800 ml of blood each minute to the skin.

Human circulatory adjustments to heat stress provide the best example of Krogh's ideas because reciprocal interaction between two large and compliant vascular beds is required. Consider regions C_{sk} and C_{sp} in Figure 6-8. The only effective strategy for compensating for the vasodilation of skin is to reduce blood flow in another highly compliant circuit, for example, the splanchnic circulation. The kidney, being a small noncompliant organ, does nothing to compensate for the shift of volume into the cutaneous vasculature. As illustrated in Figure 6-16, the consequences of diverting an increased fraction of cardiac output through the cutaneous circuit are partly compensated for by the passive shift of blood volume out of splanchnic veins when the resistance vessels upstream in the splanchnic circuit constrict. The compensation is not perfect, and central venous pressure and stroke volume fall (Figure 6-15).

The vasoconstriction in active muscle predicted previously (Rowell, 1974c, 1983) has not been observed during moderate to heavy exercise (that is, at levels at which there is still some reserve in oxygen extraction so that muscle blood flow could be reduced somewhat without sacrificing its oxygen uptake) (Savard et al., 1988). However, in a subsequent study at higher rates of oxygen uptake (60 to 70 percent of $\dot{V}o_2max$), Nielsen and colleagues (1990) again found a constant leg blood flow during exercise in cool followed by hot environmental conditions, but total oxygen uptake rose by more than 0.4 L min^{-1} in the heat. The rise in oxygen uptake (presumably in active muscle) during prolonged fatiguing exercise was not accompanied by increased leg blood flow, suggesting some vasoconstriction in muscle had indeed occurred. This is consistent with the marked increments observed in venous norepinephrine levels (presumably originating mainly from active muscle; see Chapter 7) during exercise coupled with heat stress (Figure 6-17) (Rowell et al., 1987).

Summary.   In summary, the basic idea put forward by Dastre and Morat in 1884 and also by Krogh in 1912, and others, was that, when blood flow through one compliant region increases, blood flow through another compliant region must decrease if filling pressure is to be maintained. This is borne out by findings from humans during exercise, but the compensation is not complete because ventricular filling pressure falls when skin

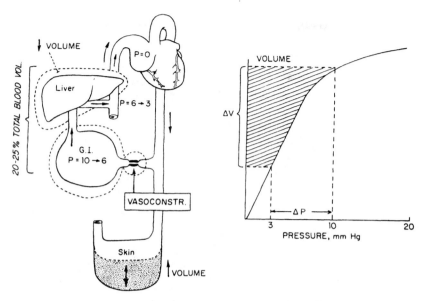

Figure 6-16   Schematic illustration of the reciprocal actions of splanchnic vasoconstriction and cutaneous vasodilation on blood volume distribution during heat stress—both at rest and during exercise. Volume is passively mobilized toward the heart by splanchnic vasoconstriction, and passively translocated into cutaneous veins by dilation of cutaneous arterioles. The rise in cardiac output lowers central venous pressure (P = 0) (Figure 6-15), increasing the initial pressure gradient from right atrium to hepatic veins. Vasoconstriction reduces pressures in hepatic veins (P = 6 → 3 [mm Hg]) and gastrointestinal (G.I.) veins (P = 10 → 6 [mm Hg]). Right panel shows steep splanchnic venous volume-pressure curve; a small decrease in venous pressure displaces a large volume of blood. (From Rowell, 1983, with permission from the American Physiological Society.)

blood flow is increased. Although sympathetic nervous activity and plasma norepinephrine concentration rise markedly, a surprise is the new finding that little of this sympathetic activity appears to be directed to skin after it is well vasodilated. Rather, a potentially hemodynamically disabling vasodilation by skin may be prevented during exercise by withdrawal of active vasodilation, whereas sympathetic vasoconstrictor outflow appears to be directed mainly to splanchnic organs and the kidneys, with skeletal muscle still in question.

Unique Importance of the Skin Circulation in Exercising Humans

A final comment about the stress imposed by rising body temperature during exercise is that humans and other primates appear to require mechanisms differing from those used by other species to protect the brain from hyperthermia during exercise. Humans appear to lack specialized structures that can make functionally significant changes in brain tempera-

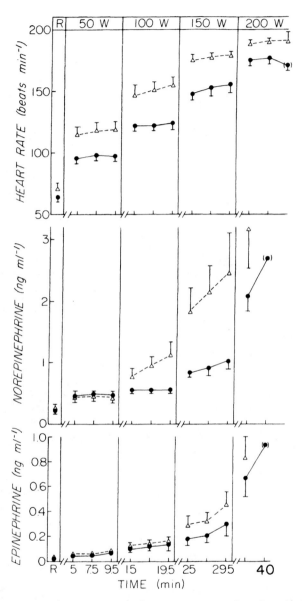

Figure 6-17   Average heart rate and plasma concentrations of norepinephrine and epinephrine in six subjects during continuous graded exercise at 50, 100, 150, and 200 watts. Solid circles show responses at neutral environmental temperature, and open triangles show responses when heat stress was added (body skin temperature held at 38°C). Increases in norepinephrine (but not epinephrine) above 50 watts were significant. Relationship between norepinephrine and heart rate was not significantly altered by heat stress. (From Rowell et al., 1987, with permission of the American Physiological Society.)

ture separate from changes in body temperature. In contrast, panting mammals possess a potent active vasodilator mechanism in the tongue where much of the heat exchange and evaporative cooling occurs. In addition, specialized vascular networks such as the carotid rete have large surface area for effective countercurrent exchange of heat between arteries and veins in the head; that is, blood going toward the brain loses its heat to cooler blood in veins flowing away from the nasopharynx. These structures minimize the rise in brain temperature during exercise, whereas body temperature may rise beyond levels tolerated by humans; that is, brain temperature is guarded at the expense of body temperature. These animals lack the body cooling provided by a humanlike cutaneous circulation.

In humans the entire burden of protecting the central nervous system from hyperthermia falls on sweating and the entire cutaneous circulation. This means *we must control brain and whole-body temperature together as a single unit.* This would explain why humans require such a great range of cutaneous blood flow under the control of a unique and powerful active vasodilator system.

There are those who disagree with the concepts stated above and argue that humans can maintain a brain temperature that is at least 1°C lower than body temperature during prolonged exercise (Cabanac, 1986). Counterarguments by Wenger (1987) and Brengelmann (1990) explain the apparently unattainable physical conditions required to achieve this large a temperature difference. Shiraki and coworkers (1988) directly measured deep brain temperature in a young patient who was receiving postsurgical therapy for a pineal tumor. When body temperature was raised by heated blankets to 38°C, cooling facial skin did not lower brain temperature as predicted by Cabanac (1986) (it did lower tympanic temperature, which is sensitive to changes in local skin temperature).

THE RENAL CIRCULATION

The renal artery branches into intralobular arteries, which give rise to the *afferent* arterioles supplying the functional units of the kidney—the nephrons. The afferent arteriole feeds into a tuft of capillaries called the glomerulus within Bowman's capsule. A nephron consists of Bowman's capsule, proximal tubule, loop of Henle, distal tubule, and collecting duct. There are about one million nephrons in each kidney. Because the emphasis here is on the control of organ blood flow, focus is on the afferent arterioles because they control the blood supply to the nephrons, which receive most of the total renal blood flow. Each glomerular capillary tuft empties into an *efferent* arteriole that supplies a network of peritubular capillaries surrounding proximal and distal tubules and collecting tubules. Again, as in the hepatic portal circulation, two capillary beds are arranged in series (i.e., a portal circulation).

Measurement of Renal Blood Flow

The measurement of renal blood flow by clearance of p-aminohippuric acid (PAH) constitutes a straightforward application of the Fick principle. PAH, together with about 20 percent of the renal plasma flow, is filtered in each pass through the glomeruli. This filtered plasma and PAH then pass through the proximal distal tubules. Nearly 80 percent of the PAH remains in the plasma as blood flows out of the glomerulus and into the network of capillaries surrouding the tubules—the peritubular capillaries. Most of this unfiltered PAH is then actively secreted from peritubular vessels into the proximal tubules and passes along with the filtered PAH into urine. In this way, about 95 percent of all PAH is removed from plasma by both filtration (approximately 20 percent) and active secretion (approximately 75 percent) in each pass through the kidney. As expressed in Equation 6-1, renal blood flow (RBF) is equal to the product of the concentration of PAH in urine (U) and the rate of urine formation in millimeters per minute (V). Ca is the concentration of PAH in arterial (or systemic venous) blood and Crv is the concentration in renal venous blood.

$$RBF = \frac{UV}{Ca - Crv} = \frac{UV}{0.95\,Ca} \qquad (6\text{-}1)$$

Because Crv is normally so close to zero, the renal vein is usually not catheterized in human subjects with normal kidneys. The method is basically sound, as demonstrated by Selkurt (1974), who simultaneously compared measurements of renal blood flow by Fick technique (PAH clearance) and by electromagnetic flow meters on the renal arteries of anesthetized dogs.

Renal Blood Flow and Blood Volume

In a supine resting human, the two kidneys normally receive 1,200 ml min^{-1} or about 20 percent of the cardiac output, making this the second largest regional circulation at rest (without heat stress). When related to the total renal mass of 300 g, blood flow is extremely high at about 400 ml 100 g^{-1} min^{-1}. Relative to total renal oxygen uptake (approximately 15 ml min^{-1}) the blood flow is still extremely high; the kidney extracts only 6 percent of the oxygen from blood so that renal arteriovenous oxygen difference is only about 1.2 ml O_2 100 ml^{-1}. Thus, like splanchnic organs and the skin, kidneys are overperfused relative to their metabolic needs.

Approximately 660 ml of plasma pass through the glomerular capillaries each minute, of which 20 percent or 130 ml min^{-1}, or 190 liters per day, are filtered and passed out of the circulation into the proximal tubule. Of this filtered volume, 188.5 liters are reabsorbed by the renal tubules each day, leaving only 1.6 L to pass into the bladder. As a consequence of this high filtration rate, our entire extracellular fluid volume is reworked or processed by filtration and reabsorption approximately 16 times per day.

The plasma volume by itself is processed about 60 times per day or once every 25 minutes (Smith, 1956).

Renal blood volume is small, ranging from only 12 to 72 ml 100 g^{-1} of kidney, depending on the methods of measurement. This volume is too small to be of hemodynamic significance.

Neural Control

Renal afferent arterioles are densely innervated by sympathetic noradrenergic nerve fibers supplied by the renal branches of the splanchnic nerves. Renal efferent arterioles, on the other hand, have sparse sympathetic innervation. In humans and other species, the renal arterioles usually receive little or no tonic vasoconstrictor nerve activity at rest. In addition, drugs that paralyze vascular smooth muscle often have minimal effects on renal blood flow under normal resting conditions (sometimes, however, vasodilation is observed). Therefore, the basal myogenic tone of renal arterioles, distended by normal levels of arterial blood pressure, appears to be slight. Accordingly, under normal resting conditions and in striking contrast to other major vascular beds, the renal circulation appears to be close to maximally dilated. The renal afferent arterioles are on the efferent arm of neural activity originating in arterial and cardiopulmonary baroreflexes, thermoregulatory reflexes, and reflexes associated with exercise and upright posture. The afferent arterioles appear also to be primarily responsible for the powerful *autoregulation* of renal blood flow when reflexes do not interfere with the intrinsic rise or fall in afferent arteriolar resistance in response to changing renal perfusion pressure (see Figure 6-20) (Knox and Spielman, 1983).

Humoral Control

The importance of the renin-angiotensin system in the control of blood volume and as an adjunct to sympathetic vasoconstriction in controlling blood pressure was emphasized in Chapter 3. Recall from Chapter 3 that the kidney is the primary source of renin, a proteolytic enzyme that initiates the formation of angiotensin I, which is subsequently converted into angiotensin II. Angiotensin II is a potent vasoconstrictor of renal and most other arterioles; it also facilitates sympathetic vasoconstriction, and it stimulates the release by the adrenal gland of aldosterone, which acts on the kidney to facilitate reabsorption of sodium, thereby playing a vital role in the regulation of plasma volume. Therefore, the renin-angiotensin system, which originates within the kidney, has a profound effect on the entire cardiovascular system.

Despite the rise in arterial pressure during exercise (a rise in pressure normally blunts adrenergically mediated renin release), plasma renin activity rises in proportion to the increases in heart rate, plasma norepinephrine concentration, and splanchnic and renal vascular resistances (Figure 3-1)

(Tidgren et al., 1991) (see Figure 6-19). Again, in exercise these changes begin when heart rate reaches approximately 100 beats min^{-1} (compare with rest in Figure 6-4). The functional importance of the renin-angiotensin system has been investigated by comparing systemic hemodynamic responses to exercise before and after preventing the formation of angiotensin II from angiotensin I by administering converting enzyme inhibitor; responses up to the level of $\dot{V}o_2max$ were, with one exception, unaffected by converting enzyme inhibitor (Fagard et al., 1982). $\dot{V}o_2max$ was also unaffected. The one exception was a slightly lower mean arterial pressure (average 7 mmHg), which was first observed when subjects sat up on the cycle ergometer. This small decrement in pressure simply persisted thereafter as a constant offset throughout each stage of exercise. An apparent orthostatic effect of converting enzyme inhibition was simply maintained, suggesting that angiotensin II does not contribute to the rise in arterial pressure with exercise. There is, however, indirect evidence suggesting that angiotensin II may be involved in the renal vasoconstriction in severe exercise (Tidgren et al., 1991) (see below).

The renin-angiotensin-aldosterone axis (Chapter 3) could play an important role during prolonged heavy exercise when renal conservation of salt and water becomes a key factor in plasma volume regulation.

Control of Renal Blood Flow During Exercise

Figure 6-18 shows the typical relationship between renal blood flow and heart rate, illustrated as well in Figures 3-1 and 6-3 (Grimby, 1965; Castenfors, 1967, 1977; Tidgren et al., 1991). Splanchnic and renal blood flows keep basically the same constant relationship to heart rate (Rowell, 1983), irrespective of whether heart rate is increased by prolonging the exercise at a given intensity, by increasing the intensity of exercise, or by superimposing heat stress on exercise. The same applies to norepinephrine concentration (Galbo et al., 1975; Rowell et al., 1987).

In a detailed investigation of renal neurohormonal responses to mild to severe dynamic exercise (supine posture) Tidgren and coworkers (1991) observed graded increases in the overflow of norepinephrine, renin, and immunoreactive neuropeptide Y into the left renal vein in normal young people (Figure 6-19). The exercise-elicited decrements in renal blood flow were similar to those observed by Grimby (1965) and Castenfors (1967, 1977), and average values are related to heart rate in Figure 6-18. Tidgren and coworkers (1991) measured renal venous outflow from the left kidney by a thermal dilution technique.

Dynamic exercise is a far more potent stimulus to sympathetic activation of the kidneys than other stresses such as mental stress, isometric exercise, or lower body suction and tilting, as judged from renal outpouring of norepinephrine, renin, and neuropeptide Y (for references, see Tidgren et al., 1991). Neuropeptide Y was released only at the highest levels of sympathetic activation. Tidgren and colleagues also observed marked

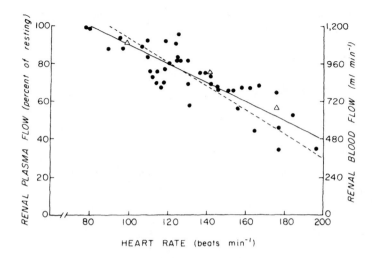

Figure 6-18 Relationship between renal plasma flow (also estimated renal blood flow) and heart rate during prolonged (45-minute) exercise at loads ranging from 25 to 150 watts. Solid line and data points from Grimby (1965) [y (renal plasma flow) = $-0.51 \times$ (heart rate) + 139, r = -0.89, n = 44]. Dashed line is from Castenfors (1977) [y = 517 $-$ 4.25 (x $-$ 114), r = -0.91, n = 47]. Renal blood flows were estimated from plasma flows with an assumed hematocrit of 48 percent. Three open triangles are average values from Tidgren and coworkers (1991), who measured renal venous blood flow by thermal dilution. Resting renal blood flow (100 percent) was taken as 1,200 ml min^{-1}. (Adapted from Rowell, 1986.)

increases in release of dopamine from the kidney; apparently human kidneys have a "subset" of dopaminergic nerves, the functional significance of which is unknown.

Most of the renal vasoconstriction during exercise is generally assumed to be caused by norepinephrine released from renal sympathetic nerves. This could be true in spite of the fact that the correlation between renal norepinephrine release and renal vascular resistance (which rose 140 percent) was poor, owing to individual variations in the relationship (much like those discussed in Chapter 4 for the relationship between muscle sympathetic nerve activity and venous norepinephrine concentration during hypoxemia).

The relationship between renal releases of renin and of norepinephrine was close, suggesting that renal sympathetic nerves initiated the renin release. At the highest work rate the sixfold increase in arterial epinephrine could also be expected to stimulate renin release; when these levels of epinephrine are reached by infusion without increased renal sympathetic nerve activity, renin levels increase (see Tidgren et al., 1991).

Angiotensin II was the variable most closely correlated with the rise in renal vascular resistance (this does not imply cause). However, Tidgren and colleagues could not determine if there was significant intrarenal

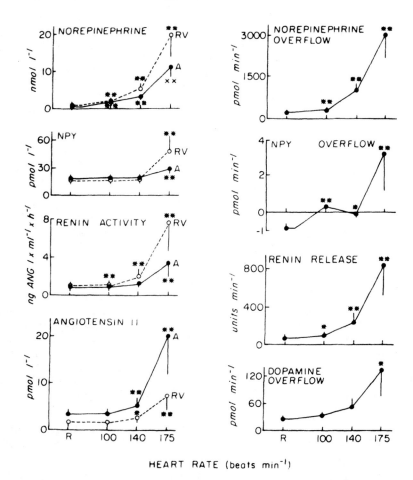

Figure 6-19 Renal neurohormonal responses to graded dynamic exercise (supine posture) in eight normal young humans. Exercise levels were 69, 132, and 188 watts. Arteriovenous differences across the kidney (*left column*) and renal overflows (*right column*) of norepinephrine, immunoreactive neuropeptide Y, renin, and dopamine are related to the average heart rates during exercise. The renal arteriovenous differences for angiotensin (*lower left*) and also for epinephrine (not shown) were positive, showing net renal uptake of these hormones. The three average values for renal blood flow at the three heart rates are in Figure 6-18. (Redrawn from Tidgren et al., 1991.)

formation of angiotensin II inasmuch as 60 percent of the angiotensin II entering the kidney via arterial blood was extracted both at rest and exercise. Neuropeptide Y (Figure 6-19) could have also contributed to the final increment in renal vascular resistance at the highest work rate when renal overflow of this peptide rose markedly.

These findings all confirm that dynamic exercise markedly increases sympathoadrenal system activity which is carried either directly via sympathetic nerves or indirectly through circulating hormones to many organs. This activation is pronounced in humans, baboons, and pigs, but much less so in dogs whose cardiac pumping capacity exceeds that of these other species.

CEREBRAL CIRCULATION

Maintenance of adequate blood flows to the brain and the heart are the most urgent tasks of the cardiovascular system. In contrast to other regions, *total* blood flow to the brain remains relatively constant under a variety of conditions. Despite this constancy of total flow, however, flows in different regions of the brain change markedly, paralleling changes in its regional activity. For reviews see Lassen (1974, 1978), Traystman (1981), and Heistad and Kontos (1983).

Cerebrovascular anatomy is extremely complex, and this complexity has contributed to the difficulties in measuring total and regional cerebral blood flow and understanding the factors that regulate it. It is clear that the brain is supplied mainly by two carotid and two vertebral arteries that eventually communicate with each other through anastomoses that form the circle of Willis. This interconnection with the circle of Willis guards cerebral perfusion when flow through a carotid artery is reduced. Another important feature of the cerebral circulation is called the "blood-brain barrier." This refers to a barrier between capillaries and cerebral interstitial fluid caused by tight junctions between capillary endothelial cells. The barrier provides the brain with a special fluid environment.

Measurement of Cerebral Blood Flow

Measurement of total cerebral blood flow in humans was based on an application of the Fick principle that employs the uptake of an inert foreign gas (commonly N_2O [nitrous oxide]). During 10 to 15 minutes of inhaling a mixture of N_2O, oxygen and nitrogen, the arterial-internal jugular venous N_2O difference is repeatedly determined until cerebral tissues are saturated with N_2O (krypton 85 or xenon 133 has also been used). After saturation, blood flow is calculated from the ratio of N_2O uptake and integrated arterial-venous N_2O difference. The method is limited by its applicability only to steady states of flow and by its inability to reveal important regional differences in cerebral flow. Another potentially serious problem is the contamination of internal jugular venous blood with blood from extracranial tissues. Although this contamination may be relatively small in humans, its greater prevalence in other species has called into question measurements of cerebral blood flow by flow meters placed on veins draining the brain. Despite the wide variety of techniques that have been applied, there is still no single method that is acceptable as a valid standard for total cerebral blood flow. The advantages and disadvantages of various methods have been reviewed by Edvinsson and MacKenzie (1977), Lassen (1974), and Heistad and Kontos (1983).

The most important methodological advance in humans is the determination of relative changes in regional cerebral blood flow by regional clearances of xenon 133 after its injection into a carotid artery. Clearances are monitored by scintillation detectors arranged around the head. This technique has allowed observers to match local blood flow with local neural activity when specific parts of the brain are involved in a task (see Lassen et al., 1981). In separate studies, the linkage between regional hyperemia and increased metabolism was demonstrated by measuring the local metabolic rate by the uptake of [^{14}C]deoxyglucose, a metabolically inert form of glucose (Sokoloff, 1977).

Blood Flow

The brain, which weighs approximately 1,400 g and is about 2 percent of body weight, receives 50 to 60 ml 100 g^{-1} min^{-1} or 750 ml min^{-1} of blood, which is 12 to 15 percent of resting cardiac output. Total cerebral oxygen uptake is 40 to 50 ml min^{-1} or 3 to 3.5 ml 100 g^{-1} min^{-1} of oxygen. This accounts for 15 to 20 percent of the basal metabolic rate. The brain is encased in a rigid cranium and therefore the tissue is essentially incompressible and total brain blood volume is constant. Large chemically or metabolically induced changes in regional and total cerebral blood flow do occur, despite the constant volume, and markedly alter the pressure-flow relationship in the autoregulatory zone for that region, but not for the brain as a whole.

Neural Control

Cerebral blood vessels are innervated by noradrenergic sympathetic nerve fibers; however, their intracranial distribution is heterogeneous and the role of these fibers in the regulation of cerebral blood flow is not well understood. One point of view is that the importance of neural control in some studies is exaggerated because the cerebral blood flow measurements included *extracranial* tissues that react strongly to increased sympathetic nervous activity. Sympathetic vasoconstrictor influences in cerebral blood vessels are thought by most to be small. Blockade of sympathetic nerves is not associated with increased cerebral blood flow, that is, there is no tonic influence. Also, maximal sympathetic nerve stimulation at 15 Hz causes only minor and transient increases in cerebral vascular resistance; this is in contrast to the maintained five- to six-fold increases in resistance observed in skeletal muscle, for example, with similar stimulation. In addition to their sympathetic nerve fibers, the surface vessels of the brain are innervated by parasympathetic cholinergic nerve fibers, which are in close proximity to the noradrenergic fibers. It has been suggested that this proximity allows acetylcholine to modulate norepinephrine release

(Vanhoutte et al., 1981). Peptidergic nerve fibers are also present and vessels also contain histamine, but the significance of these features is unknown (Duckles, 1981; Owman and Hardebo, 1981). In general, cerebral vessels have unusual neural effector mechanisms in that their α-receptors are insensitive to norepinephrine and also their dependence on calcium is different from that of other vessels.

Sympathetic nerves seem not to play a role in the overall reflex control of cerebral blood flow such as that seen in other organs. There is no cerebral vascular response to even the most powerful baroreflex. The most important function of cerebral sympathetic nerves may be to protect cerebral vessels by constricting them rapidly during sudden and extreme increases in blood pressure. They may also modulate cerebrospinal fluid formation and protect the blood-brain barrier during acute hypertension, which can physically disrupt the barrier (Heistad and Kontos, 1983).

Local Metabolic and Chemical Control

The constancy of *total* cerebral blood flow during intense mental activity originally led to the belief that metabolic regulation of cerebral vascular resistance did not occur. The newer methods for measuring regional cerebral blood flow in humans, combined with techniques for assessing regional metabolic rate (i.e., cellular uptake of [^{15}O]- or [^{14}C]deoxyglucose) clearly show that cerebral blood flow and metabolism are closely linked. Presumably the rise in blood flow to one region is compensated for by a fall in flow elsewhere so that total flow is kept essentially constant by an unknown mechanism (a relative insensitivity of methods for measuring total flow could mask small changes).

The usual list of candidates for metabolic vasodilators applies to the brain just as to skeletal muscle and other regions. It is difficult to believe that these candidates vary significantly from organ to organ despite special pleas to the contrary. The most promising candidates (discussed in more detail in Chapter 7) are Pco_2, potassium, pH, decreased Po_2, adenosine, Krebs cycle intermediates, and so on.

The cerebral circulation has a uniquely high responsiveness to changes in blood gases. This has led some to propose that these factors are the primary controllers of cerebral blood flow, a view that is no longer considered tenable under most conditions. It is clear, however, that alterations in arterial Pco_2 and Po_2 caused by various breathing patterns can have profound effects on cerebral blood flow. These reactions are important during exposure to high altitude and hypoxemia, and can also occur during hyperthermia as well as during severe exercise at sea level. Figure 6-20A shows the relationship between arterial Pco_2 and cerebral blood flow; Figure 6-20B shows the relationship between flow and arterial Po_2. In humans, inhalation of 5 percent CO_2 causes a 50 percent increase in cerebral blood flow. Inhalation of 7 percent oxygen causes a 100 percent increase in flow. The vasodilator effect of increased CO_2 concentration is

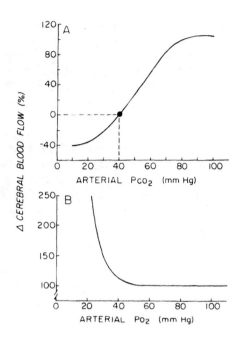

$PaCO_2 \uparrow$, $CBF\uparrow$
$PaO_2 \uparrow$, $CBF\downarrow$

Figure 6-20 (**A**) Relationship between arterial P_{CO_2} and the percent change in cerebral blood flow in dogs. (**B**) Relationship between arterial oxygen tension and cerebral blood flow as percent of resting value (100 percent) in dogs. Arterial P_{CO_2} was maintained constant. (Adapted from Rowell, 1986.)

mediated by the increase in cerebral extracellular fluid pH. Molecular CO_2 and HCO_3^- per se have little or no direct vasodilator effect (Heistad and Kontos, 1983). Lipid-soluble gases such as CO_2 pass rapidly through the blood-brain barrier, and in the cerebral extracellular fluid the CO_2 reacts with water to form H^+ and HCO_3^-. The H^+ causes the vasodilation. A rise in *arterial* H^+ concentration does not increase cerebral blood flow because H^+ crosses the relatively impermeable blood-brain barrier so slowly.

The dilation of cerebral arteries by a low partial pressure of oxygen is probably mediated by the local production of metabolites; adenosine may play an important role (Winn et al., 1981). The vasodilation is not a direct effect of oxygen on vascular smooth muscle. Prostaglandins do not appear to be involved. Cerebral blood flow (in dogs) was surprisingly insensitive to reduced oxygen tension down to an arterial P_{O_2} of about 50 mmHg; below this value, cerebral blood flow rose markedly as resistance fell (arterial P_{CO_2} was kept constant) (Figure 6-20B). Responses to reductions in arterial P_{O_2} in humans are roughly similar to those shown in Figure 6-20B (Shapiro et al., 1970). Between an arterial P_{O_2} of 68 and 49 mmHg, cerebral blood flow rose sharply. However when arterial P_{CO_2} fell to 27 mmHg, due to hyperventilation, cerebral blood flow fell back almost to prehypoxia levels. During hypoxemia, hyperventilation reduces $PaCO_2$ so that the vasoconstrictor effects of hypocapnia compete with the vasodilator effects of hypoxia. Therefore hyperventilation during severe exercise will tend to reduce cerebral blood flow, even if arterial P_{O_2} were reduced by altitude or suboptimal pulmonary function (Dempsey et al., 1975).

Hormonal Control

The blood-brain barrier restricts the influence of circulating hormones on the cerebral circulation. This barrier to water-soluble molecules and ions also insulates brain cells from rapid fluctuations in the composition of plasma. It isolates brain cells from bloodborne vasoactive agents such as epinephrine, norepinephrine, angiotensin II, and vasopressin. Thus the brain is protected from the great swings in plasma hormone levels attending severe exertion. The restraint offered by cerebral capillaries differs radically from the negligible resistance to transport imposed by most capillaries such as those in skin and skeletal muscle, for example, where transcapillary transport of water-soluble molecules is determined mainly by molecular size and the size of pores in the capillary wall.

Autoregulation

Possibly the most striking feature of the cerebral circulation is the relative constancy of blood flow over a wide range of blood pressures, called autoregulation. The cerebral pressure-flow curve as it is depicted in Figure 6-21 shows the autoregulated portion to have a definite upward slope with rising pressure. In humans there may be as much as a 6 to 7 percent decrease in flow for every 10-mmHg reduction in arterial blood pressure over the autoregulatory range (see Chapter 2) (Heistad and Kontos, 1983).

The Cushing Reflex: An "Agonal Reflex"

Reflexes that serve to solve one problem while creating an equally serious one are sometimes called "agonal" reflexes. The Cushing reflex is an excellent example. This reflex occurs in response to increased intracranial pressure caused by bleeding into the cerebrospinal fluid after a serious head injury. Here the cranium and cerebrospinal fluid behave as a "Starling resistor," as illustrated in Figure 6-22. As cerebrospinal fluid pressure increases, effective perfusion pressure or transmural pressure of cerebral

Figure 6-21 Schematic illustration of *autoregulation*. In the autoregulatory zone, blood flow rises much less with increasing driving pressure and vascular resistance rises. The range of blood pressure encompassing the autoregulatory zone varies from organ to organ. (From Rowell, 1986, with permission of Oxford University Press.)

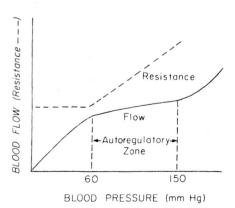

vessels decreases. At first, cerebral blood flow tends to remain constant because of autoregulatory vasodilation; then cerebrospinal fluid pressure reduces cerebral blood flow to a *threshold* level at which ischemia activates the Cushing reflex, as indicated by the bold arrows in Figures 6-23A and B. *This reflex, along with the reflex arising from active muscle when it is rendered ischemic* (Chapter 11) *are the two most powerful blood pressure-raising reflexes known.* The putative stimulus for the intense widespread vasoconstriction is a local accumulation of metabolites in the vasomotor "centers" of an ischemic medulla. This reflex accounts for the extreme hypertension seen in victims of severe head injury. It is called an "agonal reflex" because its *positive feedback* usually leads to death; that is, the hypertension increases cerebral perfusion pressure, which increases the bleeding into cerebrospinal fluid, which in turn raises cerebrospinal fluid pressure even more and further decreases cerebral blood flow in a "vicious cycle." The approach to studying such reflexes is discussed below because it is used repeatedly throughout the remainder of the book.

"Open-Loop" Experiments

Our quantitative understanding of the strength or sensitivity (often called "gain") of reflexes comes from what are called "open-loop experiments."

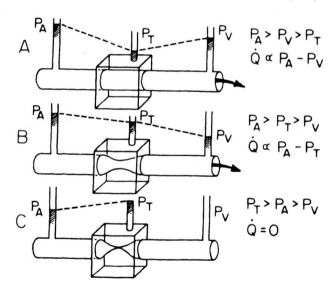

Figure 6-22 The "Starling resistor" model to show the effects of surrounding tissue pressure on arterial inflow (P_A) and venous outflow pressure (P_V) differences. In part A both P_A and P_V exceed box pressure (or tissue pressure) (P_T). So the flow (Q) is proportional to $P_A - P_V$. In part B, P_T exceeds P_V but not P_A so that $\dot{Q}$ is determined by the difference between P_A and P_T rather than P_A and P_V. When P_T exceeds P_A, $\dot{Q} = 0$; Q can only be restored by raising P_A or lowering P_T. (From Rowell, 1986, with permission of Oxford University Press.)

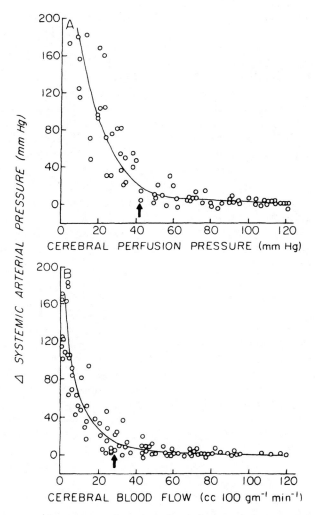

Figure 6-23 Quantification of the strength of the pressor response to cerebral ischemia (Cushing reflex) in dogs. (**A**) Rise in systemic arterial pressure in response to lowering cerebral arterial perfusion pressure. The cerebral circulation was isolated from the systemic circulation so that input was independent of output ("open-loop" experiment). Also the reflex rise in systemic pressure (pressor response) was unopposed by baroreflexes—baroreceptors were denervated. Average slope (Δ systemic pressure/Δ cerebral pressure) expresses the "open-loop" gain of the reflex above its *threshold*, marked by arrow. (**B**) Relationship between cerebral blood flow and the rise in systemic pressure from experiments on the same animals (compare with Figure 11-12). (Adapted from Sagawa et al., 1961.)

"Open-loop" means that the primary feedback loop in the reflex has been abolished or opened so that the receptors are isolated from the influence of their afferent neural output on the system; that is, they are deprived of the feedback that counteracts the stimulus.

Sagawa and colleagues (1961) quantified the sensitivity of the Cushing reflex by isolating the arterial side of the cerebral circulation from the systemic circulation. In this way, cerebral *input* pressure could be controlled at any desired level and be independent of the *output,* namely, the effect of the reflex on systemic arterial pressure. They also eliminated the negative feedback from the arterial baroreceptors on the output variable, systemic arterial pressure by denervating the carotid sinus and aortic baroreceptors. This open-loop experiment yielded a sensitivity, expressed as the change in systemic arterial pressure divided by the change in cerebral perfusion pressure, that averaged -7.7. This so-called "open-loop gain" (G_{OL}) can be expressed as the closed-loop gain (G_{CL}) that would exist in the presence of feedback that counteracts the stimulus in the following expression:

$$G_{CL} = \frac{G_{OL}}{1 - G_{OL}} = -0.89 \qquad (6\text{-}2)$$

where G_{CL} is negative because the slope relating output to input is negative. This calculation indicates that the Cushing reflex could, in theory, correct by 89 percent any mismatch between cerebral perfusion pressure and cerebral metabolism. This is a powerful emergency mechanism to protect the brain from ischemia. The experimental approach used in this study was applied later to investigate the mechanisms that protect skeletal muscle from ischemia during exercise (Chapter 11) or that protect arterial pressure (Chapter 12). The problem with the approach here is that as it is calculated, "gain" is based on changes in *pressure* rather than *flow,* or more importantly, the concentration of metabolites causing the response, that is, the error being corrected.

The preceding is one of the two best examples we have of a reflex pressor response to ischemia. The other example is the pressor reflex arising from skeletal muscle. The reason for the detail in this discussion is that both are studied as open-loop experiments, both have a threshold, and both have similar gains when competing influences of the arterial baroreflex are removed. Both raise pressure in order to restore flow. In contrast to the Cushing reflex, the reflex from ischemic muscle is a putative controller of the circulation during exercise (compare Figure 6-23 with Figure 11-12). The analogy will be revealing.

Control of Cerebral Blood Flow During Exercise

The factors presumed to have the greatest influence on *total* cerebral blood flow during exercise are blood tensions of CO_2 and oxygen (H^+ and circulating vasoactive hormones do not cross the blood-brain barrier in significant amounts). For example, hyperventilation during severe exercise lowers Pa_{CO_2} and can constrict cerebral arteries (Figure 6-20A) even if vasoconstriction is opposed by a modest fall in Pa_{O_2} (Figure 6-20B). Also a rise in arterial pressure will cause an autoregulatory vasoconstriction (Heistad and Kontos, 1983).

In the earliest studies of human cerebral blood flow, the N_2O method was used and most observers found that average blood flow through the entire brain was unaffected by exercise (see Thomas et al., 1989). Different results were obtained when cortical blood flow was determined from ^{133}Xe washout technique (Olesen, 1971).

Thomas and colleagues (1989) measured the cerebral clearance rate of ^{133}Xe in 16 normal people during rest and semirecombant cycle ergometer exercise up to 86 percent of their $\dot{V}_{O_2}$max. They observed significant *increases* in cerebral blood flow when oxygen uptake exceeded 40 percent of $\dot{V}_{O_2}$max. The increments in flow averaged 31 percent and 58 percent above resting values, depending on how the ^{133}Xe clearance data were analyzed. The increments in ^{133}Xe clearance could not be explained by temperature-induced cutaneous vasodilation on the head; cooling the scalp to reduce skin perfusion did not affect the results. Similar results from a study employing only hand movement (Olesen, 1971) suggests that the mass of muscle activated via the motor cortex was not a factor, as might be predicted from the greater cortical respresentation for the hands.

When Manohar (1987) determined regional brain blood flow via the radioactive microsphere (15μm) technique in ponies during moderate and severe exertion, he found significant work-related increases in blood flow to the cerebellar cortex. No significant increases were found in blood flow to the cerebral cortex, cerebral and cerebellar white matter, thalamus-hypothalamus, midbrain, pons, and medulla.

REFERENCES

Ashkar, E. (1973). Effects of bilateral splanchnicectomy on circulation during exercise in dogs. *Acta Physiol. Lat. Am. 23,* 171–177.
Blackmon, J.R., L.B. Rowell, J.W. Kennedy, R.D. Twiss, and R.D. Conn (1967). Physiological significance of maximal oxygen intake in pure mitral stenosis. *Circulation 36,* 497–510.
Bradley, S.E. (1963). The hepatic circulation. In W.F. Hamilton and P. Dow, eds. *Handbook of Physiology. Circulation,* sect. 2, vol. II, pp. 1387–1438. American Physiological Society, Washington, D.C.
Bradley, S.E., P.A. Parks, P.C. Reynell, and J. Meltzer (1953). The circulating splanchnic blood volume in dog and man. *Trans. Assoc. Am. Physicians 66,* 294–302.
Brengelmann, G.L. (1989). Temperature regulation. In C.C. Teitz, ed. *Scientific Foundations of Sports Medicine,* pp. 77–116. B.C. Decker, Philadelphia.
Brengelmann, G.L. (1990). Brain cooling via emissary veins: fact or fancy? [Commentary]. In: Falk, D. Brain evolution in homo: the "radiator" theory. *Behav. Brain Sci. 13.* 349–350.

Brengelmann, G.L., P.R. Freund, L.B. Rowell, J.E. Olerud, and K.K. Kraning (1981). Absence of active cutaneous vasodilation associated with congenital absence of sweat glands in humans. *Am. J. Physiol. 240 (Heart Circ. Physiol. 9)*, H571–H575.

Brengelmann, G.L., J.M. Johnson, L. Hermansen, and L.B. Rowell (1977). Altered control of skin blood flow during exercise at high internal temperature. *J. App. Physiol. (Respir. Environ. Exercise Physiol.) 43*, 790–794.

Cabanac, M. (1986). Keeping a cool head. *News Physiol. Sci. 1*, 41.

Castenfors, J. (1967). Renal function during exercise. With special reference to exercise proteinuria and the release of renin. *Acta Physiol. Scand. 70 (Suppl. 293)*, 1–44.

Castenfors, J. (1977). Renal function during prolonged exercise. In *Ann. N.Y. Acad. Sci. 301*, 151–159.

Clausen, J.-P. (1977). Effect of physical training on cardiovascular adjustments to exercise in man. *Physiol. Rev. 57*, 779–815.

Clausen, J.-P., and J. Trap-Jensen (1974). Arteriohepatic venous oxygen difference and heart rate during initial phases of exercise. *J. Appl. Physiol. 37*, 716–719.

Dastre, A.F., and J.P. Morat (1884). Influence du sang asphyxique sur l'appareil nerveux de la circulation. *Arch. Physiol. Pathol. 3 (Ser. 3)*, 1–45.

Dempsey, J.A., J.M. Thomson, S.C. Alexander, H.V. Forster, and L.W. Chosy (1975). Respiratory influences on acid-base status and their effects on O_2 transport during prolonged muscular work. In H. Howald and J.R. Poortmans, eds. *Metabolic Adapation to Prolonged Physical Exercise*, pp. 56–64. Birkhauser Verlag, Basel.

Detry J.-M.R., G.L. Brengelmann, L.B. Rowell, and C. Wyss (1972). Skin and muscle components of forearm blood flow in directly heated resting man. *J. Appl. Physiol. 32*, 506–511.

Duckles, S.P. (1981). Vasodilator innervation of cerebral blood vessels. In P.M. Vanhoutte and I. Leusen, eds. *Vasodilation*, pp. 27–37. Raven Press, New York.

Edvinsson, L., and E.T. MacKenzie (1977). Amine mechanisms in the cerebral circulation. *Pharmacol. Rev. 28*, 275–348.

Ekelund, L.-G. (1967). Circulatory and respiratory adaptation during prolonged exercise. *Acta Physiol. Scand. 70 (Suppl. 292)*, 1–38.

Fagard, R., P. Lijnen, L. Vanhees, and A. Amery (1982). Hemodynamic response to converting enzyme inhibition at rest and exercise in humans. *J. Appl. Physiol. 53*, 576–581.

Fixler, D.E., J.A. Atkins, J.H. Mitchell, and L.D. Horowitz (1976). Blood flow to respiratory, cardiac, and limb muscles in dogs during graded exercise. *Am. J. Physiol. 231*, 1515–1519.

Fox, R.H., and S.M. Hilton (1958). Bradykinin formation in human skin as a factor in heat vasodilatation. *J. Physiol. (Lond.) 142*, 219–232.

Froelich, J.W., H.W. Strauss, R.H. Moore, and K.A. McKusick (1988). Redistribution of visceral blood volume in upright exercise in healthy volunteers. *J. Nucl. Med. 29*, 1714–1718.

Galbo, H., J.J. Holst, and N.J. Christensen (1975). Glucagon and plasma catecholamine responses to graded and prolonged exercise in man. *J. Appl. Physiol. 38*, 70–76.

Greenway, C.V., and R.D. Stark (1971). Hepatic vascular bed. *Physiol. Rev. 51*, 23–65.

Grimby, G. (1965). Renal clearances during prolonged supine exercise at different loads. *J. Appl. Physiol. 29*, 1294–1298.

Haase, E.B., and A.A. Shoukas (1991). Carotid sinus baroreceptor reflex control of venular pressure-diameter relations in rat intestine. *Am. J. Physiol. 260 (Heart Circ. Physiol. 29)*, H752–H758.

Heistad, D.D., and H.A. Kontos (1983). Cerebral circulation. In J.T. Shepherd, F.M. Abboud, and S.R. Geiger, eds. *Handbook of Physiology. The Cardiovascular System: Peripheral Circulation and Organ Blood Flow*, sect. 2, vol. III, part 1, pp. 137–182. American Physiological Society, Bethesda, MD.

Hökfelt, T., O. Johansson, A. Ljungdahl, J.M. Lundberg, and M. Schultzberg. (1980). Peptidergic neurons. *Nature 284*, 515–521.

Johnson, J.M. (1986). Nonthermoregulatory control of human skin blood flow. *J. Appl. Physiol. 61*, 1613–1622.

Johnson, J.M., and L.B. Rowell (1975). Forearm skin and muscle vascular responses to prolonged leg exercise in man. *J. Appl. Physiol. 39*, 920–924.

Johnson, J.M., W.F. Taylor, A.P., Shepherd, and M.K. Park (1984). Laser-Doppler measurement of skin blood flow: comparison with plethysmography. *J. Appl. Physiol. (Respir. Environ. Exercise Physiol.) 56*, 798–803.

Katz, L.N., and S. Rodbard (1939). The integration of the vasomotor responses in the liver with those in other systemic vessels. *J. Pharmacol. Exp. Ther. 67*, 407–422.

Keatinge, W.R., and M.C. Harman (1980). *Local Mechanisms Controlling Blood Vessels*. Acadmic Press, New York.

Kellogg, D.L. Jr., J.M. Johnson, and W.A. Kosiba (1990). Baroreflex control of the cutaneous active vasodilator system in humans. *Circ. Res. 66*, 1420–1426.

Kellogg, D.L. Jr., J.M. Johnson, and W.A. Kosiba (1991a). Competition between cutaneous active vasoconstriction and active vasodilation during exercise in humans. *Am. J. Physiol. 261 (Heart Circ. Physiol. 30)*, H1184–H1189.

Kellogg, D.L., Jr., J.M. Johnson, and W.A. Kosiba (1991c). Control of internal temperature theshold for active cutaneous vasodilation by dynamic exercise. *J. Appl. Physiol. 71*, 2476–2483.

Kellogg, D.D., Jr., W.L. Kenney, J.M. Johnson, and W.A. Kosiba (1991b). Neural mechanisms of altered control of skin blood flow during prolonged exercise. *FASEB J. 5*, A774.

Kenney, W.L., C.G. Tankersley, D.L. Newswanger, and S.M. Puhl (1991). α_1-Adrenergic blockade does not alter control of skin blood flow during exercise. *Am. J. Physiol. 260 (Heart Circ. Physiol. 29)*, H855–H861.

Knox, F.G., and W.S. Spielman (1983). Renal circulation. In J.T. Shepherd, F.M. Abboud, and S.R. Geiger, eds. *Handbook of Physiology. The Cardiovascular System: Peripheral Circulation and Organ Blood Flow*, sect. 2, vol. III, part 1, pp. 183–217. American Physiological Society, Bethesda, MD.

Lassen, N.A. (1974). Control of cerebral circulation in health and disease. *Circ. Res. 34*, 749–760.

Lassen, N.A. (1978). Brain. In P.C. Johnson, ed. *Peripheral Circulation*, pp. 337–358. Wiley, New York.

Lassen, N.A., L. Henriksen, and O. Paulson (1981). Regional cerebral blood flow in stroke by [133]Xenon inhalation and emission tomography. *Stroke 12*, 284–288.

Lautt, W.W. (1980). Hepatic nerves: a review of their functions and effects. *Can. J. Physiol. Pharmacol. 58*, 105–123.

Lundberg, J., L. Norgren, E. Ribbe, I. Rosen, S. Steen, J. Thorne, and B.G. Wallin (1989). Direct evidence of active sympathetic vasodilatation in the skin of the human foot. *J. Physiol. (Lond.) 417*, 437–446.

Lynn, R.B., S.M. Sancetta, F.A. Simeone, and R.W. Scott (1952). Observations on the circulation in high spinal anesthesia. *Surgery 32*, 195–213.

Manohar, M. (1987). Regional distribution of brain blood flow during maximal exertion in splenectomized ponies. *Respir. Physiol. 68*, 77–84.

Müller, O. (1905). Über die Blutverteilung im menschichen Korper unter dem Einfluss thermischer Reize. *Arch. Klin. Med. 84*, 547–585.

Nielsen, B., G. Savard, E.A. Richter, M. Hargreaves, and B. Saltin (1990). Muscle blood flow and muscle metabolism during exercise and heat stress. *J. Appl. Physiol. 69*, 1040–1046.

Olesen, J. (1971). Contralateral focal increase of cerebral blood flow in man during arm work. *Brain 94*, 635–646.

Owman, C., and J.E. Hardebo (1981). Mechanisms of cerebral vasodilatation: amines, peptides, and the blood-brain barrier. In P.M. Vanhoutte and I. Leusen, eds. *Vasodilatation*, pp. 159–174. Raven Press, New York.

Peronnet, F., J. Cleroux, H. Perrault, D. Cousineau, J. DeChamplain, and R. Nadeau (1981). Plasma norepinephrine response to exercise before and after training in humans. *J. Appl. Physiol. (Respir. Environ. Exercise Physiol.) 51*, 812–815.

Robinson, B.F., S.E. Epstein, R.L. Kahler, and E. Braunwald (1966). Circulatory effects of acute expansion of blood volume: studies during maximal exercise and at rest. *Circ. Res. 19*, 26–32.

Roddie, I.C. (1983). Circulation to skin and adipose tissue. In J.T. Shepherd, F.M. Abboud, and S.R. Geiger, eds. *Handbook of Physiology. The Cardiovascular System: Peripheral Circulation and Organ Blood Flow*, sect. 2, vol. III, part 1, pp. 285–317. American Physiological Society, Bethesda, MD.

Rothe, C.F. (1983). Venous system: physiology of the capicitance vessels. In J.T. Shepherd, F.M. Abboud, and S.R. Geiger, eds. *Handbook of Physiology. The Cardiovascular System: Peripheral Circulation and Organ Blood Flow*, sect. 2, vol. III, part 1, pp. 397–452. American Physiological Society, Bethesda, MD.

Rowell, L.B. (1974a). Dye technique for estimating hepatic-splanchnic blood flow in man. In D.A. Bloomfield, ed. *Dye Curves: The Theory and Practice of Non-Diffusible Indicator Dilution*, pp. 209–229. University Park Press, University Park, PA.

Rowell, L.B. (1974b). The splanchnic circulation. In T.C. Ruch and H.D. Patton, eds. *Physiology and Biophysics. II. Circulation, Respiration and Fluid Balance*, pp. 215–233. W.B. Saunders, Philadelphia.

Rowell, L.B. (1974c). Human cardiovascular adjustments to exercise and thermal stress. *Physiol. Rev. 54*, 75–159.

Rowell, L.B. (1977). Competition between skin and muscle for blood flow during exercise. In E.R. Nadel, ed. *Problems with Temperature Regulation During Exercise*, pp. 49–76. Academic Press, New York.

Rowell, L.B. (1981). Active neurogenic vasodilatation in man. In P.M. Vanhoutte and I. Leusen, eds. *Vasodilatation*, pp. 1–17. Raven Press, New York.

Rowell, L.B. (1983). Cardiovascular adjustments to thermal stress. In J.T. Shepherd, F.M. Abboud, and S.R. Geiger, eds. *Handbook of Physiology. The Cardiovascular System: Peripheral Circulation and Organ Blood Flow*, sect. 2, vol. III, part 2, pp. 967–1023. American Physiological Society, Bethesda, MD.

Rowell, L.B. (1984). Reflex control of regional circulations in humans. *J. Auton. Nerv. Syst. 11*, 101–114.

Rowell, L.B. (1986). *Human Circulation: Regulation During Physical Stress.* Oxford University Press, New York.

Rowell, L.B., J.R. Blackmon, and R.A. Bruce (1964). Indocyanine green clearance and estimated hepatic blood flow during mild to maximal exercise in upright man. *J. Clin. Invest. 43*, 1677–1690.

Rowell, L.B., J.R. Blackmon, R.H. Martin, J.A. Mazzarella, and R.A. Bruce (1965). Hepatic clearance of indocyanine green in man under thermal and exercise stresses. *J. Appl. Physiol. 20*, 384–394.

Rowell, L.B., G.L. Brengelmann, J.R. Blackmon, and J.A. Murray (1970). Redistribution of blood flow during sustained high skin temperature in resting man. *J. Appl. Physiol. 28*, 415–420.

Rowell, L.B., G.L. Brengelmann, J.-M.R. Detry, and C. Wyss (1971). Venomotor responses to rapid changes in skin temperature in exercising man. *J. Appl. Physiol. 30*, 64–71.

Rowell, L.B., G.L. Brengelmann, and P.R. Freund (1987). Unaltered norepinephrine : heart rate relationship in exercise with exogenous heat. *J. Appl. Physiol. 62*, 646–650.

Rowell, L.B., J.A. Murray, G.L. Brengelmann, and K.K. Kraning II (1969). Human cardiovascular adjustments to rapid changes in skin temperature during exercise. *Circ. Res. 24*, 711–724.

Rowell, L.B., and D.R. Seals (1990). Sympathetic activity during graded central hypovolemia in hypoxemic man. *Am. J. Physiol. 259 (Heart Circ. Physiol. 28)*, H1197–H1206.

Sagawa, K., J.M. Ross, and A.C. Guyton (1961). Quantitation of cerebral ischemic pressor response in dogs. *Am. J. Physiol. 200*, 1164–1168.

Saltin, B. (1964). Aerobic work capacity and circulation at exercise in man. *Acta Physiol. Scand. 62 (Suppl. 230)*, 1–52.

Sandler, M.P., M.W. Kronenberg, M.B. Forman, O.H. Wolfe, J.A. Clanton, and C.L. Partain (1984). Dynamic fluctuations in blood and spleen radioactivity: splenic contractions and relation to clinical radionuclide volume calculations. *J. Am. Col. Cardiol. 3*, 1205–1211.

Savage, M.V., G.L. Brengelmann, A.M.J. Buchan, and P.R. Freund (1990). Cystic fibrosis, vasoactive intestinal polypeptide, and active cutaneous vasodilation. *J. Appl. Physiol. 69*, 2149–2154.

Savard, G.K., B. Nielsen, I. Laszcynska, B.E. Larsen, and B. Saltin (1988). Muscle blood flow is not reduced in humans during moderate exercise and heat stress. *J. Appl. Physiol. 64*, 649–657.

Schönung, W., C. Jessen, H. Wagner, and E. Simon (1971). Regional blood flow antagonism induced by central thermal stimulation in the concious dog. *Experientia 27*, 1291–1292.

Selkurt, E.E. (1974). Current status of renal circulation and related nephron function in hemorrhage and experimental shock. I. Vascular mechanisms. *Circ. Shock 1*, 3–15.

Shapiro, W., A.J. Wasserman, J.P. Baker, and J.L. Patterson (1970). Cerebrovascular response to acute hypocapnic and eucapnic hypoxia in normal men. *J. Clin. Invest. 49*, 2362–2368.

Shepherd, J.T. (1963). *Physiology of the Circulation in Human Limbs in Health and Disease.* W.B. Saunders, Philadelphia.

Shiraki, K., S. Sagawa, F. Tajima, A. Yokota, M. Hashimoto, and G.L. Brengelmann (1988). Independence of brain and tympanic temperatures in an unanesthetized human. *J. Appl. Physiol. 65,* 482–486.

Smith, H.W. (1956). *Principles of Renal Physiology.* Oxford University Press, New York.

Sokoloff, L. (1977). Relation between physiological function and energy metabolism in the central nervous system. *J. Neurochem. 29,* 13–26.

Thomas, S.N., T. Schroeder, N.H. Secher, and J.H. Mitchell (1989). Cerebral blood flow during submaximal and maximal dynamic exercise in humans. *J. Appl. Physiol. 67,* 744–748.

Tidgren, B., P. Hjemdahl, E. Theodorsson, and J. Nussberger (1991). Renal neurohormonal and vascular responses to dynamic exercise in humans. *J. Appl. Physiol. 70,* 2279–2286.

Traystman, R.J. (1981). Control of cerebral blood flow. In P.M. Vanhoutte and I. Leusen, eds. *Vasodilatation,* pp. 39–48. Raven Press, New York.

Tyden, G., H. Samnegard, and L. Thulin (1979). The effects of changes in the carotid sinus baroreceptor activity on splanchnic blood flow in anesthetized man. *Acta Physiol. Scand. 106,* 187–189.

Vanhoutte, P.M. (1980). Physical factors of regulation. In D.F. Bohr, A.P. Somlyo, and H.V. Sparks Jr., eds. *Handbook of Physiology. The Cardiovascular System: Vascular Smooth Muscle,* sect. 2, vol. II, pp. 443–474. American Physiological Society, Bethesda, MD.

Vanhoutte, P.M., T.J. Verbeuren, and R.C. Webb (1981). Local modulation of adrenergic neuroeffector interaction in the blood vessel wall. *Physiol. Rev. 61,* 151–247.

van Lieshout, J.J. (1989). *Cardiovascular Reflexes in Orthostatic Disorders.* Rodopi, Amsterdam.

Vatner, S.F. (1975). Effects of exercise on distribution of regional blood flows and resistances. In R. Zelis, ed. *The Peripheral Circulations,* pp. 211–233. Grune & Stratton, New York.

Victor, R.G., and W.N. Leimbach Jr. (1987). Effects of lower body negative pressure on sympathetic discharge to leg muscles in humans. *J. App. Physiol. 63,* 2558–2562.

Wade, O.L., and J.M. Bishop (1962). *Cardiac Output and Regional Blood Flow.* Blackwell, Oxford, UK.

Wade, O.L., B. Combes, A.W. Childs, H.O. Wheeler, A. Cournand, and S.E. Bradley (1956). The effects of exercise on the splanchnic blood flow and splanchnic blood volume in normal man. *Clin. Sci. 15,* 457–463.

Wenger, C.B. (1987). More comments on "keeping a cool head." *News Physiol. Sci. 2,* 150.

Whelan, R.F. (1967). *Control of the Peripheral Circulation in Man.* CC Thomas, Springfield, IL.

Winn, H.R., R. Rubio, and R.M. Berne (1981). The role of adenosine in the regulation of cerebral blood flow. *J. Cereb. Blood Flow Metab. 1,* 239–244.

7

Control of Blood Flow to Dynamically Active Muscles

This chapter focuses on the local chemical and neural control of all active muscles including the heart and respiratory muscles. Table 6-2 summarizes how blood flow is distributed to the different major vascular beds during "maximal" exercise. Figure 7-1 illustrates the progression of changes in the distribution of cardiac output away from "inactive" regions and to active muscle with increasing oxygen uptake. Skeletal muscle stands out because the small fraction of cardiac output directed to *all* of the muscles at rest, that is, about 20 percent, increases so that at $\dot{V}o_2$max approximately 85 percent of the cardiac output is distributed to skeletal muscles, only one-half of which, more or less, are active; flow to other muscles is reduced by sympathetic vasoconstriction. The fraction of the total muscle mass that is actually active is unknown.

This chapter raises some fundamental questions about sympathetic vasomotor control during exercise. Is sympathetic vasomotor outflow directed mainly to the "inactive" regions or is it directed to virtually every organ including the heart and active skeletal muscle?

Does the increased spillover of norepinephrine from the heart (Esler at al., 1990) simply reflect the chronotropic or β_1-adrenergic effects of norepinephrine released from sympathetic nerves, or does it also indicate an activation of cardiac α-adrenoceptors and some coronary vasoconstriction—or at least a potential for it? What would be gained if coronary vessels also vasoconstricted?

Does the increase in sympathetic outflow to active muscle mean that muscle blood flow during exercise is the resultant of metabolic vasodilation and completing neural vasoconstriction? If so, what is to be gained?

The idea that muscle blood flow is held in check by sympathetic nerve activity has suggested to some that muscle is a "sleeping giant" able to vasodilate to such a degree that the heart cannot perfuse it at a rate of flow necessary to maintain blood pressure. Restated, the question is: can muscle vascular conductance rise enough to outstrip the pumping capacity of the heart? If so, this would mean we could hover precariously close to the edge of arterial hypotension whenever we activate too much muscle during severe exercise.

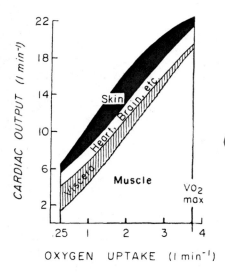

Figure 7-1 Estimated distribution of cardiac output to active skeletal muscle including respiratory muscles (*muscle*), visceral organs, heart and brain, and skin over the full range of oxygen uptake from rest to V_{O_2}max (at 3.7 L min^{-1}). Blood flow to the heart also increased. (Adapted from Rowell, 1974a).

Despite the developing evidence that both the heart and active skeletal muscle are recipients of increased sympathetic outflow during exercise, ideas about its significance have been influenced for years by a concept called "sympatholysis." This concept holds that the vasoconstrictor effects of norepinephrine are prevented or markedly blunted by an increased concentration of metabolites within the tissues. The idea is that norepinephrine release is prejunctionally inhibited by metabolites (see Chapter 4, "Hypoxemia" and "Orthostatic Intolerance"). The evidence showing that sympathetic vasoconstriction is effective in active muscles is presented.

CONTROL OF BLOOD FLOW TO THE HEART

The heart is the only organ that must provide the perfusion pressure for its own blood supply; the more blood the heart provides to other organs, the more it must provide for itself as its own metabolic costs rise with increased pumping. Like skeletal muscle, the heart depends on metabolic vasodilation for its arterial blood supply. The main issues currently concerning the control of coronary blood flow are the roles of adenosine and other local factors and also that of the sympathetic nervous system in this regulation. This field was reviewed by Berne and Rubio (1979), Klocke and Ellis (1980), Olsson (1981), and Feigl (1983); only a few of the main ideas can be touched on here.

The heart is supplied by two major coronary arteries that originate at the root of the aorta. The left coronary artery divides into the left circumflex and the anterior descending arteries which supply mainly the left ventricle. The right coronary artery divides and sends descending branches to both right and left ventricles. All of these vessels course over the epicardial surface before descending into myocardial tissue where they ultimately give rise to a dense distribution of arterioles and capillaries. Most of the heart's venous blood drains into the coronary sinus, which empties into the right atrium.

Normal human hearts contain approximately 3,000 to 4,000 capillaries per square millimeter in contrast to approximately 300 to 500 per square millimeter in skeletal muscle. In both tissues the number of capillaries per muscle fiber is approximately the same, but the diameter of the fibers is much smaller in the heart than in skeletal muscle (approximately 17 μm as opposed to 50 μm in skeletal muscle) (see Feigl, 1983). Accordingly, diffusion distances between the capillaries and the cells are much smaller in the heart and capillary exchange of small molecules is estimated to be 15 times more effective in cardiac muscle. (Note, however, that the extraction of oxygen by skeletal muscle is virtually the same as that by the heart over the full range of metabolism, indicating that something besides diffusion *distance* determines arteriovenous oxygen difference [diffusion time?].)

Measurement of Coronary Blood Flow

Coronary blood flow in humans is commonly measured from the rate of uptake of an inert foreign gas such as N_2O. This method is based on the Fick principle and is the same as that described in Chapter 6 for the cerebral circulation. The arteriovenous N_2O difference across the heart is determined from catheters introduced into an artery and into the coronary sinus. Proper placement of a catheter in the coronary sinus is essential because of the ease of contamination of samples with more oxygen-rich right atrial blood (or more oxygen-poor blood during severe exercise). The reflux of right atrial blood into the sinus during the hyperventilation associated with exercise is a major concern. In a modification of this procedure, ^{131}I antipyrine is infused intravenously at a constant rate. The rapid diffusion of antipyrine reduces the 10-minute equilibration time required for N_2O to only 2 minutes. These techniques provide *measurements mainly of left ventricular coronary blood flow* because the coronary sinus drains blood primarily from the main left coronary artery which supplies the left ventricle.

Other techniques employ the clearance rate of radioisotopes such as [85]Kr and ^{133}Xe from the heart and are measured by precordial scintillation detection. Basically the same technique are also used to measure the total and regional cerebral blood flow and the limitations are similar for both organs.

Range of Coronary Blood Flow and Oxygen Uptake

Inasmuch as the heart is always beating, there is no "resting" value for blood flow to the heart as there is for skeletal muscle. In a normal person at supine rest with a heart rate of 60 to 70 beats min^{-1}, blood flow to each 100 g of left ventricle is 60 to 80 ml min^{-1}, and the oxygen consumed is 7 to 9 ml 100 g^{-1} min^{-1}. Total coronary blood flow is approximately 250 ml min^{-1} or about 5 percent of cardiac output in a supine resting human. Most of this blood flow and oxygen uptake meets the costs of contraction. When the heart is stopped by infusion of potassium and is perfused with oxygenated blood at a normal pressure, the blood flow and oxygen uptake necessary to pay for basic living costs of cardiac cells can be determined. These costs are about one-fifth the total costs in a beating heart under basal conditions. Therefore about 80 percent of the blood flow and oxygen uptake is required for contractions under basal conditions. The coronary circulation is considered unique in that 60 to 70 percent of the available oxygen is extracted from blood in resting humans when metabolic demands on the heart are lowest; the arteriovenous difference across the heart is normally about 14 ml 100 ml^{-1} and may or may not change much with increasing cardiac oxygen consumption; that is, flow increases in direct proportion to increased demands for oxygen. We have viewed skeletal muscle as an organ that increases its extraction of oxygen in proportion to its metabolic rate. It will be shown later that when an isolated small mass of skeletal muscle becomes active, its arteriovenous oxygen difference is also about 14 ml 100 ml^{-1} and does not increase further with increased oxygen consumption (see Figures 7-13 and 7-16)—in short, *oxygen extraction by small active muscles is like that by the heart; only when the mass of active muscle is large does its oxygen extraction exceed that of the heart.*

Exercise and other stresses that raise cardiac output and heart rate increase myocardial oxygen uptake and coronary blood flow. Coronary blood flow rises linearly with increases in heart rate (see Figure 7-2). Total coronary blood flow may reach as high as 1.0 L min^{-1} in a heart weighing 300 g. Once heart rate reaches 195 beats min^{-1} cardiac output cannot increase further as long as stroke volume is also maximal so that maximal cardiac output has been reached. A recurrent question is whether myocardial oxygen uptake and coronary blood flow have also reached "maximal" values. Inability to increase coronary blood flow further might limit the ability to raise cardiac output.

What is "maximal" coronary blood flow? Inasmuch as the same question has been asked repeatedly about skeletal muscle blood flow, it is important to understand what is meant by "maximal" just as was done for total body oxygen uptake ($\dot{V}o_2$max) in Chapter 5. The $\dot{V}o_2$max has a precise physiological definition. Figure 7-3 attempts to show why the term "maximal blood flow" has no rigorous definition such as that for $\dot{V}o_2$max (Rowell, 1988). The top panel of this figure shows the relationship between muscle blood flow and some assumed driving pressures for the purpose of illustration. Two "peak values" for flow (Pk$_1$ and Pk$_2$) simply illustrate the arbitrary nature of selecting a so-called "maximal" or "peak" value inasmuch as such values depend on perfusion pressure and vascular con-

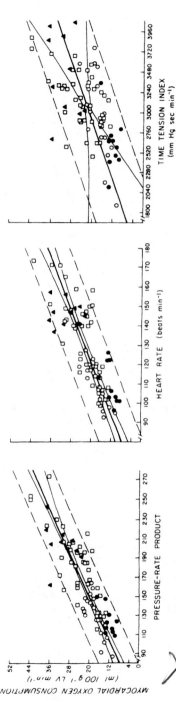

Figure 7-2 Determinants of myocardial oxygen consumption MVo$_2$ from 29 subjects during static plus dynamic exercise (*filled triangles*), dynamic exercise (*open squares*), static exercise (*filled cycles*), and dynamic exercise with β-blockade (propranolol) (*open circles*). The dashed lines show 95 percent confidence zones for individual data. Also shown are the 95 percent confidence limits for the slopes of the regression lines (Nelson et al., 1974). Regression equations were as follows:

Left panel	MVo$_2$ = 0.17 (HR × BP) − 5.31 r = .86
Middle panel	MVo$_2$ = 0.30 (HR) − 16.44 r = .82
Right panel	MVo$_2$ = 0.01 (TTI) − 13.55 r = .65

(From Rowell, 1986, with permission from Oxford University Press.)

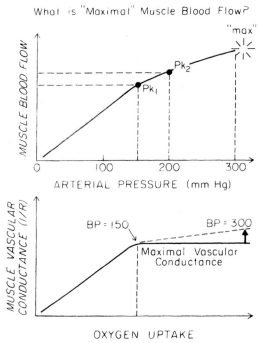

Figure 7-3 (*Top*): Hypothetical relationships between muscle blood flow and blood pressure. Blood flow rises with blood pressure until the vessel bursts—at "max" or "maximal" blood flow. "Maximal" blood flow has no meaning unless referred to some pressure and called more appropriately a "peak" value for that pressure, as in arbitrary peak values, Pk$_1$ and Pk$_2$. (*Bottom*): Relationship between muscle oxygen uptake and muscle vascular conductance. "Maximal" vascular conductance or "maximal" vasodilation would be observed as a sudden change in slope (arbitrary at 150 mmHg perfusion pressure), above which rising transmural pressure passively distends the vessels and raises conductance further—but much more gradually. (Adapted from Rowell, 1988.)

ductance. *Peak blood flow* is defined as the highest attainable flow for a specific blood pressure and a specific vascular conductance. The bottom panel of Figure 7-3 shows that initially the relationship between pressure and flow is steep until maximal vascular conductance is reached at a blood pressure of 150 mmHg (again an arbitrary value). Maximal vasodilation has occurred at this hypothetical point because further increases in oxygen uptake caused no additional vasodilation. In reality conductance can continue to increase slightly above its value at a pressure of 150 mmHg because pressure continues to rise and passively distend the blood vessels. Thus, the goal of defining a "maximal" blood flow is not really attainable unless it is referred to a specific driving pressure. So far we can only speak of *peak* values for blood flow to the heart and skeletal muscle; no well-defined maxima for either flow or conductance currently exist.

Keep in mind that because of technical limitations in the measurement of coronary blood flow in humans, only blood flow to the left ventricle is measured, and not to the entire 300 g of cardiac muscle. In dogs, values for coronary blood flow at "peak" vasodilation are reported to be 300 to 400 ml 100 g^{-1} min^{-1} of left ventricle. In humans peak coronary vasodilation induced pharmacologically with dipyradimole yields blood flows of 400 ml 100 g^{-1} min^{-1} of left ventricle. It is not known if these vasodilator drugs elicit a "maximal" value for vascular conductance. Unfortunately, we have no measurements of coronary blood flow at maximal cardiac output in humans. Coronary blood flow can reach very high values in exercising dogs; for example, measurement of *total* coronary blood flow by the radioactive microsphere technique in heavily exercised animals has in various studies yielded blood flows of 390, 400, and 424 ml 100 g^{-1} min^{-1} (see Feigl, 1983). Even under these conditions a further 50 percent increase in blood flow was obtained during reactive hyperemia after a brief coronary artery occlusion. Another group infused dipyradimole into dogs during severe exercise (heart rate 270 beats min^{-1}) and coronary blood flow rose from 424 to 618 ml 100 g^{-1} min^{-1} (Barnard et al., 1977). This means that coronary vasodilator reserve was not exhausted in these animals despite the high demand of the myocardium at a heart rate of 270 beats min^{-1}. In fact, only 63 percent of total left ventricular blood flow reserve was utilized.

An important series of experiments was carried out on normal young men by Kitamura and coworkers (1972), Jorgensen and coworkers (1973, 1977), and Nelson and coworkers (1974) (see Figure 7-2). In these men coronary blood flow averaged 280 ml 100 g^{-1} min^{-1} of left ventricle and reached as high as 390 ml min^{-1} during moderately severe exercise requiring heart rates of 165 beats min^{-1} or about 85 percent of maximal heart rate. Arterial-coronary sinus oxygen difference rose from 11 to 12 ml 100 ml^{-1} at the lowest work rate (heart rate was 104 beats min^{-1}) up to 13.5 ml 100 ml^{-1} at the highest rate of exercise.

Before a conclusion can be made concerning peak values for coronary blood flow in humans, it is necessary to consider mechanical and other factors that modify blood flow to the myocardium during a cardiac cycle (see Klocke and Ellis, 1980; Feigl, 1983).

Determinants of Myocardial Oxygen Uptake and Coronary Blood Flow

The work done by the heart, expressed as pressure times volume pumped, is not well correlated with the heart's oxygen consumption. Metabolic costs are more closely related to the development of ventricular pressure and, to a much lesser degree, the speed of contraction. Actually, the most costly portion of the cardiac cycle is the isovolumic contraction period during which ventricular pressure rises while all valves are closed. Inasmuch as this contraction is isovolumic or almost isometric, external work is zero. The three major determinants of myocardial oxygen uptake are

(1) heart rate; (2) ventricular wall stress, which is proportional to intraventricular pressure and radius of ventricular curvature (LaPlace's law) and inversely proportional to wall thickness; and (3) contractility or inotropic state—the least important of the three (Rooke and Feigl, 1982). When the velocity and strength or vigor of a contraction is increased by circulating epinephrine or by increased sympathetic nerve activity, cardiac oxygen costs are reportedly increased out of proportion to the external work performed. However, in this conclusion a constant mechanical efficiency is incorrectly assumed (Rooke and Feigl, 1982).

The three factors listed above not only determine myocardial oxygen demand, they also affect oxygen supply. Blood flow to the left ventricle is reduced or even stopped during systole, depending on the force of contraction, the intraventricular pressure, and the wall stress. These effects are smaller in the right ventricle because intraventricular pressure and wall stress are much lower. Compression of vessels in the left ventricular subendocardium is greater than in the epicardium. Ratios of subendocardial to subepicardial blood flow (studied in animals by the radioactive microsphere technique) differ from condition to condition. Some have suggested that the increase in epicardial blood flow is at the expense of the endocardium, called a "steal phenomenon" (see "Neural Control" below). In resting dogs, subendocardial blood flow exceeds subepicardial flow per unit mass of tissue by about 30 percent. In contrast, during strenuous exercise the transmural distribution of coronary blood flow equalizes so that the ratios of subendocardial to subepicardial blood flow become $1:1$.

When the heart contracts, it restricts its own blood flow because of the compression of vessels by contracting muscle. Because of this mechanical compression approximately 70 to 80 percent of coronary perfusion occurs during diastole. This percentage is probably greater during severe exercise because of the greater intravascular pressure. In humans we can determine neither wall stress nor contractility without making many assumptions. Indices such as the time-tension index (TTI) have been used to relate the metabolic demands of the heart to its oxygen supply. In animals the TTI was calculated by summing the areas of the left ventricular systolic-pressure curve for 1 minute to get a measure of the total tension developed by the left ventricle. The TTI has been approximated in humans by summing the areas of the systolic portion of an aortic pressure tracing. In their studies on humans Kitamura and colleagues (1972) and Nelson and colleagues (1974) confirmed the findings of others from dogs; the TTI was a poor index of myocardial oxygen consumption (Figure 7-2). This was especially true when cardiac contractility was altered. These investigators studied normal young men at three levels of exercise; the highest levels required 2.1 L O_2 min^{-1}, which corresponded to 56 percent of the subjects' $\dot{V}o_2$max and 85 percent of their maximal heart rates. The product of heart rate and aortic systolic pressure, called the *pressure-rate product,* correlated best with the myocardial oxygen uptake and coronary blood flow. The correlation was equally good when the aortic pressure variable used in this product was peak systolic, mean systolic, or mean pressure. However, heart rate alone correlated almost as well as is shown in Figure 7-2. Nelson and colleagues (1974) also made similar measurements in another group of subjects after they were given the β-blocking drug, propranolol. Despite the decrease in myocardial contractility and a significant lengthening of the ventricular ejection period due to decreased heart rate, the close relationship between myocardial oxygen uptake and coronary blood flow and the pressure-rate product persisted, whereas the correlation between TTI and myocardial oxygen consumption (and coronary blood flow) became much worse. Therefore, when expressed in quantities we can measure in humans, *left ventricular blood flow and oxygen consumption are best correlated to the number of times the ventricle must produce a given aortic pressure each minute.* Some animal experiments, which featured tight control of the critical variables, support this conclusion (Rooke and Feigl, 1982).

The reason myocardial oxygen uptake and/or coronary blood flow are correlated equally well with arterial pressure and heart rate during dynamic exercise is because all of these variables rise together and are strongly correlated. However, the particular importance of arterial pressure is unmasked in isometric exercise during which arterial pressure rises much more in relation to the increase in heart rate than it does during dynamic exercise (see Chapter 8). Again, the pressure-rate product correlates best with the myocardial oxygen uptake and (coronary blood flow), as summarized in Figure 7-2.

Local Metabolic Control

The candidates for metabolic vasodilators in the heart are the same as those proposed for skeletal muscle (see below) and other vascular beds. Like the brain, the heart cannot incur significant oxygen debt because its metabolism is almost entirely aerobic, and therefore it depends critically on its oxygen supply. For both the heart and the brain, oxygen appears to play an important and probably indirect role in the control of blood flow. Berne and Rubio (1979) and their colleagues have assembled convincing evidence that myocardial oxygen supply and adenosine production are closely linked, and that adenosine mediates coronary vasodilation *when oxygen supply is compromised.* The notion that adenosine is *always* the principle metabolic vasodilator that normally modulates coronary blood flow from beat to beat is not convincing (adenosine could be important in hypoxemia). For example, application of agents that block the actions of adenosine showed that neither enhanced adenosine degradation produced by administration of adenosine deaminase nor adenosine receptor blockade with 8-phenyltheophylline changed myocardial blood flow during rest or submaximal exercise (Bache et al., 1988). These findings argue against any important role for adenosine in mediating coronary vasodilation in a heavily working heart. Further, adenosine receptor blockade did not alter the relationship between cardiac oxygen consumption and coronary blood flow nor did it decrease coronary venous Po_2 during exercise (Bache et al., 1988).

Neural Control

Coronary arteries receive a rich supply of sympathetic noradrenergic and parasympathetic cholinergic nerve fibers. This innervation and its physiological role were reviewed by Feigl (1983) (see also Stone, 1983). The importance of coronary vascular innervation is questioned by those who feel that metabolic control of coronary vessels normally overpowers any neural influence. The underlying question is whether any significant role is ever played by the sympathetic and parasympathetic nervous systems in the regulation of coronary blood flow, particularly during exercise. Investigation of this problem has been impeded by the secondary inotropic and chronotropic effects of nerve stimulation on coronary blood flow. For example, stimulation of cardiac sympathetic nerves usually causes coronary vasodilation as a secondary effect of increased heart rate and contractility on myocardial oxygen consumption. The primary vasoconstrictor effects of sympathetic stimulation are unveiled only when they are abolished by α-adrenergic blockade or when the secondary metabolic effects are prevented by β-blockade.

The studies of sympathetic (and also parasympathetic) innervation of the heart reveal the *potential* for direct neural control of coronary vessels. The focus here is on tonic sympathetic control during the stress of exercise (parasympathetic effects appear to be only transient ones when secondary effects on heart rate and myocardial oxygen uptake are eliminated [Feigl, 1983]). Does sympathetic vasoconstriction compete with the powerful metabolic control of coronary blood flow? There is evidence indicating that a neurally induced coronary vasoconstriction occurs in response to carotid sinus hypotension. Mohrman and Feigl (1978) eliminated the competition between the baroreflex-induced sympathetic coronary vasoconstriction and metabolic coronary vasodilation caused by the rise in left ventricular afterload and myocardial oxygen consumption. They found that a significant α receptor-mediated coronary vasoconstriction does attend carotid sinus hypotension in dogs.

One of the most surprising findings, again from dogs, is that blockade of cardiac α-receptors increases coronary blood flow and reduces arterial-coronary sinus oxygen difference at a given level of myocardial oxygen uptake during exercise (see Feigl, 1983; Stone, 1983). This suggests that coronary vasodilation during exercise is restricted by sympathetic coronary vasoconstriction. Reductions in coronary blood flow in the order of 6 percent (Huang and Feigl, 1988), 14 percent (Heyndrickx et al., 1982), and 30 percent (Gwirtz et al., 1986) have been reported. It is difficult to imagine what advantage this vasoconstriction might offer to the animal unless the constriction were somehow localized so as to optimize the distribution of blood flow between epicardial and endocardial layers during systole, as suggested by Stone (1983) and by Huang and Feigl (1988).

When coronary arteries are dilated pharmacologically, or when the heart is electrically paced from 100 to 250 beats min^{-1}, the ratio of inner myocardial blood flow (endocardial) to outer myocardial blood flow (epicardial)—called inner/outer flow ratio—falls from 1.0 to 0.4. This suggests that myocardial contraction impedes blood flow to the inner layers of the heart (by vascular compression) more than it does to the outer layers. As heart rate increases, a greater proportion of each cardiac cycle is spent in systole so that tachycardia tends to exaggerate the effects of any transmural gradient of compression. In contrast to the situation in which coronary blood flow is increased pharmacologically, or as a result of ventricular pacing, the transmural distribution of coronary blood flow changes little in response to exercise and the inner/outer flow ratio remains at or above 1.0 (Ball and Bache, 1976; Von Restorff et al., 1977). Huang and Feigl (1988) selectively blocked the α-adrenoceptors in one region of the myocardium with phenoxybenzamine. They found the ratio of inner-layer myocardial blood flow to outer-layer blood flow tended to be better maintained in the region with α-receptors intact than in the region with those receptors blocked when myocardial oxygen consumption was increased during exercise. Although the effects were small, the authors concluded that adrenergic coronary vasoconstriction did help to maintain a more uniform transmural distribution of myocardial blood flow during exercise in spite of limiting the average transmural flow.

Although the primary control of the coronary vasculature is, as in skeletal muscle, achieved by endogenous production of metabolites, adrenergic coronary vasoconstriction appears to be a normal response to a generalized sympathetic outflow that occurs during exercise and other stresses. The reflexes that govern this sympathetic outflow to active tissues are covered in later chapters.

CONTROL OF BLOOD FLOW TO RESPIRATORY MUSCLES

The oxygen consumption of respiratory muscles increases in proportion to the work of breathing during exercise. This means that the portion of the cardiac output directed to these muscles is unavailable for the locomotive muscles. In fact, the increased costs of breathing during severe exercise have been considered a factor that limits exercise capacity because respiratory muscles take a greater and greater fraction of the cardiac output and available oxygen away from the locomotive muscles. As a consequence of this, the respiratory muscles have been viewed as a factor limiting exercise performance.

The metabolic cost of increased ventilation and exercise has traditionally been investigated by measuring the rise in total body oxygen consumption during voluntary hyperventilation. Figure 7-4 gives a typical example of the hyperbolic relationship between the rise in oxygen uptake attributed to the respiratory muscles and the rate of voluntary hyperventilation; carbon dioxide was administered in order to maintain normocapnia (Anholm et al., 1987; Aaron et al., 1992). Figure 7-4 reveals the considerable differences in estimates of ventilatory costs in different studies. The main point is that ventilation becomes expensive metabolically when values approach those observed during exercise at $\dot{V}o_2$max—commonly between 100 and 130 L min^{-1} for normal, physically active young people. Of course, much higher rates of ventilation are seen in endurance athletes whose values for $\dot{V}o_2$max reach 5 to 6 L min^{-1}.

Anholm and colleagues (1987) observed the rise in cardiac output to average 4.3 ± 1.0 L min^{-1} during maximum voluntary ventilation ranging from 127 to 193 L min^{-1} with total oxygen consumption rising by 415 ml min^{-1} (average). Figure 2-2 shows the effect of the respiratory pump on right and left ventricular outputs and suggests no net effect on cardiac

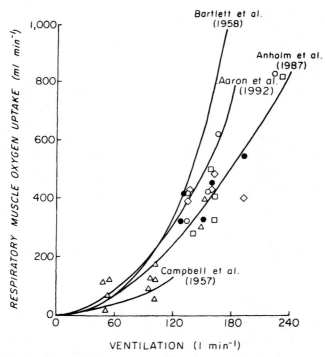

Figure 7-4 Respiratory muscle oxygen uptake measured as the rise in total oxygen uptake during maximal voluntary hyperventilation sustained for 1 minute (*open squares*), 2 minutes (*open circles*), 3 minutes (*open diamonds*), and 4 minutes (*closed circles*). Triangles represent costs for submaximal hyperventilation (from Anholm et al., 1987). Also shown are regression lines from two other earlier studies and a more recent study by Aaron et al., 1992.

output. However, Anholm and colleagues (1987) offer evidence suggesting that the speed of increase in cardiac output during the first 10 to 15 seconds of hyperventilation could indicate that approximately one-half of the rise in cardiac output is attributable to a sudden mechanical effect of the respiratory pump (see Chapter 2). The actual costs, in terms of blood flow, of hyperventilation at the observed levels might have been as low as 2.7 L min^{-1}. If so, this would still yield a reasonable calculated value for arteriovenous oxygen difference of approximately 15 ml 100 ml^{-1} across the active respiratory muscles.

A question often raised is whether the oxygen costs of ventilation rise enough during severe exercise to keep further increases from providing more oxygen to locomotive muscles; that is, all of the additional oxygen is needed for the respiratory muscles. Those who have made calculations place the upper limit of effective ventilation close to 140 L min^{-1} (for references, see Otis, 1954; Anholm et al., 1987). However, at $\dot{V}o_2$max the oxygen cost of hyperventilation has been calculated to average only 10 percent of $\dot{V}o_2$max (reaching 15 percent) (Aaron et al., 1992). Also, subjects were able to hyperventilate at this same level while at rest 3 to 10 times longer than the duration of maximal exercise. Thus requirements for oxygen are not dominated by respiratory muscles at $\dot{V}o_2$max (Aaron et al., 1992).

Are respiratory muscles vasoconstricted during moderate to heavy dynamic exercise? Inasmuch as blood vessels supplying active skeletal muscle are partially vasoconstricted by increased sympathetic vasoconstrictor activation, like those of the heart, skin, kidney, and splanchnic organs; it is probable that the blood vessels of the respiratory muscles would also become constricted. If so, this would mean that blood flow to respiratory muscles could be significantly less than the increments seen during maximal voluntary hyperventilation (assuming that lung inflation reflexes do not raise sympathetic activity significantly at rest). Currently there is no evidence to suggest that any restriction of respiratory muscle perfusion contributes to the lower levels of maximal ventilation observed during severe exhaustive exercise, as opposed to maximal voluntary hyperventilation at rest. Probably a more important factor is that the work of breathing is higher during voluntary hyperventilation than for involuntary hyperpnea during exercise (Dempsey, 1986; Johnson et al., 1992).

In achieving a given rate of air flow, the development of "excessive" pressure or effort by respiratory muscles is somehow sensed and is thereby avoided (Dempsey, 1986). This automatically regulated, efficient control system appears to be overridden by the cerebral cortex during voluntary hyperventilation. In exercise airway diameter is modulated and the pattern of breathing and the recruitment of respiratory muscles appear to be "set" *to minimize the oxygen cost of breathing* (Dempsey, 1986; Forster and Pan, 1988). Apparently we automatically "select" a breathing pattern that minimizes the total elastic and flow-resistive work during exercise. This would explain why the same expiratory flow rate is produced with much lower driving pressure and effort during whole body exercise. This economical pattern for exercise is substituted for a metabolically more expensive form of breathing during voluntary hyperventilation at rest.

The lower cost of involuntary hyperpnea during exercise suggests that a falsely low value has been set on the upper limit of effective ventilation (i.e., close to 140 L min^{-1}, see above) during exercise. The rate of ventilation at which all of the additional oxygen taken in is needed by the respiratory muscles, leaving none of that extra oxygen for locomotive muscles, may not be reached until ventilation exceeds 180 L min^{-1} (Forster and Pan, 1988); but the actual metabolic cost of ventilation *during maximal exercise* has not been measured because of some difficult methodological problems. Aaron and colleagues' (1992) estimate of ventilation requiring 10 to 15 percent of $\dot{V}o_2$max in humans is commensurate with Manohar's (1990) measurements of blood flows to all inspiratory and expiratory muscles of the abdomen and rib cage in ponies at maximal exercise. Fifteen percent of maximal cardiac output (radiolabeled microsphere technique) went to these muscles. Bear in mind these muscles also share some locomotor function as well (see also Manohar, 1986).

CONTROL OF BLOOD FLOW TO ACTIVE SKELETAL MUSCLE

Skeletal muscle comprises approximately 40 percent of the total body mass depending on age, sex, physical activity and a number of other factors. It receives 15 to 20 percent of cardiac output at rest and about 85 percent at $\dot{V}o_2$max.

Measurement of Muscle Blood Flow

The two greatest barriers to better understanding of circulatory control during exercise are our inabilities to establish how much muscle is active at a given oxygen uptake and to quantify its blood flow. Although blood flow to resting human muscle in a limb can be reliably measured by venous occlusion plethysmography or from the clearance rate of radioactive indicators injected directly into the muscle, measurement of blood flow through contracting muscles in humans has proven to be very difficult. Motion artifacts prevent plethysmographic recordings. Isotope clearances are affected by the direct exchange of isotopes between arterioles and veins, by differential solubility of labeled substances in different structural components of the muscle, by dissociation of labeled moieties from diffusible compounds which as free ions have diffusion-limited clearance, and finally by injection trauma, which alters local blood flow (for review see Lassen et al. [1983]). Further, the chances of injecting the indicator into a collection of fibers with a representative population of high and low intrinsic rates of blood flow is virtually nil. The most serious criticism of the isotope-clearance techniques is that the derived flows to active muscle are far too low to account for the increase in oxygen uptake.

The most successful approach applied to humans appears to be the constant infusion of dye or ice-cold saline through a catheter designed to provide adequate mixing (Wahren and Jorfeldt, 1973). The site of infusion must supply (if arterial) or must drain (if venous) a specifically known group of muscles and must be minimally contaminated with venous blood draining other tissues such as skin or inactive muscles (some contamination is inevitable, but it must be a small percent of muscle blood flow). The steady-state concentration of indicator must yield values of flow and calculated muscle oxygen uptake (flow times arteriovenous oxygen differences) that match the measured work output of the muscle based on the usual mechanical efficiency of human muscle of 20 to 23 percent. Again, the calculations assume that exercise is restricted to a specific muscle or muscle group of the limb, and that the conditions do not significantly raise skin blood flow in that limb (e.g., Andersen and Saltin, 1985). Bear in mind that increased skin blood flow could raise so-called "muscle blood flow" and reduce arteriovenous oxygen difference proportionally so that calculated oxygen uptake and mechanical efficiency would still be correct, but "muscle blood flow" would be falsely high (this is because skin extracts so little oxygen). More recently techniques employing bidirectional Doppler-ultrasound velocity meters, plus echo-ultrasound to determine vessel diameter, have been used to measure femoral arterial blood flow velocity and blood flow to the exercising leg (Walløe and Wesche, 1988).

The most successful method of quantifying skeletal muscle blood flow in exercising animals has been the radiolabeled microsphere technique. Microspheres (usually 15 μm) are injected into the left atrium or left ventricle and their distribution to any and all muscles and even parts of a muscle (e.g., red versus white fibers) can be determined to derive blood flow (see Armstrong and Laughlin, 1985; Musch et al., 1985).

Microcirculation

Structurally, one of the most important determinants of muscle's ability to utilize oxygen is the density of capillary networks. This density varies greatly among the two basic muscle fiber types that are present in humans (for review, see Saltin and Gollnick, 1983). The capillary surface area is estimated to be approximately 7 m^2 kg^{-1} of muscle or 210 m^2 total in a 75-kg human with 30 kg of skeletal muscle. Even on a per-gram basis, few organs have such great capacity to exchange oxygen and metabolites between capillaries and cells. Oxygen can be taken up by individual muscles at rates exceeding 300 ml kg^{-1} min^{-1}, which exceeds the resting value by nearly 50-fold.

The capillary density is highest in the fibers called red, slow-twitch, or tonic. These fibers have the highest potential for oxidative metabolism and contain approximately three times the number of capillaries per fiber (accounting for the differences in fiber size) as seen in the white fibers, which are also called fast-twitch or glycolytic fibers. The white fibers have been subdivided into groups that vary in oxidative potential. Some of these, called fast-twitch or fatigue-resistant fibers, have an oxidative capacity approaching that of the red fibers. In general, *capillary density appears to match the oxidative potential of the muscle fibers.* At rest, blood flow is highest in the red, slow-twitch fibers and is least in the white, fast-twitch (fast-fatiguing, glycolytic) fibers. For an excellent review of this topic, see Saltin and Gollnick (1983).

The arrangement of capillaries is also different with respect to muscle fiber type. Capillaries run parallel with the long axis of white fibers, but have more tortuous arrangements and form loops among red fibers, thus giving more capillary surface area for exchange of materials. Comparisons of the morphometry of capillaries and muscle fibers in cross sections of biopsy samples of vastus lateralis muscle in sedentary subjects and elite, well-conditioned mountaineers reveal some of the adaptive changes in skeletal muscle microcirculation. The ability of skeletal muscle to extract oxygen from the blood is a function of the *number of capillaries per muscle fiber;* for example, this number is 1.39 in sedentary people and 1.67 in well-conditioned mountaineers. The *number of capillaries per square millimeter of tissue* is important and the values are 387 mm^{-2} and 542 mm^{-2} in sedentary and well-conditioned subjects, respectively. The *average cross-sectional area of the muscle fiber* is 3,640 μm^2 (sedentary) and 3,108 μm^2 (well-trained); and finally the *area of tissue perfused by each capillary* is 2,300 μm^2 in sedentary subjects and only 1,939 μm^2 in well-conditioned mountaineers studied by Kayser and colleagues (1991).

Summary. In summary, the greater number of capillaries per muscle fiber, the greater capillary density, the smaller average area per muscle fiber, and the smaller area of tissue perfused by each capillary in physically conditioned people reveal the advantages for getting large quantities of oxygen to diffuse rapidly from the capillaries to the muscles. An important point to bear in mind is that, although a high capillary density fosters high oxygen extraction efficiency, the rate of blood flow through the capillaries and the mean transit time of the red blood cells can be equally important determinants of extraction.

There are no true arteriovenous shunts in skeletal muscle despite the finding that when muscles are dilated by cholinergic stimulation (in animals with cholinergic innervation), clearance of iodine 131 remains constant, oxygen uptake falls, and venous oxygen saturation rises, suggesting that blood flow bypasses the capillaries and therefore escapes tissue exchange. The explanation for these findings is that neurogenic and nonmetabolic vasodilators relax arterial smooth muscle but not precapillary sphincters, or the smallest precapillary vessels, whichever controls the number of open capillaries (see Duling, 1981). This means that despite the increase in blood flow, more capillaries are *not* open and more blood simply surges through already opened capillaries. This causes the fraction of oxygen and other substances extracted by the tissues to fall because transit times through the microcirculation become too short for effective exchange. In contrast, metabolic vasodilation opens "precapillary sphincters" or the smallest precapillary arterioles, which act as sphincters, so that the increased surface area associated with more open capillaries permits greater exchange between the blood and tissues (see Rowell, 1974b; Duling, 1981).

Blood Flow and Blood Volume

Skeletal muscle receives somewhere between 15 and 20 percent of cardiac output or about 750 to 1,000 ml min^{-1}, or from 2 to 4 ml 100 g^{-1} of muscle per minute in resting humans (See Table 6-1). Resting muscle consumes about 60 ml of oxygen each minute which is about 25 percent of resting oxygen uptake; therefore muscle extracts only about 30 percent of available oxygen at rest. The number of open capillaries per square millimeter of resting muscle is small so that transfer of oxygen from the blood to muscle cells is limited by the large diffusion distances. Another factor is both the spatial as well as temporal heterogeneity in the distribution of blood flow within a muscle, with some portions of the muscle being well perfused and others poorly perfused (Marconi et al., 1988; Grønlund et al., 1989). As a consequence, the tension and content of oxygen in veins draining resting muscle remain high, that is, two-thirds of the oxygen is "wasted" (see Figure 9-16).

Skeletal muscle and the heart have greater variations in metabolic rate than any other major organs. Inasmuch as skeletal muscle constitutes 40 percent of the total body mass, its range of blood flow is enormous. Tables 6-1 and 6-2 show that *total* muscle blood flow can increase from about 1,000 ml min^{-1} at rest to almost 22,000 ml min^{-1} in a normal person with a maximal cardiac output of 25 L min^{-1} and maximal oxygen uptake of nearly 4,000 ml min^{-1}. At $\dot{V}O_2$max arteriovenous oxygen difference in the muscles is about 18 ml 100 ml^{-1}, which represents 90 percent extraction (NOTE: this high extraction is not seen when a small mass of muscle is active by itself; see below).

Local and Neural Control of Muscle Blood Flow
Metabolic Control

The concept that intrinsic myogenic vascular tone, called *basal tone,* is inhibited by interstitial accumulation of metabolic by-products is usually credited to Gaskell in 1878, but Latschenberger and Deahna (cited by Forrester, 1981) proposed the same idea 2 years earlier. Since the classic studies of Fleisch in the 1930s (see Fleisch and Sibul, 1933), the major candidates for metabolic vasodilators of active muscle, the heart, and other organs have remained almost the same. This complex field has been ably reviewed by Sparks (1980), Shepherd (1983), Hudlicka (1985), and Vanhoutte (1988).

During contractions most substances released into the interstitial space are vasoactive. The long list includes hydrogen, potassium, phosphate ions, CO_2, adenosine, adenosine nucleotides, lactate, intermediates of the tricarboxylic acid (Krebs) cycle, vasoactive peptides, and so on. Each of these agents and a decrease in Po_2 have direct and indirect vasodilator actions. Their effects can interact in a nonadditive manner so that their combined actions far exceed their individual ones. For example, the combined effects of K^+, hyperosmolarity, and decreased Po_2 exceed their individual effects (Skinner, 1975).

There seems to be little question that changes in K^+, osmolarity, Po_2 and possibly adenosine can play some role in the *initiation* of exercise hyperemia. The problem is that these factors appear to lack any sustained influence as contraction continues. Venous and presumably interstitial concentrations of K^+ decrease because of increased activation of sodium-potassium ATPase. In fact, those metabolites measured in venous blood draining active muscle reach a peak after a few minutes of exercise and then decline to control levels within an hour as exercise continues (Morganroth et al., 1975; Sparks, 1980). Hyperosmolarity is gradually corrected by fluid exchange across the capillary so that its steady-state contribution is minimal. The vasodilator stimuli seem to disappear, whereas normal vasodilation is maintained, suggesting that we are not looking at the "right" vasodilators, or that the vasodilators at the onset of contraction are replaced by unknown ones as activity continues.

The greatest obstacle in determining the vasomotor influences of various metabolites is our inability to measure their concentration in the interstitial spaces where their actions on blood vessels occur. This has been done for K^+ by ion-specific electrodes inserted into the tissue. The increases in interstitial K^+ concentration are short-lived (Sparks, 1980; Shepherd, 1983). Concentrations of substances in venous blood often do not reflect well the interstitial concentrations even when blood flow is artificially *restricted* (the condition for most studies) so as to exaggerate the venous concentration of metabolites, blood gases, and so on.

Furchgott and Zawadzki's (1980) discovery of the role of the vascular endothelium as a modulator and sometimes initiator of vasomotor responses has opened a new chapter in this story. Some potent vasodilators exert their relaxing effects on vascular smooth muscle by stimulating the release of endothelial-derived relaxing factor (EDRF), which many now believe to be the nitric oxide radical or an unstable nitrosal compound (see Moncada et al., 1991). One of the newest findings in this exploding area of research is that in the skeletal muscle microcirculation an increase in blood flow velocity elicits a dilation of arterioles that is dependent on vascular endothelium (Koller and Kaley, 1990a). This "flow-dependent" dilation appears to be caused by the increase in shear-stress on the surface of endothelial cells; the vasodilation is mediated by substances released from the endothelium, shown in one study on skeletal muscle arterioles to be prostaglandins (Koller and Kaley, 1990b). The vasodilation can be marked and it has the effect of relieving the shear-stress on the endothelium. The prostaglandin mediation of this vasodilation (it can be blocked by several inhibitors of prostaglandin synthesis) could be unique for skeletal muscle inasmuch as the flow-sensitive vasodilation in larger arteries from other organs appears to be mediated by EDRF in some cases and by activation of ion channels in others (see Koller and Kaley, 1990b). On the other hand, Bevan and coworkers (1988) observed flow-induced vasodilation in isolated arteries from the rabbit after removal of their endothelium. Could a flow-induced local vasodilation actually maintain muscle blood flow after metabolic vasodilators are washed away? What would shut it off?

Local Neural Influences

Hilton (1959) postulated that vasodilation is spread through the arterial bed of exercising muscle by excitation of intrinsic nerves located within the blood vessel wall. Honig and Frierson (1976) found, by histochemical techniques, neuronal cell bodies in the walls of small arteries in skeletal muscle of several mammalian species (human vessels have not been similarly studied). Most of these intrinsic neurons are nonadrenergic and are thought to release peptidergic vasodilator transmitters from their endings. The still unproven hypothesis is that these intrinsic neurons initiate the rapid onset of vasodilation during contractions (metabolic vasodilation is assumed to be much slower), particularly during phasic contractions that are too brief to elicit slow metabolic vasodilation. An alternative hypothesis invokes the muscle pump and is discussed later in the chapter (see Figure 7-12).

Segal and associates (1989) proposed that the arteriolar network in the hamster cheek pouch functions much like a "syncytium" over which vasodilation can be propagated so that diverse vasomotor stimuli can be summed within the microvasculature. The propagation of vasodilation across branch points from daughter vessels into the parent vessel insures balance of local perfusion commensurate with metabolic requirements of the cells; any "steal" of flow from less dilated to more dilated vessels is minimized. Subsequent experiments ruled out rapid neural conduction by the reticulum of intrinsic vascular nerves; tetrodotoxin and calcium channel blockers did not prevent the spread of vasodilation (Segal and Duling, 1989). Putative gap junction uncouplers block the response, suggesting that vasodilation is spread by a cell-to-cell electrotonic propagation across gap junctions.

Mechanical Factors

Muscular compression of blood vessels during contraction reduces their transmural pressure and their rate of perfusion. If contractions are forceful, flow may actually be stopped. During static contractions blood flow in some muscles, depending on how fibers are aligned, is impeded if force of contraction requires more than 10 to 15 percent of maximum tension.

In other muscles with different fiber alignment, blood flow increases until 30 percent of maximum tension is developed (see Chapter 8).

During rhythmic exercise, muscle tensions appear not to exceed 20 to 30 percent of maximal tension even if the exercise is severe. Any reduction in flow during contraction is rapidly compensated by an overshoot during the relaxation phase (analogous to coronary blood flow during systole and diastole). Hobbs & McCloskey (1987) also found that muscle force development during rhythmic contractions fell sharply with small reductions in perfusion pressure and blood flow.

The *myogenic* response to a reduction in transmural pressure is relaxation of vascular smooth muscle tone or vasodilation. Thus vigorous compression of arterioles at the rate of one to three per second in the heart or once every second in skeletal muscle would be expected from a myogenic theory of autoregulation to reduce vascular resistance. Some evidence suggests that this myogenic mechanism could account for as much as one-third of the vasodilation in response to brief tetanic contraction (Mohrman and Sparks, 1974).

Of the mechanical factors, the muscle pump (discussed below) is the most important and it could represent a missing factor among those needed to account for the rise in muscle blood flow. This is discussed in a later section.

Competition Between Neural and Local "Metabolic" Control

To discover how muscle blood flow is controlled during exercise, it is necessary to determine whether the blood flow is the resultant of a competition between the dilator action of metabolites and the constrictor action of sympathetic adrenergic nerves. The term "functional sympatholysis" was coined to express the once commonly held view that metabolic vasodilation prevented the vasoconstrictor action of norepinephrine released from nerve terminals. For example, hypoxia, acidosis, potassium ions, adenosine, and hyperosmolarity can in vitro impede neural release of norepinephrine by prejunctional inhibition (see Vanhoutte et al., 1981). Some of these factors also alter norepinephrine reuptake and have direct inhibitory effects on vascular smooth muscle cells. However, a number of studies have shown conclusively that local metabolic vasodilator mechanisms in the active muscle do not override sympathetic vasoconstriction (see Donald et al., 1970; Thompson and Mohrman, 1983; Figure 7-5). In fact, the vasoconstriction can occur to such a degree in active muscle that its oxygen uptake is reduced (Thompson and Mohrman, 1983). Apparently conflicting findings such as those of Kjellmer (1965), showing that exercise blunted changes in muscle vascular resistance, may not actually be in conflict. When marked differences in baseline blood flow exist between rest and exercise, opposite conclusions can be made regarding the magnitude of vasoconstrictor response, depending on whether changes are expressed in terms of resistance or conductance.

Figure 7-5   Electrical stimulation of the lumbar sympathetic chain at a constant frequency (6 Hz, duration 30 seconds) at graded intensities of exercise shown as percent grade. Total heights of bars show leg blood flow before stimulation, and solid area alone shows flow during the last 10 seconds of nerve stimulation. The absolute reduction in blood flow was greater during exercise than at rest whereas the relative reduction (percent, at top) decreased with increasing work rate. (Adapted from Donald et al., 1970.)

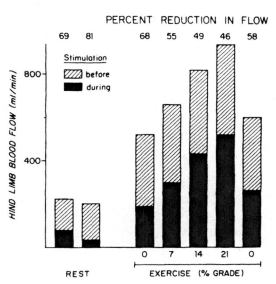

It is easy to fall victim to a polemic on the issue of whether one should quantify vasoconstriction in terms of changes in resistance or conductance. The reader is referred to three papers that deal skillfully with this issue (Lautt, 1989; O'Leary, 1991; Rowlands and Donald, 1968). Briefly, the crux of the problem is that it is easy to be seriously misled by the effects of changing baselines, as we saw when the R-R interval was used as an index of baroreflex sensitivity. For example, Kjellmer (1965) found in cats that steady-state changes in muscle vascular resistance in response to direct sympathetic nerve stimulation became smaller and smaller as blood flow increased during electrically induced exercise; however, recalculation of his data showed that changes in vascular conductance did not diminish. Figure 7-6 shows that when the same data are expressed as vascular conductance, it is clear that the vasomotor change was not blunted by metabolic vasodilation (Rowell, 1991). In short, *when muscle blood flow is high, vasocontriction causes large changes in vascular conductance and in blood pressure, but only small changes in resistance.* Conductance reflects the magnitude of active change in blood flow and vascular tone (Lautt, 1989; O'Leary, 1991). The fact that naturally occurring metabolic vasodilation and sympathetic vasoconstriction both impose large and competing effects on blood flow to active muscle is of central importance throughout the remainder of this book (see O'Leary et al., 1991).

Summary.   In summary, several points are germane. The first is that no combination or concentration of vasodilator substances infused into the arterial supply of a resting muscle can simulate the magnitude or time

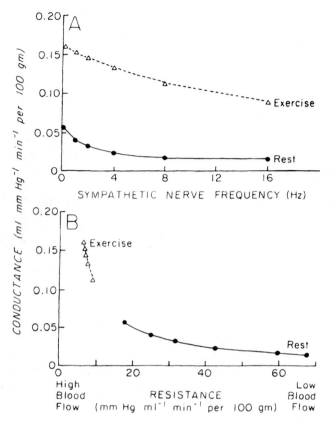

Figure 7-6 (A) Similar decrements in muscle vascular conductance in response to electrical stimulation of sympathetic nerves supplying *resting* and *active* skeletal muscle in cats (calculated from the data of Kjellmer, 1964). Values were calculated after a steady state of blood flow was achieved (initial transient effects on conductance are larger during exercise than rest). (**B**) The same level of sympathetic stimulation causes large changes in blood flow and conductance and trivial changes in resistance *during exercise* (high flow), but small changes in flow and conductance and large changes in resistance *at rest*. The point is that during exercise when muscle blood flow is high, vasoconstriction causes large changes in blood flow, blood pressure and vascular conductance and trivial changes in vascular resistance. (Adapted from Rowell, 1991.)

course of its vasodilation in response to dynamic exercise. A tacit conclusion has been that there are some missing vasodilators that must account for the remaining vasodilation. Recognition of a local flow-sensitive mechanism mediated by the endothelium adds a piece to the puzzle but may not solve it. The time courses of muscle vasodilation and changes in concentration of metabolites depend on the (1) experimental conditions, (2) type of contraction, tonic versus rhythmic, (3) intensity and duration of contraction, (4) type of muscle, white glycolytic versus red oxidative, and (5) conditions for blood flow, free versus restricted flow (see Sparks, 1980; Shepherd, 1983; Laughlin, 1987). It is suggested in the following section that the muscle pump may provide the missing factor in vasodilation. Although there is some competition between metabolic vasodilation and neurogenic vasoconstriction in active muscles, resistance vessels constrict vigorously to sympathetic stimulation. Changes in resistance are small because baseline blood flow is high, whereas changes in vascular conductance are large.

How High Can Muscle Blood Flow Go?
What is "Maximal" Muscle Blood Flow?

Figure 7-3 points out the problems of defining "maximal" muscle blood flow and shows that for any single muscle (like the heart) or small group of skeletal muscles, this value depends on the *perfusion pressure,* which sets the upper limit; cardiac pumping capacity is not a factor. If there were unlimited ability to raise blood pressure, "maximal" muscle blood flow would not be reached until the vessels burst. In practical terms we can define an upper limit for total muscle blood flow because it must be set by the maximal cardiac output. Thus any estimate of *peak* or maximal muscle blood flow must fall within this constraint and that set by the $\dot{V}O_2$max, so that the law of conservation of mass is obeyed. For example, Table 7-1 shows estimates of the *minimum* muscle blood flow required to account for measured $\dot{V}O_2$max in sedentary to endurance-trained people with body weight 75 kg and total muscle mass 30 kg. Muscle oxygen uptake is $\dot{V}O_2$max, less "resting" oxygen uptake assumed to be 250 ml min^{-1}. The key point to gain from Table 7-1 is that peak values for muscle blood flow per 100 g depend not only on $\dot{V}O_2$max and maximal cardiac output, but also on the mass of muscle engaged in exercise. Our biggest problem is that we do not know that mass. Figure 7-7 shows the calculated values for

Table 7-1 Estimates of the Minimum Muscle Blood Flow Needed to Account for Measured Oxygen Uptakes in Sedentary to Endurance-Trained Humans*

Muscle $\dot{V}O_2$ = Blood Flow × A$\dot{V}O_2$ Difference			Blood Flow/100 g Active Muscle/Min
3.5 L min^{-1}	= 19.4 L min^{-1} ×	180 ml L^{-1}	Assume 10 kg active muscle = 194 ml 100 g^{-1} min^{-1}
			Assume 15 kg active muscle = 129 ml 100 g^{-1} min^{-1}
5.0 L min^{-1}	= 27.8 L min^{-1} ×	180 ml L^{-1}	Assume 10 kg active muscle = 278 ml 100 g^{-1} min^{-1}
			Assume 15 kg active muscle = 185 ml 100 g^{-1} min^{-1}
6.13 L min^{-1}	= 34.0 L min^{-1} ×	180 ml L^{-1}	Assume 10 kg active muscle = 340 ml 100 g^{-1} min^{-1}
			Assume 15 kg active muscle = 227 ml 100 g^{-1} min^{-1}

*Body weight = 75 kg; total muscle mass = 30 kg.

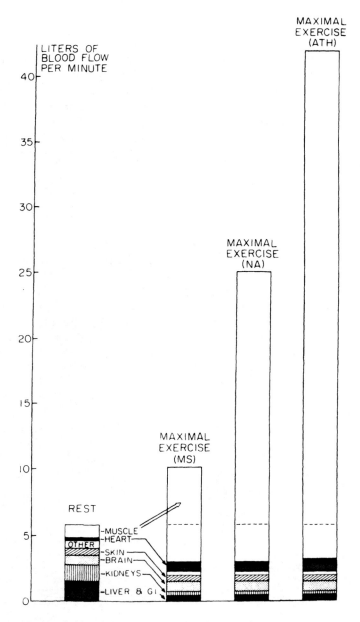

LITERS OF
BLOOD FLOW
PER MINUTE

MAXIMAL
EXERCISE
(ATH)

MAXIMAL
EXERCISE
(NA)

MAXIMAL
EXERCISE
(MS)

REST

-MUSCLE
-HEART-
OTHER
-SKIN -
-BRAIN-
-KIDNEYS-
-LIVER & GI

Figure 7-7 Total blood flow and its distribution during rest and brief exercise requiring $\dot{V}o_2$max in the three groups as depicted in Figure 5-2. Blood flow to nonmuscular regions, except the heart, is virtually the same in all three groups. The higher coronary flow in the athletes reflects the greater tissue mass, otherwise flow per 100 g of left ventricle should be similar (see text, this chapter). Cerebral blood flow should stay constant (Chapter 6). Skin blood flow would not be expected to rise during brief maximal exercise (Chapter 6). The maximal reductions in splanchnic and renal blood flows are well established and flow to "other" regions (bone, connective tissue, etc.) is estimated. (From Rowell, 1986, with permission from Oxford University Press.)

maximal *total* muscle blood flow in the patients with pure mitral stenosis (MS), normally active (NA), and athletic (ATH) subject groups discussed in Chapter 5. The regional vasoconstriction discussed in Chapter 6 provides an additional (approximately) 3 L min^{-1} of blood flow to the active muscles in each group.

Most measurements of peak blood flow per 100 g of active muscle come from isolated muscle, and the values are in fundamental disagreement with those presented in Table 7-1. This long-standing disagreement (e.g., Rowell, 1974a) was the subject of a provocative review by Laughlin (1987) and a 1988 symposium (see Armstrong, 1988; Musch, 1988; Rowell, 1988; Stainsby and Andrew, 1988; and Terjung and Engbretson, 1988). These publications compare the values for peak muscle blood flow during contractions in situ with those in in vivo conditions.

Traditionally, peak values for blood flow to isolated mammalian skeletal muscle range from 40 to 120 ml 100 g^{-1} min^{-1} for various muscles in different species. These values depend partly on whether contractions were generated by increasing twitch stimulation frequencies or rhythmic tetanic stimulations (for references, see Terjung and Engbretson, 1988; Armstrong, 1988). The most commonly accepted values for peak flows were between 50 and 80 ml 100 g^{-1} min^{-1}; peak power outputs of the isolated muscle were 7 to 8 W kg^{-1} (Stainsby and Andrew, 1988). In short, if the highest attainable muscle blood flow and power output were as low in the intact animal as found in isolated muscle, the values for $\dot{V}O_2$max observed in dogs and in humans could never be reached.

Range of Peak Blood Flows in Active Muscle

Figure 7-8 shows the blood flows to various muscles of the hind limb as determined from the distribution of radioactive microspheres while dogs (sedentary Foxhounds) ran at $\dot{V}O_2$max (Musch, 1988). Values for peak muscle blood flow range between 100 ml 100 g^{-1} min^{-1} to over 300 ml 100 g^{-1} min^{-1} in the various exercising muscle groups of rats, pigs, ponies, horses, and steers with values approaching 500 ml 100 g^{-1} min^{-1} in rats (see Laughlin, 1987; Armstrong, 1988).

Differences Within and Between Muscles at Peak Exercise. The differences between muscles shown in Figure 7-8 can be attributed to their relative number of fast-twitch red (oxidative) and white (glycolytic) fibers and slow-twitch red fibers as illustrated in Figure 7-9. A general relationship exists between peak muscle blood flow and the inherent capacity for oxidative metabolism in a particular muscle fiber group as well as that group's capillary density and mitochondrial volume. In the rat gastrocnemius (Figure 7-9) peak flows through fast-twitch white muscle with its low-oxidative capacity were only one-fourth of the peak flows through fast-twitch red muscle, which has high oxidative capacity. Armstrong (1988) observed fivefold differences in peak blood flows of deep red fibers and superficial white fibers *of the same muscle* (vastus lateralis muscle) of a

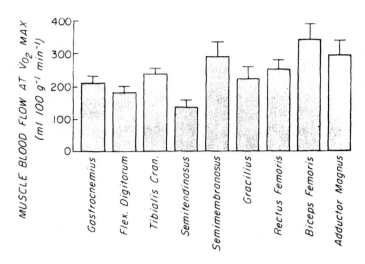

Figure 7-8   Blood flows to individual muscles of the hindlimbs of sedentary fox-hounds as measured by radioactive microsphere technique during maximal exercise. (Adapted from Musch, 1988.)

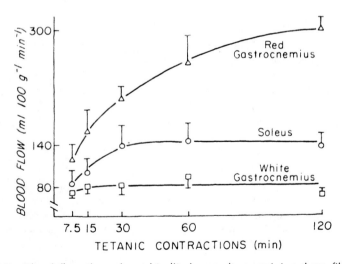

Figure 7-9   Blood flow through rat hindlimb muscle containing three fiber types during isometric tetanic contractions (each 100 msec at 100 Hz). Fast-twitch red oxidative fibers of the gastrocnemius have the highest blood flow and comprise one-third of the gastrocnemius mass. Fast-twitch white glycolytic fibers have the lowest blood flow and comprise two-thirds of the total. The soleus muscle is composed of slow-twitch red fibers. (Adapted from Mackie and Terjung, 1983.)

rat during a treadmill exercise at maximal speed. The data are presented to reveal the difficulty in expressing average values of peak muscle blood flow for the entire animal. Clearly values from one group of muscles cannot be simply extrapolated to others to derive a total.

Importance of Natural Muscle Pumping Action in Generating High Peak Blood Flows. Laughlin (1987) argued convincingly that artificially induced contraction cannot generate the peak flows seen when muscles are activated in natural running movements. The main thrust of Laughlin's argument is in Figure 7-10, which compares peak flows to three types of rat muscle during three types of activation from the original studies of Mackie and Terjung (1983) and Armstrong and Laughlin (1985). The first point is that the highest vascular conductances in *resting* muscle attained by papaverine infusion are far below those attained during contractions (resting flows are not shown in the bottom panel of Figure 7-10 because they were measured at different perfusion pressures than during exercise). Low flows at rest may be the consequence of (1) poor intramuscular distribution of the dilator (diffusing from arteries *outward* rather than from tissues *inward*), (2) the large outward filtration from capillaries caused by increased capillary pressure is unopposed by the high tissue pressure in contracting muscle, and (3) the lack of effective mechanical pumping on blood flow.

Peak muscle flows are always greatest during running, except for fast-twitch white fibers (Figure 7-10). Laughlin's main hypothesis (also discussed in Chapters 1 and 5) is *that the muscle pump increases blood flow across the muscle at any given arterial perfusion pressure.* In order to separate this effect from that of perfusion pressure, Laughlin described what could be called a *virtual* ''conductance''—called virtual because a simple ohmic conductance does not exist across a pump that directly imparts energy to the system. Also the pump does not increase the diameter of the resistance vessels. Laughlin contends that the normal sequential pattern of motor unit recruitment in voluntary locomotion could provide a wavelike pumping action that is enhanced by the active lengthening and shortening of muscles during the stride. Both Laughlin (1987) and Stegall (1966) (Stegall's data were from human legs) estimated that approximately one-third of the calculated energy for muscle perfusion is generated by the muscle pump (this would be approximately 30 to 50 mmHg in the experiments of Laughlin). The pump could work effectively even without the high venous pressures caused by gravity that are seen in humans. That is, when muscle relaxes rapidly, the sudden release of a high compressive force could, by elastic recoil, pull open empty veins making their transmural pressure negative with a proportional increase in pressure gradient across the muscle (in humans the pump greatly enhances muscle perfusion by momentarily reducing muscle venous pressure to zero while the hydrostatic effect on arterial driving pressure persists). Figure 7-11 provides a dramatic illustration of the action of muscle pumping on femoral arterial

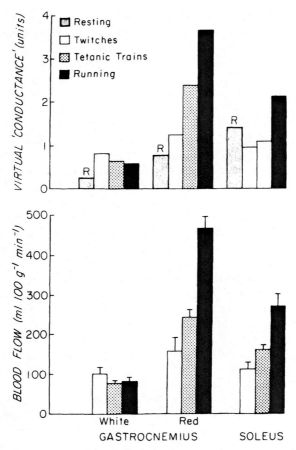

Figure 7-10 Virtual vascular "conductances" (at a perfusion pressure of 130 mmHg) in hindlimb muscles of the rat during so-called "maximal" vasodilation at rest (*shaded bars, R*), by papaverine infusion and during exercise induced by twitch stimulations (*open bars*), rhythmic tetanic stimulations (*stippled bars*) (from Mackie and Terjung, 1983). The contrast with "conductance" at rest reveals the influence of contractions on muscle blood flow at a given perfusion pressure. Electrically stimulated oxidative muscles have lower peak blood flows than muscle voluntarily activated during running when the muscle pump is presumably most effective (*solid bars*). (From Armstrong and Laughlin, 1985.) The bottom panel shows *blood flows* from the same experiments. Resting blood flows were measured at a different perfusion pressure and are not shown. (Adapted from Laughlin, 1987.)

blood flow and cardiac output in a supine subject exercising on a cycle ergometer (Eriksen et al., 1990).

Sheriff (unpublished) postulated that the immediate increase in vascular conductance in response to exercise, shown in Figure 7-12, in a dog with autonomic ganglionic blockade (hexamethonium) could be due to the

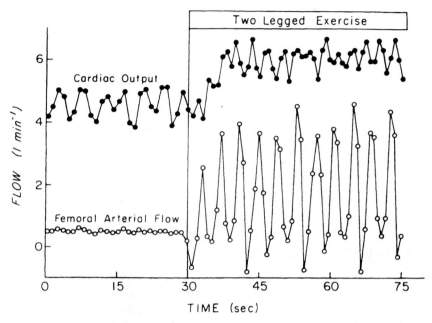

Figure 7-11 Simultaneous measurements of ascending aortic and right femoral arterial blood flows by bidirectional Doppler ultrasound velocity meter (flow calculated from vessel cross-sectional areas) in a supine subject during mild leg exercise (two-legged cycling). During each contraction the skeletal muscle pump caused marked oscillations in femoral blood flow. When maximal flow was observed in one femoral artery, minimum flow was observed in the other. (Adapted from Eriksen et al., 1990.)

muscle pump. It seems to occur too fast to be a metabolically linked event. The speed of increase in muscle blood flow led others to postulate a neural mechanism (see ''Local Neural Influences,'' above).

Summary.   In summary, Laughlin (1987) lists six factors that have large influences on what has been loosely and often erroneously referred to as ''maximal'' muscle blood flow:

1. The type of stimulation used to elicit contraction
2. The type of voluntary exercise, especially the force (e.g., static versus dynamic) and magnitude of muscle length changes
3. Muscle fiber type and deep versus superficial location of fibers
4. Vascular arrangement within the muscles
5. Adequacy of venous valves
6. Effects of gravity on muscle pumping

Results from several studies reveal that the degree of vasodilation obtainable in resting muscle by infusion of vasodilators is far less than can be

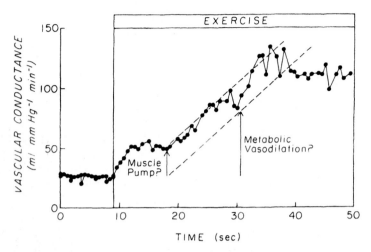

Figure 7-12   The time course of muscle vasodilation in response to sudden onset of moderate exercise (treadmill running) in a dog with ganglionic blockade by hexamethonium. The first and rapid phase of the rise in vascular conductance appears to be too rapid for metabolic vasodilation and may represent the action of the muscle pump. Metabolic vasodilation may begin after 8 or 9 seconds (at 18 seconds). The difference between upper and lower slopes (dashed lines) represents an hypothetical constant upward bias on conductance caused by the muscle pump. (Unpublished data kindly provided by D.D. Sheriff.)

obtained when the muscle is electrically stimulated to make brief tetanic contractions. But the greatest vasodilation is seen when muscles contract rhythmically during voluntary exercise. The latter is attributed to the possible enhancement of muscle pumping action by a normal sequential pattern of motor unit recruitment. The muscle pump may also increase the "virtual" vascular conductance across the muscle by lowering post-capillary venous pressures during their elastic recoil after each contraction.

Is There a Mismatch Between the Capacities of the Heart to Deliver and the Muscle to Receive Blood?

Many estimates of peak muscle blood flow or maximal *total* flow appear *not* to obey conservation laws being either too low to provide a $\dot{V}o_2max$ or too high to be supplied by the heart. The problems surface when one attempts to normalize blood flow to a unit mass of muscle. Unless we know the peak blood flow per 100 g of muscle and the mass of active muscle, we cannot predict whether cardiac output can supply the total oxygen requirements of a large active muscle mass. If the demands of 10 or 15 kg of muscle for blood flow outstrip the pumping capacity of the heart, the rise in total vascular conductance will cause arterial pressure to fall unless there is sufficient vasoconstriction to counteract it. Table 7-1 shows what the average *minimum* blood flow per 100 g of muscle would have to be at a given $\dot{V}O_2$max if 10 kg and 15 kg (30 percent and 50 percent of total muscle mass) were active.

Terjung and Engbretson (1988) calculated that the peak muscle blood flows they observed during tetanic contractions could just barely be supplied by the maximal cardiac output of the rat. Their calculations assumed for the whole body the distribution of red and white muscle fibers within the rat gastrocnemius (Figure 7-9). However, the demonstration that peak flows are higher during running than tetanic stimulation (see Laughlin, 1987) suggests that the rise in total vascular conductance might overwhelm the pump.

The calculations for humans in Table 7-1 simply point out that the more muscle mass we activate during severe exertion, the less blood flow is available for each 100 g of active muscle, because of the fixed upper limit for cardiac output. For example, in the sedentary individual in Table 7-1, whose maximal *total* muscle blood flow is 19.4 L min^{-1} (85 percent of maximal cardiac output of 22.8 L min^{-1}) and whose peak muscle blood flow is 194 ml 100 g^{-1} min^{-1}, activation of 15 kg of muscle would raise the demand for total muscle blood flow to 29.1 L min^{-1}. Inasmuch as this demand cannot be met, the 1.5-fold rise in total vascular conductance would cause arterial pressure to fall from 120 to 80 mmHg. Alternatively, muscle blood flow could be reduced from 194 to 129 ml 100 g^{-1} min^{-1} by sympathetic vasoconstriction (e.g., arterial baroreflex) so that blood pressure would remain at 120 mmHg.

Two key points emerge from this discussion:

1. It is not possible to determine the peak muscle blood flow per 100 g of a muscle by measuring muscle blood flow when other muscles are heavily engaged during whole-body exercise. Neural control of the muscle vasculature will compete with metabolic control and reduce muscle blood flow by vasoconstriction.

2. In order to observe an upper limit for muscle blood flow, unimpeded by reflexes, the mass of muscle maximally activated must be too small to tax the pumping capacity of the heart.

In order to bypass cardiac limitations on muscle blood flow, and thus any reflex vasoconstriction, Andersen and Saltin (1985) measured femoral venous blood flow (thermal dilution) during exercise that was confined to the knee extensors (quadriceps femoris muscle). Figure 7-13 shows the average responses. Blood flow reached a peak value of 5.7 L min^{-1} and oxygen uptake of the leg reached 800 ml min^{-1} or 35 ml 100 g^{-1} min^{-1} (calculated weight of the quadriceps was 2.3 kg). Mechanical efficiency was 22 to 24 percent. Of the total femoral venous blood flow, 0.5 L min^{-1} was assumed to go to inactive regions of the thigh giving an estimated total quadriceps blood flow of 5.2 L min^{-1}, or 226 ml 100 g^{-1} min^{-1}. If this number is applied to Table 7-1, it is obvious that only the endurance-

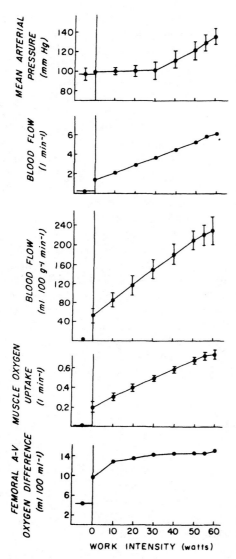

Figure 7-13 Average hemodynamic responses during mild to "peak" exercise confined to extensors of the knee. Exercise was accompanied by marked increases in arterial pressure. The blood flow of almost 6 L min^{-1} was high considering active muscle mass was only 2 to 3 kg, giving a flow per 100 g of muscle of up to 200 ml min^{-1} and oxygen uptake of 0.8 L min^{-1}. Some of the increase in blood flow can be explained by the rise in pressure plus a small fraction to inactive tissue of the thigh (see text). Once exercise began, increasing demands for oxygen were met primarily by increasing flow; oxygen extraction tended to remain constant. These data reveal the high flow capacity, or vascular conductance, of active human muscles. Because of their small mass (and conductance) relative to the total, the knee extensors were not subject to limitations of cardiac pumping capacity. That is, the heart could supply as much as they could receive at a given pressure (Andersen and Saltin, 1985). (From Rowell, 1986, with permission from Oxford University Press.)

trained individual could maximally activate 15 kg of muscle and generate a minimum total muscle blood flow of 34 L min^{-1}. An unanswered question is how well the quadriceps femoris represents the other muscles of the body.

Figure 7-13 reveals a tendency for leg vascular conductance to level off at 30 watts or approximately 160 ml O$_2$ 100 g^{-1} min^{-1}, suggesting that "maximal" vasodilation (as depicted in Figure 7-3) may have occurred at that power output, with further increases in leg blood flow to 226 ml kg^{-1} min^{-1} being caused by increased blood pressure, which reached 135 mmHg. Normally blood pressure rises to approximately 110 mmHg during maximal whole-body exercise (pressure increases much more during severe exercise with small muscle groups). If we reduce quadriceps blood flow to the value that would exist if blood pressure were 110 mmHg rather than 135 mmHg, peak muscle blood flow would be 183 ml 100 g^{-1} min^{-1}. This would mean that our sedentary subject in Table 7-1 could maximally activate 10.6 kg of muscle (10.6 kg $\times$ 1.83 L kg^{-1} min^{-1} = 19.4 L min^{-1}), but not 15 kg, without either a fall in arterial pressure or a vasoconstriction to reduce muscle blood flow. The point is that there appears to be an upper limit to how much muscle we can activate without causing a mismatch between cardiac output and vascular conductance. We do not know what that upper limit is.

Two observations that would confirm a mismatch between muscle vasodilation and cardiac output during severe exercise with large muscle groups would be either (1) a fall in blood pressure, or (2) vasoconstriction and reduced blood flow in active muscle (preventing a fall in pressure). The latter, but not the former, has been observed. Blood flow to active muscle in humans is reduced during exercise by increased sympathetic nervous outflow; the spillover of norepinephrine from active muscle increases markedly with increased severity of exercise (Savard et al., 1987, 1989; Esler, 1990). Figure 7-14 shows the spillover of norepinephrine from the heart, kidneys, and active muscle in normal young people during moderately heavy supine exercise (approximately 60 to 70 percent of "maximum"). Although percentage increments from muscle were less than those from other organs, muscle is nevertheless the main source of norepinephrine in plasma because of its large mass. Figure 7-15 shows that the spillover of norepinephrine from the active quadriceps muscle increases when the mass of other muscles that are simultaneously activated is increased (Savard et al., 1989). Also, if we compare the arterial-femoral venous oxygen difference during running (see Figure 5-15) with that measured during exercise with only the quadriceps (Figure 7-16),

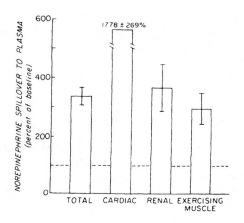

Figure 7-14 Spillover of radio-labeled norepinephrine into plasma from all organs (total), the heart, kidneys, and exercising muscle during *supine* exercise for 10 to 15 minutes at 60 to 70 percent of "maximal" working capacity. Sympathetic outflow to the heart increased 16-fold, whereas outflow to the body as a whole and the kidneys and working muscle tripled. Because of its mass and high flow, muscle had the greatest effect on the total spillover. (Adapted from Esler et al., 1990.)

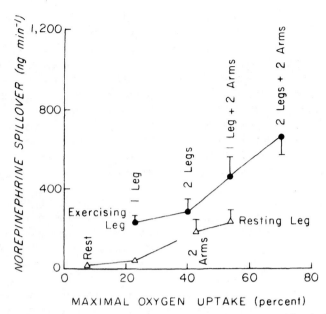

Figure 7-15 Spillover of norepinephrine into femoral venous blood draining the active quadriceps muscles of one leg and into the femoral vein draining inactive muscles of the contralateral leg. Dynamic quadriceps exercise increased norepinephrine spillover from the contralateral resting quadriceps (*open triangles*) probably by a flow-related washout owing to the passive rise in muscle blood flow caused by increased arterial pressure. Exercise increased norepinephrine spillover from the active quadriceps and this spillover increased in proportion to the rise in oxygen uptake caused by adding more and more active muscle (*solid circles*). Spillover from the active muscles represents an increase in muscle sympathetic nerve activity. (Adapted from Savard et al., 1989.)

whose oxygen extraction is approximately constant at 14 ml 100 ml^{-1}, extraction is much higher when more muscles are engaged in running. Presumably blood flow to active legs is reduced by vasoconstriction. The higher circulating concentrations of norepinephrine support this suggestion.

PERIPHERAL VASCULAR ADJUSTMENTS TO PHYSICAL CONDITIONING

The increase in the capacity of the central circulation to transport oxygen to the working muscle normally accounts for approximately 50 percent of the increase in $\dot{V}o_2$max during physical conditioning; the remainder is achieved by widening the systemic arteriovenous oxygen difference.

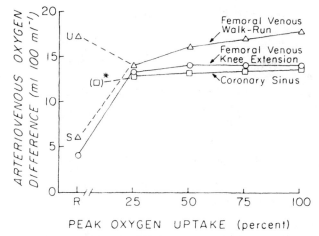

Figure 7-16 Arteriovenous oxygen difference across the heart (coronary sinus, *open squares*), extensors of the knee (or quadriceps femoris, *open circles*) during repeated knee extensions at loads of 20 to 60 watts (Andersen and Saltin, 1985) and across the entire leg during upright rest (U, *open triangle*) and supine rest (S, *open triangle*) and walking and running to $\dot{V}_{O_2}$max. Oxygen extraction by the heart and quadriceps muscles remains virtually constant over their full range of metabolism whereas extraction approaches 90 percent when large masses of muscle become severely active (see Figure 5-15).

How Does Systemic Arteriovenous Oxygen Difference Increase?

There are three possibilities to explain the approximately 7 to 10 percent increase in total extraction of oxygen that normally attends physical conditioning (Rowell, 1974a; Clausen, 1977; Saltin and Rowell, 1980);

1. *The content of oxygen in arterial blood could increase.* It does not and in fact, the tendency is for arterial oxygen content to *decrease* and capacity to *increase* slightly during 2 to 3 months of conditioning (Rowell et al., 1964).
2. *Greater vasoconstriction in inactive regions would increase total oxygen extraction.* This does not occur; vasoconstriction is essentially maximal at $\dot{V}_{O_2}$max before and after physical conditioning. The relationships among visceral organ blood flow, heart rate, the percent of $\dot{V}_{O_2}$max required, and plasma norepinephrine concentration during exercise remain unchanged by the adaptation. *The scale over which the sympathetic nervous activity increases is expanded, but indices of its activity at any particular fraction of $\dot{V}_{O_2}$max remain constant.*
3. *Increased extraction of oxygen by the active muscles could occur in two ways.*

a. By directing exclusively the increase in cardiac output with conditioning to the active muscles, meaning that they receive a greater *percent* of maximal cardiac output, as illustrated in Figure 7-17. This is what occurs. Longitudinal studies showed that total leg blood flow (dye infusion technique) during "maximal" exercise increased in parallel with the rise of $\dot{V}o_2$max. Also, femoral arteriovenous oxygen difference is significantly wider after conditioning (Saltin and Rowell, 1980).

b. Through structural and metabolic changes within the muscle.

These are discussed in the next section.

Adjustments in Skeletal Muscle

Two questions are answered in this section: What adjustments in the muscle accommodate the increase in perfusion? Does the efficiency of oxygen extraction by the muscle increase and if so, by what mechanisms?

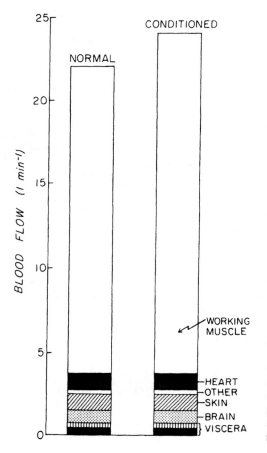

Figure 7-17 The distribution of cardiac output at $\dot{V}o_2$max in normal young people before and after 2 to 3 months of endurance conditioning. Available evidence indicates that blood flow to the heart (the pressure-rate product and cardiac mass are not changed) and visceral organs is virtually the same at $\dot{V}o_2$max irrespective of how much $\dot{V}o_2$max has been increased by physical conditioning (this includes endurance athletes). Accordingly skeletal muscle is the only organ whose blood flow is significantly increased by conditioning.

Muscle Blood Flow: Greater Vasodilation or Less Vasoconstriction?

Inasmuch as we do not know what maximal blood flow or vascular conductance is in human skeletal muscle, it is difficult to say whether physical conditioning increases the intrinsic ability of muscle to dilate its resistance vessels. Arterial blood pressure at a given fraction of $\dot{V}o_2$max (including 100 percent) is not altered by physical conditioning so that the increase in maximal cardiac output is accommodated by a rise in total vascular conductance. This must occur within the active muscles that are the site of approximately 85 percent of the total vascular conductance at $\dot{V}o_2$max (see Figure 5-12). (Keep in mind this is a virtual conductance, see Figure 5-13.)

Could this rise in muscle vascular conductance result from a local release of vasdilator metabolites in the muscle that increases vasodilator capacity in parallel with its expanded oxidative capacity? Alternatively, is this rise in vascular conductance caused by a decrease in vasoconstrictor outflow to the active muscles? One important adjustment to physical conditioning appears to be a reduction in vasoconstrictor outflow to the active muscles which "permits" their conductance to rise further. Accordingly, the rise in cardiac output can occur without any rise in arterial pressure. A withdrawal of sympathetic vasoconstriction is suggested by the finding that plasma norepinephrine levels remain constant at a given heart rate and fraction of $\dot{V}o_2$max before and after physical conditioning despite the fact that the absolute rate of work is much higher; that is, relative to absolute work intensity, sympathetic outflow appears to be lower (see Galbo, 1983). More detailed evidence follows.

Experiments Suggesting That Physical Conditioning Modifies Sympathetic Control of Muscle Blood Flow

One key to understanding how physical conditioning alters the capacity of the muscles to increase their peak vascular conductance rests on studies in which the adaptation is confined to the peripheral vasculature. This is achieved by conditioning a mass of muscle that is too small to elicit any adaptation of the central circulation, for example; maximal cardiac output does not increase. In this context two experiments demonstrated the inability of the unadapted central circulation to keep pace with local adaptations in skeletal muscle when conditioning was confined to a small muscle mass. Davies and Sargeant (1975) conditioned both legs, one at a time, and observed that peak oxygen uptake during "maximal" one-legged exercise was increased by approximately 0.5 L min^{-1} in each leg, whereas the increase in $\dot{V}o_2$max during two-legged exercise was only 0.14 L min^{-1}. Klausen and colleagues (1982) provided an explanation. They trained subjects in essentially the same manner and saw that when "maximal exercise" was confined to one unconditioned leg, the capacity of that leg to vasodilate and increase its oxygen uptake exceeded that which could occur when both legs were simultaneously "maximally" active. Peak blood flow, peak oxygen uptake, and vascular conductance of that active leg *fell* when additional muscles were made active as it continued to exercise. That is, *the active muscle vasoconstricted.* Thus the local adaptations in muscle were opposed by a vasoconstriction that was required to maintain blood pressure. Therefore, a fixed maximal cardiac output after conditioning prevented the central circulation from taking advantage of the locally created potential for increased muscle blood flow during "maximal exercise" with large muscle groups.

The experiments just described lead to two conclusions: *First,* in order to increase $\dot{V}o_2$max and muscle blood flow, one adjustment must be a withdrawal of some vasoconstrictor outflow to the working muscle, permitting a further rise in its vascular conductance. *Second,* the other essential adjustment in conditioning has to be an increase in pumping capacity of the heart in order to raise muscle blood flow and prevent a fall in blood pressure. The adjustments proceed as though blood pressure were the regulated variable.

How Does Extraction of Oxygen by the Muscle Increase?

Saltin and Gollnick (1983) pointed to the increase in capillary density of the muscle as the major factor permitting increased oxygen extraction. Figure 7-18 shows the relationship between the number of capillaries per muscle fiber and $\dot{V}o_2$max. The findings of Kayser and coworkers (1991), discussed earlier in this chapter, reveal that the number of capillaries per muscle fiber, the number of capillaries per unit area of tissue, the area of

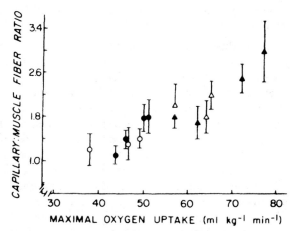

Figure 7-18 The number of capillaries per muscle fiber increases in proportion to $\dot{V}o_2$max expressed per kg of body weight. Circles are from men, triangles from women. Closed symbols indicate electron microscopy and open circles, light microscopy and staining techniques (Saltin and Gollnick, 1983). (From Rowell, 1986, with permission from Oxford University Press.)

muscle tissue perfused by each capillary are greater in well-conditioned mountain climbers than in sedentary people. Also, wild animals have greater muscle capillary density than their domestic relatives. Longitudinal studies on animals (see Hudlicka, 1985) and on young human subjects (Andersen and Henriksson, 1977) confirm that these differences can be generated acutely during several months of conditioning (and this number declines during inactivity) (Figure 7-19). Capillary density, leg blood flow, and $\dot{V}o_2$max all increase in similar proportion after several months of physical conditioning (Saltin and Rowell, 1980).

On the surface it would appear that the reduction in diffusion distances between the capillary and the muscle fibers must enable the muscle to extract more oxygen from each milliliter of blood. Nevertheless, Figure 7-16 shows less oxygen extraction by the heart over its full range of metabolism than by the muscles of the legs during maximal exercise. Yet capillary density in the heart is much greater than in skeletal muscle.

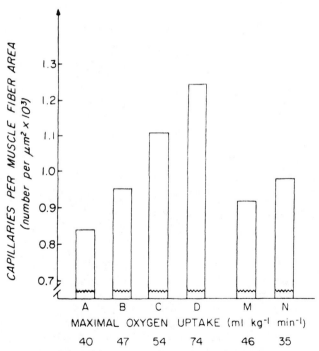

Figure 7-19 Average values for the number of capillaries per 1,000 μm^2 of muscle fiber area in relation to maximal oxygen uptake in milliliters per kilogram shown below each bar. Bars A and B show values for two groups of sedentary subjects. Bar C shows the result of conditioning the group in Bar B for 8 weeks. Bar D shows the capillary density in well-conditioned subjects. Bars M and N show values for athletes recovering from knee surgery (Saltin and Rowell, 1980). (From Rowell, 1986, with permission from Oxford University Press.)

Another factor that determines oxygen extraction is the *mean transit time* (flow divided by volume) of the red blood cells through the capillaries. The longer this time, the greater the exchange of material across the capillary. The increase in the number of capillaries in the conditioned muscles could promote greater oxygen extraction by counteracting any reduction in the mean transit time caused by the increase in muscle blood flow. Figure 7-20 shows that as long as muscle capillary blood volume rises as more capillaries open, the fall in mean transit time is minimized and venous oxygen tension and content continue to fall. When all capillaries are open and their volume is at a maximum, further increases in flow will *raise venous* oxygen content because the transit time is too short to

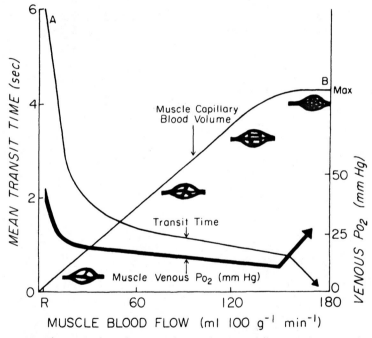

Figure 7-20   Theoretical explanation for inadequate diffusion of oxygen from red blood cells to active muscle during severe exercise. Line A shows how estimated mean transit times for red cells through muscle capillaries decreases with increasing blood flow. Line B shows the relative rise in muscle capillary blood volume caused by recruitment of more capillaries with increasing metabolism and blood flow. As long as capillary blood volume increases with blood flow, mean transmit time will be long enough to permit equilibration of oxygen between capillaries and muscle fibers. When all capillaries are open and capillary volume can no longer increase, any further increases in blood flow will reduce mean transit time so that time to *unload* oxygen is too brief. Consequently, oxygen extraction falls, and *venous oxygen content rises.* The same can occur in the lung, as shown in Chapter 9. The effect there, however, is a *fall* in pulmonary venous and arterial oxygen content when mean transit time is too brief. (Redrawn from Rowell, 1990.)

permit equilibration of oxygen between capillaries and muscle fibers. This could explain the higher venous oxygen content in the heart or in the relatively overperfused quadriceps muscle during knee extension (Figure 7-16). Therefore *there must be a fine balance between the increase in muscle blood flow and the minimum mean transit time needed to effect the most efficient extraction of oxygen.* Accordingly, one fortuitous effect of vasoconstriction in active muscle could be to reduce flow velocity enough to maintain the mean transit time required to permit maximum extraction of oxygen.

A reduction in hemoglobin-oxygen affinity via the Bohr effect within the muscle capillaries would enable a greater widening of arteriovenous oxygen difference across these vessels at $\dot{V}o_2$max after conditioning. There is no reasoin to expect lower pH in the capillaries of conditioned muscle at $\dot{V}o_2$max (Saltin et al., 1977), but the higher rate of work required to elicit $\dot{V}o_2$max could elevate intramuscular temperature. Although a greater Bohr effect has been observed after conditioning, it is though to be of minor importance to the adaptation (see Rowell, 1974a).

An increase in the content myoglobin in the muscle may also contribute to the greater extraction of oxygen. When rats are physically conditioned, muscle content of myoglobin and oxidative enzymes increase in similar proportions (Booth and Thomason, 1991). Myoglobin releases its oxygen to cells at very low partial pressures of oxygen, and it facilitates diffusion of oxygen within the muscle.

An increase in the activity of oxidative enzymes in the muscle does not always accompany physical conditioning (one exception is the fox-hound) and does not normally contribute to the increase in oxygen extraction by the muscle or in $\dot{V}o_2$max. The greater reliance on oxidative metabolism to provide energy, however, has a great impact on endurance (i.e., *performance* increases much more than *capacity*). Treatment of this topic is postponed until Chapter 9 and the discussion of factors that limit $\dot{V}o_2$max.

Finally, the spatial and temporal heterogeneity of blood flow which causes some portions of the muscle to be poorly perfused while other portions are well perfused (Marconi et al., 1988; Grønlund et al., 1989) might be lessened by the microcirculatory adjustments attending physical conditioning. This will also be discussed further in Chapter 9.

Summary. In summary, the most important peripheral circulatory adjustments to physical conditioning are the increase in muscle blood flow and in its extraction of oxygen at $\dot{V}o_2$max. The rise in peak muscle blood flow appears to be achieved by withdrawal of vasoconstrictor tone; evidence of an increase in the intrinsic ability of muscle vessels to dilate is lacking. The increase in muscle capillary density is the main factor permitting the rise in maximal oxygen extraction by muscle. This improvement in extraction plus the higher percentage of maximal cardiac output going to the active muscles after conditioning explain the widened systemic

arteriovenous oxygen difference. The latter accounts for 50 percent of the
rise in $\dot{V}O_2$max during this adaptation.

REFERENCES

Aaron, E.A., K.C. Seow, B.D. Johnson, and J.A. Dempsey (1992). Oxygen cost
    of exercise hyperpnea: implications for performance. *J. Appl. Physiol. 72*,
    1818–1825.
Andersen P., and J. Henriksson, (1977). Capillary supply of the quadriceps femoris
    muscle of man: adaptive response to exercise. *J. Physiol. (Lond.) 270*,
    677–691.
Andersen, P., and B. Saltin (1985). Maximal perfusion of skeletal muscle in man.
    J. Physiol. (Lond.) 366, 233–249.
Anholm, J.D., R.L. Johnson, and M. Ramanathan (1987). Changes in cardiac
    output during sustained maximal ventilation in humans. *J. Appl. Physiol.
    63*, 181–187.
Armstrong, R.B. (1988). Magnitude and distribution of muscle blood flow in con-
    scious animals during locomotory exercise. *Med. Sci. Sports Exer. 20*,
    S119–S123.
Armstrong, R.B., and M.H. Laughlin (1985). Rat muscle blood flows during high-
    speed locomotion. *J. Appl. Physiol. 59*, 1322–1328.
Bache, R.J., X.-Z. Dai, J.S. Schwartz, and D.C. Homans (1988). Role of adenosine
    in coronary vasodilation during exercise. *Circ. Res. 62*, 846–853.
Ball, R.M., and R.J. Bache (1976). Distribution of myocardial blood flow in the
    exercising dog with restricted coronary artery inflow. *Circ. Res. 38*, 60–66.
Barnard, R.J., H.W. Duncan, J.J. Livesay, and G.D. Buckberg (1977). Coronary
    vasodilator reserve and flow distribution during near-maximal exercise in
    dogs. *J. Appl. Physiol. (Respir. Environ. Exercise Physiol.) 43*, 988–992.
Berne, R.M., and R. Rubio (1979). Coronary Circulation. In R.M. Berne, N.
    Sperelakis, and S.R. Geiger, eds. *Handbook of Physiology: The Heart*,
    sect. 2, vol. 1, pp. 873–952. American Physiological Society, Bethesda,
    MD.
Bevan, J.A., E.H. Joyce, and G.C. Wellman (1988). Flow-dependent dilation in a
    resistance artery still occurs after endothelium removal. *Circ. Res. 63*,
    980–985.
Booth, F.W., and D.B. Thomason (1991). Molecular and cellular adaptation of
    muscle in response to exercise: perspectives of various models. *Physiol.
    Rev. 71*, 541–585.
Clausen, J.P. (1977). Effect of physical training on cardiovascular adjustments to
    exercise in man. *Physiol. Rev. 57*, 779–815.
Davies, C.T.M., and A.J. Sargeant (1975). Effects of training on the physiological
    responses to one- and two-leg work. *J. Appl. Physiol. 38*, 377–381.
Dempsey, J.A. (1986). Is the lung built for exercise? *Med. Sci. Sports Exer. 18*,
    143–155.
Donald, D.E., D.J. Rowlands, and D.A. Ferguson (1970). Similarity of blood flow
    in the normal and the sympathectomized dog hind limb during graded
    exercise. *Circ. Res. 26* 185–199.
Duling, B.R. (1981). Coordination of microcirculatory function with oxygen de-
    mand in skeletal muscle. In A.G.B. Kovach, J. Hamar, and L. Szabo, eds.

Advances in Physiology. Cardiovascular Physiology: Microcirculation and Capillary Exchange, vol. 7, pp. 1–16. Akademiai Kaido, Budapest.

Eriksen, M., B.A., Waaler, L. Walløe, and J. Wesche (1990). Dynamics and dimensions of cardiac output changes in humans at the onset and at the end of moderate rhythmic exercise. *J. Physiol. (Lond.) 426,* 423–437.

Esler, M., G. Jennings, G. Lambert, I. Meredith, M. Horne, and G. Eisenhofer (1990). Overflow of catecholamine neurotransmitters to the circulation: source, fate, and functions. *Physiol. Rev. 70,* 963–985.

Feigl, E.O. (1983). Coronary physiology. *Physiol. Rev. 63:* 1–205.

Fleisch, A. and I. Sibul, (1933). Über nutritive Kreislaufregulierung. II. Die Wirkung von pH, intermediären Stoffwechselprodukten und anderen biochemischen Verbindung. *Pflugers Arch. 231,* 787–804.

Forrester, T. (1981). Adenosine or adenosine triphosphate? In P.M. Vanhoutte and I. Leusen, eds. *Vasodilatation,* pp. 205–229. Raven Press, New York.

Forster, H.V., and L.G. Pan (1988). Breathing during exercise: demands, regulation, limitations. *Adv. Exp. Med. Biol. 227,* 257–276. (*Oxygen Transfer From Atmosphere to Tissues* [N.C. Gonzales and M.R. Fedde, eds.]). Plenum Press, New York.

Furchgott, R.F. and Zawadzki, J.V. (1980). The obligatory role of endothelial cells in the relaxation of arterial smooth muscle by acetylcholine. *Nature 288,* 373–376.

Galbo, H. (1983). *Hormonal and Metabolic Adaptation to Exercise.* Thieme-Stratton, New York.

Grønlund, J., G.M., Malvin, and M.P. Hlastala (1989). Estimation of blood flow distribution in skeletal muscle from inert gas washout. *J. Appl. Physiol. 66,* 1942–1955.

Gwirtz, P.A., S.P. Overn, J.H. Mass, and C.E. Jones (1986). α-Adrenergic constriction limits coronary flow and cardiac function in running dogs. *Am. J. Physiol. 250 (Heart Circ. Physiol. 19),* H1117–H1126.

Heyndrickx, G.R., P. Muylaert, and J.L. Pannier (1982). α-Adrenergic control of oxygen delivery to myocardium during exercise in conscious dogs. *Am. J. Physiol. 242 (Heart Circ. Physiol. 11)* H805–H809.

Hilton, S.M. (1959). A peripheral arterial conducting system underlying dilation of femoral artery and concerned with functional dilation in skeletal muscle. *J. Physiol. (Lond.) 149,* 93–111.

Hobbs, S.F., and D.I. McCloskey (1987). Effects of blood pressure on force production in cat and human muscle. *J. Appl. Physiol. 63,* 834–839.

Honig, C.R. and J.L. Frierson (1976). Neurons intrinsic to arterioles initiate postcontraction vasodilation. *Am. J. Physiol. 230,* 493–507.

Huang, A.H., and E.O. Feigl (1988). Adrenergic coronary vasoconstriction helps maintain uniform transmural blood flow distribution during exercise. *Circ. Res. 62,* 286–298.

Hudlicka, O. (1985). Regulation of muscle blood flow. Editorial. *Clin. Physiol. 5,* 201–229.

Johnson, B.D., K.W. Saupe, and J.A. Dempsey (1992). Mechanical constraints on exercise hyperpnea in endurance athletes. *J. Appl. Physiol. 73,* (August).

Jorgensen, C.R., F.L. Gobel, H.L. Taylor, and Y. Wang (1977). Myocardial blood flow and oxygen consumption during exercise. In P. Milvy, ed. *The Marathon: Physiological, Medical, Epidemiological, and Psychological Studies,* pp. 213–223. The New York Academy of Sciences, New York.

Jorgensen, C.R., K. Wang, Y. Wang, F.L. Gobel, R.R. Nelson, and H.L. Taylor (1973). Effect of propranolol on myocardial oxygen consumption and its hemodynamic correlates during upright exercise. *Circulation 48*, 1173–1182.

Kayser, B., H. Hoppeler, H. Claassen, and P. Cerretelli (1991). Muscle structure and performance capacity of Himalayan Sherpas. *J. Appl. Physiol. 70*, 1938–1942.

Kitamura, K., C.R. Jorgensen, F.L. Gobel, H.L. Taylor, and Y. Wang (1972). Hemodynamic correlates of myocardial oxygen consumption during upright exercise. *J. Appl. Physiol. 32*, 516–522.

Kjellmer, I. (1965). On the competition between metabolic vasodilation and neurogenic vasoconstriction in skeletal muscle. *Acta Physiol. Scand 63*, 450–459.

Klausen, K., M.H. Secher, J.P. Clausen, O. Hartling, and J. Trap-Jensen (1982). Central and regional circulatory adaptations to one-leg training. *J. Appl. Physiol. 52*, 976–983.

Klocke, F.J., and A.K. Ellis (1980). Control of coronary blood flow. *Annu. Rev. Med. 31*, 489–508.

Koller, A., and G. Kaley, (1990a). Endothelium regulates skeletal muscle microcirculation by a blood flow velocity sensing mechanism. *Am. J. Physiol. 258 (Heart Circ. Physiol. 27)*, H916–H920.

Koller, A., and G. Kaley, (1990b). Prostaglandins mediate arteriolar dilation to increased blood flow velocity in skeletal muscle microcirculation. *Circ. Res. 67*, 529–534.

Lassen, N.A., O. Henriksen, and P. Sejersen (1983). Indicator methods for measurement of organ and tissue blood flow. In J.T. Shepherd, F.M. Abboud, and S.R. Geiger, eds. *Handbook of Physiology. The Cardiovascular System: Peripheral Circulation and Organ Blood Flow*, sect. 2, vol. III, part 1, pp. 21–63. American Physiological Society, Bethesda, MD.

Laughlin, M.H. (1987). Skeletal muscle blood flow capacity: role of muscle pump in exercise hyperemia. *Am. J. Physiol. 253 (Heart Circ Physiol. 22)*, H993–H1004.

Lautt, W.W. (1989). Resistance or conductance for expression of arterial vascular tone. *Microvasc. Res. 37*, 230–236.

Mackie, B.G., and R.L. Terjung (1983). Blood flow to different skeletal muscle fiber types during contraction. *Am. J. Physiol. 245 (Heart Circ. Physiol. 14)*, H265–H275.

Manohar, M. (1986). Blood flow to the respiratory and limb muscles and to abdominal organs during maximal exertion in ponies. *J. Physiol. (Lond.) 377*, 25–35.

Manohar, M. (1990). Inspiratory and expiratory muscle perfusion in maximally exercised ponies. *J. Appl. Physiol. 68*, 544–548.

Marconi, C., N. Heisler, M. Meyer, H. Weitz, D.R. Pendergast, P. Cerretelli, and J. Piiper (1988). Blood flow distribution and its temporal variability in stimulated dog gastrocnemius muscle. *Respir. Physiol. 74*, 1–14.

Mohrman, D.E., and E.O. Feigl (1978). Competition between sympathetic vasoconstriction and metabolic vasodilation in the canine coronary circulation. *Circ. Res. 42*, 79–86.

Mohrman, D.E., and H.V. Sparks, (1974). Myogenic hyperemia following brief tetanus of canine skeletal muscle. *Am. J. Physiol. 227*, 531–535.

Moncada, S., R.M. Palmer, and E.A. Higgs (1991). Nitric Oxide: Physiology, Pathophysiology, and Pharmacology. *Pharmacol. Rev. 43*, 109–142.

Morganroth M.L., D.E. Mohrman, and H.V. Sparks (1975). Prolonged vasodilation following fatiguing exercise of dog skeletal muscle. *Am. J. Physiol. 229*, 38–43.

Musch, T.I. (1988). Skeletal muscle blood flow in exercising dogs. *Med. Sci. Sports Exer. 20.*, S104–S108.

Musch, T.I., G.C. Haidet, A.G. Ordway, J.C. Longhurst, and J.H. Mitchell (1985). Dynamic exercise training in foxhounds. I. Oxygen consumption and hemodynamic responses. *J. Appl. Physiol. 59*, 183–189.

Nelson, R.R., F.L. Gobel, C.R. Jorgensen, K. Wang, Y. Wang, and H.L. Taylor (1974). Hemodynamic predictors of myocardial oxygen consumption during static and dynamic exercise. *Circulation 50*, 1179–1189.

O'Leary, D.S. (1991). Regional vascular resistance vs. conductance: which index for baroreflex responses? *Am. J. Physiol. 260 (Heart Circ. Physiol. 29)*, H632–H637.

O'Leary, D.S., L.B. Rowell, and A.M. Scher (1991). Baroreflex-induced vasoconstriction in active skeletal muscle of conscious dogs. *Am. J. Physiol. 260 (Heart Circ. Physiol. 29)*, H37–H41.

Olsson, R.A. (1981). Local factors regulating cardiac and skeletal muscle blood flow. *Annu. Rev. Physiol. 43*, 385–395.

Otis, A.B. (1954). The work of breathing. *Physiol. Rev. 34*, 449–458.

Rooke, G.A., and E.O. Feigl (1982). Work as a correlated of canine left ventricular oxygen consumption, and the problem of catecholamine oxygen wasting. *Circ. Res. 50*, 273–286.

Rowell, L.B. (1974a). Human cardiovascular adjustments to exercise and thermal stress. *Physiol. Rev. 54*, 75–159.

Rowell, L.B. (1974b). Circulation to skeletal muscle. In T.C. Ruch and H.D. Patton, eds. *Textbook of Physiology and Biophysics*, 20th ed., vol. II, pp. 200–214. W.B. Saunders, Philadelphia.

Rowell, L.B. (1986). *Human Circulation: Regulation During Physical Stress.* Oxford University Press, New York.

Rowell, L.B. (1988). Muscle blood flow in humans: how high can it go? *Med. Sci. Sports Exer. 20*, S97–S103.

Rowell, L.B. (1990). Exercise physiology. In R.M. Berne and M.N. Levy, eds. *Principles of Physiology*, part IX, pp. 618–645. CV Mosby, St. Louis, MO.

Rowell, L.B. (1991). Control of the circulation during exercise. In J.P. Gilmore and I.H. Zucker, eds. *Reflex Control of the Circulation*, pp. 795–828. CRC Press, Boca Raton, FL.

Rowell, L.B., H.L. Taylor, Y. Wang, and W.S. Carlson (1964). Saturation of arterial blood with oxygen during maximal exercise. *J. Appl. Physiol. 19*, 284–286.

Rowlands, D.J., and D.E. Donald (1968). Sympathetic vasoconstrictive responses during exercise- or drug-induced vasodilation. *Circ. Res. 23*, 45–60.

Saltin, B. and P.D. Gollnick (1983). Skeletal muscle adaptability: significance for metabolism and performance. In L.D. Peachey, R.H. Adrian, and S.R. Geiger, eds. *Handbook of Physiology: Skeletal Muscle*, sect. 10, pp. 555–631. American Physiological Society, Bethesda, MD.

Saltin, B., J. Henriksson, E. Nygaard, E. Jansson, and P. Andersen (1977). Fiber types and metabolic potentials of skeletal muscles in sedentary man and endurance runners. *Ann. NY Acad. Sci. 301,* 3–29.

Saltin, B., and L.B. Rowell (1980). Functional adaptations to physical activity and inactivity. *Fed. Proc. 39,* 1506–1513.

Savard, G.K., E.A. Richter, S. Strange, B. Kiens, N.J. Christensen, and B. Saltin (1989). Norepinephrine spillover from skeletal muscle during exercise in humans: role of muscle mass. *Am. J. Physiol. 257 (Heart Circ. Physiol. 26),* H1812–H1818.

Savard, G., S. Strange, B. Kiens, E.A. Richter, N.J. Christensen, and B. Saltin (1987). Noradrenaline spillover during exercise in active versus resting skeletal muscle in man. *Acta Physiol. Scand. 131,* 507–515.

Segal, S.S., D.N. Damon, and B.R. Duling (1989). Propagation of vasomotor responses coordinates arteriolar resistances. *Am. J. Physiol. 256 (Heart Circ. Physiol. 25),* H832–H837.

Segal, S.S., and B.R. Duling (1989). Conduction of vasomotor responses in arterioles: a role for cell-to-cell coupling? *Am. J. Physiol. 256 (Heart Circ. Physiol. 25),* H838–H845.

Shepherd, J.T. (1983). Circulation to skeletal muscle. In J.T. Shepherd, F.M. Abboud, and S.R. Geiger, eds. *Handbook of Physiology. The Cardiovascular System: Peripheral Circulation and Organ Blood Flow,* sect 2, vol. III, part 1, pp. 319–370. American Physiological Society. Bethesda, MD.

Skinner, N.S., Jr. (1975). Skeletal muscle blood flow: metabolic determinants. In R. Zelis, ed. *The Peripheral Circulation,* pp. 57–78. Grune & Stratton, New York.

Sparks, H.V. Jr. (1980). Effect of local metabolic factors on vascular smooth muscle. In D.F. Bohr, A.P. Somlyo, H.V. Sparks Jr., and S.R. Geiger, eds. *Handbook of Physiology. The Cardiovascular System: Vascular Smooth Muscle,* sect. 2, vol. II, pp. 475–513. American Physiological Society, Bethesda, MD.

Stainsby, W.N., and G.M. Andrew (1988). Maximal blood flow and power output of dog muscle *in situ. Med. Sci. Sports Exer. 20,* S109–S112.

Stegall, H.F. (1966). Muscle pumping in the dependent leg. *Circ. Res. 19,* 180–190.

Stone, H.L. (1983). Control of the coronary circulation during exercise. *Annu. Rev. Physiol. 45,* 213–227.

Terjung, R.L., and B.M. Engbretson (1988). Blood flow to different rat skeletal muscle fiber type sections during isometric contractions in situ. *Med. Sci. Sports Exer. 20,* S124–S130.

Thompson, L.P., and D.E. Mohrman (1983). Blood flow and oxygen consumption in skeletal muscle during sympathetic stimulation. *Am. J. Physiol. 245 (Heart Circ. Physiol. 14),* H66–H71.

Vanhoutte, P.M. (ed.) (1988). *Vasodilatation. Vascular Smooth Muscle, Peptides, Autonomic Nerves, and Endothelium.* Raven Press, New York.

Vanhoutte, P.M., T.J. Verbueren, and R.C. Webb (1981). Local modulation of adrenergic neuroeffector interaction in the blood vessel wall. *Physiol. Rev. 61,* 151–247.

Von Restorff, W., J. Holtz, and E. Bassenge (1977). Exercise induced augmentation of myocardial oxygen extraction in spite of normal coronary dilatory capacity in dogs. *Pflugers Arch. 372,* 181–185.

Wahren, J., and L. Jorfeldt (1973). Determination of leg blood flow during exercise in man: an indicator-dilution technique based on femoral venous dye infusion. *Clin Sci. 45*, 135–146.

Walløe, L., and J. Wesche (1988). Time course and magnitude of blood flow changes in the human quadriceps muscles during and following rhythmic exercise. *J. Physiol. (Lond.) 405*, 257–273.

8

Cardiovascular Adjustments to Isometric Contractions

The purpose of this chapter is to discuss the cardiovascular adjustments to isometric contractions—also called isometric or static exercise—and to contrast these adjustments with those already described for dynamic exercise. This will provide background and set the stage for later chapters dealing with the reflexes that govern the cardiovascular responses to dynamic exercise (Chapters 10–12).

It is customary to think of "exercise" in terms of the movement provided by the active shortening of skeletal muscles. In *isometric* or static contractions, muscles do not shorten (except for internal shortening of more elastic elements) and no net work is done. The total energy transformation within the muscle (E) can be described approximately as the energy connected with activation and production of force (A) and the energy appearing as external work (W) (or the "Fenn-effect"). In the equation,

$$E = A + kW, \tag{8-1}$$

when contraction is truly isometric, work is zero, so that for a given force production, $E = A$, meaning that the oxygen cost is less than that for an isotonic contraction at the same force over the same time (Asmussen, 1981).

Figure 8-1 contrasts the oxygen uptake at a given tension × time for isometric versus isotonic contraction, showing the much lower energy cost of the former. Thus for a given force, the cardiovascular demands for isometric contractions are much less than for dynamic ones. Nevertheless, the cardiovascular responses to a given force × time are far greater for dynamic exercise than for isometric contractions.

The striking differences in responses to the two forms of exercise are ascribable to their effects on blood flow through the active muscle. For example, the pumping action of rhythmic isotonic contractions increases muscle blood flow at any given perfusion pressure. Conversely, during isometric contractions, the swelling and stiffening of the active fibers raises

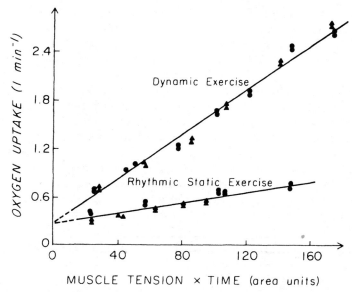

Figure 8-1   Dynamic exercise (bicycling) requires much more oxygen than rhythmic static or isometric contractions. Comparisons were based on the same total area under curves for tension × time during the two forms of exercise. The data are from two subjects. (Adapted from Asmussen, 1981.)

intramuscular pressure, which is transferred to blood vessels and reduces muscle blood flow, despite the rise in arterial pressure. Therefore there is not only an absence of muscle pumping, but also an active *impedance* to blood flow by the contracting muscle as well. *The cardiovascular response to isometric contractions is characterized by its failure to secure adequate blood flow for the contracting muscles* once their force exceeds 10 to 15 percent of the maximal force they can develop.

Inasmuch as the mechanical impedance to muscle blood flow at high levels of contraction force cannot be overcome by increased perfusion pressure, the large cardiovascular responses in a sense constitute an overreaction or a failure of regulation. A dramatic rise in cardiac output serves no useful purpose in overperfusing regions whose requirements for blood flow are not increased. When muscle blood flow can no longer be increased by even the most severe hypertension, we have what might be similar to an open-loop condition such as described for the Cushing reflex in Chapter 6. If the "reflex" (see Chapter 11) that serves to restore muscle blood flow originates from within the muscle, then the "receptors" for the reflex are isolated from their efferent neural output on the system and are thereby deprived of the feedback (increased blood flow) that counteracts the stimulus. Another analogy is the rise in systemic arterial pressure in response to decreased pressure within the isolated carotid sinus; the systemic hypertension can do nothing to restore carotid sinus pressure. A *negative* feedback within the system that serves to counteract the rise in cardiac output and blood pressure during isometric contractions at high levels of force is the fall in ventricular filling pressure and stroke volume. It is argued that this is caused by driving high blood flow through resting, nonpumping organs.

Many investigations of the reflexes thought to control the cardiovascular system during all forms of muscular activity have focused on the responses to isometric contractions. In many ways these contractions have provided a valuable tool, particularly in understanding how the cardiovascular system is "turned on" by exercise. Nevertheless there is a danger in using a form of muscular activity (isometric) in which changes in blood flow, metabolism, and vascular conductance are *not matched* in order to study control in another form of activity (dynamic exercise) in which blood flow, metabolism and vascular conductance *are well matched*. In short, the autonomic nervous system can correct the regulatory problems associated with dynamic exercise, but cannot correct those presented by sustained isometric contractions.

BLOOD FLOW TO ACTIVE MUSCLES

Gaskell (1877) proposed that the blood flow to an active muscle is a compromise between two opposing events: first, the dilation of its vasculature to provide increased blood flow and second, the impedance of this dilation by the mechanical compression of the vessels. Lindhard (1920) appears to have been among the first to record cardiovascular and respiratory responses to isometric contractions. He found that strong contractions of the arms were accompanied by relatively small increases in oxygen uptake, but by large increases after the contraction had stopped. He concluded that blood flow to the muscles must have been impeded by mechanical compression. This was supported by the observation of Dolgin and Lehmann (1930) that durations of strong isometric contractions were unaffected when the investigators occluded arterial inflow (i.e., the contraction must have also stopped blood flow) whereas this occlusion procedure markedly reduced the duration of weaker contractions, which did not stop flow. The idea that there was mechanical occlusion of vessels was also supported by measurements of intramuscular pressures of 150 to 300 mmHg which would exceed arterial pressure and collapse the vessels (Sejersted et al., 1984). The model to keep in mind is that of a Starling resistor illustrated in Figure 6-22.

How Is Muscle Blood Flow Reduced?

Barcroft and Millen (1939) determined that blood flow through human calf muscles was stopped when contractions of these muscles were sustained at tensions that required only 20 percent of the maximal tension that they could develop, referred to hereafter as a percent of maximal voluntary contraction (MVC). Subsequent evidence indicated that the impedance to flow may have been caused by "nipping" or "twisting and shearing" of the vessels and not simply by the effect of the compression on vascular radius and resistance. For example, Gray and colleagues (1967) made direct observations showing that both "nipping" or twisting and vascular narrowing by compression occurred predominantly in the larger arteries and veins as they entered and exited the muscle (electrically stimulated dog hindlimb); capillaries were not compressed. Others have emphasized the importance of venous compression, which has been demonstrated by application of positive pressure to the muscle externally (this may not mimic pressures occurring during a contraction). For example, Reneman and colleagues (1980) found that when an external positive pressure of only 25 mmHg was applied to a resting muscle, the veins within it were completely collapsed. Figure 8-2 shows the relationship between external positive pressure, applied to a resting human leg, and the clearance of ^{133}Xe from the muscle—an index of its blood flow (Nielsen, 1983). For contrast, the top of this figure shows the effects of the same levels of positive pressure on the blood flow to the leg when the muscle pump is

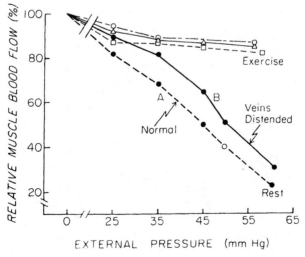

Figure 8-2   Effects of external positive pressure on blood flow (percent changes in ^{133}Xe clearance) in muscles of a resting leg (lines A and B) with veins distended (line B), and without distension (normal, dashed line A). Positive pressure reduced leg blood flow by collapsing intra- and extramuscular veins. This external pressure at which venous collapse began was shifted to higher external pressures by distending the veins by partial occlusion with a cuff proximal to the site of applied positive pressure. Activation of the muscle pump by dynamic contractions (lines at top designated "exercise") opened the veins and greatly reduced the effects of positive external pressure on estimated leg blood flow. (From Rowell et al., 1991.)

active in dynamic exercise (changes in blood flow were estimated from changes in oxygen consumption and in femoral arteriovenous oxygen difference [Rowell et al., 1991]). Again, the major effect of the external pressure was thought to be venous compression and this, in addition to the twisting of arteries observed by Gray and colleagues (1967), would be expected to impede blood flow during an isometric contraction.

By How Much Is Muscle Blood Flow Reduced?

Figure 8-3 shows the total blood flow through 100 ml of forearm tissue (active plus inactive muscle, skin, bone, and connective tissue) during isometric contractions (handgrip) at the various percentages of MVC (Lind and McNicol, 1967). Forearm blood flows appear to reach peak values at approximately 30 to 40 percent of MVC; at higher tensions flow *decreases*

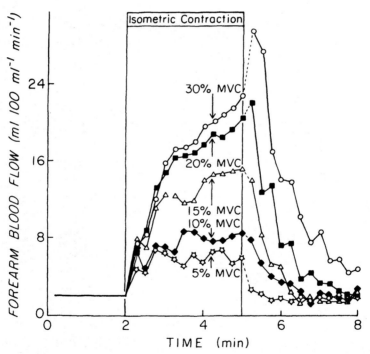

Figure 8-3   Effect of isometric contraction on the forearm (handgrip) on blood flow through the active forearm at five levels of force development expressed as percent of maximal voluntary contraction (MVC). The first indication of inadequate matching of blood flow and metabolism occurs at 20 percent MVC; fatigue develops rapidly and there is a postcontraction hyperemia which becomes marked at 30 percent MVC and above. Above 30 or 40 percent MVC blood flow is reduced below the highest levels shown in this figure, approaching zero flow at 70 percent of MVC. (Adapted from Lind and McNicol, 1967.)

below these peak values in inverse proportion to the increasing percent of MVC and blood flow ultimately approaches resting values (note that measurement of forearm blood flow by plethysmography in an isometrically contracting muscle is very difficult). When a force of approximately 70 percent of MVC or less is reached in the *forearm,* its blood flow approaches zero (Humphreys and Lind 1963). This is not the case in other muscles (see below); for example, it takes much less of a relative increase in tension to reduce blood flow through the quadriceps muscle.

Figure 8-3 shows that a time-dependent increase in forearm blood flow occurs when force of contraction exceeds 10 to 15 percent of MVC. Humphreys and Lind (1963) asked if this increase in perfusion was directed to the contracting muscle or to the inactive tissue of the forearm. They identified active muscles by electromyography and their temperatures were recorded from thermocouple needles as they contracted. A rise in their temperatures signified an increase in perfusion with warm blood (the arm was cooled in a bath before the contraction so that the rise in temperature would be easier to see). Inasmuch as temperatures of active muscles rose much more than temperatures of the inactive muscles, it was concluded that blood flow was directed preponderantly to active tissue. This may not be correct as a far more complex situation for blood flow exists within and between muscles than recognized heretofore (see Iversen and Nicolaysen, 1989). There is little guarantee from the temperature measurements of Humphreys and Lind (1963) that the active regions of a particular muscle were not underperfused. In fact, there is evidence that even 10 to 15 percent of MVC, some regions of the contracting quadriceps muscle may be underperfused so that even within a given muscle the distributions of the contracting fibers and their blood supply is complex (Saltin et al., 1981, Sjøgaard et al 1986, Wesche, 1986). Thus only part of the rise in blood flow may supply active portions of the muscle.

The complexity of the distribution of intramuscular pressures during a static contraction was described by Sejersted and colleagues (1984). They investigated the intramuscular fluid pressure at various depths in the vastus medialis muscle at four different fractions of MVC in human subjects. Intramuscular fluid pressure was a linear function of contraction force, and at any given contraction force, a linear function of depth. Intramuscular pressure was greatest deep within the muscle and least close to the muscle surface (Figure 8-4). At 100 percent of MVC, pressure deep within the vastus medialis, close to the femur, sometimes exceeded 500 mmHg.

Varying Effects of Contraction on Blood Flow in Different Muscles

The high intramuscular pressures in the quadriceps could explain why its blood flows appear to be lower than those of the forearm muscles, both at the same percent of MVC. Similar measurements of intramuscular pressure for forearm muscles were not found. Comparison of Figure 8-3 to

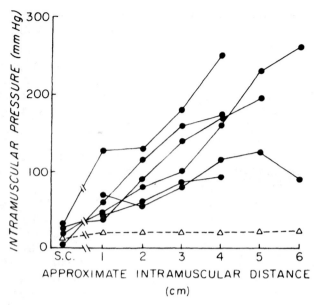

Figure 8-4 Depth-dependent increase in intramuscular fluid pressure in the vastus medialis muscles in seven normal young men. Open circles are controls for pressure at various depths in the *resting* muscle and closed symbols show pressures at these depths during voluntary isometric contraction at 50 percent of maximal voluntary contraction (MVC). Data show the relationship of intramuscular pressure to approximate depth within the muscle. Slit catheters were withdrawn from close to the femur in 1-cm steps and pressure recorded at each step until the muscle surface (subcutaneous tissue [SC]) was reached. (Adapted from Sejersted et al., 1984.)

Figure 8-5 reveals that already at 15 percent of MVC, quadriceps blood flow falls below values observed at 5 percent of MVC. Also, the duration of a contraction to the point of fatigue is lower at 15 percent of MVC than at 5 percent of MVC. Blood flow was markedly reduced at 25 percent of MVC, and at 50 percent of MVC flow appears to be virtually nil following a transient increase (blood flows were estimated from multiple bolus injections of ice-cold saline into the femoral vein, which carries venous drainages from other tissues in the region [Sjøgaard et al., 1988; Gaffney et al., 1990]).

Wesche's (1986) measurements of femoral arterial flow velocity (by pulsed bidirectional Doppler-ultrasound flowmetry) suggest that relatively small increases in blood flow occurred during isometric contractions of the human quadriceps at 10 percent of MVC. The marked reactive hyperemia shown in Figure 8-6 after such a low-force contraction suggests that the blood flow was not low simply because the force was low, but rather, the contraction had caused a hypoperfusion relative to metabolic rate somewhere within the quadriceps muscle. (Note that

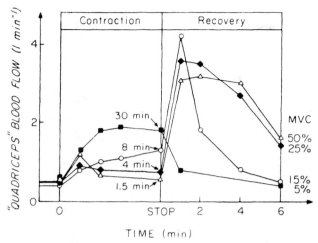

Figure 8-5   Femoral venous blood flow (from dilution of bolus injection of ice-cold saline into the femoral vein) during isometric contraction of the qradriceps (knee extension) at four percentages of maximal voluntary contraction (MVC). Time scale is arbitrary—average duration of contraction at each force is shown as time in minutes with contraction at 50 percent MVC being the shortest at 1.5 minutes, and contraction at 5 percent of MVC for 30 minutes being the longest. Note in contrast to Figure 8-3 (forearm blood flow), quadriceps blood flow at 15 percent of MVC is already reduced below the highest flow at 5 percent of MVC. Marked postcontraction hyperemia after 15 percent of MVC contraction signifies inadequate blood flow (data from Sjøgaard et al., 1988 and Gaffney et al., 1991). (Adapted from Sjøgaard et al., 1988.)

the change in velocity will slightly underestimate the rise in blood flow because increased perfusion pressure will distend the femoral artery a little.) Figure 8-3 shows that such a marked reactive hyperemia is not seen after a forearm muscle contraction until that contraction force exceeds 20 percent of MVC. The different fiber orientation of the two groups of muscles may explain the different effects of contraction force on their blood flows.

Spatial and Temporal Heterogeneity of Muscle Blood Flow

Saltin and coworkers (1981) observed a transient rise in femoral venous lactate concentration even after a 5-minute contraction of the quadriceps at only 10 percent of MVC. At this low fraction of MVC the intramuscular pressure appears to be well below both systolic and diastolic pressures (Sejersted et al., 1984), but again the spatial distribution of intramuscular pressure, like the heterogeneous intramuscular distribution of blood flow (e.g., Iversen and Nicolaysen, 1989), is complex. This rise in lactate seen by Saltin and coworkers (1981) suggests that, even at this low force, there are small regions within the muscle to which flow is impeded. At the

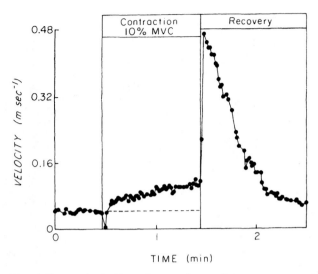

Figure 8-6   Blood flow velocity in a human femoral artery measured by pulsed bidirectional Doppler-ultrasound velocimetry during and after a single 60-second isometric contraction of the quadriceps muscles at *10 percent of MVC*. Flow velocity is transiently reduced to zero at the onset of contraction (also see Gray et al., 1967) and then increases gradually over 6 seconds and is immediately followed by marked reactive hyperemia when contraction stops. Calculated femoral arterial flow rates agreed with thermal dilution values of Gaffney et al. (1991) during hyperemia. Contrast with Figure 8-3. (Adapted from Wesche, 1986.)

slightly higher force of 15 percent of MVC, there was not only a marked increase in lactate release after the contraction but the release was increased during the contraction as well.

The data in Figure 8-7 reinforce the idea that spatial and temporal heterogeneity of muscle blood flow complicate our understanding of the relationship between muscle blood flow and metabolism in isometrically contracting muscle. This figure reveals the presence of brief spontaneous decrements and increments in electromyographic activity and intramuscular pressure in different regions of the knee extensors during one hour of maintained contraction at a *constant force* of 50 N (5 percent of MVC). Note the spontaneous fall in intramuscular pressure from 30 to 35 mmHg down to 15 mmHg and subsequent rise to 50 mmHg 40 seconds later. Sejersted and colleagues (1984) also recorded spontaneous oscillations in intramuscular pressure of similar magnitude at a rate of approximately 1 or 2 per minute during 20 minutes of vastus medialis contraction at 15 percent of MVC. These observations suggest that some cycling of contractions occurs within portions of the muscle so that a constant force is maintained by alternating recruitment patterns. This unearths an old thesis

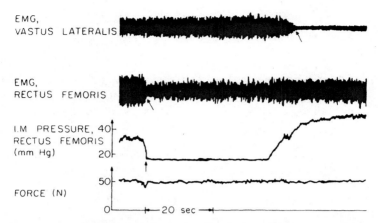

Figure 8-7 Spontaneous reductions (*arrows*) in electromyographic (EMG) activity (measured via surface electrodes) in both the vastus lateralis and rectus femoris, and in intramuscular pressure in the rectus femoris during a sustained isometric contraction of the quadriceps at 5 percent of maximal voluntary contraction (MVC) for 1 hour during which total force generation remained constant at 50 N. These observations suggest a cycling of contractions by alternating recruitment patterns as originally suggested by Forbes (1922). (Adapted from Sjøgaard et al., 1986.)

about selective activation of motor units that has never been fully confirmed (Forbes, 1922).

Summary. In summary, isometric contractions begin to interfere with muscle blood flow at levels of force development that are low relative to the maximum tension that the muscle can develop. The relative force at which interference with blood flow becomes obvious varies greatly between different muscle groups, depending on structural characteristics of the muscle such as muscle fiber orientation, thickness, curvature of the muscle fibers, and so on. Although it has been generally assumed that the rise in muscle blood flow, especially at relatively low levels of contraction force, is directed to the active muscles or active portions of those muscles, there are clearly regions within these muscles that are poorly perfused judging from the hyperemia and lactate washout immediately after their contraction ceases. There appears to be substantial heterogeneity of blood flow, both spatial and temporal, in the active as well as the inactive muscles. Even during lengthy, nonfatiguing contractions at constant force (5 to 15 percent of MVC), sudden spontaneous changes in local electromyographic activity and intramuscular pressure suggest the possibility of an alternating recruitment of various portions of the muscle that alleviates fatigue during prolonged contraction. Adequate perfusion of all parts of the isometrically contracting muscle never seems to be assured.

CENTRAL CIRCULATORY RESPONSES

The onset of an isometric contraction is characterized by rapid increases in arterial pressure, heart rate, and cardiac output as shown in Figure 8-8. The overall cardiovascular responses to isometric contractions have been well summarized and analyzed in excellent reviews by Asmussen

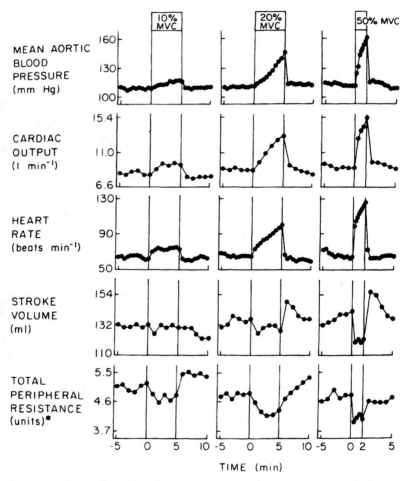

Figure 8-8 Hemodynamic data from one subject before, during, and after isometric contractions of the forearm (handgrip) at 10, 20, and 50 percent of maximal voluntary contraction (MVC). Cardiac output reached 15.4 L min^{-1} in this subject after a 2-minute contraction at 50 percent of MVC (the average for four subjects was 13.0 L min^{-1}). All subjects showed marked decreases in stroke volume at 50 percent of MVC. Note also the decrements in total peripheral resistance (units are dyne sec^{-1} per cm^5 × 10^3). (Adapted from Lind et al., 1964.)

(1981), Lind and coworkers (1966, 1983), and in a 1981 symposium (see Shepherd et al., 1981).

Arterial Blood Pressure

From the earliest studies, it was obvious that isometric contractions cause far greater increments in arterial blood pressure than does dynamic exercise; mean arterial blood pressure commonly exceeds 150 mmHg at fatigue. This pressor response is what first attracted physiologists' attention to isometric contractions. In one of the earliest reports, Lindhard (1920) explained the "peculiar" physiological response (i.e., arterial hypertension) as simply the mechanical consequence of the contracted muscles blocking their own blood flow. However, Lindhard's simple explanation could only apply when arteries were compressed in a mass of muscle large enough to significantly decrease total vascular conductance. Given such a fall in total vascular conductance, arterial blood pressure would rise only if cardiac output flow were maintained. The puzzle to both physiologists and clinicians for nearly a century has been the cause of the persistence of such high cardiac output and blood pressure in the face of powerful compensatory mechanisms, such as the arterial baroreflex (see Chapter 11). This compensatory reflex could quickly restore blood pressure by reducing heart rate (as in Figure 2-11).

The rate of rise of arterial pressure is proportional to the isometric contraction force expressed as percent of MVC. The greater the force, the faster the rise in pressure (Lind et al., 1964; Funderburk et al., 1974). For example, arterial pressure rose to its average peak value of approximately 145 mmHg in 1.3 minutes (60 percent of MVC), 2.3 minutes (40 percent of MVC), and 9.6 minutes (20 percent of MVC) at three forces of contraction in descending order (Funderburk et al., 1974). The end point of each contraction was the inability to maintain the tension owing to fatigue. The most interesting finding was that *at fatigue, arterial pressure reached the same level at all three tensions,* only the rates of rise differed. However, the rise in heart rate and presumably cardiac output was not the same at the three muscle tensions; heart rate rose most at 60 percent of MVC (75 to 125 beats min^{-1}) and least at 20 percent of MVC (75-110 beats min^{-1}). If we assume that heart rate and cardiac output rose together, this would mean that the rise in arterial pressure required more of an increase in peripheral vascular resistance at 20 percent of MVC than at 60 percent of MVC. This would appear to be in conflict with the findings of Lind and coworkers (1964), illustrated in Figure 8-8, which shows the rise in blood pressure to be due solely to the rise in cardiac output (but this was not the case in all of their subjects).

There is an interesting parallel between the findings of Funderburk and colleagues (1974) and those of Seals and Enoka (1989); results of the latter study are shown in Figure 8-9. Three separate contractions, all at the same percent of MVC, were held to an end point of fatigue. The duration of

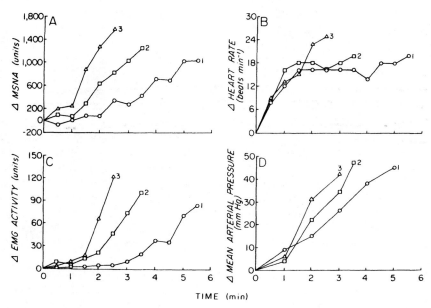

Figure 8-9   Responses of one subject to three successive isometric contractions at 30 percent of maximal voluntary contraction (MVC) to an end point of muscle fatigue (inability to maintain force). The increase in electromyographic activity (EMG) was used as an index of fatigue. The close relationship between increases in muscle sympathetic nerve activity (MSNA) and EMG suggest a link between the development of fatigue and increase in MSNA. Note that mean arterial pressure rose by the same amount at fatigue despite the different durations of contraction. This was not the case for either MSNA or heart rate. Other aspects of this important figure are discussed in Chapter 10. (Adapted from Seals and Enoka, 1989.)

contraction decreased with each repetition, but the rise in arterial pressure was always the same (Seals and Enoka, 1989). The point is that in addition to the force of contraction, fatigue is an important but nonquantifiable factor determining the responses.

Arterial Pressure and Muscle Mass

Mass of contracting muscle is another factor, in addition to duration of contraction and fatigue, that may bear importantly on the magnitude of rise in arterial pressure (Mitchell et al., 1980). Lind and McNicol (1967), Freyschuss (1970) and McCloskey and Streatfeild (1975), had found that the rise in pressure at a given percent of MVC was independent of the muscle mass. They argued that at 50 percent of MVC, for example, the rise in arterial pressure caused by contraction of 2.5 kg of quadriceps would be the same as that generated by a few grams of contracting finger muscle despite the enormous difference in the absolute force generated. In contrast, Mitchell and coworkers (1980) observed a strong dependency of the pressor responses on muscle mass and absolute force generation. The problem rests in the time dependency of the rise in arterial pressure. Mitchell and coworkers (1980) found, correctly, that over a fixed and relatively short time, the rise in arterial pressure was greater when the muscle mass was larger than when the mass was small. Lind (1983) agreed with this result, but argued that the rate of rise in arterial pressure depends on the muscle's endurance time (for example, see Figure 8-9). In some studies, at least (Reindl et al., 1977), the endurance time of a muscle depended on its mass. If correct, then it takes a small muscle longer than a large muscle to cause the same rise in arterial pressure. The key in this dispute seems to rest on the decision of what end point is appropriate. Although it now seems clear that if the contraction is taken to an end point of fatigue the rise in arterial pressure tends to be independent of the muscle mass (Williams, 1991), the issue of mass dependency is still not fully resolved.

The importance of this discussion of the effect of muscle mass on the rise in arterial pressure will become obvious in Chapter 11, when it is revealed that blood pressure-raising *reflexes arising from muscle are muscle-mass dependent.*

Cardiac Output

In one of the earliest studies of the hemodynamic responses to isometric contraction, carried out in 1938 by Asmussen and Hansen (Asmussen, 1981), cardiac output rose to 11 to 12 L min^{-1} with only a doubling of resting oxygen consumption. If anything, calculated arteriovenous oxygen difference fell slightly (calculated from the uptake of acetylene in a rebreathing technique). Later the rapid rise in cardiac output in response to isometric contraction was shown to be due almost entirely to the rise in heart rate caused by vagal withdrawal (e.g., Freyschuss, 1970; Martin et al., 1974). The subsequent sympathetic activation of the heart increases its contractile force (e.g., Perez-Gonzalez et al., 1981).

Figure 8-8 presents results from one of four subjects of a detailed hemodynamic study by Lind and colleagues (1964). Results from another subject were the same, but the other two showed less fall in peripheral vascular resistance (resistance rose at 50 of percent of MVC in one subject). The measurements of cardiac output were obtained by right atrial injection of dye and proximal aortic sampling.

(NOTE: Aortic sampling assures that the area beneath the dilution curve in a non-steady state of aortic blood flow provides a valid flow average during the brief period of sampling. Sampling from a vessel branching from the aorta would not do so because of the uneven temporal distribution of dye with changing flow.)

Stroke volume fell markedly during the contraction at 50 percent of MVC in all subjects. One explanation for this decline could be that the high aortic pressure or left ventricular afterload would, through its negative effect on the force-velocity relationship, depress left ventricular stroke volume. It will be shown later that the blood pressure-raising reflexes arising from muscle ischemia have powerful inotropic effects on the heart that prevent increased afterload from reducing stroke volume (Chapter 11).

An alternative explanation for the fall in stroke volume during a strong isometric contraction (50 percent of MVC) is that the large increase in cardiac output, exceeding 5 L min^{-1}, would be expected to reduce central venous pressure (direct measurements during static contractions appear not to have been made). A fall in stroke volume is not a consistent response at lower isometric contraction forces in which increments in cardiac output are much smaller (see Kilbom and Brundin, 1976).

Figure 6-8 shows that an increase in blood flow to nonpumping regions (such as skin or splanchnic) during dynamic exercise will reduce central venous pressure and as a result, stroke volume, just as it does at rest. This is because of the high compliance of nonmuscular regions and the augmentation of their vascular volume by increased blood flow. Therefore, the expected effect of raising cardiac output during a static contraction would be to shift the relationship between ventricular filling pressure and cardiac output (Figure 6-8A) from an *increased* filling pressure with *increased* cardiac output (line 1) to a *decreased* filling pressure with increased output (line 2). In addition, the marked rise in arterial pressure during isometric contractions will raise arterial volume somewhat, causing a fall in venous volume and pressure (this effect is small relative to that of increased flow, [Chapter 2]). The sensitivity of central venous pressure to changes in cardiac output during rest and exercise (dynamic in this case) is illustrated in Figure 8-10.

It is now clear that little, if any, of the increase in cardiac output goes to the active muscles, particularly when the mass is small. At low levels of isometric forearm contraction (18 percent of MVC) the 2.4-L min^{-1} increase in cardiac output was unaccompanied by any change in pulmonary arterial oxygen content and arteriovenous oxygen difference so that in terms of oxygen the increase in flow was partially wasted (Kilbom and Brundin, 1976). Figure 8-8 shows cardiac output reaching 15.4 L min^{-1} during a forearm contraction at 50 percent of MVC. The average cardiac output at this muscle tension was 13.0 L min^{-1}. The rise in cardiac output was far in excess of the metabolic needs of the forearm muscles so that calculated systemic arteriovenous oxygen difference fell on the average from 4.0 ml 100 ml^{-1} at rest to 3.6 ml 100 ml^{-1} during the contraction. Clearly, inactive regions were overperfused. The next question is: to what organs are these increments in cardiac output directed?

PERIPHERAL VASCULAR RESPONSES

A consensus is that the rise in arterial pressure during isometric contractions is due almost entirely to the rise in cardiac output (e.g., Shepherd et

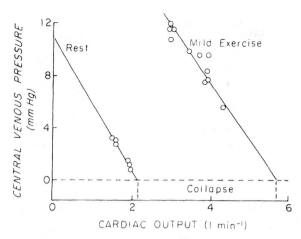

Figure 8-10   The relationship between central venous pressure (ventricular filling pressure) and cardiac output when cardiac output and blood flow through inactive regions is artificially decreased or increased by ventricular pacing during rest and dynamic exercise. An increase in blood flow through non-pumping organs will increase their volume; the consequent reduction in filling pressure and stroke volume serves as a self-limiting negative feedback which limits the rise in cardiac output, and in arterial pressure (data kindly provided by D.D. Sheriff).

al., 1981). On the average, total vascular conductance was higher at the end of each isometric contraction in the study of Lind and colleagues (1964). Martin and colleagues (1974) observed no significant changes in total vascular conductance, and this is more or less consistent across a number of studies. These results seem to be incompatible with Lind's (1983) conclusion that there is "mild but widespread sympathetic vasoconstriction" during isometric contractions. There would appear to have been *net* vasodilation instead (this does not mean there was no vasoconstriction anywhere).

Regional Blood Flow

An only partially solved mystery concerns the sites that receive the marked increases in cardiac output. Little goes to active muscle. According to Lind and colleagues (1964), neither splanchnic nor renal blood flow increased during isometric contractions, but these results have never been published. Kilbom and Brundin (1976) measured cardiac output, splanchnic blood flow (hepatic clearance and extraction of indocyanine green), and blood flow to one leg (femoral venous dye infusion) during a sustained isometric forearm contraction at 20 percent of MVC. Although cardiac output increased by 2.3 L min^{-1} on the average (Lind and colleagues [1964] observed the same increase at 20 percent of MVC), there were no significant increments in blood flows to either the splanchnic region or the resting leg. Splanchnic vascular conductance must also have fallen inasmuch as blood pressure rose from 90 to 126 mmHg during the contraction. Calculated leg vascular conductance decreased, and this was seen also by Rusch and coworkers (1981). Gaffney and coworkers (1990) observed an initial rise in femoral venous blood flow draining the resting leg during an isometric contraction of the quadriceps (20 to 25 percent of MVC) in the contralateral leg; but after 1 minute, vascular conductance fell in the resting leg, presumably because of vasoconstriction.

In contrast to the findings of Kilbom and Brundin (1976), Chaudhuri and associates (1991) observed a 30 percent *decrease* in superior mesenteric arterial blood flow, which supplies a major proportion of the splanchnic region. Flow velocity was determined by a pulsed Doppler ultrasound method with real-time imaging of arterial diameter for determination of volume flow. The conflicting results from different studies compound the mystery.

Two of the first reports of any marked vasodilation during sustained isometric contractions were by Eklund and Kaijser (1976) and by Rusch and coworkers (1981), who observed marked vasodilation in a nonexercising forearm. In disagreement with Eklund and Kaijser who saw no rise in electromyographic activity, Lind (1983) attributed the vasodilation to unconscious activation of resting forearm muscle. Inasmuch as the forearm vasodilation could be blocked by a β-blocker, the marked increase in circulating epinephrine normally observed during isometric contractions (see Galbo, 1983) could be responsible, but release would have to be very rapid. The mechanism for this putative β-adrenergic vasodilation also remains a mystery. Parenthetically, the existence of cholinergic vasodilation in human skeletal muscle is not well supported by the evidence (Chapter 4).

One of Kilbom and Brundin's (1976) most interesting observations, shown in Figure 8-11, was of the contrasting effects of isometric and dynamic exercise on the cutaneous circulation and the temperature of mixed venous blood. As expected, pulmonary arterial temperature rose rapidly and by a large amount (approximately 0.5°C) during dynamic leg exercise at 100 watts (Figure 8-11B), whereas subcutaneous temperature on the thorax initially fell and then rose, suggesting a fall and then a rise in skin blood flow. Panel A shows a continuous increase in subcutaneous temperature and a continuous reduction in pulmonary arterial temperature during an isometric contraction at 20 percent of MVC. The fall in pulmonary arterial temperature of 0.13°C means that skin blood flow rose proportionally more than heat production (which rose from 1.5 to 2.1 kcal min^{-1}) so that body heat was lost via the skin. The increase in skin blood flow needed to cause these changes is far less than the 2.3-L min^{-1} rise in cardiac output, but at least it accounts for a portion of it. In subsequent studies, Taylor and colleagues (1989) came to the same conclusion. They showed by laser-Doppler velocimetry that skin blood flow in the forearm

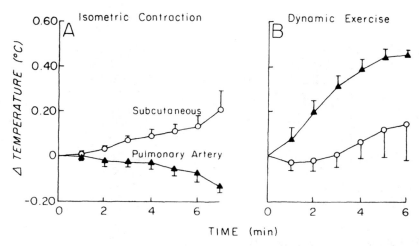

Figure 8-11 (**A**) Evidence showing significant cutaneous hyperemia during an isometric forearm contraction at 20 percent maximal voluntary contraction (MVC) indicated by a rise in subcutaneous temperature on the thorax owing to increased skin blood flow and a significant *fall* in pulmonary arterial blood temperature (filled triangles) caused by excessive heat loss from skin due to its increased blood flow. (**B**) In contrast, the increased heat production during dynamic leg exercise (bicycling 100 watts) raised pulmonary arterial blood temperature and also subcutaneous temperature after it declined initially. (Adapted from Kilbom and Brundin, 1976.)

and the chest rose an estimated 25 to 30 percent during an isometric forearm contraction at 30 percent of MVC.

Therefore skin, together with the vasodilation observed in some but not all resting skeletal muscle, may be sites that receive significant portions of the increase in cardiac output. Increased blood flow to respiratory muscles and to the heart should require only a small fraction of this increase in blood flow. The change in ventilation is relatively small and probably exceeded by the cardiac costs, which are elevated by the high arterial pressure.

If Lind and colleagues (1964) were correct about the kidneys, then we are still faced with the mystery of what regions received a sizeable fraction of the 30 percent increase (2.3-L min^{-1}) in cardiac output. If one-half of this increase goes to the regions mentioned above, then it is possible that a 15 percent increase in blood flow might escape detection if it were uniformly distributed throughout the body; an increase of this magnitude is within the error of measurement of blood flow to some organs.

Figure 8-8 provides an idea about the magnitude of vasodilation needed to accommodate the rise in cardiac output at higher levels of isometric contraction force. Parenthetically, the short endurance time at forces exceeding 20 to 25 percent of MVC makes good measurements of regional blood flow difficult in humans. In the subject shown in Figure 8-8, cardiac output rose from 8.8 L min^{-1} at an arterial pressure of 110 mmHg at rest to 15.4 L min^{-1} at 160 mmHg during a contraction at 50 percent of MVC. Total vascular conductance rose from 0.0800 to 0.0963 L min^{-1} mmHg^{-1} during contraction. This rise in conductance of 0.0163 L min^{-1} mmHg^{-1} means that vasodilation was sufficient to accommodate a flow increase of 2.6 L min^{-1} at 160 mmHg arterial pressure.

$$\frac{\Delta flow = \Delta conductance \times pressure}{2.6\ L\ min^{-1} = 0.0163\ L\ min^{-1}\ mmHg^{-1} \times 160\ mmHg} \quad (8\text{-}2)$$

Were it feasible to measure regional blood flows at contraction forces as high as 50 percent of MVC, it would be even more surprising if we failed to see blood flow increase; the cardiovascular system must accommodate a 6.6-L min^{-1} rise in cardiac output.

Sympathetic Nervous Activity

Although Lind's (1983) proposal that sympathetic vasoconstriction plays an important role in the pressor response to an isometric contraction is not supported by the findings of decreased or unchanged total vascular conductance, it is supported by the following observations: *First,* blood flow to some regions remains constant when blood pressure rises during an isometric contraction, indicating that vasoconstriction has occurred. *Second,* plasma concentration of norepinephrine increases during contractions; however, the increase is far less than that seen during moderate isotonic exercise (see Galbo, 1983; Seals and Victor, 1990). *Third,* directly measured sympathetic nerve traffic to resting muscle (MSNA; see Chapter 3) increases in proportion to the relative tension once this tension exceeds 15 percent of MVC, as illustrated in Figure 8-12 (Seals et al., 1988). Also, at any given relative force of contraction, the mass of contracting muscle appears to be an important determinant of the degree to which MSNA increases—*over a fixed time* (Seals, 1989). However, the data in Figure 8-9 suggest that any dependency of MSNA on muscle mass could diminish or disappear if the contractions were prolonged to fatigue (MSNA increases markedly as fatigue approaches) (Seals and Enoka, 1989).

Sympathetic nerve traffic to skin of the resting forearm also increases during isometric contractions of the contralateral forearm at 30 percent of MVC. In contrast to the ramp increase in MSNA, skin sympathetic activity increased in a step along with sweating, and both remained elevated throughout the contraction in a more or less rectangular response pattern (Saito et al., 1990). The traffic in the sympathetic fibers to skin appears to have been dominated by sudomotor activity rather than vasoconstrictor activity; skin blood flow (laser-Doppler velocimetry) increased.

The most obvious examples of the importance of sympathetically mediated vasoconstriction during isometric contractions are seen when the ability to increase cardiac output rapidly is blocked by atropine (Freyschuss, 1970), or when ability to increase heart rate and contractile force

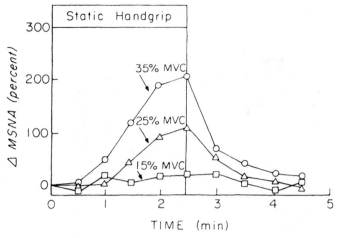

Figure 8-12   Average increases in muscle sympathetic nervous activity in response to a fixed duration (2.5 minutes) of isometric contraction of the forearm (handgrip) in eight subjects. A nonfatiguing contraction of the forearm at 15 percent of maximal voluntary contraction (MVC) caused no significant increase in muscle sympathetic nerve activity (MSNA). (Adapted from Seals et al., 1988.)

is blunted by β-adrenergic blockade (Freyschuss, 1970; Martin et al., 1974; Perez-Gonzalez et al., 1981). When the normally predominant mechanism for raising blood pressure, that is, increased cardiac output, is blocked, a normal rise in arterial pressure still occurs. This rise is achieved by vasoconstriction. Also, a normal increase in arterial pressure during isometric contraction occurs in patients who have had heart transplants and thus have completely denervated ventricles (Haskell et al., 1981). An important point is that cardiovascular reflexes continue to raise blood pressure by a fixed amount for a given relative force of isometric contractions despite the loss of one mechanism of control. The signals and reflexes that achieve this are covered in Chapters 10 and 11.

Vasoconstriction in the Active Muscle?

If we assume for now that the rise in cardiac output and blood pressure and the increased sympathetic nerve activity during isometric contractions stem from a reflex originating in an underperfused active muscle, an increase in sympathetic outflow to this muscle and further reduction in its blood flow would be highly undesirable. The teleological argument for the value of a hypertensive response to isometric contractions is the same as that offered for the Cushing reflex (Figure 6-23). In isometric contractions, the rise in blood pressure should improve blood flow through the mechanically impeded muscle circulation. In the case of the Cushing reflex accompanying a head injury, the increased blood pressure should improve blood flow through cerebral vessels whose transmural pressure and blood flow are reduced by the increase in cerebrospinal fluid pressure caused by bleeding. However, the extreme hypertension simply increases the bleeding into the cerebrospinal fluid and causes a further reduction in cerebral blood flow and a further rise in blood pressure in a vicious cycle. The same positive feedback cycle would attend further restriction of blood flow to isometrically contracting muscle by vasoconstriction; vasoconstriction further reduces its blood flow, which further augments sympathetic nervous outflow to the heart and active muscle (and elsewhere?) in another vicious cycle. This applies to forces of isometric contraction that do not arrest blood flow, but merely reduce it. The fall in stroke volume puts a self-limiting negative feedback on the ability to increase cardiac output, the primary mechanism for raising arterial pressure. This will end the vicious cycle (arterial baroreflexes may also counteract the pressor response; see Chapter 12). Vasoconstriction in active muscle during isometric contraction has been reported (Williams et al., 1981; Gaffney et al., 1990). If it occurs, it constitutes a serious failure in regulation and would make the pressor response to isometric contraction appear like other "agonal" reflexes by exacerbating rather than ameliorating an existing regulatory problem.

SUMMARY

In summary, the active muscles do not receive adequate perfusion during isometric contractions above a certain level of force development. This threshold level could be as high as 20 to 30 percent of MVC in the forearm muscles and below 10 percent MVC in the quadriceps—based on the magnitudes of reactive hyperemia after the contractions. The pressor response to contraction depends on the duration of contraction but probably not on the mass of active muscle if contractions are taken to fatigue. Sympathetic nerve activity to resting muscles also increases as fatigue develops. The rise in arterial pressure is believed to be caused almost exclusively by the rise in cardiac output; in general total vascular conductance tends to remain constant or may rise a little. Inasmuch as virtually the entire increase in cardiac output goes to inactive (i.e., noncontracting) regions, the fall in stroke volume at high percents of MVC probably stems from a fall in central venous pressure caused by increasing blood flow through noncontracting organs. Later chapters will suggest that increased afterload is not the major cause of the fall in stroke volume. The organs that receive the increased cardiac output are skin (sympathetic sudomotor activity and blood flow increase) and probably resting muscle (despite increased sympathetic traffic to them). So far no increases in blood flow have been observed in other organs (e.g., splanchnic, kidneys). Some evidence suggests that blood flow to the *contracting muscles* is decreased further, by sympathetic vasoconstriction; this is added onto the decrease caused by contraction when force development is low. Such positive feedback would produce a vicious cycle of hypertension that is probably counteracted by the negative feedback on arterial pressure stemming from the fall in stroke volume (and also arterial baroreflexes). Isometric contractions provide a useful tool for investigating the factors that activate the cardiovascular and sympathetic nervous systems during an unsuccessful attempt to move. If movement occurs then the responses *during isometric* contractions no longer represent what happens *during dynamic* exercise when increased muscle blood flow compensates for reduced peripheral resistance so that blood pressure rises very little.

REFERENCES

Asmussen, E. (1981). Similarities and dissimilarities between static and dynamic exercise. *Circ. Res. 48 (Suppl. 1)*, 3–10.

Barcroft, H., and J.L.E. Millen (1939). The blood flow through muscle during sustained contraction. *J. Physiol. (Lond.) 97*, 17–31.

Chaudhuri, K.R., T. Thomaides, P. Hernandez, and C.J. Mathias (1991). Noninvasive quantification of superior mesenteric artery blood flow during sympathoneural activation in normal subjects. *Clin. Auton. Res. 1*, 37–42.

Dolgin, P., and G. Lehmann (1930). Ein Beitrag zur Physiologie der statischen Arbeit. *Arbeitsphysiologie 2*, 248–252.

Eklund, B., and L. Kaijser (1976). Effect of regional α- or β-adrenergic blockade on blood flow in the resting forearm during contralateral isometric handgrip. *J. Physiol. (Lond.) 262*, 39–50.

Forbes, A. (1922). The interpretation of spinal reflexes in terms of present knowledge of nerve condition. *Physiol. Rev. 2*, 361–414.

Freyschuss, U. (1970). Elicitation of heart rate and blood pressure increase on muscle contraction. *J. Appl. Physiol. 28*, 758–761.

Funderburk, C.F., S.G. Hipskind, R.C. Welton, and A.R. Lind (1974). Development of and recovery from fatigue induced by static effort at various tensions. *J. Appl. Physiol. 37*, 392–396.

Gaffney, F.A., G. Sjøgaard, and B. Saltin (1990). Cardiovascular and metabolic responses to static contraction in man. *Acta Physiol. Scand. 138*, 249–258.

Galbo, H. (1983). *Hormonal and Metabolic Adaptation to Exercise*. Thieme-Stratton, New York.

Gaskell, W.H. (1877). On the changes of the blood stream in muscles through stimulation of the nerves. *J. Anat. (Lond.) 11*, 360–402.

Gray, S.D., E. Carlsson, and N.C. Staub (1967). Site of increased vascular resistance during isometric muscle contraction. *Am. J. Physiol. 213*, 683–689.

Haskell, W.L., N.M. Savin, J.S. Schroeder, E.A. Alderman, N.B. Ingles, G.T. Daughters, and E.A. Stinson (1981). Cardiovascular responses to handgrip isometric exercise in patients following cardiac transplantation. *Circ. Res. 48 (Suppl. 1)*, 156–161.

Humphreys, P.W., and A.R. Lind (1963). The blood flow through active and inactive muscles of the forearm during sustained hand-grip contractions. *J. Physiol. (Lond.) 166*, 120–135.

Iversen, P.O., and G. Nicolaysen (1989). Heterogeneous blood flow distribution within single skeletal muscles in the rabbit: role of vasomotion, sympathetic nerve activity and effect of vasodilation. *Acta Physiol. Scand. 137*, 125–133.

Kilbom, A., and T. Brundin (1976). Circulatory effects of isometric muscle contractions, performed separately and in combination with dynamic exercise. *Eur. J. Appl. Physiol. 36*, 7–17.

Lind, A.R. (1983). Cardiovascular adjustments to isometric contractions: static effort. In J.T. Shepherd, F.M. Abboud, and S.R. Geiger, eds. *Handbook of Physiology. The Cardiovascular System: Peripheral Circulation and Organ Blood Flow*, sect. 2, vol. III, pp. 947–966. American Physiological Society, Bethesda, MD.

Lind, A.R., and G.W. McNichol (1967). Local and central circulatory responses to sustained contractions and the effect of free or restricted arterial inflow on post-exercise hyperaemia. *J. Physiol. (Lond.) 192*, 575–593.

Lind, A.R., G.W. McNicol, and K.W. Donald (1966). Circulatory adjustments to sustained (static) muscular activity. In K. Evang, ed. *Physical Activity in Health and Disease*, pp. 38–63. Universitets Forlaget, Oslo, Norway.

Lind, A.R., S.H. Taylor, P.W. Humphreys, B.M. Kennelly, and K.W. Donald (1964). The circulatory effects of sustained voluntary muscle contraction. *Clin. Sci. 27*, 229–244.

Lindhard, J. (1920). Untersuchungen über statischer Muskelarbeit I. *Skand Arch. Physiol. 40*, 145–195.

McCloskey, D.I., and K.A. Streatfeild (1975). Muscular reflex stimuli to the cardiovascular system during isometric contractions of muscle groups of different mass. *J. Physiol. (Lond.) 250*, 431–441.

Martin, C.E., J.A. Shaver, D.F. Leon, M.E. Thompson, P.S. Reddy, and J.J. Leonard (1974). Autonomic mechanisms in hemodynamic responses to isometric exercise. *J. Clin. Invest. 54*, 104–115.

Mitchell, J.H., F.C. Payne, B. Saltin, and B. Schibye (1980). The role of muscle mass in the cardiovascular response to static contraction. *J. Physiol. (Lond.) 309*, 45–54.

Nielsen, H.V. (1983). External pressure-blood flow relations during limb compression in man. *Acta Physiol. Scand. 119*, 253–260.

Perez-Gonzalez, J.F., N.B. Schiller, and W.W. Parmley (1981). Direct and noninvasive evaluation of the cardiovascular response to isometric exercise. *Circ. Res. 48 (Suppl. 1)*, 138–148.

Reindl, A.M., R.W. Gotshall, J.A. Peinki, and J.J. Smith (1977). Cardiovascular responses of human subjects to isometric contraction of large and small muscle groups. *Proc. Soc. Exp. Biol. Med. 154*, 171–174.

Reneman, R.S., D.W. Slaaf, L. Lindbom, G.J. Tangelder, and K.-E. Arfors (1980). Muscle blood flow disturbances produced by simultaneously elevated venous and total muscle tissue pressure. *Microvasc. Res. 20*, 307–318.

Rowell, L.B., M.V. Savage, J. Chambers, and J.R. Blackmon (1991). Cardiovascular responses to graded reductions in leg perfusion in exercising humans. *Am. J. Physiol. 261 (Heart Circ. Physiol. 30*, H1545–H1553.

Rusch, N.L., J.T. Shepherd, R.C. Webb, and P.M. Vanhoutte (1981). Different behavior of the resistance vessels of the human calf and forearm during contralateral isometric exercise, mental stress, and abnormal respiratory movements. *Circ. Res. 48 (Suppl. 1)*, 118–130.

Saito, M., M. Naito, and T. Mano (1990). Different responses in skin and muscle sympathetic nerve activity to static muscle contraction. *J. Appl. Physiol.* *69*, 2085–2090.

Saltin, B., G. Sjogaard, F.A. Gaffney, and L.B. Rowell (1981). Potassium, lactate, and water fluxes in human quadriceps muscle during static contractions. *Circ. Res. 48 (Suppl. 1)*, 18–24.

Seals, D.R. (1989). Influence of muscle mass on sympathetic neural activation during isometric exercise. *J. Appl. Physiol. 67*, 1801–1806.

Seals, D.R., P.B. Chase, and J.A. Taylor (1988). Autonomic mediation of the pressor responses to isometric exercise in humans. *J. Appl. Physiol. 64*, 2190–2196.

Seals, D.R., and R.M. Enoka (1989). Sympathetic activation is associated with increases in EMG during fatiguing exercise. *J. Appl. Physiol. 66*, 88–95.

Seals, D.R., and R.G. Victor (1990). Regulation of muscle sympathetic nerve activity during exercise in humans. In J. Holloszy, ed. *Exercise and Sport Sciences Reviews*, vol. 19, pp. 313–349. Williams & Wilkins, Baltimore.

Sejersted, O.M., A.R. Hargens, K.R. Kardel, P. Blom, O. Jensen, and L. Hermansen (1984). Intramuscular fluid pressure during isometric contraction of human skeletal muscle. *J. Appl. Physiol. (Respir. Environ. Exercise Physiol.) 56*, 287–295.

Shepherd, J.T., C.G. Blomqvist, A.R. Lind, J.H. Mitchell, and B. Saltin (1981). Static (isometric) exercise; retrospection and introspection. *Circ. Res. 48 (Suppl. 1)*, 179–188.

Sjøgaard, G., B. Kiens, K. Jorgensen, and B. Saltin (1986). Intramuscular pressure, EMG and blood flow during low-level prolonged static contraction in man. *Acta Physiol. Scand. 128*, 475–484.

Sjøgaard, G., G. Savard, and C. Juel (1988). Muscle blood flow during isometric activity and its relation to muscle fatigue. *Eur. J. Appl. Physiol. 57*, 327–335.

Taylor, W.F., J.M. Johnson, W.A. Kosiba, and C.M. Kwan (1989). Cutaneous vascular responses to isometric handgrip exercise. *J. Appl. Physiol. 66*, 1586–1592.

Wesche, J. (1986). The time course and magnitude of blood flow changes in the human quadriceps muscles following isometric contraction. *J. Physiol. (Lond.) 377*, 445–462.

Williams, C.A. (1991). Effect of muscle mass on the pressor response in man during isometric contractions. *J. Physiol. (Lond.) 435*, 573–584.

Williams, C.A., J.G. Mudd, and A.R. Lind (1981). The forearm blood flow during intermittent hand-grip isometric exercise. *Circ. Res. 48 (Suppl. 1)*, 110–117.

9

Limitations to Oxygen Uptake During Dynamic Exercise

What factors limit the uptake of oxygen during dynamic exercise? Claims have been laid at each of the steps that have the greatest potential to limit the transfer of oxygen from the air to the mitochondria. Nevertheless, it is unlikely that any single step could be *the* limiting factor inasmuch as three determinants of $\dot{V}o_2$max are expressed in the Fick equation; namely, cardiac output, arterial oxygen content, and mixed venous oxygen content, each of which can adjust during chronic activity or inactivity (Chapters 5 and 7).

At $\dot{V}o_2$max, 90 percent of the oxygen that moves by forced convection and by diffusion through the pulmonary and cardiovascular systems is consumed by active skeletal, respiratory, and cardiac muscles. The transfer of oxygen from the atmosphere via the lung to the skeletal muscle mitochondria has distinct physical or anatomical barriers along its route of transport. There are barriers that limit the diffusive transfer of oxygen at two locations. There are also two steps that involve convective transfer and these also impose potential limitations in the transfer of oxygen. These four potentially limiting steps are summarized as follows:

Step 1: *Convective transfer* of oxygen from the atmosphere to the alveolus by pulmonary ventilation.

Step 2: *Diffusive transfer* of oxygen across the alveolar membrane to the red blood cells.

Step 3: *Convective transfer* of oxygen via the blood that is pumped by the heart away from the alveoli to the capillaries of all organs.

Step 4: *Diffusive transfer* of oxygen across the capillary, cellular, and mitochondrial membranes.

Weibel and Taylor (1981) and Taylor and colleagues (1987) put together a well-developed synthesis of how these functional and structural features operate in an integrated manner in the multiple steps of the oxygen cascade. Figure 9-1 is adapted from their treatise on the design of the mammalian respiratory system (Taylor et al., 1987). It summarizes the four steps just outlined and emphasizes both *functional* and *structural* limitations. Some structural barriers in the oxygen cascade are illustrated in Figure

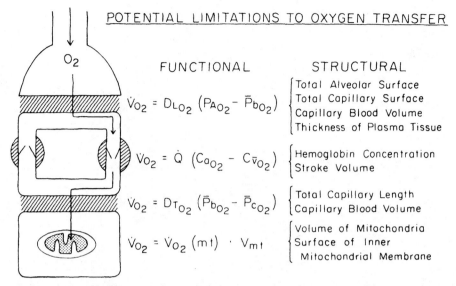

Figure 9-1 Summary of functional and structural factors that impose potential limitations on the transfer of oxygen from the alveolus (*top*) to the muscle cell mitochondria (*bottom*). Functional limitations in *convection* are expressed as variations of the Fick principle shown via equations in which

D_{LO_2} = diffusive conductance for oxygen in the lung
$P_{AO_2} - P_{bO_2}$ = alveolar P_{O_2} − mean pulmonary capillary P_{O_2}
$\dot{Q}$ = cardiac output or pulmonary blood flow
$C_{aO_2} - C_{\bar{v}O_2}$ = arterial − mixed venous oxygen content
D_{TO_2} = diffusive conductance for oxygen in the tissue
$\bar{P}_{bO_2} - \bar{P}_{cO_2}$ = mean tissue capillary P_{O_2} − mean intracellular P_{O_2}
$\dot{V}_{O_2}$ (mt · Vmt) = oxygen uptake per mitochondria × total volume of mitochondria

Structural limitations are as listed on the right. (Adapted from Taylor et al., 1987.)

9-2. These are the diffusion barriers for oxygen, which are determined mainly by surface areas, thicknesses, and solubilities.

Traditionally the cause of the upper limit to oxygen consumption during severe exercise has been sought in the following:

1. The *respiratory system* and the limitations in pulmonary function; this includes the ability to maintain adequate arterial P_{O_2} and capillary P_{O_2} in the working muscle.
2. The *heart* and its capacity to pump blood.
3. The *peripheral circulation* and the extent to which blood vessels of active muscle can vasodilate and receive blood flow without an excessive rise in blood pressure (such as occurs in static contractions). [Also, the optimization of blood flow distribution to active as opposed to inactive regions, that is, not only throughout the

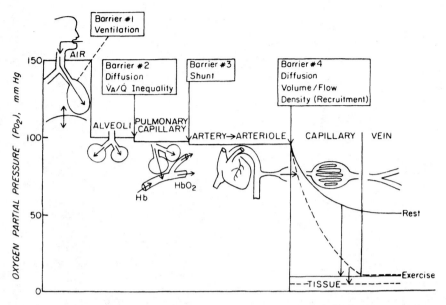

Figure 9-2 The "oxygen cascade" illustrates the progressive decline in PO_2 of air passing from the mouth through the airways to the alveoli (called barrier 1). At rest, barrier 2, which is diffusional or due to $\dot{V}_A/\dot{Q}$ inequality, is small, as is the potential barrier 3, due to postpulmonary arteriovenous shunts. The large drop in PO_2 from arterial to venous capillary at barrier 4 is related to diffusion distances, mean transit time (volume/time) and capillary-cell-mitochondrial distances (see text). These decrements in PO_2 throughout the entire respiratory and cardiovascular systems are commonly seen in resting (supine) humans. (Adapted from West, 1974.)

entire cardiovascular system but within the muscle itself as well, is required to provide the maximal utilization of oxygen. Within the muscle, the number of open capillaries and the distances for diffusion of oxygen to the mitochondria are critical factors.]

4. The *metabolic capacity* of the active muscles, namely, the oxidative capacity of the mitochondrial enzymes.

Each of these potential limitations is discussed in separate sections of this chapter. They are summarized in Figure 9-3.

A central question, raised in Chapter 5 is: Is $\dot{V}O_2$max really a measure of the capacity of the cardiovascular system to transport oxygen to the tissues in normal humans? This question accepts that there are several potential limitations in cardiovascular transport of oxygen, and many physiologists today would answer this question in the affirmative. There are also many who would not so answer because of the growing evidence that pulmonary gas exchange can *sometimes* pose a significant limitation in normal endurance athletes with exceptionally high maximal cardiac outputs (such a limitation clearly exists in patients with pulmonary dis-

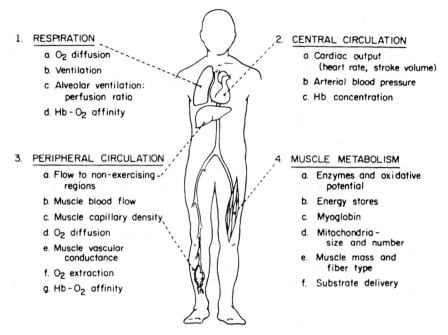

1. RESPIRATION
    a. O_2 diffusion
    b. Ventilation
    c. Alveolar ventilation:
       perfusion ratio
    d. Hb - O_2 affinity

2. CENTRAL CIRCULATION
    a. Cardiac output
       (heart rate, stroke volume)
    b. Arterial blood pressure
    c. Hb concentration

3. PERIPHERAL CIRCULATION
    a. Flow to non-exercising
       regions
    b. Muscle blood flow
    c. Muscle capillary density
    d. O_2 diffusion
    e. Muscle vascular
       conductance
    f. O_2 extraction
    g. Hb - O_2 affinity

4. MUSCLE METABOLISM
    a. Enzymes and oxidative
       potential
    b. Energy stores
    c. Myoglobin
    d. Mitochondria -
       size and number
    e. Muscle mass and
       fiber type
    f. Substrate delivery

Figure 9-3   Summary of possible limitations to oxygen consumption within the major systems involved in transport and consumption of oxygen during exercise. See text for discussion. (From Rowell, 1986, with permission from Oxford University Press.)

ease). The fact that serious limitations in pulmonary gas exchange are not common in normal people is not relevant to this discussion. What is important from a mechanistic viewpoint is that such limitations do exist in normal people. The prevalence of such limitations in the racehorse amplifies the point.

The most active debate concerning what restricts oxygen uptake once centered on the conflicting views that $\dot{V}o_2max$ is, on the one hand, limited by factors associated with oxygen transport and transfer, and, on the other hand, $\dot{V}o_2max$ is limited by the capacity of the active muscle to consume oxygen owing to functional limitations in its oxidative enzyme capacity. The conclusion was soon reached by most that $\dot{V}o_2max$ is limited by the oxygen transport system because skeletal muscle appeared to possess a far greater potential for oxidative metabolism than could be met by the cardiovascular and respiratory systems (e.g., Saltin and Gollnick, 1983).

This debate has been reopened by Weibel and Taylor (1981) and Taylor and colleagues (1987), who have investigated this problem from a combined morphological and physiological perspective across a range of species. Some groups of animals differed over orders of magnitude in their body mass (allometric variation); other animal groups differed only in $\dot{V}o_2max$ (adaptive variation) rather than in body mass. A hypothesis called by Weibel and Taylor (1981) "symmorphosis" was defined as "a state of structural design commensurate to functional needs resulting from regulated morphogenesis." In their scheme, every part of the respiratory system (i.e., lungs, cardiovascular system, and muscle mitochondria) is closely matched functionally to every other part so that there are no specific weak links in the chain of oxygen delivery and utilization. Therefore the system has "economic design," meaning that during an adaptation such as physical conditioning *all parts of the system must increase their function in proportion to the increase in* $\dot{V}o_2$max.

This hypothesis of symmorphosis appears to reflect rather diverse views about the functional "design" of the body. Perhaps a physiologist "designs," in his or her mind, oxygen delivery systems that permit cells and mitochondria to develop (physiologists usually do not think in these terms). Conversely, a morphologist might design a system in which the cells and their mitochondria determine the development of the supply system. The hypothesis of symmorphosis is essentially deterministic in nature so that if a part of it is found not to hold, then the hypothesis collapses. Weibel and Kayar (1988) conclude from their studies of the pulmonary system that the hypothesis does *not* hold for the pulmonary system in animals adapted to high metabolic rates. The hypothesis is clearly inapplicable to the human pulmonary system because of its failure to improve its function along with cardiovascular function during physical conditioning (Dempsey, 1986). It is also argued that the capacity of the cardiovascular system to transport oxygen is not matched to the metabolic capacity of skeletal muscle in humans, dogs, and possibly some other species. In short, a body of evidence refutes the idea that all animals have well-matched capacities to transfer oxygen by ventilation, alveolar diffusion, blood flow, and capillary diffusion, and to consume oxygen in the mitochondria.

LIMITATIONS IN THE RESPIRATORY SYSTEM

Ventilation

The lung has been viewed as being well down on the list in the hierarchy of factors that limit $\dot{V}o_2$max. The pulmonary system is seen as being sufficiently "well designed" and regulated so as to provide optimal movement of oxygen from surrounding air to the gas-blood interface even during the most severe metabolic demands. However, Dempsey (1986) and Whipp and Pardy (1986) and, more recently, Johnson and coworkers (1992), have pointed out definite limitations in the ability of the respiratory system to move air in and out of the lungs in highly conditioned individuals during maximal exercise.

Increased demands for oxygen must be met by increased alveolar ventilation. The pulmonary system must meet two specific demands:

1. It must move enough air to supply the necessary oxygen to all working muscles, including respiratory muscles.
2. It must move air as economically as possible so that the share of oxygen used by the respiratory muscles is not so great that it jeopardizes the supply of oxygen to the locomotive muscles.

The second demand (above) that ventilation be as efficient as possible bears on work *performance* and not on $\dot{V}o_2$max or oxygen uptake capacity (even though the high cost of peak ventilation is often cited as a limitation to $\dot{V}o_2$max). The respiratory muscles do not limit $\dot{V}o_2$max, but rather are a part of it just as are any other muscles used during exercise. Inasmuch as the heart's pumping capacity is limited, the more blood that is directed to the respiratory muscles the less blood is available for locomotive muscles. Excessive oxygen utilization by respiratory muscles would simply lower the exercise intensity required to elicit $\dot{V}o_2$max—just as adding arm exercise to leg exercise reduces work performance time but does not change $\dot{V}o_2$max. (Raising the cost of ventilation could only change variables in the Fick equation—and thus reduce $\dot{V}o_2$max—if the oxygen were not as efficiently extracted by respiratory muscles as it is by locomotive muscles.)

All indications are that oxygen uptake is not limited by pulmonary ventilation in normally active young people exercising at $\dot{V}o_2$max—at sea level. The functional capabilities of the lungs and respiratory muscles are thought to be well in excess of the demands placed on them up to maximal levels of exercise. This judgement is based on the criteria for adequate pulmonary gas exchange; namely, during severe exercise the modest hyperventilation reduces alveolar Pco_2 by 10 to 15 mmHg and it increases alveolar Po_2, with arterial Po_2 and oxygen content being maintained close to resting level (Holmgren and Linderholm, 1958; Asmussen, 1965; Dejours, 1965).

The main point of this discussion is that a modest hyperventilation is needed to reduce alveolar Pco_2 so as to increase alveolar Po_2 enough to raise the driving pressure for alveolar to pulmonary capillary diffusion of oxygen. When alveolar Pco_2 is not reduced, and alveolar Po_2 is not maintained, the reduced driving pressure for diffusion of oxygen leads to hypoxemia and reduced $\dot{V}o_2$max.

Does Alveolar Ventilation Ever Limit Oxygen Uptake in Normal Individuals?

In 1919, Harrop observed that "exhausting" exercise could reduce the oxygen saturation of arterial blood to 85 percent. Subsequently, several investigators observed a rise in oxygen uptake when they increased inspired Po_2 during severe exercise. The rise in oxygen uptake was thought to be a consequence of reducing the arterial hypoxemia present during severe exercise at normal ambient oxygen tension (see Rowell et al., 1964). That is, the rise in oxygen uptake was in some cases too large to be explained by the relatively small increases in physically dissolved oxygen, meaning that hemoglobin saturation would appear to have been reduced (Rowell, 1974). Holmgren and Linderholm (1958) observed an average arterial P_{O_2} of 78.8 mmHg in 13 normal subjects during exhausting exercise. This corresponded to an average oxygen saturation of 94 percent (arterial pH was 7.35). However, four of their subjects exhibited arterial P_{O_2} values as low as 57 and 64 mmHg up to 72 mmHg. Rowell and colleagues (1964) found arterial saturation to be 90 to 94 percent in four normal young men at $\dot{V}_{O_2}$max; 3 months of endurance conditioning raised their $\dot{V}_{O_2}$max by 15 percent but reduced arterial oxygen saturation of each man by 2 to 3 percent at $\dot{V}_{O_2}$max. A more extreme arterial oxygen desaturation was seen in four highly conditioned endurance athletes ($\dot{V}_{O_2}$max close to 5 L min^{-1} and ventilation averaged 140 L min^{-1} STPD); oxygen saturation fell to 85 percent, with arterial P_{O_2} estimated to be 65 mmHg (based on measurements of pH and temperature in other subjects at $\dot{V}_{O_2}$max) (Rowell et al., 1964).

The first systematic investigation of arterial hypoxemia during severe exercise was carried out on 16 well-conditioned endurance athletes ($\dot{V}_{O_2}$ = 72 ± 2 ml kg^{-1} min^{-1}) by Dempsey and coworkers (1984) (Dempsey had for nearly 20 years energetically disputed the existence of an "exercise hypoxemia," but his ultimate resort to experimentation was rewarded by the results shown in Figure 9-4). Dempsey and coworkers (1984) observed that the most severe hypoxemia occurred in subjects showing little or no alveolar hyperventilation; alveolar P_{CO_2} exceeded 35 mmHg and alveolar P_{O_2} fell to 60 mmHg, with two individuals having values below this level. Their alveolar-arterial (Aa) P_{O_2} differences exceeded 40 mmHg, which is nearly twice the normal difference at $\dot{V}_{O_2}$max (see below). Figure 9-4 emphasizes the authors' conclusion that the relative magnitude of the ventilatory response was an important determinant of the exercise-induced hypoxemia. Usually, *but not always,* the most marked hypoxemia was unattended by any significant hyperventilation and hypocapnia.

Thoroughbred racehorses, like some well-conditioned humans, also become hypoxemic during severe exercise, as illustrated in Figure 9-5. Figure 9-6 emphasizes the point made earlier by Dempsey and colleagues (1984) that, when hypoxemia accompanies severe exercise, a truly compensatory hyperventilatory response to heavy exercise is often not achieved. Bayly and colleagues (1989) concluded that hypoxemia is the consequence of the animals' inability to provide the high rates of air flow needed to move the extreme volumes of CO_2 produced each minute, that is, 82 L CO_2 min^{-1}. They also found an excessively widened Aa P_{O_2} difference.

One consequence of the arterial hypoxemia is that it cancels the beneficial effects of increased hemoglobin concentration and oxygen carrying capacity on arterial oxygen content, and thus on $\dot{V}_{O_2}$max as well. Arterial hemoglobin concentration increases 10 to 15 percent during severe exercise because plasma water is lost into active muscle cells and interstitial

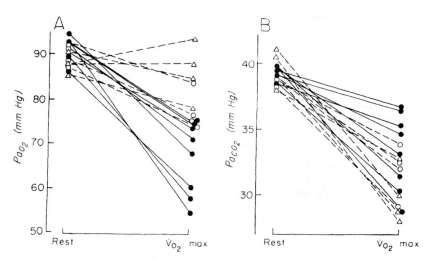

Figure 9-4 The fall in PaO$_2$ from rest to exercise, requiring V̇O$_2$max, tends to be related to the fall in, or lack thereof, in PaCO$_2$. In general, endurance athletes who show the least hyperventilation tend to show the lowest PaO$_2$, but not always. For example, subjects represented by open triangles experience less than a 10-mmHg fall in PaO$_2$; the fall was 10 to 15 mmHg in those shown by open circles, and was 21 to 35 mmHg in those shown by solid circles. All but four showed significant desaturation. (Adapted from Dempsey et al., 1984.)

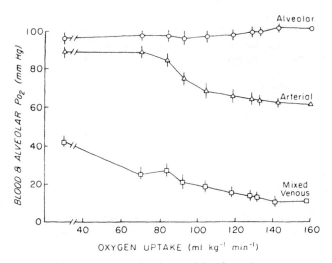

Figure 9-5 Arterial hypoxemia in the thoroughbred racehorse with average values during exercise up to and including those requiring V̇O$_2$max (in nine animals, Bayly et al., 1989). The progressive decline in arterial PO$_2$ was accompanied by rising alveolar PCO$_2$ and a marked widening of the Aa PO$_2$ difference to 40 mmHg. The fall in mixed venous PO$_2$ confirms the approach to V̇O$_2$max and maximal arteriovenous oxygen difference in these horses. (Adapted from Bayly et al., 1989.)

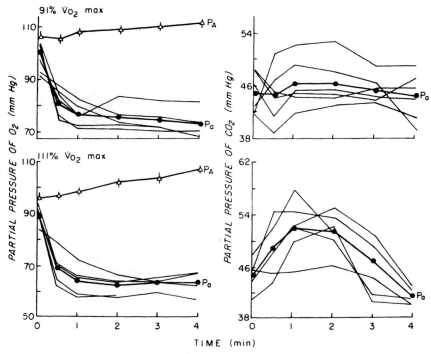

Figure 9-6 Failure to achieve adequate compensatory hyperventilation in five thoroughbred racehorses during 4 minutes of exercise at 91 percent $\dot{V}O_2$max (*top*) and supramaximal exercise calculated to be at 111 percent $\dot{V}O_2$max (*bottom*). At 91 percent $\dot{V}O_2$max, $PaCO_2$ does not decrease and PaO_2 falls markedly. At 111 percent $\dot{V}O_2$max, PaO_2 falls even more and $PaCO_2$ actually *rises* temporarily, but then falls without affecting PaO_2 (see text). Hypercapnia is not long tolerated by the system and ventilation must be driven to extremes that compromise skeletal muscle perfusion and work performance in order to decrease PaO_2 at 111 percent $\dot{V}O_2$max. (Adapted from Bayly et al., 1989.)

fluid as the concentration of osmotically active particles in the muscle rises. In normally active subjects arterial oxygen-carrying capacity rose from 19.7 at rest to 21.9 at $\dot{V}O_2$max while oxygen content rose from 18.8 to 20.1 L ml 100 ml^{-1} so that the change in oxygen saturation was small, that is, from 96 percent at rest to 93 percent at $\dot{V}O_2$max. Although the effect of $\dot{V}O_2$max is small compared to that seen in the athletes (Rowell et al., 1964), the small desaturation reduced arterial oxygen content by 1.8 ml 100 ml^{-1}. This could lower their $\dot{V}O_2$max from 3.4 to 3.0 L min^{-1} (12 percent) by narrowing arteriovenous oxygen difference.

Small changes in arterial oxygen content at the high maximal cardiac outputs of endurance athletes have large effects on oxygen delivery. In the athletes, arterial oxygen capacity was 21.33 ml 100 ml^{-1} at $\dot{V}O_2$max, but oxygen content was only 18.18 ml 100 ml^{-1}, and average oxygen saturation was only 85 percent (Rowell et al., 1964). This reduction in arterial oxygen content reduced the maximal potential to widen arteriovenous oxygen difference by 3.15 ml 100 ml^{-1}. At a cardiac output of 30 L min^{-1}, the maximal oxygen *transport* (cardiac output times arterial oxygen content) without this desaturation would have been 6,400 ml min^{-1} (30,000 × 21.33 ml 100 ml^{-1}) but because of the desaturation, maximal oxygen transport was reduced to 5,454 ml min^{-1}. In this example, if total oxygen extraction were 85 percent, then $\dot{V}O_2$max would have been reduced from 5,439 ml min^{-1} (cardiac output × [0.85 × 21.33 ml 100 ml^{-1}]) to 4,636 ml min^{-1} by the arterial desaturation. For example, when Powers and coworkers (1989) restored arterial oxygen saturation to 96 percent in endurance athletes whose saturations fell to 90.6 percent at $\dot{V}O_2$max, their values for $\dot{V}O_2$max rose from 5 to 5.7 L min^{-1} (14 percent) (saturation was restored by giving 26 percent oxygen).

These differences between arterial oxygen content and capacity are far more spectacular in the racehorse. The contraction of the horse's enormous spleen during severe exercise increases arterial oxygen capacity to 34 ml 100 ml^{-1}, whereas the exercise-induced hypoxemia reduces oxygen saturation to 77 percent and oxygen content to 26 ml 100 ml^{-1} (Bayly et al., 1989). The maximal oxygen transport in the horse (maximal cardiac output = 286 L min^{-1}) would be 97.2 L min^{-1} without the fall in oxygen saturation; the hypoxemia reduces this value to 74.4 L min^{-1}.

Why Does Ventilation Become "Inadequate"?

The word "inadequate" applies to those conditions in which alveolar P_{CO_2} does not fall, or falls very little during exercise, thus contributing to a lower alveolar P_{O_2}. In no case has arterial P_{CO_2} been observed to increase *above resting values* in exercising humans (it does increase temporarily in the horse—see below). Keep in mind that some human athletes showed marked lowering of arterial P_{O_2} despite a normal ventilatory response to exercise; that is, the usual reductions in arterial and alveolar P_{CO_2} were observed (Dempsey et al., 1984).

Dempsey (1986) proposed that when some individuals raise $\dot{V}O_2$max by physical conditioning, the primary changes are in the cardiovascular system with little adaptation in the pulmonary system. In his view, the capacity of the pulmonary system for oxygen transport in these individuals no longer matches that of the cardiovascular system; "arterial blood gas and acid-base homeostasis fail and the lungs become a significant limitation ..." (to $\dot{V}O_2$max and performance). This occurrence is clearly counter to the hypothesis called "symmorphosis," even if the incidence is low. However, the incidence is still unknown because not enough athletes have been studied.

What Adaptation in the Pulmonary System Was Needed to Prevent Hypoxemia?

A major limitation has been sought in the complex mechanical properties of the lung and chest wall (Dempsey, 1986, 1988; Whipp and Pardy, 1986; Forster and Pan, 1988). One idea is that the ventilatory control is mediated by mechanoreceptive and proprioceptive feedback from the chest wall (sensing stretch, tension, and velocity) and from the lung (sensing variables related to flow, pressure, volume and impedence). In order to achieve the alveolar ventilation required at $\dot{V}o_2$max, there must be precise control of respiratory frequency, tidal volume, respiratory muscle recruitment, and also control of airway diameter to minimize resistance to air flow (Dempsey, 1986, 1988; Forster and Pan, 1988). We appear to select breathing patterns that minimize the total elastic and flow-resistant work of breathing, a hypothesis called the "minimum work hypothesis" (see Whipp and Pardy, 1986; Dempsey, 1986; Chapter 7 in this book).

Why Do Some Endurance Athletes—Including Racehorses—Hypoventilate During Severe Exercise?

The attenuated hyperventilation observed in some athletes by Dempsey and colleagues (1984) was reversed during severe exercise by suddenly switching the subjects to a gas mixture containing 20 percent oxygen balanced with 80 percent helium. The reduction in inspired gas density contributed by helium reduced mechanical resistance to air flow in the lung by approximately 40 percent. As a consequence, arterial Po_2 rose and Pco_2 fell toward the values normally observed, during mild exercise (see Figure 9-7). Later Hussain and colleagues (1985) and Pan and colleagues (1987) observed a sudden drop in diaphragmatic electromyographic activity when an oxygen-helium gas mixture was inspired during severe exercise. They proposed that prior to exchanging the gases, ventilation was inhibited by the mechanoreceptive and proprioceptive feedback from the chest wall in response to an excessive resistive load.

The idea evolved that in well-conditioned humans, ventilation in excess of 150 L min^{-1} may approach the mechanical limits of the pulmonary system so that gas exchange is compromised because it is too expensive metabolically to maintain the necessary ventilation (Forster and Pan, 1988). Dempsey's (1986) argument for this proposal is based on three observations:

1. The ventilation necessary to keep alveolar Pco_2 close to 30 mmHg and alveolar Po_2 at 115 mmHg with CO_2 production equal to 3 to 4 L min^{-1} would be 120 L min^{-1}. In contrast, if CO_2 production were 5 to 6 L min^{-1} the requirement for ventilation would be an unreachable 240 L min^{-1}.
2. Air flow and lung volume during tidal breathing are often at the maximal limits of the expiratory flow-volume loop (see Grimby et al., 1971; Whipp and Pardy, 1986).

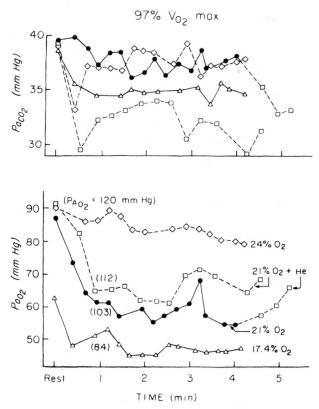

Figure 9-7   Effect of changing density on oxygen tension of inspired gas on $Paco_2$ (*top*) and Pao_2 (*bottom*) during exercise requiring 97 percent of $\dot{V}o_2$max in one subject. *Reducing gas density* (21 percent oxygen in helium) *increased ventilation and reduced $Paco_2$, but this did not prevent the fall in Pao_2, meaning that hypoxemia was not caused primarily by "hypoventilation" in this individual (the fall in Pao_2 was reduced somewhat). Conversely, raising inspired oxygen concentration by only 3 percent, from 21 to 24 percent, prevented most of the fall in Pao_2, but $Paco_2$ did not decline, suggesting that hypoxemia was caused by restricted alveolar-arterial diffusion; hypoxemia was not caused by arterial-venous shunting.* (Adapted from Dempsey et al., 1984.)

3. The ventilatory response to severe exercise appears, at least for a short time (see Figure 9-6), to become dissociated from the powerful chemical stimuli of increased Pco_2 and elevated concentrations of hydrogen ion and norepinephrine. Nevertheless, a sudden reduction in mechanical impedance by reducing inspired gas density with helium permits a prompt increase in ventilation, suggesting it had been limited by mechanical factors, otherwise it would have responded to chemical stimulation.

In a more recent study, Johnson and colleagues (1992) concluded that highly conditioned endurance athletes ($\dot{V}o_2$max $= 73$ ml kg^{-1} min^{-1}) reach their mechanical limits for generating expiratory air flow and inspiratory pleural pressure during exercise at $\dot{V}o_2$max. These athletes could not increase their ventilation at $\dot{V}o_2$max even when 4 to 6.9 percent CO_2 was inspired or when they were made hypoxemic by inspiring 16 percent oxygen.

An impressive example of relative hypoventilation is seen in the galloping racehorse whose breathing becomes so entrained with stride that alveolar ventilation is no longer sufficient to eliminate CO_2 and maintain normal alveolar Po_2 (Bayly et al., 1989). Entrainment of breathing with stride appears to be a physical requirement because of the pistonlike effect of shifting abdominal contents on the diaphragm and lung volume with acceleration and deceleration of the horse accompanying each stride. There is also a mechanical interaction between forelimb extension and rib cage enlargement.

Figure 9-5 shows the horse's very high $\dot{V}o_2$max (per kg body weight), the progressive fall in arterial Po_2 with a marked increase in the Aa Po_2 difference during 2 minutes of exercise. Figure 9-6 shows the time course of these changes and also an unexplained lowering of alveolar Pco_2 (but not arterial Po_2) during the most severe exercise when the duration was extended to 4 minutes. The latter suggests that something else in addition to a mechanical limitation has restricted ventilation and that something other than failure to lower Pco_2 keeps arterial Po_2 low. Keep in mind that not all endurance athletes who experience hypoxemia at $\dot{V}o_2$max do so as a consequence of blunted hyperventilation. The marked increase in Aa Po_2 difference points toward a diffusion limitation at the lung.

The horse provides so far the only example in which the hypoventilation actually leads to true hypercapnia during exercise, but it is short-lived. Probably the increased Pco_2 activates arterial chemoreceptors with such intensity that ventilation is increased at great cost in terms of its excessive requirements for blood flow and oxygen. This means that *performance* (not $\dot{V}o_2$max) must become sharply curtailed by the competition between locomotive and respiratory muscles for blood flow. Parenthetically, these studies on human and equine athletes raise some fascinating questions about the putative importance of CO_2 in the control of breathing during severe exercise.

The pony and the thoroughbred racehorse provide the same contrast in ventilatory responses to severe exercise that are sometimes seen in unconditioned and endurance-trained humans. The pony at $\dot{V}o_2$max (122 ml kg^{-1} min^{-1} or 19.8 L min^{-1}) maintains arterial Po_2 at 90 mmHg while reducing arterial Pco_2 to 27 mmHg and raising Aa Po_2 difference to about 30 mmHg (Bayly et al., 1989) (see Manohar, 1986). Figures 9-5 and 9-6 reveal the contrast with the racehorse which on the average raised alveolar Pco_2 to 41 mmHg, Aa Po_2 difference increased to 44 mmHg, and arterial

Po$_2$ fell to 64 mmHg at the highest work rate (11 percent above that required to elicit $\dot{V}o_2$max).

Why does the horse "hypoventilate"? Elimination of CO_2 is a formidable job for the horse with rates of production exceeding 80 L min^{-1} in contrast to ~20 L min^{-1} in ponies. Mixed venous Pco$_2$ is 116 mmHg in the horse and 55 mmHg in the pony (Bayly et al., 1989). Despite the fact that the horse's $\dot{V}co_2$ exceeds that of the pony by fourfold, the ventilation of the horse is only two times greater. The main constraint could be the excessive ventilation required to eliminate CO_2. The observed maximal alveolar ventilation of 1,500 L min^{-1} would require a tidal volume of approximately 80 to 90 percent of vital capacity, but the alveolar ventilation required to provide the same alveolar Pco$_2$ observed in the pony would be about 3,000 L min^{-1}, which is unattainable.

The conclusion is that, in some endurance-trained animals, ventilation becomes inadequate because the requirements for alveolar ventilation can exceed the functional limits of the pulmonary system. As a consequence, arterial Po$_2$ and oxygen content fall and this constitutes a limit in oxygen transport. Such limitations are not observed in well-conditioned foxhounds, whose $\dot{V}o_2$max per kilogram of body weight equals that of the racehorse (see Musch et al., 1985). This reemphasizes the point that pulmonary limitations are not universal.

The next section explores the potential limitation in exchange of oxygen between the alveoli and the red blood cells, and the factors that might cause any restriction.

ALVEOLAR TO ARTERIAL OXYGEN TRANSFER

Figure 9-2 shows what has been called the "oxygen cascade" (West, 1974). This diagram illustrates the potential barriers between the lung and the muscle cells that reduce in stepwise fashion the initial high driving pressure for oxygen. The data are representative of the resting state. In the normally active young person the Aa Po$_2$ difference commonly increases from 5 to 10 mmHg at rest to about 25 mmHg at $\dot{V}o_2$max. Figure 9-8 illustrates the changes in Po$_2$ across the various potential barriers to oxygen transfer in normally active young people during "maximal" exercise. Arterial Po$_2$ remains close to the resting value. In these individuals the following conditions are thought to be met:

1. Alveolar-capillary diffusion distances are maintained.
2. The mean transit time of red blood cells through the pulmonary capillaries remains within approximately one-half of the resting transit time.
3. Ventilation : perfusion ratios in the lung are high (four : five) and fairly uniformly distributed, and arterial Po$_2$ is maintained at resting values.

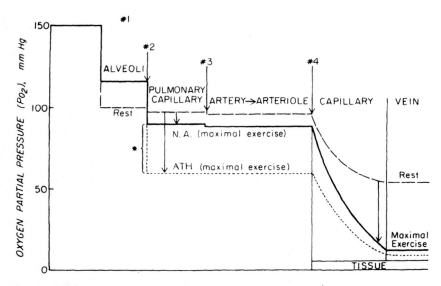

Figure 9-8 The "cascade for oxygen" during exercise at $\dot{V}O_2$max in a normally active (N.A.) individual indicated by *heavy line* and in an endurance athlete (ATH) indicated by a *dotted line*. Values are compared with those at rest shown as a *dashed line*. The alveolar PO_2 is higher during exercise than rest (Figure 9-2) owing to hyperventilation in normally active individuals; alveolar PO_2 is not shown for the athletes because of the marked differences in PO_2 associated with different degrees of hyper- or relative hypoventilation. Normally the alveolar-arterial or Aa PO_2 difference increases by approximately 25 mmHg at $\dot{V}O_2$max, but this gradient can reach or exceed 40 mmHg in endurance athletes, owing in part to lower alveolar PO_2 and higher alveolar PCO_2 stemming from relative hypoventilation.

Thus, the question is: Which of these variables might change enough to contribute, along with reduced hyperventilation when it occurs, to the hypoxemia attending severe exercise in endurance-trained people and racehorses?

Is There a Limitation in Alveolar-Arterial Gas Exchange?

The study of Dempsey and colleagues (1984) shows that, although the alveolar PO_2 remained near 110 mmHg (alveolar PO_2 was also well maintained in racehorses [Bayly et al., 1989]), the Aa PO_2 difference increased from approximately 25 to 33 mmHg on the average and up to 40 mmHg in those who become the most hypoxemic (arterial $PO_2 < 60$ mmHg). Figure 9-8 shows also how endurance conditioning can dramatically alter the drop in oxygen driving pressure along the oxygen cascade. The fall in arterial PO_2 could originate from postpulmonary arteriovenous shunts, from a limitation in alveolar to end-capillary diffusion, or from inequalities in matching alveolar ventilation to pulmonary capillary blood flow, called $\dot{V}_A/\dot{Q}$ mismatching or inequality.

Postpulmonary Arteriovenous Shunts

An increase in inspired oxygen fraction from 20.9 to 23.9 percent virtually corrected the hypoxemia as shown in Figure 9-7 for one subject during repeated bouts of exercise at 97 percent of $\dot{V}_{O_2}max$. This means that shunting of oxygen was not the primary cause of the fall in arterial P_{O_2}; otherwise little or no restoration of arterial P_{O_2} would have occurred. Note also in Figure 9-7 that alveolar P_{CO_2} did not change when arterial P_{O_2} was maintained so that the hypoxemia was not caused by relative hypoventilation in this individual. Furthermore, the improvement in ventilation attending the breathing of a helium-oxygen mixture did not improve this subject's arterial P_{O_2} very much, but it did raise alveolar ventilation as indicated by the fall in alveolar P_{CO_2}. Thus something other than blunted hypoventilation and postpulmonary arteriovenous shunts caused the hypoxemia in this individual.

Gledhill and colleagues (1977) point out that a minor part of this widening of the Aa P_{O_2} difference could be explained by a small postpulmonary venoarteriolar shunt that is approximately 1 to 1.5 percent of the cardiac output. A caution to bear in mind is that such a shunt would not be included in the estimation of $\dot{V}_A/\dot{Q}$ mismatch, but would be falsely included in the diffusion estimate.

Diffusion

The basis for the large leeway we have in maintaining adequate alveolar-capillary oxygen diffusion during rest and exercise was reviewed by Piiper (1988). A deficit in diffusive equilibration or a diffusion limitation is expressed by the ratio of differences between alveolar (P_A) and arterial gas tensions (Pa) and alveolar to mixed-venous ($P\overline{v}$) gas tension as follows:

$$P_A - \frac{Pa}{P_A} - P\overline{v}.$$

This limitation increases as the ratio of pulmonary diffusion capacity (D) to pulmonary blood flow ($\dot{Q}$) times effective solubility of the gas (β). D is related to surface area and the thickness ratio by a constant, and β is the "solubility" of oxygen in blood or actually the slope of the dissociation curve, so that

$$P_A - \frac{Pa}{P_A} - P\overline{v} = e^{-D/\dot{Q}\beta}. \tag{9-1}$$

This relationship shows that the incompleteness of blood-gas equilibration, expressed as the alveolar-arterial partial pressure difference related to the alveolar-mixed venous difference, is determined by the ratio of two conductances, diffusion capacity (D) and perfusion ($\dot{Q}\beta$) (Piiper, 1988).

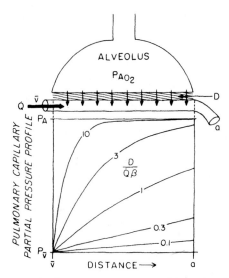

Figure 9-9   The speed at which oxygen is transported from the alveolus to pulmonary capillary is dependent on pulmonary diffusion capacity (D), pulmonary blood flow ($\dot{Q}$), and "solubility" of oxygen in blood, or actually the slope of the dissociation curve (β). The greater the diffusion capacity relative to blood flow and solubility, the more rapidly blood at $P\bar{v}O_2$ equilibrates with PAO_2 along the distance of the capillary as shown by the rate of rise of lines originating at Pv and approaching PAO_2. Complete equilibration is shown as convergence of the line representing the ratio $D/\dot{Q}\beta$ with the horizontal line labeled PA (e.g., $D/\dot{Q}\beta = 10$). When this ratio exceeds 3, oxygen transfer is limited by blood flow; the higher the flow, the sooner the transfer is complete in the capillary, for example, $D/\dot{Q}\beta = 10$. When flow is high and PO_2 is low (e.g., hypoxia), $D/\dot{Q}\beta$ falls below 3 and oxygen transfer from alveolus to capillary is limited by both diffusion and blood flow. $D/\dot{Q}\beta$ also must fall when $\dot{Q}$ becomes extremely high at $\dot{V}O_2$max in athletes. (Adapted from Piiper, 1988.)

Figure 9-9 reveals the significance of the ratio $D/\dot{Q}\beta$. The "speed" with which PO_2 of mixed venous blood ($P\bar{v}O_2$) approaches alveolar PO_2 (PAO_2) is expressed by this ratio so that when $D/\dot{Q}\beta > 3$, gas transfer is limited by *perfusion*. In hypoxia, because of high $\dot{Q}$ and low PO_2, $D/\dot{Q}\beta$ falls well below 3, and, in this case, oxygen transfer is limited by both *perfusion and diffusion*.

Our question of whether any diffusion limitation exists for oxygen across the alveoli seems answered when we see a high alveolar PO_2 (>100 mmHg), an arterial PO_2 of 60 mmHg or less, and a mixed-venous PO_2 of 10 coupled with an extremely high pulmonary blood flow during maximal exercise. Also, Piiper (1988) and others have shown the main diffusive resistance to oxygen transfer from the alveolus to the red blood cells is outside the red cells; reuptake or release of oxygen by red cells is so rapid that a reaction limitation seems unlikely. The remaining possibility, a $\dot{V}_A/\dot{Q}$ mismatch is discussed below.

Inequalities in Alveolar Ventilation: Perfusion Ratios ($\dot{V}_A/\dot{Q}$)

Wagner and colleagues (1986) used the multiple inert-gas washout technique to estimate the degree of mismatch in the $\dot{V}_A/\dot{Q}$ ratio and along with this, the degree to which alveolar–end-capillary diffusion limitation existed during various levels of oxygen uptake up to and including $\dot{V}_{O_2}$max. This technique reputedly distinguishes among $\dot{V}_A/\dot{Q}$ mismatch and diffusion limitation for oxygen and shunt as potential causes for an increased Aa P_{O_2} difference. Distinction is based on the fact that washout of all gases is equally affected by $\dot{V}_A/\dot{Q}$ inequalities and shunt whereas the inert gases have unequal degrees of diffusion limitation. Thus measures of dispersion of gas washout are evaluated. Some data from their subjects are summarized in Figure 9-8, which, again, shows a rise in Aa P_{O_2} difference from 8 to 25 mmHg and a small fall in arterial P_{O_2} from 94 to 91 mmHg between zero load exercise and $\dot{V}_{O_2}$max (3.72 L min^{-1}).

Figure 9-10 shows average findings from Wagner and coworkers (1986) and several studies done by this group at sea level. The line labeled $\dot{V}_A/\dot{Q}$ is the Aa P_{O_2} difference predicted from the degree of $\dot{V}_A/\dot{Q}$ mismatch. Up to an oxygen uptake of approximately 2 L min^{-1}, the small increments in the Aa P_{O_2} difference due to diffusion limitation and $\dot{V}_A/\dot{Q}$ inequalities were approximately the same. At higher oxygen uptakes most of the increase in Aa P_{O_2} difference at sea level was attributable to an alveolar–end-capillary diffusion limitation. Dempsey and colleagues (1984) concluded that owing to the high $\dot{V}_A/\dot{Q}$ ratios (4:6) and the fact that arterial P_{O_2} could be corrected with slight hyperoxia, the hypoxemia is unlikely to be caused by nonuniformity in $\dot{V}_A/\dot{Q}$.

Wagner and coworkers (1989) viewed the mechanisms of hypoxemia in horses during severe exercise to be as follows:

1. An elevation in arterial P_{CO_2} owing to relative hypoventilation lowered arterial P_{O_2} by 6 to 7 mmHg.
2. A mild $\dot{V}_A/\dot{Q}$ inequality accounted for 25 percent of the total Aa P_{O_2} difference (a large postpulmonary shunt of 8 percent would also explain this gradient). In contrast to humans, the $\dot{V}_A/\dot{Q}$ inequality that existed at rest in the horse did not worsen with exercise.
3. An alveolar–end-capillary diffusion disequilibration accounted for approximately 75 percent of the Aa P_{O_2} difference.

Thus in horses, as in humans, diffusion limitation of oxygen transport was the major cause of hypoxemia.

The $\dot{V}_A/\dot{Q}$ mismatch might be attributable in part to increased pulmonary arterial pressure. Wagner and colleagues (1986) observed the high

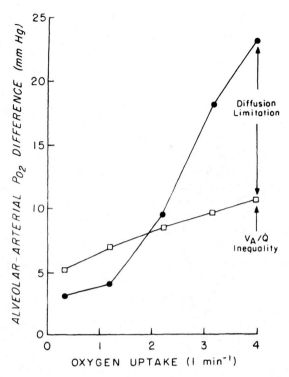

Figure 9-10 Estimates of the relative contributions of alveolar-pulmonary capillary diffusion limitation and $\dot{V}_A/\dot{Q}$ inequality to the widening of the Aa P_{O_2} difference when oxygen uptake increases from resting to maximum. Measurement of washouts of multiple inert gases from the lungs (*open squares*) show that about one-half of the small increase in Aa P_{O_2} difference during exercise requiring less than 2 L O_2 min^{-1} is due to $\dot{V}_A/\dot{Q}$ inequality. The increase in Aa P_{O_2} difference due to limited alveolar diffusion of oxygen (*closed circles*) is calculated from the observed increase in Aa P_{O_2} difference minus the portion of this difference caused by $\dot{V}_A/\dot{Q}$ mismatch. Above 2 L O_2 min^{-1} the gradient is increased mainly by a diffusion limitation, which explains approximately two-thirds of the Aa P_{O_2} difference at $\dot{V}_{O_2}$max. (Adapted from Hammond et al., 1988 and Wagner et al., 1986.)

correlation between the $\dot{V}_A/\dot{Q}$ mismatch and pulmonary arterial pressure when they pooled and analyzed data from their subjects exercising up to maximal levels at sea level, 3,000 m and 4,500 m. However, the correlation between $\dot{V}_A/\dot{Q}$ inequalities and ventilation was equally good. Other possible causes of nonuniform $\dot{V}_A/\dot{Q}$ at altitude are (asymptomatic) interstitial pulmonary edema owing to the high (40 mmHg) pulmonary arterial pressure and also nonuniform (hypoxia-induced) pulmonary vasoconstriction. Parenthetically, the latter was not a cause at sea level because hyperoxia (100 percent oxygen) did not alter the indices of $\dot{V}_A/\dot{Q}$. Also the high pulmonary arterial pressure in the horse (~90 mmHg) in the face of maintained relatively small $\dot{V}A/\dot{Q}$ mismatch in this animal at severe exercise argues against the importance of high pulmonary artery pressure and edema in the deterioration of $\dot{V}A/\dot{Q}$ matching.

The preceding studies lend credence to Dempsey's hypothesis expressed in Figure 9-11. The hypothesis is that the extra widening of the Aa Po_2 difference in the endurance athletes stems from an increase in pulmonary blood flow beyond the point at which pulmonary capillary blood volume can increase owing to limitations in capillary structure. As a consequence transit time of the red blood cells through the pulmonary capillaries falls precipitously with further increase in cardiac output and pulmonary blood flow.

In normally active people the transit time of the red blood cells through the pulmonary capillaries, although reduced at high cardiac outputs, remains sufficient for virtually complete exchange of oxygen (Figure 9-12).

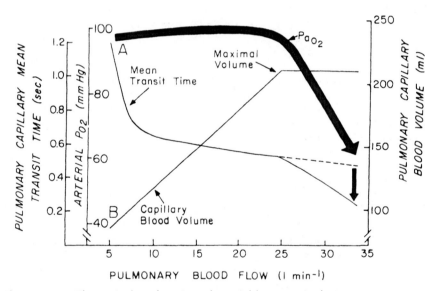

Figure 9-11 Theoretical explanation of arterial hypoxemia during severe exercise in endurance athletes. Line A shows computed mean transit times for red cells through pulmonary capillaries with increasing pulmonary blood flow. Line B shows estimated average pulmonary capillary blood volume with increasing blood flow. As long as capillary blood volume increases with pulmonary blood flow, mean transit time is sufficient to permit alveolar-capillary oxygen equilibration. In some athletes flow increases beyond the point at which capillary volume can increase (shown here at 25 L min⁻¹), causing mean transit time to fall suddenly (*smaller arrow*). Heavy line at top (labeled PaO_2) shows the decline in PaO_2 that accompanies the sudden decline in mean transit time. In this scheme hypoxemia is caused by a diffusion limitation caused by very brief mean transit times. (Adapted from Dempsey and Fregosi, 1985.)

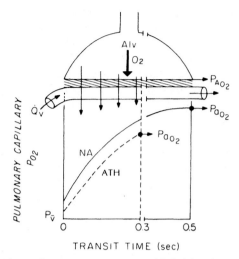

TRANSIT TIME (sec)

Figure 9-12 Hypothetical time course over which blood at mixed venous P_{O_2} ($P\bar{v}_{O_2}$) reached Pa_{O_2} during maximal exercise in normally active (NA) individuals and in endurance athletes (ATH). In the athletes $P\bar{v}_{O_2}$ is lower at $\dot{V}_{O_2}$max and pulmonary mean transit time is shorter (~0.3 seconds) owing to higher pulmonary blood flow. The transit time is not sufficient for pulmonary capillary P_{O_2} and Pa_{O_2} to reach PA_{O_2}. The figure does not illustrate the additional effect of reduced rate of rise in pulmonary capillary P_{O_2} owing to the lower $D/\dot{Q}\beta$ in the athlete (see Figure 9-9). In NA individuals, the lower pulmonary blood flow, longer transit time, and also faster rate of rise in P_{O_2} (i.e., larger $D/\dot{Q}\beta$ ratio) brings pulmonary capillary and arterial P_{O_2} closer to PA_{O_2}.

Any reduction in pulmonary capillary mean transit time is minimized by the three-fold expansion of pulmonary capillary volume accompanying increased pulmonary blood flow and transmural pressure. Accordingly, mean transit time is thought to remain adequate at approximately 0.5 seconds to insure gas equilibration in unconditioned young people. Volume expansion of pulmonary capillaries not only insures adequate equilibration of alveolar gas tension with that of red blood cells, it also fosters more uniform distribution of pulmonary blood flow and better $\dot{V}A/\dot{Q}$ matching and also expansion of the surface between alveolus and capillary. Despite these adjustments, the Aa P_{O_2} difference normally increases four to five times in going from rest to severe exercise.

Figures 9-11 and 9-12 summarize what is thought to happen in endurance athletes when pulmonary blood flow continues to increase after pulmonary capillary blood volume has expanded maximally. An additional point is that the precipitous fall in mean transit time comes at a time when the rate of equilibration of mixed venous P_{O_2} with alveolar P_{O_2} requires more, not less, time for the red blood cells to transit through the pulmonary capillaries. This equilibration time depends on the slope of the hemoglobin-oxygen dissociation curve between mixed venous ($\bar{P}v$) and end-pulmonary capillary blood. The closer the alveolar Po_2 is to the steep region of the oxygen dissociation curve, and the lower the mixed venous Po_2, the longer the capillary transit time needed for oxygen equilibration. The higher alveolar Pco_2 and lower alveolar Po_2 of the athletes, plus their very low mixed venous Po_2 (approximately 15 mmHg) means that those individuals who hypoventilate need approximately 30 percent longer capillary transit times than they have (Dempsey, 1986).

Summary

Expressed in terms of the Fick principle, the first clear limitation in oxygen uptake is a reduction in the arterial oxygen content, which reduces $\dot{V}o_2$max in proportion to the narrowing of arteriovenous oxygen difference. Arterial oxygen desaturation is slight in normally active individuals and is attributable to the rise in hemoglobin concentration and oxygen-carrying capacity which is unaccompanied by any significant change in oxygen content. Arterial Po_2 is well maintained by the increase in alveolar Po_2 in the face of a four- to fivefold increase in the Aa Po_2 difference caused mainly by a small alveolar to end-pulmonary capillary diffusion limitation (two-thirds of the effect) and an even smaller nonuniformity in $\dot{V}A/\dot{Q}$ (one-third of the effect). In contrast, human and equine endurance athletes who have greater hemoconcentration and increased oxygen-carrying capacity sometimes show marked arterial desaturation and a fall in arterial Po_2 at $\dot{V}o_2$max; even arterial oxygen content falls below resting levels in some cases. This arterial hypoxemia is accompanied by a seven- to eight-fold increase in the Aa Po_2 difference (up to 40 mmHg) again caused mainly by a diffusion limitation with a possible small contribution from $\dot{V}A/\dot{Q}$ mismatch. In some cases a relative hypoventilation fails to lower alveolar Pco_2 and the consequent lowering of alveolar Po_2 contributes further to the fall in arterial Po_2. Inasmuch as the hypoxemia is corrected by slight hyperoxia, the hypoxemia is not caused by arteriovenous shunting. Relative hypoventilation is especially pronounced in racehorses whose ventilation is entrained to locomotion. The principal cause in both humans and horses appears to be an attainment of mechanical limits for breathing. A sudden shift to a low-density oxygen-helium gas mixture, which lowers mechanical resistance to air flow in the lung and raises ventilation, often does not restore arterial Po_2 so that factors other than hypoventilation can lead to hypoxemia. Most of the hypoxemia is caused by a diffusion limitation which is related to the high pulmonary blood flow and short pulmonary mean transit time, which limits time for oxygen transfer between alveoli and red blood cells.

The observation that the structure of the pulmonary system is not well suited to the needs of the other systems in the chain of oxygen transport and consumption is damaging to a deterministic hypothesis such as symmorphosis, which holds that structure determines function, and the two are ideally matched. It would also be destructive to the hypothesis to find at the other end of the oxygen cascade that the oxidative capacity of the muscle exceeded the capacity of the cardiovascular delivery system.

CARDIAC OUTPUT AS A LIMITATION TO OXYGEN UPTAKE

In preceding chapters, the ability of humans to raise cardiac output is treated as an important limitation to $\dot{V}o_2$max. In summary, the main points of evidence are as follows:

1. $\dot{V}o_2$max in humans is achieved by intense activation of only about 50 percent of the total muscle mass. During exercise at the $\dot{V}o_2$max, addition of more active muscle causes no further increase in cardiac output or in oxygen uptake, that is, both are at their maximal values. In short, the heart cannot provide enough blood flow for all of the muscles.
2. When additional muscles are activated at $\dot{V}o_2$max, total vascular conductance and arterial pressure are maintained by vasoconstriction in active muscle.
3. The capacity of the muscles to consume oxygen each minute exceeds what the heart can deliver. Although the evidence provided in Chapter 7 supports this idea for humans, it has not been clear that this applies to other mammals such as the dog or horse, whose cardiac pumping capacities per kilogram of body weight exceed that of humans by two- to threefold.

If skeletal muscles of humans, dogs, and horses had essentially the same range of vascular conductances (per 100 g muscle) (this is not known), then the mismatch between cardiac pumping capacity and peak conductances of skeletal muscle in humans would far exceed that of mammals such as dogs and horses, whose cardiac pumping capacities per kilogram of body weight so far exceed ours. Nevertheless, Figure 9-13 demonstrates that oxygen transport also limits the $\dot{V}o_2$max in the foxhound, an endurance animal with a $\dot{V}o_2$ kg^{-1} min^{-1} equal to that of the thoroughbred racehorse (approximately 150 ml kg^{-1} min^{-1}). Maximal cardiac output and oxygen uptake were established in these dogs before and after pericardectomy (Stray-Gundersen et al., 1986). The pericardectomy removed a mechanical constraint on stroke volume and thereby enabled the heart to respond to the high filling pressure at maximal exercise. Stroke volume increased by 14 percent and as a consequence, maximal cardiac output rose by 17 percent. The figure shows that $\dot{V}o_2$max rose less than the 17 percent that would be predicted from the rise in cardiac output because hemoglobin concentration fell following thoracotomy. In these dogs and also in sham-operated (control) dogs (thoracotomy without pericardectomy) $\dot{V}o_2$max was reduced in proportion to the fall in hemoglobin concentration. However, the main point is that the $\dot{V}o_2$max rose

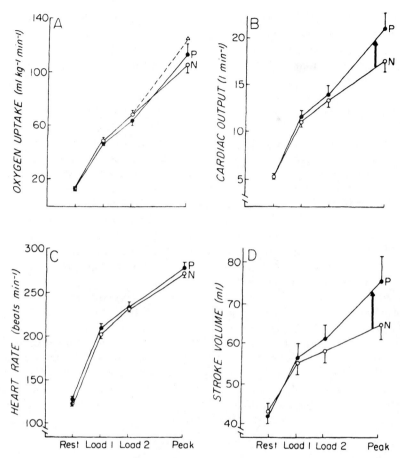

Figure 9-13 Cardiac responses to graded exercise up to "maximal" levels (heart rate and cardiac output reached plateaus) before (N) and after (P) pericardectomy. All exercise intensities were the same before and after the surgery. Removal of pericardial constraints permitted higher maximal stroke volume, thereby permitting higher maximal values for cardiac output and oxygen uptake. $\dot{V}O_2$max rose by only 8 percent rather than by 17 percent as predicted (panel A, *dashed line and open triangle*) because surgery reduced arterial hemoglobin concentration. The acute increase in $\dot{V}O_2$max reveals that oxygen uptake was limited by blood flow and not by the oxidative capacity of the active muscles. (Adapted from Stray-Gundersen et al., 1986.)

significantly (8 percent) and would have risen 17 percent had hemoglobin concentration not fallen.

An equally convincing demonstration of the limitation in oxygen consumption by cardiac output in the foxhound was made in a joint study by Musch and colleagues (1985) and Parsons and colleagues (1985). The 28 percent increase in $\dot{V}O_2$max that accompanied physical conditioning was attributable to the increase in stroke volume and cardiac output. There were no significant changes in oxygen extraction or in the oxidative capacity of the conditioned muscles as measured by a battery of biochemical determinations that assess this function (this is an unusual response for normally both increase). Thus, in an animal noted for its high cardiovascular and metabolic capacity, the ability of the muscles to consume oxygen is limited by the ability of the heart to supply them with oxygen.

Summary.   In summary, the ability of humans to raise cardiac output is not sufficient to supply oxygen to more than a fraction of the active muscles during exhausting exercise. That fraction is unknown but may be 50 to 60 percent of the total mass. Thus $\dot{V}o_2$max is not muscle-mass dependent once a critical mass is active. When this mass is exceeded, muscle blood flow is actively reduced by sympathetic vasoconstriction, as indicated by a widening of arteriovenous difference across the muscle and also by a marked rise in its spillover of norepinephrine into plasma. In foxhounds $\dot{V}o_2$max can be increased acutely along with maximal cardiac output (i.e., to a new maximum) by cutting the pericardium and allowing stroke volume to increase further. Further physical conditioning increases $\dot{V}o_2$max in these animals simply by increasing maximal cardiac output. Extraction of oxygen by the conditioned muscles did not change, nor did any biochemical indices of their oxidative capacity (this may be unique to foxhounds and possibly other high-endurance animals). All of these findings are inconsistent with the Weibel-Taylor hypothesis called symmorphosis, which holds that the oxidative capacity of the muscles is closely matched functionally to the capacity of the cardiovascular system to transport oxygen. In terms of the variables in the Fick expression,

$$\dot{V}o_2max = \dot{Q}max \, (Cao_2 - C\bar{v}o_2), \qquad (9\text{-}2)$$

the italic variables ($\dot{Q}max$ or maximal cardiac output and Cao_2 or arterial oxygen content) represent clear limitations to $\dot{V}o_2$max. A modest increase in Cao_2 by increasing inspired oxygen tension or, in some cases, by raising hemoglobin concentration (this is more controversial [Rowell, 1974, 1986]) will *raise* $\dot{V}o_2$max, again indicating that muscle metabolism is not limiting.

TRANSFER OF OXYGEN FROM MUSCLE CAPILLARY
TO MITOCHONDRIA

Another variable in the Fick expression to consider as a potential limitation to $\dot{V}o_2$max is mixed venous oxygen content ($C\bar{v}o_2$). More specifically, what determines its reduction to as low a value as possible in order to gain a maximal widening of arteriovenous oxygen difference? Reduction in muscle venous oxygen content clearly constitutes another limitation in $\dot{V}o_2$max in humans because it is lower after physical conditioning and its reduction appears to *explain the entire increase in systemic arteriovenous oxygen difference.* Recall that in normally active young people the widening of systemic arteriovenous oxygen difference accounts for one-half of the adaptation that increases $\dot{V}o_2$max during conditioning (Rowell, 1974, 1986).

Possibilities that could explain a reduction in mixed venous oxygen content and widening of arteriovenous oxygen difference are (1) increased oxygen extraction by inactive regions, or (2) increased oxygen extraction by active muscles. The second possibility is the only choice. The first option is dismissed because at $\dot{V}o_2$max blood flow to inactive regions appears to be reduced to the same degree before and after conditioning. Thus the entire increase in maximal cardiac output caused by conditioning goes to the active muscles. This in itself would lower mixed venous oxygen content if the oxygen content in veins draining the muscle were lower than that of veins draining the rest of the body, that is, a greater fraction of the total venous return has lower oxygen content.

Adjustments within the muscle that could explain the greater oxygen extraction include the following: (1) an increase in capillary density providing more capillaries per muscle fiber, (2) greater number of capillaries per area of tissue, and (3) greater area of muscle tissue perfused by each capillary. In short, distances for diffusion of oxygen between capillaries and cells are reduced. After physical conditioning capillary density, leg blood flow and $\dot{V}o_2$max all increase in similar proportions (Chapter 7), while venous oxygen content and Po_2 of blood draining the muscles are reduced; these adjustments explain the reduction in $C\bar{v}o_2$. Another important point is that there must be a delicate balance between the increase in muscle blood flow and the mean transit time needed to maximize the extraction of oxygen (Chapter 7). The increase in capillary density entails a rise in capillary blood volume which minimizes the fall in capillary transit times that would otherwise attend the higher blood flow after conditioning. These points all suggest that another important limitation in the transport of oxygen is its diffusion from the capillaries to the mitochondria of the active muscles.

In thinking about the possible limitations to oxygen transfer from the capillaries to the mitochondria in the muscle, we can apply the same thinking used to explain the limitations in oxygen *loading* or the transfer of oxygen from the alveoli to the red blood cells in the pulmonary capillaries. On the one hand, we consider the factors at the lung that interfere with oxygen loading and reduce *arterial* Po_2. On the other hand, at the muscle we must consider those factors that would interfere with oxygen *unloading* from capillaries to the mitochondria and *raise muscle venous* Po_2. To increase oxygen unloading, the Po_2 gradient from the muscle capillaries to the mitochondria ($Pco_2 - Pmito_2$) must be increased.

In the lung arterial hypoxemia is caused by

1. Decreased inspired Po_2
2. Hypoventilation

3. Diffusion limitation
4. Arteriovenous shunt
5. $\dot{V}_A/\dot{Q}$ inequalities or mismatch

Some analogous factors that might be expected to keep muscle venous Po_2 elevated in severe exercise would be

1. Increased arterial Po_2
2. Hyperperfusion
3. Diffusion limitation
4. Blood flow inhomogeneities
5. $\dot{V}o_2/\dot{Q}$ inequalities or mismatch

In order to dissect out these factors at the muscle capillary interface, some fundamental obstacles need to be overcome. Samples of average capillary Po_2 and oxygen content at the muscle are not directly attainable as are samples of mixed alveolar Po_2 and oxygen concentrations at the lung. The same applies to the mixed venous Po_2 in the muscle veins in contrast to the easily obtainable mixed pulmonary venous blood leaving the lungs as arterial blood. The analysis we need at the tissues is essentially the reverse of that carried out by Piiper (1988) at the lung and illustrated in Figure 9-9. The data are not available and evidence for diffusion limitation for oxygen at the muscle is still indirect. Again, the basic question being asked here is what might explain the existence of values for muscle venous Po_2 and oxygen content at $\dot{V}o_2$max that are well above the theoretical minimum needed to keep the efficiency of oxygen extraction by the muscle as high as possible (e.g., ~90 percent)?

Are Muscle Oxygen Uptake and $\dot{V}o_2$max Limited by Diffusion of Oxygen into the Muscle?

Increased Arterial Oxygen Content

Hyperoxia not only raises arterial oxygen content but it also raises femoral venous oxygen content at $\dot{V}o_2$max to higher values than observed at $\dot{V}o_2$max under normoxic conditions (Pirnay et al., 1972). Despite the higher $\dot{V}o_2$max allowed by the increased arterial oxygen content, the increase in arteriovenous oxygen difference across the muscle is small because of the rise in venous oxygen content. It is as though oxygen transfer from the capillaries to the cell were limited.

Hyperperfusion

A second factor that could lead to higher muscle venous Po_2 is hyperperfusion of the active muscle. Andersen and Saltin (1985) maximally exercised the quadriceps muscle so that perfusion of a small muscle mass was unrestricted by any limitations in cardiac output. As quadriceps muscle oxygen uptake reached a surprisingly high peak value of 350 ml kg^{-1} min^{-1} at exhausting exercise, Figure 9-14 shows that the femoral arteriovenous

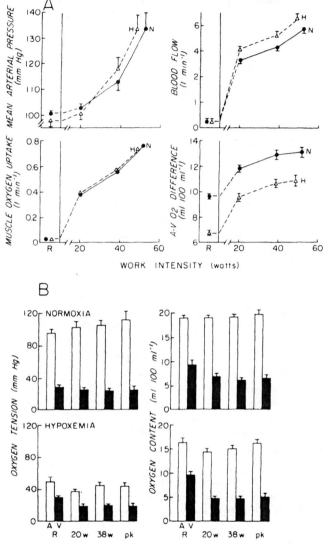

Figure 9-14 (**A**) Hemodynamic responses to moderate to peak power output of human knee extensors (quadriceps femoris) during normoxia (N, *solid circles*) and hypoxemia (inspired oxygen = 10 to 11 percent) (H, *open triangles*). Hypoxemia raised quadriceps blood flow and reduced femoral arteriovenous oxygen difference. Note the constancy of this arteriovenous difference in both conditions. (**B**) shows arterial (A, *open bars*) and femoral venous (V, *solid bars*) values for oxygen content and PO_2. Note than in normoxia femoral venous PO_2 and oxygen content remains nearly constant with increasing power output but with values much higher than seen during peak exercise of all muscles in both legs. Even in hypoxemia both femoral venous PO_2 and oxygen content remain constant and at higher values than seen during total leg exercise. (Adapted from Rowell et al., 1986.)

oxygen difference across the muscle, was much narrower than the femoral arteriovenous oxygen difference observed in severe whole-body exercise (even when subjects were made hypoxemic by breathing 10 to 11 percent oxygen) (Figure 7-16). Figure 9-14 shows that in both normoxia and hypoxemia the muscle venous oxygen content and Po_2 remained surprisingly high (Rowell et al., 1986). The high blood flows must have caused such short transit times for red blood cells through muscle capillaries that there was limited time for diffusion of oxygen. Keep in mind that in whole-body exercise, transit time may never decrease to this critical point because muscle blood flow per unit mass of muscle cannot increase that much.

Diffusion Limitation

Any diffusional barrier between the red blood cell and the muscle cell would keep muscle venous oxygen pressure and content higher than needed to provide maximal extraction. Wagner (1988) points to the fact that the venous blood draining muscle is rarely depleted of its oxygen at $\dot{V}o_2$max. He postulates that a limitation to the diffusion of oxygen from the muscle capillary to the mitochondria always exists at high levels of oxygen uptake. The muscle capillary Po_2-mitochondrial Po_2 (Pco_2 − $Pmito_2$) gradient is in effect widened, which is analogous to the widening of the alveolar-pulmonary capillary Po_2 gradient.

The principal observation suggesting that a tissue diffusion limitation for $\dot{V}o_2$max exists at the capillary-muscle cell interface is the linear relationship between $\dot{V}o_2$max and muscle venous oxygen content (or Po_2) that passes through the origin or close to it (e.g., Wagner, 1988; Roca et al., 1989). Further, when arterial Po_2 and oxygen content were changed by altering inspired gas concentrations, the points relating $\dot{V}o_2$max to venous Po_2 still fell together on a straight line passing close to the origin. In accordance with Fick's first law of diffusion we predict a linear relationship between oxygen uptake, mixed venous Po_2, femoral venous Po_2 and mean capillary Po_2 (derived by Bohr integration) (Dto_2 is tissue diffusion capacity for oxygen, and $P\bar{v}o_2$ and $Pmito_2$ are muscle venous and muscle mitochondrial Po_2 values, respectively) (Wagner et al., 1989)

$$\dot{V}o_2 = Dto_2(P\bar{v}o_2 - Pmito_2). \qquad (9-3)$$

In Wagner's (1988) scheme, as venous Po_2 decreases, calculated oxygen uptake must decrease because the pressure gradient that drives the diffusion of oxygen from the capillary to the mitochondria is reduced.

The hypothesis predicts that the rate of oxygen delivery (flow times arterial oxygen content) determines mean capillary Po_2 so that, for example, increased delivery of oxygen would increase both the mean capillary Po_2 and the capillary-mitochondrial diffusion gradient for oxygen so that $\dot{V}o_2$max would increase. This concept is discussed in more detail below (see Figure 9-18). Hogan and coworkers (1989) tested this idea in the isolated (in situ) dog gastrocnemius and showed that under rigorously controlled conditions for constant oxygen delivery with altered blood flow and arterial oxygen content (controlled by the investigator) results consistent with the hypothesis of tissue diffusion limitation could be obtained.

Blood Flow Inhomogeneities and Perfusion: Oxygen Uptake ($\dot{Q}/\dot{V}O_2$) Inequalities

These two inseparable (so far) factors are the fourth and fifth factors cited above that could interfere with the reduction in muscle venous oxygen content to values that would provide the greatest extraction of oxygen by the muscle. Two crucial assumptions in Wagner's analysis are that in humans at $\dot{V}O_2$max, perfusion : oxygen uptake ($\dot{Q}/\dot{V}O_2$) heterogeneity and both perfusional and diffusional shunting are negligible. It is clear that muscle perfusion per unit mass during exercise is heterogeneous (e.g., Sparks and Mohrman, 1977; Piiper and Haab, 1991) (see Chapter 7). What is not known is the extent of $\dot{Q}/\dot{V}O_2$ mismatching and if this mismatching becomes greater (as it does for $\dot{V}A/\dot{Q}$ in the lung in humans) or smaller with increasing oxygen uptake. Figure 9-15 simply illustrates schematically an inhomogeneous distribution of regional oxygen consumptions and blood flow through a muscle and how this might alter local venous oxygen values throughout the muscle without affecting the oxygen content of "mixed" venous effluent from the muscle. Some sections within the muscle have high metabolic activity (black regions) and are relatively underperfused ($Cvo_2 = 2$ mmHg, $Pvo_2 = \sim 10$ mmHg), whereas other regions are so overperfused relative to oxygen uptake that they are virtual shunts (e.g., white region $Cvo_2 = 16$ ml 100 ml^{-1}, $Pvo_2 = 62$ mmHg). Keep in mind that even though total flow through the muscle is constant, changes in the distribution of flow between sections of the muscle could also change the average venous oxygen content ($C\overline{v}o_2$) and Po_2 as well as $\dot{V}o_2$ if some metabolically active regions were underperfused so that oxygen needs could not be met. This would be analogous to a shunt (i.e., decreased $\dot{V}o_2$ and increased Cvo_2 in the lumped Fick equation for the whole muscle).

Honig and colleagues (1984) examined the sequential barriers to oxygen transport from red blood cells in the muscle capillary to the mitochondria by rapidly "trapping" oxygen gradients by quick-freezing the muscle and then determining myoglobin saturation in frozen slices of the muscle by a spectrophotometric technique. In agreement with others, they found the red cell membrane not to be a significant barrier for diffusion (e.g., Piiper, 1988). The main barrier or "resistance" to oxygen diffusion resides in the narrow layer of plasma between the red cell and the endothelium, in the endothelium itself, and the extracellular space before the muscle cell membrane. Red blood cell transit times through muscle in severe exercise were found to be shorter than the minimum time required to release oxygen; otherwise Honig and colleagues (1984) conclude that oxygen extraction would be greater than it is and the necessary oxygen could be

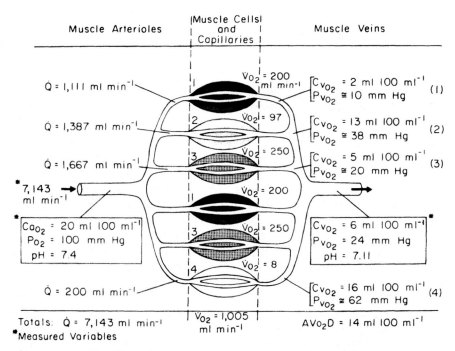

Figure 9-15 Hypothetical heterogeneous distribution of blood flow, oxygen up-takes, and muscle venous oxygen contents and P_{O_2} values within one active muscle. Asterisks and box enclosures show average measured blood flow and arterial and venous values for the entire muscle group. This illustrates the potential *blood flow inhomogeneity and* $\dot{V}_{O_2}/\dot{Q}$ *inequality* that could exist within an active muscle and thereby influence the P_{O_2} gradient between muscle capillary blood and muscle cells. Darkest muscle cell regions represent relatively underperfused regions and less shaded regions are those less underperfused; unshaded regions are overperfused. Increasing blood flow to dark regions would have the greatest effects on muscle venous P_{O_2} and oxygen content; these effects would be smallest in underperfused regions. An array of changes in blood flow are possible with or without changes in average muscle C_{VO_2} or P_{O_2}. Rates of diffusion of oxygen from muscle capillary to mitochondria would be lowest where capillary P_{O_2} is lowest and greatest where it is highest. Note P_{VO_2} values are estimates based on estimated changes in pH and temperature of the different regions.

supplied at lower flow. They view the muscle venous oxygen content at exercise as a reflection of a *"convective shunt" attributable to a diffusional barrier at the capillary.* This is illustrated in Figure 9-16 which shows in isolated muscle a progressive fall in venous oxygen saturation with increasing muscle oxygen uptake and blood flow caused by increasing twitch frequency. Note that a point is reached at which venous oxygen saturation starts to rise with further increases in muscle blood flow and oxygen consumption (Honig et al., 1984); mean transit time becomes too short to maintain oxygen transfer by diffusion.

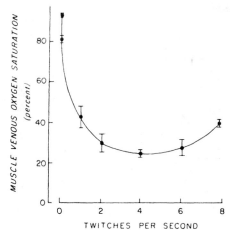

Figure 9-16   Decrements in muscle venous oxygen saturation during twitch contractions of the dog gracilis muscle. Venous oxygen saturation fell with increasing muscle oxygen uptake and blood flow up to 4 twitches sec^{-1}. Above 4 twitches sec^{-1} and at higher $\dot{V}O_2$ and blood flow, venous oxygen saturation rose despite lower muscle myoglobin saturation and cell PO_2. This rise in venous oxygen saturation offered evidence that the muscle capillary is a functional oxygen barrier. Mean transit time became too short to maintain oxygen transfer by diffusion so there is in effect a "convective shunt" for oxygen amounting to approximately one-third of the total oxygen consumed by the muscle. (Adapted from Honig et al., 1984.)

Myoglobin with its P_{50} (partial pressure at 50 percent saturation) of only 5.3 mmHg (compared to 27 mmHg for normal hemoglobin at pH 7.4, 37°C) is well-suited to stabilize (analogous to the action of a buffer) tissue PO_2 well below capillary PO_2. That is, the myoglobin maximizes the transcapillary PO_2 gradient. Honig and colleagues (1984) found low PO_2 and low myoglobin saturation throughout muscle cells, irrespective of capillary location. The PO_2 values within a given cell were surprisingly uniform and were unrelated to the distance of the muscle cells from the nearby capillaries as illustrated in Figure 9-17. Effective intracellular stabilization of oxygen by the myoglobin minimized intracellular PO_2 gradients. This contradicts what would be predicted from Krogh's cylinder model shown in Figure 9-17. Thus, resistance to oxygen transport within the cell appears to be small relative to the resistance to oxygen transfer from the muscle capillary to the cell.

Adjustments in Tissue Diffusion Capacity

The relationship between oxygen uptake and muscle venous PO_2 illustrated schematically in Figure 9-18 shows the expected relationship between

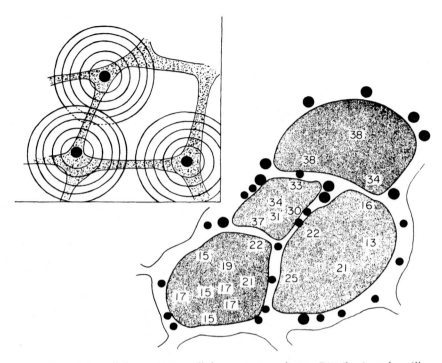

Figure 9-17   Intracellular and intercellular oxygen gradients. Distribution of capillaries around muscle cells and intracellular myoglobin oxygen saturations at various sites of measurement. Muscles were suddenly frozen during tetanic contractions; capillary distribution and intracellular myoglobin oxygen saturations (*encircled numbers*, spectrophotometric technique) were measured in frozen slices by Honig et al. (1984). Krogh's cylinder model (*left*) predicts a uniform radial distribution of myoglobin saturations, an index of intracellular P_{O_2}. This model of oxygen diffusing uniformly from a point source into a uniform sink is not supported by the data of Honig et al. (1984). Note the similarity of myoglobin saturations within a given cell irrespective of distance from the capillaries. (Adapted from Honig et al., 1984).

these variables with the *negative* slope representing the oxygen uptake values calculated from the Fick principle ($\dot{V}_{O_2} = \dot{Q}[Ca_{O_2} - C\bar{v}_{O_2}]$) as a function of muscle venous P_{O_2} with constant flow and arterial oxygen content (assume blood flow or cardiac output is maximal). The *positive* slope represents the oxygen uptake values calculated from Fick's law of diffusion based upon a muscle venous P_{O_2} equal to a mean capillary P_{O_2} times estimated tissue diffusion capacity (mitochondrial P_{O_2} is usually assumed to be zero). $\dot{V}_{O_2}$max is at the point of the intersection of the two lines (e.g., point A); that is, the point at which oxygen diffusion limits any further increase in oxygen uptake that might be made by moving up the negative (Fick) slope, from point A to point C. That is, oxygen uptake cannot increase by increasing only $\dot{Q}$ or $Ca_{O_2} - C\bar{v}_{O_2}$ because the transfer

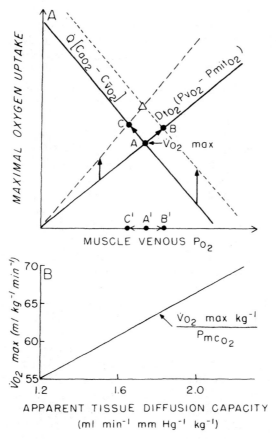

Figure 9-18   Relationship between maximal oxygen uptake and muscle venous P_{O_2} is determined by the interaction between *convective delivery* of oxygen to the muscle, represented by the negative slope for $\dot{V}_{O_2} = \dot{Q}[CaO_2 - C\bar{v}_{O_2}]$ (Fick principle), and the *diffusion* of oxygen from the capillary to muscle cell represented by the positive slope for $\dot{V}_{O_2} = Dt_{O_2} [Pv_{O_2} - Pmit_{O_2}]$ (after Fick's law of diffusion). $Dt_{O_2} =$ tissue diffusion capacity. The scheme is by Wagner (1988). $\dot{V}_{O_2}$max is at the intersection of these two slopes (point A) and at muscle venous P_{O_2} (point A' on x-axis). An increase in convective delivery of oxygen (e.g., by increased cardiac output) would shift $\dot{V}_{O_2}$max and muscle venous P_{O_2} to point B on the new slope (*dashed line*) for $\dot{Q}[CaO_2 - C\bar{v}_{O_2}]$. The higher muscle venous P_{O_2} (point B') reflects the diffusion limitations set by $Dt_{O_2} [Pv_{O_2} - Pmit_{O_2}]$. It is not possible to increase $\dot{V}_{O_2}$max and muscle venous P_{O_2} to point C' without first increasing the slope of $Dt_{O_2} [Pv_{O_2} - Pmit_{O_2}]$. The response to physical conditioning is represented by the open triangle at the intersection of the two dashed lines showing both increased convection and diffusion. The higher $\dot{V}_{O_2}$max and lower muscle venous P_{O_2} accompanying physical conditioning is accompanied by increases in both cardiac output and Dt_{O_2}. (Adapted from Wagner, 1988.) Panel B shows the relationship betwen $\dot{V}_{O_2}$max and an apparent tissue diffusion capacity estimated from calculated mean capillary P_{O_2} in athletes. The higher the $\dot{V}_{O_2}$max the greater the tissue diffusion capacity. (Adapted from Roca et al., 1989.)

of oxygen to muscle is limited (in this model) by diffusion. Without a marked increase in the positive slope of the line depicting diffusion limitation (i.e., to the dashed line), the predicted effect of an increase in maximal cardiac output and $\dot{V}o_2$max with physical conditioning would be *a rise* in muscle venous Po_2 (i.e., points A to B in Figure 9-18). That is, driving pressure would have to increase to permit increased diffusion and increased $\dot{V}o_2$max. Actually the converse occurs; the rise in $\dot{V}o_2$max with physical conditioning is accompanied by a *reduction* in muscle venous Po_2 and oxygen content (e.g., Saltin et al., 1968; Shappell, 1971) meaning that the *rise in cardiac output with conditioning must be accompanied by a marked increase in* Dto_2. This is shown as an increased slope of the "Diffusion" line in Figure 9-18. The increase in Dto_2 alone (no change in $\dot{Q}(Cao_2 - C\bar{v}o_2)$ would raise $\dot{V}o_2$max from points A to C and reduce muscle venous Po_2 from A' to C'. Therefore the best depiction of the adjustment to physical conditioning in Figure 9-18 would be the upward shift from point A to the delta illustrating the rise in $\dot{V}o_2$max that would be caused by increased cardiac output, increased tissue diffusion capacity, and reduced muscle venous oxygen content.

Roca and associates (1989) observed a positive relationship between $\dot{V}o_2$max and an index of apparent tissue diffusion capacity ($\dot{V}o_2$max/estimated mean capillary Po_2). This estimate of diffusion capacity (shown in panel B in Figure 9-18) was nearly twice as large in individuals with $\dot{V}o_2$max of 70 ml kg^{-1} min^{-1} as those with $\dot{V}o_2$max of 55 ml kg^{-1} min^{-1}. The adjustments that permit this increase would, from Honig and colleagues' findings, be expected to occur at the capillary-muscle cell interface where the greatest resitance to oxygen transfer exists. The simplest proposal is that the proliferation of muscle capillaries during the adaptation to conditioning would not only reduce diffusion distances, but would also increase total capillary blood volume. This increase in capillary blood volume after conditioning would increase mean transit time of red blood cells through the capillaries and permit more time for transfer of oxygen to the cell, despite the higher blood flow.

This analysis leaves unaddressed some very large assumptions about the control of muscle blood flow and the factors that determine the $\dot{V}o_2/\dot{Q}$ relationship in inhomogeneously perfused muscle. Another point to hold in mind is that there are *active, reflex* changes in muscle blood flow during severe exercise which can superimpose their own separate effects on muscle perfusion and oxygen transfer.

LIMITATIONS IN SKELETAL MUSCLE METABOLISM

The remaining variable in the Fick expression to consider as a possible limitation to $\dot{V}o_2$max is "$\dot{V}o_2$" itself; that is, oxygen uptake could be limited by the oxidative capacity of skeletal muscle.

Experimental Constraints

It has not been difficult to demonstrate experimentally that oxygen uptake of active muscle can be limited by the oxidative capacity of its mitochondrial enzymes. For example, some have studied the factors that limit a so-called "$\dot{V}o_2$max" of an electrically stimulated animal limb to which the investigator can control blood flow externally. There are two points. *First:* $\dot{V}o_2$max for a muscle or a limb cannot be objectively defined; there are no functional criteria of a maximum. The accepted definition of $\dot{V}o_2$max includes maximal cardiac output and maximal arteriovenous oxygen difference. *Second:* once the investigator separates from the active muscle any constraints normally imposed by the limited pumping capacity of the heart and the sympathetic nervous system, then the limitations are those set by the investigator rather than by the animal. The outgrowth of this has been that physiologists and biochemists sometimes have difficulty communicating their ideas about the potential limitations to muscle metabolism. The physiologist often thinks of large active muscles whose oxidative metabolism during severe exercise can easily be limited by an oxygen supply system which has a relatively low capacity pump. In contrast, the biochemist may base arguments on results from either an isolated muscle or a small mass of active muscle both of which may have a virtually unlimited supply of oxygen. The conclusions reached by the two investigators are in opposition, but each is correct because the models are different. The key to any dispute of this topic is to consider first when the oxygen transport system could be limiting and when it could not be. The peak oxygen uptake of an active finger or a single forearm muscle in humans is clearly not limited by the oxygen delivery system.

Arguments Against a Metabolic Limitation to $\dot{V}o_2$max

The main arguments against a limitation in $\dot{V}o_2$max imposed by restrictions in the oxidative capacity of the muscles have been mentioned in some of the preceding chapters and described elsewhere (Rowell, 1974, 1986; Saltin and Rowell, 1980; Saltin and Gollnick, 1983). In summary, the three main arguments against this idea are as follows. *First:* Were $\dot{V}o_2$max limited by the metabolic capacity of skeletal muscle to consume oxygen, then at any level of oxygen uptake, including $\dot{V}o_2$max, the addition of more active muscle should raise oxygen uptake in proportion to the total power output. For example, during submaximal leg exercise, the addition of arm exercise raises total oxygen uptake in proportion to the increase in total power output. At or near $\dot{V}o_2$max, addition of arm exercise will not raise oxygen uptake further. *Second:* An increase in arterial oxygen content raises $\dot{V}o_2$max. If $\dot{V}o_2$max had been limited by the oxidative capacity of the active muscle, oxygen uptake would not have risen further. In these experiments, arterial oxygen content was raised either by increasing hemoglobin concentration (see Kanstrup and Ekblom, 1984) or by increasing the partial pressure of oxygen in inspired air (Fagraeus, 1974). Keep in mind that in the latter approach, part of the rise in oxygen uptake could be simply due to improved pulmonary diffusion of oxygen owing to the higher alveolar Po_2. This would not be a factor when arterial oxygen content was raised by increasing hemoglobin concentration. *Third:* One can examine the highest rates of metabolism by some individual muscles and calculate the total oxygen uptake if one-half or if all of the body's muscles were similarly active. This, of course, assumes a similarity in the metabolic capacity of different muscles. For the human quadriceps, Andersen and Saltin (1985) estimated the peak oxygen uptake to be 350 ml kg^{-1} min^{-1}. This would extrapolate to the unobtainable oxygen uptake (in their subjects) of 5,250 ml min^{-1} if 15 kg of muscle (50 percent of total) were heavily active.

For the sake of perspective, clear examples can be offered to show that the oxidative capacity of human skeletal muscle can become low enough to reduce $\dot{V}o_2$max. For example, patients with muscle glycogen phosphorylase deficiency (McArdle's disease) (Lewis and Haller, 1986) or those having phosphofructokinase deficiency (Lewis et al., 1991), have severe substrate limitations in oxidative metabolism, and they are characterized by their low work capacity and low $\dot{V}o_2$max. Both deficiencies prevent the utilization of muscle glycogen, which is the dominant fuel for exercise at levels requiring more than 50 percent of $\dot{V}o_2$max. Patients with defective long-chain fatty acid oxidation associated with deficiencies of the enzymes carnitine palmitoyl transferase and acyl-CoA dehydrogenase (Lewis and Haller, 1989), and others with electron transport defects such as muscle cytochrome c-oxidase deficiency (Haller et al., 1989), all have low values for both $\dot{V}o_2$max and work capacity. As we will see later, endurance or work capacity is affected much more by changes in muscle oxidative enzyme activity than is $\dot{V}o_2$max (e.g., Saltin and Rowell, 1980).

An Argument Favoring Muscle Oxidative Capacity as One Determinant of $\dot{V}o_2$max: Symmorphosis

Most of the ideas presented so far on metabolic limitations to $\dot{V}o_2$max are counter to those of Weibel, Taylor, and their colleagues (Weibel, 1984; Taylor et al., 1987). Their thinking is based on experiments carried out on animals differing widely in body mass, and they also compared species with similar body mass and great differences in $\dot{V}o_2$max. Although the topic of skeletal muscle metabolism is somewhat beyond the scope of this book, the following provides a brief summary of some findings that were stimulated by the hypothesis called *symmorphosis*. The purpose here is to present another point of view.

According to Weibel (1984), all parts of the respiratory system (including the muscle mitochondria) "should be adjusted to the needs of maintaining the oxygen flow required for oxidative phosphorylation, and they should all be adjusted to each other." For example, at $\dot{V}o_2max$, oxygen is consumed per kilogram of body weight by the mitochondria of a 30-g mouse at a rate four times greater than in a 300-kg cow. This is called "allometric variation," which is attributable to differences in body mass. On the other hand, at $\dot{V}o_2max$ far more oxygen is consumed per kilogram of body weight in a physically active, 28-kg dog than in a 30-kg sedentary goat. This they called "adaptive variation" (Weibel and Kayar, 1988). Their underlying question was whether these "allometric variations" or "adaptive variations" in oxygen uptake are related to more mitochondria per unit of muscle mass, or to higher rates of oxidative phosphorylation within a given volume of mitochondria, or both. Hoppeler and colleagues (1987) calculated that "the total volume of muscle mitochondria increases with body size with approximately the same scaling factor as $\dot{V}o_2max$." That is, $\dot{V}o_2max$ is also set by the total mitochondrial volume or actually total mitochondrial oxidative capacity when muscles of 30-g mice and 300-kg cows are compared (allometric variation). It was assumed that the quantity of oxidative enzymes within the individual mitochondria were essentially the same so that total mitochondrial volume provides an estimate of the total amount of oxidative enzymes (Taylor et al., 1988).

When dogs and goats or ponies and calves were compared, adaptation to chronic physical activity made $\dot{V}o_2max$ two to three times greater per kilogram of body weight in dogs than in goats (body weight 28 versus 30 kg) and two to three times greater in ponies than in calves (body weight 170 versus 140 kg). It was concluded that the higher $\dot{V}o_2max$ per kilogram of the dog and pony was due "entirely" to their greater mitochondrial volume; $\dot{V}o_2max$ per unit volume of mitochondria was constant; oxidative capacity of the mitochondria was invariant (Weibel and Kayar, 1988). In their view, therefore, in order to increase $\dot{V}o_2max$ by physical conditioning, it is necessary to grow more mitochondria; the adaptation is structural. An additional part of the structural adaptation was seen in the increased capillary density which permitted approximately one-half of the higher $\dot{V}o_2max$ through widening of arteriovenous oxygen difference (reduced diffusion limitation). The other half of the increased $\dot{V}o_2max$ was permitted by the oxygen transport system through increased hemoglobin concentration (this is a unique observation in that hemoglobin concentration and arterial oxygen content often decrease with physical conditioning [Rowell, 1974]).

The data relating mitochondrial volume and mitochondrial $\dot{V}o_2$ per unit body mass were linear and appeared somewhat invariant on a log-log scale. With such scaling, the small acute effects on $\dot{V}o_2max$ of increasing maximal cardiac output by pericardectomy (Figure 9-13) would be invisible as would the 28 percent increase in $\dot{V}o_2max$ that attended physical conditioning with no change in muscle oxygen extraction or oxidative enzyme capacity (Parsons et al., 1985). But the latter are deterministic experiments which show that $\dot{V}o_2max$ can increase without an increase in muscle mitochondrial volume or oxidative capacity. According to the hypothesis of symmorphosis, no rise in $\dot{V}O_2$max would have been observed in the foxhounds. This chapter is about these relatively small magnitudes of normal physiological adjustment in $\dot{V}O_2$max that are commonly seen with acute (months) adaptation to physical conditioning. This does not mean that a 200 to 300 percent increase in $\dot{V}O_2$max (visible in logarithmic plots) would not require the mitochondrial adaptation described by Weibel and Kayar (1988)—nor is it the point.

Thus it is the conclusion of Weibel, Taylor, and their colleagues that cardiovascular and metabolic function are so well matched that $\dot{V}O_2$max cannot increase without increased function in the two systems. The opposite conclusion has been reached by those who have studied oxidative enzyme activities in human muscle.

Estimates of Muscle Oxidative Capacity in Human Muscle

It is granted that comparison of the different studies on different species using different approaches is a problem. Also, quantification of mitochondrial oxidative capacity and muscle enzyme capacity is difficult. In vitro enzyme assays can show relative changes in enzyme activities, that is, relative to those of other enzymes. The assays rarely reflect the actual activity in situ (Saltin and Gollnick, 1983). Estimation of maximal oxidative capacity of mixed human muscle based on activities of citrate synthase and succinate dehydrogenase yield values that exceed peak metabolic rates measured in intact human quadriceps by threefold (see Andersen and Saltin, 1985). Conversely, values for peak oxygen consumption of muscle based on the respiration of isolated mitochondria appear insufficient to account for observed muscle oxygen uptakes, meaning that isolation of the mitochondria reduces their oxidative function. The latter problem may contribute importantly to the discrepancies between the findings of Weibel and his colleagues and Saltin and Gollnick.

Would the Matching of Structure and Function Represent Optimal "Design"?

A final comment about symmorphosis is stimulated by the remark of Taylor and colleagues (1988) that the putative match between structure and function (i.e., of all parts of the respiratory system) is a "common sense prediction of economic design". This is debatable if we focus on the claim that $\dot{V}O_2$max is a function of the total number of mitochondria in all of the muscles. In this case, the fraction of $\dot{V}O_2$max that an individual muscle could consume would depend on what fraction of the total mitochondria is contained in that muscle. For example, it is possible to reach 70 percent of $\dot{V}O_2$max by severe cycle ergometer exercise of one leg. Clearly this does not mean that the remaining muscles must contain only 30 percent of the total mitochondria. In effect, Taylor's proposal is that the maximal metabolic rate of each muscle represents a fixed percentage of the total metabolic rate because the oxidative capacity of its mitochondria is a fixed percentage of the total oxidative capacity. This would mean that the highest power output at which we could saw a board or cut meat with the muscles of one arm is limited to a power output that is a fixed percentage of the total power output; in short, the same maximal power output that could also exist when all other muscles were maximally active. Strong evidence against this idea abounds and is most obviously seen in those cases in which the peak oxygen consumption of small muscles is far greater when they are active by themselves than when they are similarly active along with other large muscles (e.g., Clausen, 1977; Klausen et al., 1982; Andersen and Saltin, 1985). That is, *our muscles are supplied with enough mitochondria to permit them to consume oxygen at rates far out of proportion to their fraction of total muscle mass.* Therefore, the idea that $\dot{V}o_2$max is a function of the metabolic capacity of the skeletal muscle system fits neither a large body of scientific data nor with the experiences of everyday life.

A primary reason for rejecting the concept of symmorphosis in this chapter is the clear evidence that both functional and structural *limitations* exist in some parts of the systems for oxygen delivery and metabolism, whereas in other parts of these systems there may be excesses. Thus, in a scheme that predicts no single limitation or excess, both exist and are more obvious in some species than in others. The objections of Garland and Huey (1987) to the hypothesis of symmorphosis, both on functional grounds and on analytical grounds, are particularly cogent.

Oxidative Capacity of Skeletal Muscle as a Determinant of Work Capacity or Endurance

Although the oxidative capacity of muscle mitochondria, or their mass, appears to be unrelated to human $\dot{V}o_2$max, it is clearly related to the work capacity or endurance of the individual.

First, the distinction between $\dot{V}o_2$max, a measure of functional capacity, and work capacity, a measure of performance capacity, should be reemphasized (cf. Chapter 5). The concept that $\dot{V}o_2$max is a measure of functional capacity has been discussed. In contrast, performance criteria describe the ability to perform work or develop power at specific rates and durations—often called endurance. Over a rather broad range, $\dot{V}o_2$max can be unrelated to work capacity. For example, $\dot{V}o_2$max can be unaffected by a number of stresses that impair work capacity as well as by some that improve work capacity (Rowell, 1974, 1986). The important point is that the metabolic adjustments in skeletal muscle determine the great improvements (e.g., 300 percent) in work capacity seen with physical conditioning, whereas cardiovascular changes dictate the much smaller increments (15 to 30 percent) in $\dot{V}o_2$max.

Within the magnitudes of acute (over weeks and months) adjustment of $\dot{V}o_2$max to physical conditioning we are accustomed to seeing in mammals, it is clear that mitochondrial density need not increase in order to raise $\dot{V}O_2$max by 15 to 30 percent. Nevertheless, despite this common conclusion many, including those who made it, observed that physical conditioning can markedly increase the quantity of mitochondrial enzymes in human muscle (Gollnick and Saltin, 1982; Saltin and Gollnick, 1983). Gollnick and Saltin (1982) were apparently the first to perceive the significance of this adjustment. In accordance with Michaelis-Menton kinetics, the increased enzyme activity increases the enzyme reaction velocity. For example, a doubling of enzyme concentration will double the velocity of the reaction at any substrate concentration. Thus, with high enzyme levels it is possible to attain high rates of substrate fluxes at low substrate concentrations so that metabolic control is improved. This increase in the content of oxidative enzymes and the enhanced metabolic potential of conditioned muscle is what permits the dramatic increases in work capacity (Gollnick and Saltin, 1982; Gollnick et al., 1985). The enzyme changes have two effects:

1. A greater fraction of the pyruvate formed during glucose metabolism can be oxidized in the mitochondria (lactate production is markedly reduced in conditioned humans during submaximal exercise).
2. A greater fraction of the active acetate needed for the oxidative reactions of the tricarboxilic acid cycle can be provided by β-oxidation of free-fatty acids.

These effects lead to a sparing of muscle glycogen (muscle glycogen content increases only slightly with physical conditioning) during prolonged exercise and enhanced ability of the conditioned muscles to oxidize greater quantities of free-fatty acids (Dudley et al., 1987). The lipids represent the major fraction of the body energy stores whereas glycogen stores are relatively small. Also, because these biochemical adaptations occur in slow-twitch and to a greater extent in fast-twitch fibers, the oxidative potential is more uniformly distributed between the two fiber types after physical conditioning. Therefore, these fast-fatiguing fiber types acquire greater metabolic reserve (for review see Gollnick, et al., 1985).

SUMMARY

In summary, the close coupling between $\dot{V}O_2$max and the oxidative capacity of skeletal muscle mitochondria predicted by the hypothesis called symmorphosis is not observed in humans and dogs. In these mammals the capacity of skeletal muscle to consume oxygen exceeds the capacity of the cardiovascular and respiratory systems to transport oxygen to the muscle. Increases in muscle oxidative enzyme activities associated with physical conditioning increase speed and efficiency of metabolic reactions in the muscle and permit large increases in endurance or work capacity. These factors do not improve $\dot{V}O_2$max because they did not limit $\dot{V}O_2$max in the first place. In contrast, both $\dot{V}o_2$max and work capacity can be severely limited by muscle metabolism when substrate oxidation is impaired in patients with inborn errors of metabolism.

The hypothesis of symmorphosis brings two quotations to mind: "It is more important that a proposition be interesting than it be true" (Alfred North Whitehead, 1861–1847). "No one believes an hypothesis except its originator, but everyone believes an experiment except the experimenter" (W.I. Beveridge, 1908). An interesting and well-presented hypothesis like symmorphosis has intrinsic value; it leads to thoughtful discussion and debate. A conclusion that a hypothesis is not valid should not negate its potential value.

REFERENCES

Andersen, P., and B. Saltin (1985). Maximal perfusion of skeletal muscle in man. *J. Physiol. (Lond.) 366,* 233–249.

Asmussen, E. (1965). Muscular Exercise. In W.O. Fenn and H. Rahn, eds. *Handbook of Physiology: Respiration,* sect. 3, vol. II, pp. 939–978. American Physiological Society, Washington, D.C.

Bayly, W.M., D.R. Hodgson, D.A. Schulz, J.A. Dempsey, and P.D. Gollnick (1989). Exercise-induced hypercapnia in the horse. *J. Appl. Physiol. 67,* 1958–1966.

Clausen, J.P. (1977). Effect of physical training on cardiovascular adjustments to exercise in man. *Physiol. Rev. 57,* 779–815.

Dejours, P. (1965). Control of respiration in muscular exercise. In W.O. Fenn and H. Rahn, eds. *Handbook of Physiology: Respiration,* sect. 3, vol. I, pp. 631–648. American Physiological Society, Washington, D.C.

Dempsey, J.A. (1986). Is the lung built for exercise? *Med. Sci. Sports Exerc. 18,* 143–155.

Dempsey, J.A. (1988). Problems with the hyperventilatory response to exercise and hypoxia. *Adv. Exp. Med. Biol. 227,* 277–291. (*Oxygen Transfer From Atmosphere to Tissues* [N.C. Gonzalez and M.R. Fedde, eds.]). Plenum Press, New York.

Dempsey, J.A., and R.F. Fregosi (1985). Adaptability of the pulmonary system to changing metabolic requirements. *Am. J. Cardiol. 55,* 59D–67D.

Dempsey, J.A., P. Hanson, and K. Henderson. (1984). Exercise induced arterial hypoxemia in healthy humans at sea level. *J. Physiol. (Lond.) 355,* 161–175.

Dudley, G.A., P.C. Tullson, and R.L. Terjung (1987). Influence of mitochondrial content on the sensitivity of respiratory control. *J. Biol. Chem. 262,* 9109–9114.

Fagraeus, L. (1974). Cardiorespiratory and metabolic functions during exercise in the hyperbaric environment. *Acta Physiol. Scand. (Suppl. 414),* 1–40.

Forster, H.V., and L.G. Pan (1988). Breathing during exercise: demands, regulation, limitations. *Adv. Exp. Med. Biol. 227,* 257–276 (*Oxygen Transfer From Atmosphere to Tissues* [N.C. Gonzalez and M.R. Fedde, eds.]). Plenum Press, New York.

Garland, T. Jr., and R.B. Huey (1987). Testing symmorphosis: does structure match functional requirements? *Evolution 41,* 1404–1409.

Gledhill, N., A.B. Forese, and J.A. Dempsey (1977). Ventilation to perfusion distribution during exercise in health. In J.A. Dempsey and C.E. Reed., eds. *Muscular Exercise and the Lung,* pp. 325–342. University of Wisconsin Press, Madison.

Gollnick, P.D., M. Riedy, J.J. Quintinskie, and L.A. Bertocci (1985). Differences in metabolic potential of skeletal muscle fibres and its significance for metabolic control. *J. Exp. Bio. 115,* 191–199.

Gollnick, P.D., and B. Saltin (1982). Significance of skeletal muscle oxidative enzyme enhancement with endurance training. *Clin. Physiol. 1,* 1–12.

Grimby, G., B. Saltin, and L.W. Helmsen (1971). Pulmonary flow-volume and pressure-volume relationships during submaximal and maximal exercise in young well-trained men. *Bull. Physiol. Pathol. Respir. 7,* 157–168.

Haller, R.G., S.F. Lewis, R.W. Estabrook, S. DiMauro, S. Servidei, and D.W. Foster (1989). Exercise intolerance, lactic acidosis, and abnormal cardiopulmonary regulation in exercise associated with adult skeletal muscle cytochrome c oxidase deficiency. *J. Clin. Invest. 84,* 155–161.

Hammond, M.D. (1988). Limitations to the efficiency of pulmonary gas exchange during exercise in man. *Adv. Exp. Med. Biol. 227,* 67–74 (*Oxygen Transfer From Atmosphere to Tissues* [N.C. Gonzalez and M.R. Fedde, eds.]). Plenum Press, New York.

Hogan, M.C., J. Roca, J.B. West, and P.D. Wagner (1989). Dissociation of maximal O_2 uptake from O_2 delivery in canine gastrocnemius in situ. *J. Appl. Physiol. 66,* 1219–1226.

Holmgren, A., and H. Linderholm (1958). Oxygen and carbon dioxide tensions of arterial blood during heavy and exhaustive exercise. *Acta Physiol. Scand. 44,* 203–215.

Honig, C.R., T.E.J. Gayeski, W. Federspiel, A. Clark, Jr., and P. Clark (1984). Muscle O_2 gradients from hemoglobin to cytochrome: new concepts, new complexities. *Adv. Exp. Med. Biol. 169,* 23–38.

Hoppeler, H., S.R. Kayar, H. Claassen, E. Uhlmann, and R.H. Karas (1987). Adaptive variation in the mammalian respiratory system in relation to energetic demand. III. Skeletal muscles: setting the demand for oxygen. *Resp. Physiol. 69,* 27–46.

Hussain, S.N.A., R.L. Pardy, and J.A. Dempsey (1985). Mechanical impedance as determinant of inspiratory neural drive during exercise in humans. *J. Appl. Physiol. 59,* 365–375.

Johnson, B.D., K.W. Saupe, and J.A. Dempsey (1992). Mechanical constraints on exercise hyperpnea in endurance athletes. *J. Appl. Physiol. 73,* (August).

Kanstrup, I., and B. Ekblom (1984). Blood volume and hemoglobin concentration as determinants of maximal aerobic power. *Med. Sci. Sports Exerc. 16,* 256–262.

Klausen, K., N.H. Secher, J.P. Clausen, O. Hartling, and J. Trap-Jensen (1982). Central and regional circulatory adaptations to one-leg training. *J. Appl. Physiol. (Respirat. Environ. Exerc. Physiol.) 52,* 976–983.

Lewis, S.F., and R.G. Haller (1986). The pathophysiology of McArdle's disease: clues to regulation in exercise and fatigue. *J. Appl. Physiol. 61,* 391–401.

Lewis, S.F., and R.G. Haller (1989). Skeletal muscle disorders and associated factors that limit exercise performance. In *Exerc. Sport Sci. Rev. 17,* 67–113.

Lewis, S.F., S. Vora, and R.G. Haller (1991). Abnormal oxidative metbolism and

O$_2$ transport in muscle phosphofructokinase deficiency. *J. Appl. Physiol.* 70, 391–398.

Manohar, M. (1986). Blood flow to the respiratory and limb muscles and to abdominal organs during maximal exertion in ponies. *J. Physiol. (Lond.)* 377, 25–35.

Musch, T.I., G.C. Haidet, G.A. Ordway, J.C. Longhurst, and J.H. Mitchell (1985). Dynamic exercise training in foxhounds. I. Oxygen consumption and hemodynamic responses. *J. Appl. Physiol.* 59, 183–189.

Pan, L.G., H.V. Forster, G.E. Bisgard, T.F. Lowry, and C.L. Murphy (1987). Role of carotid chemoreceptors and pulmonary vagal afferents during helium : O$_2$ breathing in ponies. *J. Appl. Physiol.* 62, 1020–1027.

Parsons, D., T.I. Musch, R.L. Moore, G.C. Haidet, and G.A. Ordway (1985). Dynamic exercise training in foxhounds. II. Analysis of skeletal muscle. *J. Appl. Physiol.* 59, 190–197.

Piiper, J. (1988). Pulmonary diffusing capacity and alveolar-capillary equilibration. *Adv. Exp. Med. Biol.* 227, 19–32 (*Oxygen Transfer From Atmosphere to Tissues* [N.C. Gonzalez and M.R. Fedde, eds.]). Plenum Press, New York.

Piiper, J., and P. Haab (1991). Oxygen supply and uptake in tissue models with unequal distribution of blood flow and shunt. *Respir. Physiol.* 84, 261–271.

Pirnay, F., M. Lamy, J. Dujardin, R. Deroanne, and J.M. Petit (1972). Analysis of femoral venous blood during maximum muscular exercise. *J. Appl. Physiol.* 33, 289–292.

Powers, S.K., J. Lawler, J.A. Dempsey, S. Dodd, and G. Landry (1989). Effects of incomplete pulmonary gas exchange on Vo$_2$max. *J. Appl. Physiol.* 66, 2491–2495.

Roca, J., M.C. Hogan, D. Story, D.E. Bebout, P. Haab, R. Gonzales, O. Ueno, and P.D. Wagner (1989). Evidence for tissue diffusion limitation of Vo$_2$max in normal humans. *J. Appl. Physiol.* 67, 291–299.

Rowell, L.B. (1974). Human cardiovascular adjustments to exercise and thermal stress. *Physiol. Rev.* 54, 75–159.

Rowell, L.B. (1986). *Human Circulation. Regulation During Physical Stress.* Oxford University Press, New York.

Rowell, L.B., B. Saltin, B. Kiens, and N.J. Christensen (1986). Is peak quadriceps blood flow in humans even higher during exercise with hypoxemia? *Am. J. Physiol.* 251 (Heart Circ. Physiol. 20), H1038–H1044.

Rowell, L.B., H.L. Taylor, Y. Wang, and W.S. Carlson (1964). Saturation of arterial blood with oxygen during maximal exercise. *J. Appl. Physiol.* 19, 284–286.

Saltin, B., G. Blomqvist, J.H. Mitchell, R.L. Johnson, Jr., K. Wildenthal, and C.B. Chapman (1968). Response to exercise after bed rest and after training. *Circulation 38 (Suppl. 7)*, 1–78.

Saltin, B., and P.D. Gollnick (1983). Skeletal muscle adaptibility: significance for metabolism and performance. In L.D. Peachey, R.H. Adrian, and S.R. Geiger, eds. *Handbook of Physiology: Skeletal Muscle*, sect. 10, pp. 555–631. American Physiological Society, Bethesda, MD.

Saltin, B., and L.B. Rowell (1980). Functional adaptations to physical activity and inactivity. *Fed. Proc.* 39, 1506–1513.

Shappell, S.D., J.A. Murray, A.J. Bellingham, R.C. Woodson, J.C. Detter, and C. Lenfant (1971). Adaptation to exercise: role of hemoglobin affinity for oxygen and 2,3-diphosphoglycerate. *J. Appl. Physiol.* 30, 827–832.

Sparks, H.V., and D.E. Mohrman (1977). Heterogeneity of flow as an explanation of the multi-exponential washout of inert gas from skeletal muscle. *Micro-vasc. Res. 13,* 181–184.

Stray-Gunderson, J., T.I., Musch, G.C. Haidet, D.P., Swain, G.A. Ordway, and J.H. Mitchell (1986). The effect of pericardiectomy on maximal oxygen consumption and maximal cardiac output in untrained dogs. *Circ. Res. 58,* 523–530.

Taylor, C.R., R.H., Karas, E.R. Weibel, and H. Hoppeler (1987). Adaptive variation in the mammalian respiratory system in relation to energetic demand. *Resp. Physiol. 69,* 1–127.

Taylor, C.R., K.E. Longworth, and H. Hoppeler (1988). Matching O_2 delivery to O_2 demand in muscle. II. Allometric variation in energy demand. *Adv. Exp. Med. Biol. 227,* 171–181 (*Oxygen Transfer From Atmosphere to Tissues* [N.C. Gonzalez and M.R. Fedde, eds.]). Plenum Press, New York.

Wagner, P.D. (1988). An integrated view of the determinants of maximum oxygen uptake. *Adv. Exp. Med. Biol. 227,* 245–256 (*Oxygen Transfer From Atmosphere to Tissues* [N.C. Gonzalez and M.R. Fedde, eds.]). Plenum Press, New York.

Wagner, P.D., G.E. Gale, R.E. Moon, J.R. Torre-Bueno, B.W. Stolp, and H.A. Saltzman (1986). Pulmonary gas exchange in humans exercising at sea level and simulated altitude. *J. Appl. Physiol. 61,* 260–270.

Wagner, P.D., J.R. Gillespie, G.L. Landgren, M.R. Fedde, B.W. Jones, R.M. DeBowes, R.L. Pieschel, and H.H. Erickson (1989). Mechanism of exercise-induced hypoxemia in horses. *J. Appl. Physiol. 66,* 1227–1233.

Weibel, E.R. (1984). *The Pathway for Oxygen. Structure and Function in the Mammalian Respiratory System.* Harvard University Press, Cambridge, MA.

Weibel, E., and S.R. Kayar (1988). Matching O_2 delivery to O_2 demand in muscle. I. Adaptive variation. *Adv. Exp. Med. Biol. 227,* 159–169 (*Oxygen Transfer From Atmosphere to Tissues* [N.C. Gonzalez and M.R. Fedde, eds.]). Plenum Press, New York.

Weibel, E.F., and C.R. Taylor (1981). Design of the mammalian respiratory system. *Respir. Physiol. 44,* 1–164.

West, J.B. (1974). *Respiratory Physiololgy: The Essentials.* William & Wilkins, Baltimore, MD.

Whipp, B.J., and R.L. Pardy (1986). Breathing during exercise. In P.T Macklem and J. Mead, eds. *Handbook of Physiology. The Respiratory System: Mechanics of Breathing,* vol. III, sect. 3, Part 1, pp. 605–629. American Physiological Society, Bethesda, MD.

10

What Signals Govern the Cardiovascular Responses to Exercise? Role of Central Command

The nature of the signals that initiate and maintain the close matching between blood flow and metabolism during exercise is still not well understood. The question of how the cardiovascular system is "informed" about the oxygen requirements of active muscle has challenged physiologists for nearly 100 years. The final three chapters of this book are about this question. They put forward three main ideas about the origin of the signals that activate the autonomic nervous system and control the cardiovascular system during exercise.

Chapter 10 is about the hypothesis called "central command." Zuntz and Geppert (1886) and Johansson (1895) were apparently the first to suggest that motor outflow from the cerebral cortex during exercise could somehow interact with the central neuron pools that regulate the cardiovascular responses to exercise. "Central command" refers specifically to this motor outflow, often called centrally generated motor command signals.

Chapter 11 deals with another hypothesis that also originated with Zuntz and Geppert (1886), which is currently called the *muscle chemoreflex* hypothesis. Their suggestion was that a reflex might originate directly from chemosensitive afferent nerve fibers in the active muscle, the suspected stimulus being an accumulation of its metabolites within the interstitial fluid. One underlying idea is that "the signal" originates from a mismatch between blood flow and muscle metabolism that is corrected by the autonomic nervous system via its augmentation of muscle blood flow. A second idea is that reflexes might also originate from mechanosensitive afferents in the active muscle. These afferents could feed back to the central nervous system information about magnitude, duration, and rates of tension development by muscle fibers. These mechanical events should be related to metabolic rate of the muscle.

Chapter 12 examines a third hypothesis, which is that the "exercise reflex" originates from a mismatch between cardiac output and vascular conductance—a "pressure error." This mismatch or "error signal" is corrected by the activation of the arterial baroreflex. The chapter also deals with the recognition that none of these three hypotheses, by itself, is likely to provide a full explanation for the cardiovascular responses to exercise. Therefore, the major objective of Chapter 12 is to provide a synthesis of the most important findings from the preceding chapters and to put together a hypothetical scheme that might explain which signals govern the cardiovascular system during exercise. Although the scheme is a hypothesis, it is a testable one.

WHAT IS CENTRAL COMMAND?

This question can only be partly answered because "central command" is still a poorly understood part of a hypothetical scheme for cardiovascular control. Nevertheless, the attention this idea has received is warranted because the experimental support for it, albeit indirect, is quite strong.

The question has many answers and they vary in specificity and detail. To make things simpler, this question is dealt with in the stages that have grown from the increasing sophistication of the ideas and experimental approaches directed to the understanding of central command. Some of the original ideas are presented first. These were derived mainly from observations on humans that were consistent with the original central command hypothesis stated above, but they did not prove it. Also most of the investigations of central command have used isometric contractions because of the greater ease in making measurements, in quantifying muscle contraction force, and in acquiring some index of perceived effort. As a consequence, it is common to think of the central command signal as one that raises arterial pressure during an isometric contraction. Fewer studies have been made using dynamic exercise during which blood pressure may not rise significantly at first; in that setting heart rate has been used instead as an indicator of central command.

Some Original Ideas

The idea of a central command signal originated from the observations of Johansson (1895) and Krogh and Lindhard (1913, 1917) that heart rate and ventilation increase almost immediately at the onset of voluntary exercise. Johansson (1895) observed that the immediate increase in heart rate could not be induced in rabbits either by passive movements of the limb muscles or by electrically stimulating them. He therefore concluded that the responses must originate centrally, arguing that chemical feedback from the periphery would be much less rapid. Later Krogh and Lindhard (1917) compared responses to voluntary and electrically induced exercise and found a slower onset of tachycardia in response to the latter. Thus they also concluded that responses to voluntary exercise were central in origin, whereas responses to electrically induced exercise were presumed to be peripheral in origin. In short, it was the *speed* of the cardiovascular and respiratory responses to exercise that prompted the notion that a centrally generated neural command signal might initiate them.

When Zuntz and Geppert (1886) and Johansson (1895) suggested that the motor outflow from the cerebral cortex during exercise might somehow interact with the central neuron pools that regulate the cardiovascular system, their underlying idea was that central command would simultaneously activate both somatomotor systems and the autonomic nervous system. This central process was seen by Krogh and Lindhard as being an "irradiation" of descending motor impulses onto cardiovascular control centers. The word "irradiation" has had important connotations because it has suggested a diffuse outflow of motor traffic to these centers, rather than the existence of discrete neural pathways to somatomotor and cardiovascular motor centers.

Many questioned this rather vague hypothesis because central command was not defined explicitly in terms of measured variables and because it was presumed that no signals are fed back to the "centers" that regulate the cardiovascular system (i.e., according to the original hypothesis). In engineering terms, regulation is by a "feed-forward" controller rather than the more familiar feedback controller. A feed-forward controller generates "commands" without using continuous negative feedback so that its moment-by-moment operations are, in effect, "open-loop" (i.e., without feedback) (Houk, 1988). Therefore the question became how such fine regulation of the cardiovascular (or respiratory) system could be achieved with presumably no information fed back to the central nervous system about how poorly or how well blood flow, for example, had met the needs for oxygen delivery. In essence, this control scheme was viewed as one lacking any error signal (despite this objection, feed-forward control systems do exist and can function effectively with and without conventional feedback control; for a concise treatment of these concepts, see Houk [1988]).

Indirect Evidence from Human Studies

Experiments Employing Motor Paralysis and Partial Neuromuscular Blockade

If centrally generated motor command signals simultaneously activate cardiovascular and somatomotor systems in humans, then an unsuccessful attempt to contract paralyzed muscles should nevertheless be accompanied by a cardiovascular response. This suggests that a pure central command influence can exist without any feedback from active skeletal muscle. That is, inasmuch as the muscles do not contract there is no chemical, metabolic, or mechanical feedback. For example, Freyschuss (1970) blocked forearm muscle contraction peripherally by brachial arterial injection of succinylcholine, a depolarizing neuromuscular blocking agent. When her subjects were fully blocked, their unsuccessful attempts to make voluntary isometric forearm muscle contractions were still accompanied by approximately one-half of the normal increase in arterial pressure and heart rate. That is, these responses were approximately one-half of those observed in these same subjects during voluntary isometric contractions before neuromuscular blockade. Central command is thought to cause the rise in arterial pressure.

If profound muscular weakness is caused by partial neuromuscular blockade, a much greater centrally generated motor command signal will be required in order to maintain a given force of muscle contraction; this should cause an exaggerated cardiovascular response. That is, the greater the motor weakness, the greater the central command signal. Asmussen and colleagues (1965) observed that partial neuromuscular blockade by tubocurarine caused heart rate and arterial pressure to increase as the degree of perceived effort increased during dynamic exercise at a constant rate of work. This result is characteristic of a number of experiments which followed, with some important refinements (Hobbs, 1982; Leonard et al., 1985; Victor et al., 1989). For example, with a partial neuromuscular blockade, which reduced maximal voluntary contraction force (MVC) by 50 percent, arterial pressure rose much more during contractions at a given absolute force (Hobbs, 1982; Leonard et al., 1985). However, increments in arterial pressure were similar when comparisons were made at the same *relative* force or same percent of MVC (Leonard et al., 1985), but heart rate responses have been much more variable (cf., Leonard et al., 1985; Victor et al., 1989). The reason for this variation is not known (see "How Does Central Command Exert Its Effects on the Cardiovascular System" later in this chapter.)

Experiments That Eliminated Feedback from Contracting Muscle

Cardiovascular responses to muscle contraction can still be elicited by central command when sensory feedback from the active muscles is absent.

Patients who have by disease lost neural feedback from muscles provide a critical test of the hypothesis that cardiovascular responses to dynamic exercise and isometric contractions can be elicited without muscle reflexes (Chapter 11). The presumption is that the responses are governed by central command. There are published reports from four patients with sensory neuropathies who had lost sensation but retained some motor function in at least one limb (Alam and Smirk, 1938; Lind et al., 1968; Duncan et al., 1981). With the puzzling exception of one patient with syringomyelia (Lind et al., 1968) (whose cardiovascular responses were highly variable; R.A. Bruce, personal communication), arterial pressure rose in all subjects during isometric contractions and in one subject (also apparently with unilateral syringomyelia) during dynamic exercise with the circulation to the leg arrested (Figure 10-1) (Alam and Smirk, 1938). In all patients the rise in heart rate in response to muscle contractions was normal.

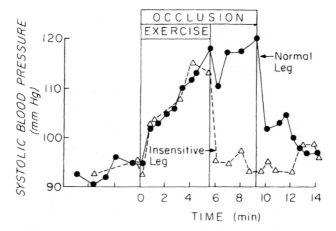

Figure 10-1   Pressor responses to muscle ischemia in response to circulatory occlusion during and after dynamic exercise with either a normal leg (*solid line*) or an insensitive leg (*dashed line*). Sensory loss, caused by a spinal cord lesion (probably syringomyelia), eliminated the pressor response after exercise but not during. (Adapted from Alam and Smirk, 1938; reproduced from Rowell, 1986, with permission from Oxford University Press.)

A way to experimentally maintain muscle contractions without sensory feedback from the muscle in normal humans has been to create temporary sensory loss by differential blockade of the small muscle afferents, leaving as many of the large motor fibers intact as possible (Freund et al., 1979). This approach has proven to be very difficult owing to the overlapping effects of the local anesthetic on the small sensory fibers and the large motor fibers (Freund et al., 1979). In order to achieve sufficient sensory blockade to eliminate the afferent feedback that arises from active muscle when it is rendered ischemic, overlapping blockade of the large motor fibers also occurs. Although the confounding effects of muscle reflexes on arterial pressure are eliminated by the blockade, this causes profound weakness and presumably exaggerates central command (Freund et al., 1979; Rowell and O'Leary, 1990). This in turn exaggerates the rise in both arterial pressure and heart rate. Nevertheless, the results add to those employing total motor paralysis and reveal that central command can raise heart rate and blood pressure without sensory feedback from the active muscles.

The above findings suggest that central command by itself can cause arterial pressure and heart rate to rise. The greater-than-normal rise in arterial pressure and heart rate during mild dynamic exercise in subjects with small sensory fiber blockade plus profound motor weakness probably paralleled augmented central command signals. Cardiovascular responses appeared to parallel the subjects' perception of effort and probably paralleled also the need to recruit more muscle motor units (see below) in order to carry out the task (Freund et al., 1979).

Experiments That Alter the Putative Command Signal but Not Muscle Force Generation

Central command can be experimentally manipulated so that responses to exercise parallel the changes in central command when the command signal or actually the perception of effort is increased or decreased at a given intensity of exercise. In an ingenious experiment Goodwin and colleagues (1972) took advantage of the fact that motor neurons can be facilitated or inhibited by exciting muscle spindles with high-frequency vibration. When they applied vibration directly to the contracting muscle, its motor neurons were facilitated so that perceived effort and motor command were reduced. When vibration was applied to the antagonist muscle, motor neurons of the agonist muscle were inhibited so that perceived effort and motor command were increased. In this way they varied the central motor command required to achieve a *constant force* of isometric contraction. Despite the maintenance of constant muscle contraction force, heart rate and arterial pressure were altered roughly in accordance with the subjects' perception of effort and with the predicted level of motor command. Heart rate and arterial pressure were reduced when the contracting muscle was vibrated and these variables were augmented when the antagonist muscle was vibrated.

Experiments That Bypass the Central Command Signal

Direct electrical stimulation of the muscle or its motor nerves causes contraction without any centrally generated motor command signals. The question is how do the cardiovascular responses compare in the same individual with those obtained during voluntary contraction at the same levels of force (note, an assumption is that electrical stimulation of the muscles will not activate muscle afferents that might initiate some central motor signal). Asmussen and colleagues (1943) measured heart rate, cardiac output, and ventilation in two subjects (one was Professor Asmussen) at multiple levels of oxygen uptake (up to 1,300 ml min^{-1}) during voluntary and during electrically induced dynamic exercise. The other subject had motor weakness and marked sensory loss from the legs owing to tabes dorsalis (it was not known exactly what sensory feedback from the legs was absent or diminished). Steady-state responses to the two forms of exercise were virtually identical in both subjects. Asmussen and colleagues (1943) concluded that "cortical impulses play no part in the regulation of circulation in the steady state of muscular work." Regulation was assigned to reflexes from working muscles despite the sensory deficit in the patient with tabes dorsalis. This experiment has always been difficult to interpret and it probably reveals the importance of multiple control systems during exercise. The results of Asmussen and colleagues (1943) suggest that normal cardiovascular (and respiratory) responses to dynamic exercise can occur without a central command signal. However, these experiments revealed nothing about possible effects of central command or its absence on the *time course* of the exercise response. Also keep in mind that any direct electrical activation of muscle afferents, along with reversal of normal muscle recruitment patterns, could affect responses.

Summary. In summary, the experiments reviewed above show five important results:

1. A "central command signal" by itself, that is, an attempt to exercise without any exercise, will cause a cardiovascular response.
2. When the effort required to make a muscle contraction is increased without a commensurate change in contraction force, the cardiovascular responses will increase.
3. When the central command signal is equated with perceived effort and the latter is experimentally increased or decreased during a given constant level of contraction force, cardiovascular responses and perceived effort change in the same direction.
4. When sensory feedback from active muscles (which can also raise heart rate and arterial pressure) is eliminated either by sensory neuropathies or by local anesthetic, normal increments in arterial pressure and heart rate can occur with exercise—presumably governed by central command.
5. Finally, when central command is eliminated or bypassed by direct rhythmic electrical stimulation of the muscles, a "normal" cardiovascular response may still be obtained during the steady state. This suggests that there is redundancy in the mechanisms of control.

Evidence from Studies on Nonhuman Species

Experiments on animals require a very different approach than those executed on humans because the degree of effort or the relative strength of a central command signal cannot be assessed in nonhuman species. For example, isometric contractions have proven useful in humans because a "maximal voluntary contraction" (MVC) can be established as full scale for the degree of effort, a putative index of the strength of the central command signal. Clearly experiments on animals require different approaches to manipulate and evaluate central command signals. For example, one approach has been to assess the strength of the command signal by recording motor nerve activity during "fictive locomotion" (contraction is blocked pharmacologically).

A Hypothetical Scheme

It is difficult to talk about the experimental generation of central command signals in animals without some kind of neuroanatomical map. For the purpose of this discussion a rather simple map of central organization of motor outflow is presented in Figure 10-2. This figure illustrates some possible patterns of neural organization for central cardiovascular command (Hobbs, 1982). *Pathway 1* is the traditional view (Krogh and Lindhard, 1913) in which motor signals act directly on brainstem centers and autonomic preganglionic cells that control the heart and blood vessels. *Pathway 2* activates the subthalamic regions that are discussed below (see Smith et al., 1960a; Eldridge et al., 1985) and also the cerebellum and fastigial nuclei, which may also play a role (Dormer and Stone, 1982; Dormer, 1984). This pathway indicates there is modulation of tonically active afferent pathways (e.g., baroreceptors) involved in cardiovascular control. *Pathway 3* expresses the idea mentioned earlier, that cardiovascular command may be independent of motor command but that the two may share a common origin. Hobbs (1982) suggested: "... as the motor

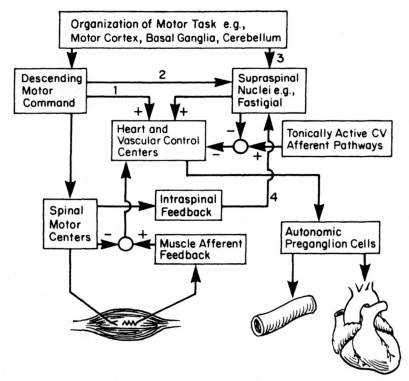

Figure 10-2 Schematic illustration by Hobbs (1982) of four probable pathways of parallel central motor command and central cardiovascular command signals. Pathway 1 is the traditional view (Krogh and Lindhard, 1913), whereas pathways 2, 3 and 4 represent more recent views about how central command may act on neurons that control the heart and blood vessels. One pathway introduces the notion that feedback from the spinal cord may be an important part of the central motor and cardiovascular command process. See text for details. (Adapted from Hobbs, 1982; reproduced from Rowell, 1986, with permission from Oxford University Press.)

cortex, thalamus, cerebellum, basal ganglia, and other integrative nuclei develop the integrated behavior response to an external cue, they may develop separate command signals for the motor and cardiovascular systems." The key to Hobbs' scheme in Figure 10-2 may be *Pathway 4,* which introduces a spinal loop that could be involved with either the generation or modulation, or both, of the command signal. It introduces the notion that feedback from the spinal cord may be an important part of central motor and cardiovascular command processes. In short, we begin with the proposition that central command is a feed-forward controller of the circulation, but will end with some newer ideas that there may be some modulation of central command by feedback from the muscle.

Electrically Induced Central Command: Animal Studies

Electrically induced "central command signals" (if we can call them that) will elicit cardiovascular responses without exercise. One hypothesis underlying such studies has been that cardiovascular command signals descend from supramedullary centers to cardiovascular centers over discrete pathways that are separate from those carrying motor command signals to skeletal muscle (Hobbs, 1982). If the hypothesis is true, stimulation of appropriate supramedullary centers should evoke cardiovascular responses whereas damaging these centers should abolish these responses without affecting motor control of the muscles.

It has been repeatedly demonstrated (see Smith et al., 1960b; Smith, 1974; Dormer and Stone, 1976; Ordway et al., 1989) that electric stimulation of supramedullary sites in the brain can cause both heart rate and arterial blood pressure to increase markedly. This, of course, does not signify that any of these sites are involved in cardiovascular and/or respiratory responses to exercise. A site, which when stimulated would cause both locomotor-like muscle contraction and increases in heart rate and arterial pressure would have a better prospect of actually being involved in the "exercise response." Smith and colleagues (1960b) proposed that such a site may exist in the posterior hypothalamus near the fields of Forel (a specific anatomical site in this region). Electrical stimulation of this area caused heart rate, left ventricular systolic pressure, left ventricular *dp/dt* and ventilation all to increase. In some cases there were "running-type movements" or rhythmic and tonic muscle contractions as well. Eldridge and associates (1985) obtained similar results when they electrically stimulated the hypothalamic motor regions in decorticate cats. Waldrop and coworkers (1986) also observed vasoconstriction in inactive vascular beds (and local vasodilation in active muscles) during central electrical stimulation of the subthalamic locomotor region.

The cardiovascular responses of the dogs as they voluntarily exercised on a treadmill were directionally similar to the responses to electrical stimulation of electrodes chronically implanted in the fields of Forel (Smith et al., 1960b). The responses to stimulation persisted after muscles were paralyzed by a neuromuscular blocking agent, meaning that these responses did not depend on muscle contraction or metabolic changes. Finally, Smith and colleagues (1960a) showed the normal cardiovascular responses to voluntary exercise could be abolished by destroying those locations in the hypothalamus that, when stimulated, caused "exercise-like" responses (they placed bilateral electrolytic lesions in the H_2 fields of Forel).

Hobbs (1982) placed bilateral lesions in the subthalamus of five baboons trained to perform voluntary isometric contractions. Prior to making the lesions, electrical stimulation of the subthalamic sites increased heart rate, arterial pressure and arm movement. The electrolytic lesions abolished the pressor responses to electical stimulation and to two levels of static contraction in one baboon without altering the animals' ability to exercise or to increase arterial pressure when startled. This condition persisted until the animal was sacrificed 4 weeks later. Unfortunately the loss, or attenuation of, cardiovascular responses to contraction did not persist more than a few days in the other baboons. Nevertheless, these experiments did leave open the possibility that distinct and separate pathways could exist for centrally generated command signals from subthalamic nuclei to both somatomotor and cardiovascular centers, and that interrupting one pathway will not disturb the other.

These technically demanding, central lesioning experiments have been extremely difficult to perform. As a consequence, "successful" results have been obtained from only two or three animals (Smith et al., 1960a; Hobbs, 1982).

The importance of the "fields of Forel" in cardiovascular control during exercise was reexamined by Ordway and colleagues (1989). They essentially repeated the experiments of Smith and colleagues (1960a, 1960b) when they studied nine dogs at rest and at four levels of dynamic exercise before and after making bilateral electrolytic lesions in the hypothalamus in the region of the fields of Forel. These lesions abolished the cardiovascular responses to electrical stimulation of the hypothalamus so that the lesions were deemed complete. But the cardiovascular responses to dynamic exercise, ranging from mild to heavy, were not significantly affected by the ablation of these hypothalamic sites, as shown in Figure 10-3. The cause of the discrepancy with the earlier findings of Smith and colleagues (1960a, 1960b) from one dog is not known. The results of Ordway and coworkers (1989) (as the authors also concluded) do not mean that these lesioned hypothalamic sites were not normally involved in cardiovascular control during exercise. This returns us to the matter of redundancy in cardiovascular control, not only in the feedback mechanisms, but possibly in the feed-forward or motor command mechanisms as well. The maintained responses after lesioning speak as well for the plasticity of the central nervous system.

A landmark investigation of centrally generated command signals was conducted by Eldridge and coworkers (1985). They compared some circulatory and respiratory responses in normal cats as they walked or ran

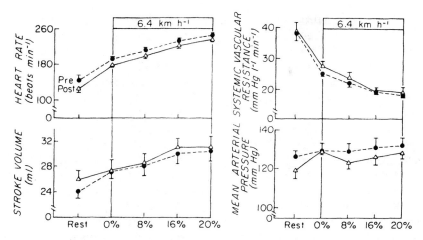

Figure 10-3 Persistence of normal cardiovascular responses to mild to heavy treadmill exercise at 6.4 km h^{-1} at grades of 0 to 20 percent in nine beagles after bilateral electrolytic lesions in the hypothalamus in the region of the fields of Forel. Responses shown before and after the lesions in the same dogs reveal no significant effects of these lesions on normal cardiovascular responses. The lesions did, however, abolish these cardiovascular responses only when they were evoked by electrical stimulation of the hypothalamic sites. (Adapted from Ordway, et al., 1989.)

spontaneously on a treadmill with responses of cats in which locomotion was induced by electrical or chemical stimulation of hypothalamic motor regions. They also investigated responses to so-called "fictive" locomotion which consisted of measuring locomotory activity in the motor nerves to the legs in which muscles were pharmacologically paralyzed. This motor nerve activity became the "exercise response" in place of actual movement. Again, this ploy eliminated any component of muscle feedback. The cats included (1) those with intact brains that were anesthetized, (2) those that were unanesthetized and *decorticate* and could develop locomotion both spontaneously and after stimulation of the hypothalamic motor region, and, finally (3) those that were unanesthetized and *decerebrate*, but still developed locomotion after stimulation of the mesencephalic locomotor region. The use of picrotoxin to elicit highly localized neural excitation meant that current spread to adjacent fiber tracts such as occurs during electrical stimulation was not causing the responses to locomotion.

Eldridge and colleagues (1985) showed that locomotor activity and proportional increases in respiration and arterial pressure that "mimic those of natural exercise" can occur in the three experimental groups of cats described above. Responses among the different animal preparations were similar irrespective of whether locomotion was spontaneous (intact and hypothalamic cats) or induced by electrical and chemical stimulation of the hypothalamic or mesencephalic regions. On the other hand, abolition

of hypothalamic drive by acute midcollicular decrebration abolished locomotion and reduced respiration and arterial pressure. Eldridge and colleagues (1985) concluded that locomotion and associated respiratory and
cardiovascular responses can be initiated from a common origin in the
suprapontine brain. In their view the command signal for exercise appears
to originate in the hypothalamic locomotor region. At least we can say
that these cells appear to be involved with the command signal.

Inasmuch as microinjections of γ-aminobutyric acid (GABA) antagonists into the posterior hypothalamus elicit locomotion along with increases in cardiovascular and respiratory activity, the suggestion is that a
"GABAergic" mechanism in the hypothalamus tonically inhibits neurons
that modulate locomotion and cardiovascular and respiratory functions
(Waldrop et al., 1988, 1991). Conceivably disinhibition of these hypothalamic neurons could provide a potential neural mechanism responsible for
the central command signal during exercise. In addition to GABA and
probably among numerous other neurotransmitters and neuropeptides,
corticotropin-releasing factor (CRF) has effects when injected into the
lateral ventricle not unlike those of GABA, whereas pharmacological
blockade of CRF compromises the cardiovascular adjustments to exercise
(Kregel et al., 1990).

Summary.   In summary, it appears that there are groups of hypothalamic
cells that play a role in turning on the cardiovascular system at the onset
of isometric contractions or dynamic exercise. At this stage the distinction
among forms of exercise is irrelevant. Under some rigidly controlled experimental conditions destruction of these cells can reduce or even prevent
cardiovascular responses to exercise. Does this mean that the source of
the central command signal has been isolated and identified? Probably not.
Although we are still a long way from understanding how central command
actually works, the case for an important role continues to grow.

HOW DOES CENTRAL COMMAND EXERT ITS EFFECTS ON THE CARDIOVASCULAR SYSTEM?

If we speak of isometric contractions, a more specific question is how does
central command increase blood pressure at the onset of a contraction—by
increased heart rate and cardiac output or by increased sympathetic vasoconstriction, or by both?

Cardiac Parasympathetic and Sympathetic Nerve Activity

The current thinking about the autonomic responses to central command
is summarized in Figure 10-4. Disregard for now the portions of this figure
that deal with reflexes from muscle; the discussion of this scheme will be
expanded in Chapter 11. Figure 10-4A schematically illustrates the changes

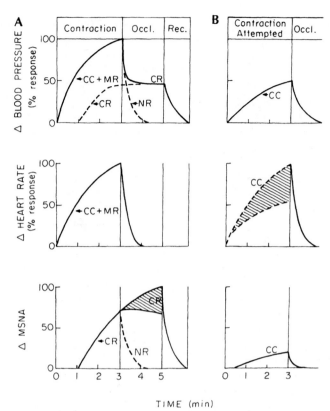

TIME (min)

Figure 10-4 Schematic illustration to demonstrate relative responses to central command (CC), muscle chemoreflex (CR), and muscle mechanoreflex (MR) during a powerful isometric contraction (A) and to an attempted contraction during complete neuromuscular blockade (B). Normal rise in *arterial pressure* is acheived initially by central command (some mechanoreflex component?). After about 1 minute, CR may contribute to rise in pressure. Time course of CR is derived from ΔMSNA (muscle sympathetic nerve activity) (arbitrary units) in bottom panel. Total vascular occlusion (Occl.) at end of contraction prevents normal recovery (NR) of pressure. *This is the test for a muscle chemoreflex.* Pressure drops approximately 50 percent when CC ceases and is kept elevated by CR as long as ischemia persists. *Heart rate* is raised by CC (some MR?) and vagal withdrawal. MSNA is presumably increased by CR and remains elevated during postexercise ischemia (shaded region reveals variations in response). During attempted contractions (panel B) CC raises arterial pressure to approximately 50 percent of normal; the heart rate response is more variable (shaded region) and the rise in MSNA is small. Occlusion had no effects because there was no contraction (no chemoreflex). (From Rowell and O'Leary, 1990, with permission from American Physiological Society.)

in arterial pressure, heart rate, and sympathetic nerve activity directed to muscle (ΔMSNA) in response to a powerful isometric contraction. The immediate rise in arterial pressure and heart rate is thought to be due almost exclusively to central command (some involvement of reflexes from active muscle has been proposed, thus the label MR along with CC for central command in Figure 10-4). The present concept is that heart rate is increased initially, during the first few seconds, by central command, which acts to withdraw tonic vagal outflow. This initial tachycardia is blocked by atropine and not by propranolol (Freyschuss, 1970; Martin et al., 1974; Maciel et al., 1987; Victor et al., 1989). The almost immediate rise in arterial pressure is attributable to the immediate increase in cardiac output stemming from the rise in heart rate (Martin et al., 1974). Heart rate and cardiac output rise together when muscle contraction expresses blood from muscle veins, and (initially in isometric contraction) cardiac filling pressure increases and permits the rise in cardiac output. In dynamic exercise the muscle pumping its continuous.

It is important to reconsider here the earlier discussion (see Figure 5-5) of the potentially high speed of parasympathetically mediated cardiac responses, which can take less than 1 second, as opposed to the relatively slow (10 to 20 seconds) sympathetically mediated responses. Clearly, if central command withdrew cardiac vagal outflow and increased sympathetic efferent traffic at the same time, the initial increase in heart rate over the first 10 to 20 seconds would still be mediated by vagal withdrawal. The latency between a muscle contraction and the rise in heart rate is in the order of 0.5 seconds (Martin et al., 1974; Maciel et al., 1987). The effects of any simultaneously activated sympathetic efferents would not be seen for approximately 10 to 15 seconds.

There is a biphasic heart rate response to a forceful isometric contraction and the durations of the parasympathetic and sympathetic phases will change as contraction force increases. For example, Martin and coworkers (1974) found that the initial 30 seconds of the tachycardia was mediated by withdrawal of vagal activity because the response was blocked by atropine. Maciel and coworkers (1987) observed that parasympathetic blockade acted only during the first 10 seconds of very severe isometric contractions at 50 and 75 percent of MVC, whereas sympathetic blockade modified the heart rate response after 10 seconds. The continued rise in heart rate after the initial 30 seconds was found to be sympathetically mediated because it was unaffected by atropine and prevented by propranolol. They concluded that sympathetic stimulation was a secondary mechanism for raising heart rate.

As shown in Chapter 8, the rise in arterial pressure during an isometric contraction is normally due to the increase in cardiac output; systemic vascular conductance is unchanged. However, after the administration of the β-adrenergic-blocking drug propranolol, isometric contraction raised arterial pressure by decreasing systemic vascular conductance along with a diminished increase in cardiac output. When the heart rate response to isometric contraction is reduced by β-blockade or combined β-adrenergic and parasympathetic blockade, arterial pressure is still raised as before (but presumably is delayed), but now by sympathetically mediated vaso-constriction (Macdonald et al., 1966; Martin et al., 1974). Arterial pressure also rises to a normal level in patients who have had their hearts denervated by transplant surgery (Haskell et al., 1981). In short, the *autonomic ner-vous system finds a "strategy"* for raising arterial pressure when at least one effector mechanism is available. This important observation has been made repeatedly and it strongly implies that some centrally integrated process provides such a "strategy." When both autonomic pathways are interrupted, as in diabetic patients with autonomic neuropathy, both arterial pressure and heart rate responses to isometric contractions are reduced.

Sympathetic Vasomotor Nerve Activity

The generally held assumption that central command signals play an im-portant role in the activation of the sympathetic nervous system (e.g., Lind, 1983) has been challenged by Mark and coworkers (1985) and by Victor and coworkers (1989), as well as by the observation that total vascular conductance often remains unchanged during a contraction (Chapter 8). Victor and colleagues directly measured muscle sympathetic nerve activity (MSNA) (see Chapter 3) in subjects who performed isomet-ric forearm contractions at 15 and 30 percent of MVC, and then attempted to do the same after they were partially neuromuscularly blocked by systemic administration of tubocurarine. Figure 10-5 shows the responses before and during blockade when near-maximal motor effort generated almost no force. In agreement with earlier studies (see Figure 10-4B), the rise in arterial pressure was reduced by approximately one-half during the most severe paralysis whereas the rise in heart rate was not reduced during a near-maximal attempt to contract. As shown in Figure 10-4, heart rate responses under such conditions are quite variable; they have less effect on cardiac output because there is no compression of muscle veins in the absence of muscle contraction. Attempted contractions increased MSNA by only 25 percent, and only when the attempts were maximal and little force could be generated. The conclusion was that *central command has a large influence on parasympathetic outflow to the heart and very little effect on MSNA.* This finding appears to disagree with that of an earlier study by Mark and colleagues (1985) in which central command was thought to *decrease* MSNA. They observed higher MSNA in a resting leg muscle during involuntary electrically induced contractions of the forearm muscle than during voluntary contractions. This may reflect the effect of direct electrical activation of muscle afferents along with reversal of nor-mal recruitment patterns. Also, a sympathetic spinal reflex could be acti-vated by electrical stimulation of the arm to raise MSNA in the leg, lending the impression that MSNA had been reduced when the arm is *voluntarily*

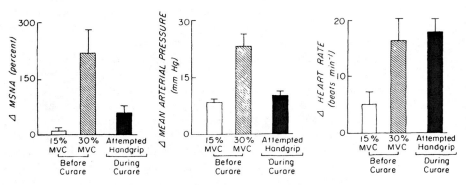

Figure 10-5   Responses to isometric contractions (handgrip) at 15 and 30 percent of MVC in eight normal subjects before neuromuscular blockade with tubocurarine chloride, and to attempted contractions in which near-maximal effort yielded almost no force. The intent to contract (central command) caused significant but much smaller increases in MSNA than measured during contractions before blockade. The increase in heart rate during an attempted contraction after curare was blocked by atropine. The results suggest a major role for central command in parasympathetic control of heart rate and a minor role in activating sympathetic outflow to skeletal muscle. (Adapted from Victor et al., 1989.)

rather than involuntarily active (see Wallin et al., 1989). The reason for the discrepancy is still not clear.

IS CENTRAL COMMAND EXCLUSIVELY A FEED-FORWARD MECHANISM?

One of the earliest objections to the basic hypothesis of central command as a feed-forward mechanism was that such precise and predictable matching between cardiac output and oxygen uptake, for example, would be unlikely without some feedback to "inform" the cardiovascular system about the adequacy of its responses. Do we achieve the "correct" cardiac output and muscle blood flow during exercise by feedback modulation of the central command signal, or, conversely, is the feedback directed instead to autonomic neurons involved directly in the control of heart rate, cardiac output, and vascular conductance? This latter scheme, which is the subject of Chapter 11, could presumably achieve the same result as the feedback modulation of central command.

"Central Command" and Motor Unit Recruitment

One hypothesis is that the magnitude of the central command signal could somehow be related to the number of motor units activated during a voluntary isometric contraction. Presumably mechanical feedback from the muscle to the central nervous system (see Chapter 11) modulates the command signal (Schibye et al., 1981; Hobbs, 1982).

The hypothesis is illustrated schematically in Figure 10-6. Experimentally, the basic idea can be tested by increasing the number of motor units recruited for a contraction maintained at *constant force* by weakening the muscle with a neuromuscular blocking agent. The hypothesis in Figure 10-6 predicts the effects of partial neuromuscular blockade on arterial pressure during a light-load contraction that requires, for simplicity, three motoneurons and six muscle fibers. The comparison is with a heavy-load contraction that requires five motoneurons and ten muscle fibers. After partial neuromuscular blockade the same light-load contraction force requires activation of all five motoneurons to contract the six muscle fibers because four of the ten fibers are now blocked. If the arterial pressure response to contraction is proportional to motor unit recruitment, then the rise in pressure during the light-load contraction after neuromuscular blockade should equal that during the normal heavy-load contraction. Figure 10-6 illustrates schematically the typical findings from five baboons who were operantly conditioned to carry out voluntary isometric contractions at two loads (Hobbs, 1982). When contraction force, muscle blood flow, and thus muscle metabolism as well were all constant, the need to recruit more motor units after neuromuscular blockade in order to maintain force caused a greater rise in heart rate and arterial pressure.

McCloskey (1981) conducted experiments similar to those just described, but on human subjects whose motor strength was reduced by

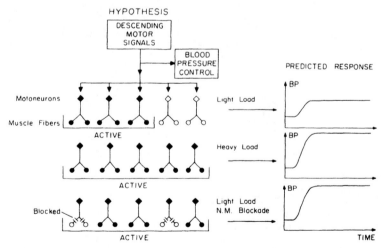

Figure 10-6 Schematic diagram of a central command hypothesis that directly relates cardiovascular command to raise blood pressure to motor command to recruit motor units (Hobbs, 1982). The scheme predicts that recruitment of more motor units at constant force will raise blood pressure because of parallel activation of the two systems. (From Rowell, 1986, with permission from Oxford University Press.)

local infusion of curare (Figure 10-7) The absolute force of contraction was kept constant throughout, but the relative force increased from 20 to 86 percent of maximum voluntary contraction (MVC) after neuromuscular blockade. Arterial pressure rose in proportion to the percent of MVC and to the augmented motor command and motor unit recruitment required to maintain constant force. Similar experiments were subsequently conducted by Secher, Mitchell, and colleagues (see Mitchell, 1990).

Schibye and colleagues (1981) took a different experimental approach to examine any link between central command and motor unit recruitment. Their experimental model is based on the idea that as individual motor units or muscle fibers fatigue during a sustained isometric contraction, recruitment of additional fresh motor units will require increasingly greater central command. The results from their well-designed experiments are shown in Figure 10-8. First, prolonged isometric knee extension at constant force was accompanied by parallel increases in electromyographic (EMG) activity, arterial pressure, and heart rate. Force was maintained constant by visual feedback and not by perception of effort which would increase over time. In contrast, when the subjects received visual feedback so that they could keep EMG activity constant during the contraction, their contraction force declined by nearly one-half. These experiments support the idea that an important portion of the rise in arterial pressure during a sustained isometric contraction could be attributed to the increase in motor unit recruitment.

Although the perception of effort was thought to be constant during experiments with constant EMG activity, arterial pressure and heart rate

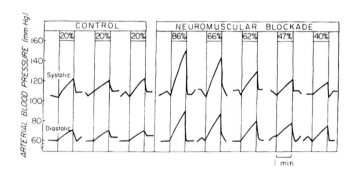

Figure 10-7 Systolic and diastolic pressures during a single series of 1-minute isometric handgrips at constant absolute force in one subject before (control) and during neuromuscular blockade by local injection of d-tubocurarine. Control handgrips were all at 20 percent of maximum voluntary contraction force (shown as percent maximal voluntary contraction [MVC]). After blockade MVC was reduced so that contractions required greater fractions of MVC and thus larger motor command. The rise in blood pressure paralleled motor command which waned together with diminishing effects of blockade. (Adapted from McCloskey, 1981; reproduced from Rowell, 1986, with permission from Oxford University Press.)

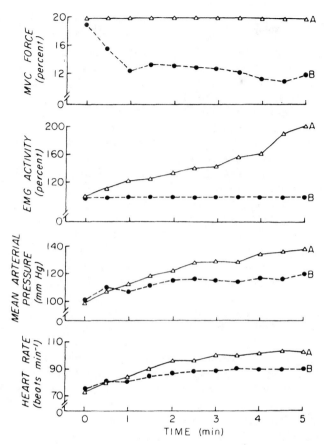

Figure 10-8 Average responses to 5-minute contraction of the knee extensors in five subjects who either maintained *constant force* at 20 percent of MVC (A) while EMG activity rose, or maintained, *constant EMG activity* (B) (and presumably constant motor command) while force and percent MVC declined (Schibye et al., 1981). Mean arterial pressure and heart rate tended to parallel EMG activity, but some rise in both variables persisted when EMG activity was kept constant. (From Rowell, 1986, with permission from Oxford University Press.)

still rose, but less than before. Neither the constant EMG activity nor perception of effect mean that central command was precisely constant. Motor neuron output at a given level of effort can be facilitated or inhibited by reflex feedback from contracting muscles. So far we have no way around this problem experimentally. The residual rise in arterial pressure and heart rate could mean that motoneuron output was inhibited by reflexes from the muscle.

The idea that motor unit recruitment might be the link between centrally generated motor activity and cardiovascular responses reintroduces the question raised in Chapter 8 about the significance of muscle mass.

The puzzle has been whether cardiovascular responses to a given relative force of isometric contraction are or are not proportional to the mass of contracting muscle. Based on a proportionality between the number of active motor units and the rise in arterial pressure, what would be the expected relationship between arterial pressure and the mass of the isometrically contracting muscle? If, for example, the number of motor units activated in an isometrically contracting forearm is the same as the number activated in the contracting knee extensors at the same percent of MVC, then the central command signal and the cardiovascular responses should be the same. This would be so despite the marked difference in the absolute force generated per motor unit in the two different muscle groups. This is consistent with the findings discussed in Chapter 8 (for example, by Lind and his colleagues [see Lind, 1983]) that the rise in arterial pressure at any given percent of MVC is independent of muscle mass. This latter finding is also consistent with the data suggesting that the smaller the muscle, the greater the number of motor units per gram of muscle (Granit, 1970). The dependency of the pressor response on mass observed by others (see Mitchell and colleagues in Chapter 8) does not support this thinking. Reasons for this dispute and some reasons for thinking that pressor responses are probably more or less *independent* of muscle mass were discussed in Chapter 8. This issue is significant because of the claim that a muscle chemoreflex (Chapter 11), rather than central command, may raise arterial pressure during isometric contractions; the strength of this muscle reflex is unquestionably proportional to muscle mass, because the rise in arterial pressure it elicits is mass-dependent. If, on the other hand, the strength of the central command signal is *not* proportional to muscle mass, then neither should the rise in arterial pressure be mass-dependent. Unfortunately this matter is not fully resolved. When it is, the distinction may help to determine whether arterial pressure is raised by central command or by a reflex from active muscle.

Importance of the Spinal Cord in Central Command

Some experimental findings suggest that disruption of spinal cord function by disease or by anesthetic blockade may prevent cardiovascular responses to centrally generated motor command. For example, Freund and colleagues (1979) observed no rise in arterial pressure in response to an attempted maximal isometric contraction of knee extensors when all motor function was blocked by peridural anesthesia. Lind and colleagues (1968) studied one subject with unilateral syringomyelia with extensive spinal cord damage extending from the medulla to the lower thoracic region (with possible involvement of vasomotor centers). Attempts by this subject to make strong isometric contractions of a forearm were usually unaccompanied by any significant rise in arterial pressure. In contrast, the normal cardiovascular *responses to attempted isometric contractions persist when motor function is blocked peripherally rather than centrally* (Freyschuss, 1970; Hobbs and Gandevia, 1985).

Hobbs (1982) proposed that there may be a spinal feedback loop that is involved with either the generation or modulation (or both) of the central motor command signal. This proposal prompted a study on normal and paraplegic subjects by Hobbs and Gandevia (1985). The paraplegic subjects had recent complete transection of the spinal cord at levels T-8 to T-12 and no other neural defects. When these paraplegic subjects attempted to contract their paralyzed leg muscles, no cardiovascular response was observed. In contrast, attempted contractions of an arm temporarily paralyzed by local anesthesia or anoxia always elicited significant increases in heart rate and arterial pressure in both their normal control subjects and their paraplegic subjects. In all subjects, normal or paraplegic, the sense of effort in an unsuccessful attempt to contract a paralyzed limb was greater than the sense of effort during isometric contraction of the normal (unblocked) forearm. Both subject groups showed normal cardiovascular changes in response to contraction of the unblocked forearm. Thus, as with spinal anesthesia, spinal transection abolished the cardiovascular response to a central motor command to the legs; in contrast, paralysis of the arms by a peripheral blockade does not abolish the cardiovascular response. Hobbs and Gandevia (1985) concluded that neural pathways to and from the spinal cord below the lesion (or at the site of epidural blockade) must be involved in transmitting central command, relaying signals to cardiovascular neurons. A more detailed scheme is presented in Figure 10-2.

Modulation of Subthalamic Locomotor Output

Waldrop and Stremel (1989) saw that in addition to initiating locomotor signals, some neurons in the subthalamic locomotor region of the posterior hypothalamus might also be involved in modulating the cardiovascular and respiratory responses to feedback from active muscles. They showed that neurons in this hypothalamic region increased their discharge frequency during isometric and rhythmic contractions of hindlimb muscles in anesthetized cats. These contractions were induced by electrical stimulation of ventral roots, which presumably eliminated central command and any direct electrical activation of muscle afferents (there are, however, a few afferents in the ventral roots). The muscle contractions evoked two types of excitatory neuronal responses in these posterior hypothalamic neurons; one was immediate and then quickly decayed, and the other response had delayed onset and then increased gradually. The significance of these responses is discussed in Chapter 11. The point to grasp here is that these responses had temporal patterns that characterize two well-known reflexes from active muscle, the former the muscle mechanoreflex, and the latter the muscle chemoreflex (Figure 11-2). The inference is that neural feedback from the active muscles may be directed to cells that initiate locomotor signals. This suggests a modulation of central command by muscle reflexes (see Waldrop and Stremel, 1989; Waldrop et al., 1991).

There is no direct evidence yet that feedback from muscle afferents actually evoked the firing patterns observed among the neurons in the posterior hypothalamus described by Waldrop and Stremel (1989). Nor is it actually known that these particular hypothalamic neurons play any role in initiating cardiovascular or respiratory responses to exercise. Waldrop and colleagues (1991) also suggested that the firing of these hypothalamic neurons has a temporal relationship to sympathetic nerve activity. However, evidence presented in previous sections indicates that centrally generated command signals in humans are not related in either time or magnitude to increases in sympathetic nerve activity.

The experiments of Waldrop and his colleagues (1989) offer support to the idea that central command signals could be modulated by feedback from the muscles and from other structures such as arterial baroreceptors, for example. The idea that central command is not an exclusively feed-forward control mechanism has some support.

SUMMARY

In summary this chapter surveys the evidence from studies on humans and other species that centrally generated motor command signals, called central command, activate both somatomotor and cardiovascular motor systems at the onset of exercise. The speed of cardiovascular and also respiratory responses has been viewed as too fast for a reflex initiation. Therefore a feed-forward controller of the circulation is proposed. There is some evidence that there may be separate activation of somatomotor and cardiovascular motor systems by parallel central command neural pathways. Central command is today seen as the signal that withdraws tonic vagal outflow to the heart and initiates the sudden increase in heart rate. Central command signals appear to have minimal effect on the sympathetic nervous system as judged by their very small effect on directly recorded muscle sympathetic nerve activity or on regional vascular resistance. Sympathetic outflow to the heart increases after a delay and then gradually during a sustained isometric contraction, but this activity may be due to other, reflex influences. In short, central command appears to act on the parasympathetic nervous system, whereas reflexes generated during exercise act on the sympathetic nervous system.

Recent neurophysiological studies on animals show that both locomotor and cardiovascular-respiratory responses, much like those to exercise, can be induced by either electrical or chemical stimulation of cells in the hypothalamic motor regions. Lesions in these cells can blunt or even abolish exercise responses, but this finding is not uniform and suggests a high degree of plasticity in the central nervous system. Finally, there is evidence to suggest that central command does not act exclusively as a feed-forward control mechanism. Its close relationship to the number of motor units recruited in the active muscle suggests an important role for mechanical feedback from the muscle. Such feedback may require a spinal feedback loop that is involved either in generation or modulation of the central command signal. There is also growing evidence that neurons in the subthalamic locomotor region of the posterior hypothalamus may receive feedback from active muscles. Therefore, the effectiveness of central command signals as feed-forward controllers of the cardiovascular system during exercise may be enhanced through their modulation by feedback signals from active muscles—and from other reflexes.

REFERENCES

Alam, M., and F.H. Smirk (1938). Unilateral loss of a blood pressure raising, pulse accelerating, reflex from voluntary muscle due to a lesion of the spinal cord. *Clin Sci. 3*, 247–252.

Asmussen, E., S.H. Johansen, M. Jorgensen, and M. Nielsen (1965). On the nervous factors controlling respiration and circulation during exercise. Experiments with curarization. *Acta Physiol. Scand. 63*, 343–350.

Asmussen, E., M. Nielsen, and G. Wieth-Pedersen (1943). On the regulation of the circulation during muscular work. *Acta Physiol. Scand. 6*, 353–358.

Dormer, K.J. (1984). Modulation of cardiovascular response to dynamic exercise by fastigial nucleus. *J. Appl. Physiol. (Respir. Environ. Exerc. Physiol.) 56*, 1369–1377.

Dormer K.J., and H.L. Stone (1976). Cerebellar pressor response in the dog. *J. Appl. Physiol. 41*, 574–580.

Dormer, K.J., and H.L. Stone (1982). Fastigial nucleus and its possible role in the cardiovascular response to exercise. In O.A. Smith, R.A. Galosy, and S.M. Weiss, eds. *Circulation, Neurobiology and Behavior*, pp. 201–215. Elsevier, New York.

Duncan, G., R.H. Johnson, and D.G. Lambie (1981). Role of sensory nerves in the cardiovascular and respiratory changes with isometric forearm exercise in man. *Clin. Sci. Lond. 60*, 145–155.

Eldridge, R.L., D.E. Milhorn, J.P. Kiley, and T.G. Waldrop (1985). Stimulation by central command of locomotion, respiration, and circulation during exercise. *Respir. Physiol. 59*, 313–337.

Freund, P.R., L.B. Rowell, T.M. Murphy, S.F. Hobbs, and S.H. Butler (1979). Blockade of the pressor response to muscle ischemia by sensory nerve block in man. *Am. J. Physiol. 236 (Heart Circ. Physiol. 6)*, H433–H439.

Freyschuss, U. (1970). Cardiovascular adjustment of somatomotor activation. *Acta Physiol. Scand. 342 (Suppl. 1)*, 1–63.

Goodwin, G.M., D.I. McCloskey, and J.H. Mitchell (1972). Cardiovascular and respiratory responses to changes in central command during isometric exercise at constant muscle tension. *J. Physiol. (Lond.) 226*, 173–190.

Granit, R. (1970). *The Basis of Motor Control*. Academic Press, London.

Haskell, W.L., N.M. Savin, J.S. Schroeder, E.A. Alderman, N.B. Ingles, G.T. Daughters, and E.A. Stinson (1981). Cardiovascular responses to handgrip isometric exercise in patients following cardiac transplantation. *Circ. Res.* *48 (Suppl. 1),* 156–161.

Hobbs, S.F. (1982). Central command during exercise: parallel activation of the cardiovascular and motor systems by descending command signals. In O.A. Smith, R.A. Galosy, and S.M. Weiss, eds. *Circulation, Neurobiology and Behavior,* pp. 217–232. Elsevier, New York.

Hobbs, S.F., and S.C. Gandevia (1985). Cardiovascular responses and the sense of effort during attempts to contract paralysed muscles: role of the spinal cord. *Neurosci. Lett. 57,* 85–90.

Houk, J.C. (1988). Control strategies in physiological systems. *FASEB J. 2,* 97–107.

Johansson, J.E. (1895). Über die Einwirkung der Muskelthätigkeit auf die Athmung und die Herzthätigkeit. *Skand. Arch. Physiol. 5,* 20–66.

Kregel, K.C., J.M. Overton, D.R. Seals, C.M. Tipton, and L.A. Fisher (1990). Cardiovascular responses to exercise in the rat: role of corticotropin-releasing factor. *J. Appl. Physiol. 68,* 561–567.

Krogh, A., and J. Lindhard (1913). The regulation of respiration and circulation during the initial stages of muscular work. *J. Physiol. (Lond.) 47,* 112–136.

Krogh, A., and J. Lindhard (1917). A comparison between voluntary and electrically induced muscular work in man. *J. Physiol. (Lond.) 51,* 182–201.

Leonard, B., J.H. Mitchell, M. Mizuno, N. Rube, B. Saltin, and N.H. Secher (1985). Partial neuromuscular blockade and cardiovascular responses to static exercise in man. *J. Physiol. (Lond.) 359,* 365–379.

Lind, A.R. (1983). Cardiovascular adjustments to isometric contractions: static effort. In J.T. Shepherd, F.M. Abboud, and S.R. Geiger, eds. *Handbook of Physiology. The Cardiovascular System: Peripheral Circulation and Organ Blood Flow,* sect. 2, vol. III, pp. 947–966. American Physiological Society, Bethesda, MD.

Lind, A.R., G.W. McNicol, R.A. Bruce, H.R. Macdonald, and K.W. Donald (1968). The cardiovascular responses to sustained contractions of a patient with unilateral syringomyelia. *Clin. Sci. 35,* 45–53.

Macdonald, H.R., R.P. Sapru, S.H. Taylor, and K.W. Donald (1966). Effect of intravenous propranolol on the systemic circulatory response to sustained handgrip. *Am. J. Cardiol. 18,* 333–343.

Maciel, B.C., L. Gallo, Jr., J.A. Marin Neto, and L.E.B. Martins (1987). Autonomic nervous control of the heart rate during isometric exercise in normal man. *Pflugers Arch. 408,* 173–177.

Mark, A.L., R.G. Victor, C. Nerhed, and B.G. Wallin (1985). Microneurographic studies of the mechanisms of sympathetic nerve responses to static exercise in humans. *Circ. Res. 57:* 461–469.

Martin, C.E., J.A. Shaver, D.F. Leon, M.E. Thompson, P.S. Reddy, and J.J. Leonard (1974). Autonomic mechanisms in hemodynamic responses to isometric exercise. *J. Clin. Invest. 54,* 104–115.

McCloskey, D.I. (1981). Centrally-generated commands and cardiovascular control in man. *Clin. Expt. Hypertension 3,* 369–378.

Mitchell, J.H. (1990). Neural control of the circulation during exercise. *Med. Sci. Sports Exerc. 22,* 141–154.

Ordway, G.A., T.G. Waldrop, G.A. Iwamoto, and B.J. Gentile (1989). Hypothalamic influences on cardiovascular response of beagles to dynamic exercise. *Am. J. Physiol. 257 (Heart Circ. Physiol. 26),* H1247–H1253.

Rowell, L.B., and D.S. O'Leary (1990). Reflex control of the circulation during exercise: chemoreflexes and mechanoreflexes. *J. Appl. Physiol. 69,* 407–418.

Schibye, B., J.H. Mitchell, F.C. Payne III, and B. Saltin (1981). Blood pressure and heart rate response to static exercise in relation to electromyographic activity and force development. *Acta Physiol. Scand. 113,* 61–66.

Smith, O.A. (1974). Reflex and central mechanisms involved in the control of the heart and circulation. *Ann. Rev. Physiol. 36,* 93–124.

Smith, O.A. Jr., S.J. Jabbur, R.F. Rushmer, and E.P. Lasher (1960b). Role of hypothalamic structures in cardiac control. *Physiol. Rev. 40,* 136–141.

Smith, O.A. Jr., R.F. Rushmer, and E.P. Lasher (1960a). Similarity of cardiovascular responses to exercise and to diencephalic stimulation. *Am. J. Physiol. 198,* 1139–1142.

Victor, R.G., S.L. Pryor, N.H. Secher, and J.H. Mitchell (1989). Effects of partial neuromuscular blockade on sympathetic nerve responses to static exercise in humans. *Circ. Res. 65,* 468–476.

Waldrop, T.G., R.M. Bauer, and G.A. Iwamoto (1988). Microinjection of GABA antagonists into the posterior hypothalamus elicits locomotor activity and a cardiorespiratory activation. *Brain Res. 444,* 84–94.

Waldrop, T.G., R.M. Bauer, G.A. Iwamoto, and R.W. Stremel (1991). Hypothalamic modulation of cardiovascular, respiratory and locomotor activity during exercise. In H.P. Koepchen and T. Houpaniemi, eds. *Cardiorespiratory and Motor Coordination* pp. 208–214. Springer-Verlag, Berlin.

Waldrop, T.G., M.C. Henderson, G.A. Iwamoto, and J.H. Mitchell (1986). Regional blood flow responses to stimulation of the subthalamic locomotor region. *Respir. Physiol. 66,* 215–224.

Waldrop, T.G., and R.W. Stremel (1989). Muscular contraction stimulates posterior hypothalamic neurons. *Am. J. Physiol. 256 (Regulatory Integrative Comp. Physiol. 25),* R348–R356.

Wallin, B.G., R.G. Victor, and A.L. Mark (1989). Sympathetic outflow to resting muscles during static handgrip and postcontraction muscle ischemia. *Am. J. Physiol. 256 (Heart Circ. Physiol. 25),* H105–H110.

Zuntz, N., and J. Geppert (1886). Über die Natur der normalen Atemreize und den Ort ihrer Wirkung. *Pflugers Arch. 38,* 337–338.

11

What Signals Govern the Cardiovascular Responses to Exercise? Reflexes from Active Muscles

This chapter asks if the control of the cardiovascular system during exercise is governed by reflexes arising from active muscles. Two reflexes are considered: (1) *chemoreflexes* caused by chemical stimulation of small sensory fibers originating in the muscles, and (2) *mechanoreflexes* caused by mechanical stimulation of muscle afferent fibers. Emphasis is directed mainly to the the former because more is known about them and they appear to be the more important; but mechanoreflexes may also play a role and cannot be ignored.

Is the primary error signal governing the cardiovascular response to exercise a mismatch between muscle blood flow and its metabolism, that is, a blood flow error? The hypothesis underlying this question was originally expressed by Zuntz and Geppert (1886) who apparently had the respiratory system in mind. Their thinking was that if muscle blood flow fell below some particular level, metabolites would accumulate within the muscle. Their hypothetical scheme required the presence of afferent nerve fibers within the muscle that would ''sense'' the increased concentration of these metabolites. No such fibers were known to exist at that time. In essence, the basic idea was, and still is, that the increased concentration of metabolites within the muscle would increase firing of its afferent nerve fibers. Their centrally directed traffic would in turn act on cardiovascular neurons that control sympathetic nervous outflow to the cardiovascular system (of course, Zuntz and Geppert were not so specific, inasmuch as they preceded W.B. Cannon and his work on the sympathetic nervous system). The role of the sympathetic nervous system is presumed to be that of restoring muscle blood flow and the intramuscular concentration of metabolites to some optimal level by raising arterial pressure and cardiac output.

Ideally a metabolic ''error signal'' could be continuously corrected by the autonomic nervous system if the muscle chemoreflex were tonically active during exercise. Inasmuch as 80 to 90 percent of the total cardiac output can be directed to working muscle, a feedback from some ''metabolic sensor'' in the muscles would be an ideal way to activate continuously the cardiovascular reflexes that govern arterial pressure and blood flow during exercise. This idea has had enough appeal to make it the focus of much of the research on cardiovascular control during exercise (for reviews see Rowell, 1980; Mitchell et al., 1981; Lind, 1983; Mitchell and Schmidt, 1983; Rowell, 1986; Mitchell, 1990).

For this general hypothesis to be valid, the following requirements must be met:

1. Trapping of metabolites within the muscles at the cessation of exercise should sustain or even increase the cardiovascular response to that exercise.
2. Chemical stimulation of the isolated resting muscle should activate some sensory nerves originating within that muscle.
3. The specific afferent fibers responding to chemical stimulation should be capable of eliciting cardiovascular reflex responses.
4. Substances liberated from active muscles should activate these afferent fiber groups.

Before reviewing briefly the neurophysiological evidence for the existence of muscle chemoreflexes, covered in requirements 2 through 4 above, requirement 1 is put forward here as the most basic one. It was also the first to be satisfied and was done so in 1937 in a simple but ingenious experiment by Alam and Smirk (1937). Their original results from human subjects were redrawn in Figure 11-1. They arrested the circu-

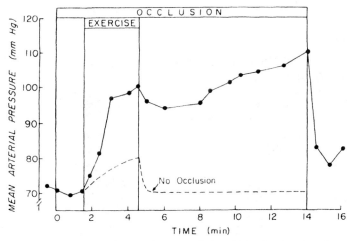

Figure 11-1 Mean arterial pressure during and after dynamic exercise of one forearm with its circulation arrested. Dashed line (no occlusion) shows the estimated response with normal circulation. Pressure rose markedly during exercise with circulatory occlusion and the elevation persisted (and even increased) for as long as blood flow was arrested. (Adapted from Alam and Smirk, 1937; reproduced from Rowell, 1986 with permission from Oxford University Press.)

lation to a dynamically exercising limb either by inflation of a blood pressure cuff or by immersion of the limb in a bath of mercury. Their key finding was that the entrapment of metabolites within the limb *after* exercise, when there was no central command or mechanical activity, prevented the fall in arterial pressure and in most cases prompted a further rise. Arterial pressure remained elevated for as long as the blood vessels were occluded and metabolites remained entrapped within the muscles.

This rise in arterial pressure caused by muscle ischemia during postexercise occlusion became the hallmark of the muscle chemoreflex. The rise in pressure could be graded in proportion to the degree of muscle ischemia or oxygen deficiency (Rowell et al., 1976) and also in proportion to muscle mass (Freund et al., 1978), that is, the strength of the muscle chemoreflex was proportional to the mass of ischemic muscles (Rowell et al., 1981) in apparent contrast to the rise in pressure caused by isometric contractions. Inasmuch as the circulation to a limb constitutes a small percentage of total vascular conductance, the rise in arterial pressure must be a reflex rather than a passive effect of vascular occlusion on arterial pressure (the reflex component was not actually proved until 1971 [Coote et al., 1971]; see below).

Occlusion of *resting* muscles for periods of up to 1 hour or more was without effect on arterial pressure, except for the small mechanical effect if the mass of occluded muscle was large (see Rowell et al., 1976). It became evident that the muscle must be metabolically active in order to elicit this reflex (Rowell et al., 1981; Shepherd et al., 1981; Rowell, 1986). The pressor responses to postexercise muscle ischemia became the most important test for the presence of, or the absence of, a muscle chemoreflex.

NEUROPHYSIOLOGICAL EVIDENCE FOR MUSCLE CHEMOREFLEXES AND MECHANOREFLEXES

Originally, the thinking about muscle mechanoreflexes focused on those mechanoreflexes or proprioceptive reflexes that originate in muscle spindles and Golgi tendon organs, whose afferent nerve fibers are the large, fast-conducting group I and group II units. These mechanoreceptors were thought to be well suited to provide important feedback to the central nervous system about duration, magnitude, and rates of tension development. Today, these mechanoreflexes are no longer thought to be important in the regulation of the circulatory or respiratory systems. For example, there are no significant cardiovascular or respiratory responses to muscle vibration—a potent stimulus to muscle spindles (McCloskey et al., 1972). Furthermore, selective blockade of group I and II afferents at the dorsal roots does not abolish the pressure-raising reflexes that originate in skeletal muscle (McCloskey and Mitchell, 1972). Finally, groups I and II muscle afferents lack any appreciable direct access to the autonomic nervous system (Sato and Schmidt, 1973). These findings do not rule out an important role for muscle mechanoreflexes that originate among the free nerve endings of the small group III and group IV muscle afferents.

The neurophysiological evidence for the existence of chemo- and mechanosensitive muscle afferents that can raise arterial pressure developed along the three lines covered under the three subheadings that follow.

Nerve Recordings During Chemical and Mechanical Activation of Muscle Afferents

Because of their overlapping functions, both chemo- and mechanoreflexes are discussed in this section. Substantial fractions of mechanosensitive afferents in the muscle are also chemosensitive, and, conversely, many chemosensitive afferents respond to mechanical stimulation as well (Kaufman et al., 1983, 1988).

The afferent arms of the muscle chemo- and mechanoreflexes are the small, slow-conducting fibers classified as group III (myelinated) and the smaller, more slowly conducting fibers classified as group IV (Unmyelinated C fibers). These small groups III and IV afferent fibers outnumber the larger ones by a factor of 4. They tend to be polymodal, responding often to mechanical, chemical, and thermal stimulation (Kalia et al., 1981; Kniffki et al., 1981; Mitchell and Schmidt, 1983).

The polymodal groups III and IV afferents have been arbitrarily classified either as *ergoreceptors* (ergo = work) or *nociceptors* (pain receptors). The main distinction is that ergoreceptors respond to nonnoxious stimuli associated with actual muscle contraction whereas nociceptors commonly respond to noxious stimulation, for example, by injected algesic substances such as bradykinin, serotonin, capsaicin, or potassium (Kniffki et al., 1981; Mitchell and Schmidt, 1983). They also respond to extreme mechanical distortion not encountered in normal contraction (e.g., strong pinching, twisting at high tension). Approximately 40 percent of the group III fibers respond to muscle contraction in a graded fashion at forces as low as 20 percent of maximum. Their activity reflects both the amplitude and time course of contraction. These fibers may be involved in the initiation of autonomic reflexes and thus appear to be the best candidates for true ergoreceptors (Kniffki et al., 1981; Mitchell and Schmidt, 1983). Again, the distinction between the sensory modalities of groups III and IV afferents is arbitrary because both groups respond to a variety of chemical and mechanical stimulations.

A potentially important point that has received little attention is that group III afferent fibers are *thermosensitive* (Mense, 1978; Kniffki et al., 1981). Increases in muscle temperature over a nonnoxious range between 24 and 44°C elevated the firing rates of both groups III and IV afferents by more than 50 percent. Muscle temperature, which is normally well below 37°C in the limbs, can increase beyond 40°C during severe exercise; thus, the temperature sensitivity of group III afferents incorporates the range over which muscle temperature increases during exercise. Their thermal sensitivity may represent a link between the metabolic rate or heat production of the muscle and its afferent nerve fiber activity, but this has not yet been systematically explored.

Reflex Effects of Chemical and Mechanical Activation of Muscle Afferents

All of the chemical and mechanical stimuli summarized above that increased the discharge of groups III and IV afferents also caused a rise in arterial pressure. Coote and colleagues (1971) first proved that the rise in arterial pressure was of reflex origin by abolishing the pressor response to muscle contraction (induced by stimulation of the distal end of cut ventral roots in anesthetized cats) by severing the dorsal (sensory) roots. Then McCloskey and Mitchell (1972) used differential nerve blockade at the dorsal roots to separate out the effects of groups III and IV fiber activity from those of the large myelinated fibers (groups I and II). Anodal block of large fibers did not abolish the rise in pressure associated with muscle contraction whereas the response was abolished during a transient period in which mainly the small fibers were thought to be blocked by application of lidocaine to the mixed nerves.

The rise in arterial pressure caused by the activation of groups III and IV fibers is achieved in anesthetized animals primarily by activation of sympathetic vasoconstriction (Mitchell and Schmidt, 1983; Rowell, 1986). These reflexes have much less effect on ventilation and heart rate than they have on arterial pressure. The small effect on heart rate has been important to the well-established view that sympathetic activity and heart rate are controlled differently during exercise. This view is challenged later in this chapter.

What Substances Liberated from Active Muscle and What Mechanical Stimuli Might Activate Muscle Afferent Fiber Groups?

Chemosensitivity

The activation of groups III and IV afferents by algesic substances (see above), with the exception of potassium, clearly does not establish their normal function as so-called "metaboreceptors." The expected stimulus for a muscle chemoreflex would be a metabolic by-product of muscle contraction. Until recently there was no neurophysiological evidence that substances normally produced by active muscle could stimulate groups III and IV nerve endings (see Kniffki et al., 1981). Recent studies in which lactate (Thimm et al., 1984; Rotto and Kaufman, 1988), phosphate and adenosine were infused into the arterial supply of muscle also revealed either little (Thimm et al., 1984) or no activation of these afferents (Rotto and Kaufman, 1988). In contrast, infusions containing lactic acid (rather than lithium or sodium lactate), arachidonic acid, or potassium all activate equal percentages of groups III and IV afferents (Rotto and Kaufman,

1988). Potassium, which has often been proposed as a key link between metabolic activity and muscle afferent nerve activity, increases the discharge of groups III and IV units (Thimm et al., 1984), but the effect is only transient even when interstitial potassium activity is maintained at elevated levels by potassium infusion (Rybicki et al., 1985; Kaufman and Rybicki, 1987).

Lactic acid and some cyclo-oxygenase products are likely causes of the pressor response because they can activate groups III and IV afferents during electrically induced contractions. Effects of lactic acid appear most powerful because they cannot be matched by equal molar infusions of hydrochloric acid. Somehow, lactate ions appear to potentiate the effects of hydrogen ions (Thimm et al., 1984; Rotto et al., 1989b). Bradykinin, which binds to kinin receptors of vascular endothelium, releases prostaglandins. Injection of bradykinin reflexly raises blood pressure and this response is reduced by inhibition of prostaglandin synthesis with indomethacin; the pressor response is restored by prostaglandin E_2 infusion (Stebbins and Longhurst, 1985).

Mechanosensitivity

Nonnoxious mechanical stimulation of receptor fields with fingers and blunted forceps activated the majority of group III afferents and about one-third of the group IV afferents (Kaufman and Rybicki, 1987). Either stretching or compressing muscle can reflexly increase arterial pressure by activating groups III and IV afferents (Stebbins et al., 1988). For example, activation of these afferents by passive, graded elevations in muscle tension (from 500 g up to 8 kg in cat triceps surae) elicited graded increments in arterial pressure as did compression of the muscle by graded increases in external pressures ranging from 125 to 300 mmHg.

A fraction of groups III and IV afferents is activated by electrically induced isometric contractions. The immediate onset and rapid recovery of group III activity, as illustrated in Figure 11-2, are consistent with mechanoreceptor function. Figure 11-2 also shows in contrast a slower onset and more sustained activity by the group IV afferents. This is consistent with a chemoreceptive function caused by a gradual buildup of metabolites within the muscle (Kaufman et al., 1983, 1988).

Responses to Electrically Induced Muscle Contractions

The metabolic changes best correlated with the rise in arterial pressure during electrically induced isometric contractions are the increases in muscle venous lactate concentration and P_{CO_2} and the fall in venous pH (Stebbins and Longhurst, 1989). However, potentiation of this pressor reflex by muscle ischemia could not be fully explained by any further increases in these variables (Stebbins and Longhurst, 1989). Bradykinin and prostaglandins may contribute significantly to the rise in blood pressure (and group IV afferent activity) during static contractions. Ischemia further increases their production (Kaufman et al., 1984). Blockade of

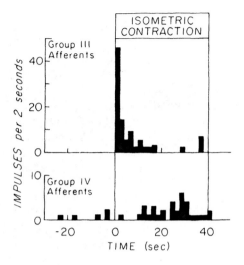

Figure 11-2 Discharge patterns of group III and group IV muscle afferents during isometric contraction of cat triceps surae (via electrical stimulation of the ventral roots). The discharge of group III afferents is highest at the onset of contraction and wains quickly and is consistent with mechanosensitivity. In contrast, the discharge of group IV afferents is delayed and tends to increase during contraction. This is consistent with chemosensitivity. (Adapted from Kaufman et al., 1983.)

bradykinin production significantly reduced the pressor responses to contraction (Stebbins and Longhurst, 1986) and blockade of prostaglandin synthesis reduced the pressor response to contraction by 76 percent; it was restored by exogenous prostaglandins. In addition, the converting enzyme inhibitor captopril, which inhibits the breakdown of bradykinin, increased the pressor response even after blockade of prostaglandins, indicating that bradykinin itself can exert an effect on arterial pressure (Stebbins and Longhurst, 1986). Isometric contraction more than doubled the levels of the prostaglandin precursor, arachidonic acid, in the muscle (Rotto et al., 1989a). Both cyclo-oxygenase and lipo-oxygenase products of arachidonic acid sensitized group III mechanosensitive afferents during contraction. Arachidonic acid administration increased discharge rates by 265 percent and indomethacin reduced them (Rotto et al., 1990).

At this point a tentative scheme might be that chemosensitive groups III and IV muscle afferents are activated whenever blood flow is restricted during a muscle contraction so that both delivery of oxygen and washout of metabolites are reduced. Lactic acid appears to be the substance most closely associated with the pressor response. In contrast, the mechanosensitive afferents appear to be sensitized by cyclo-oxygenase and lipo-oxygenase products of arachidonic acid whenever the force of contraction and restriction in blood flow foster their release. A concern here is the likelihood that the abnormal patterns of muscle contraction and force development during electrical stimulation might contribute to an abnormal release of bradykinin and prostaglandins. For example, even though electrical stimulation of muscle is not always painful in humans, the subsequent muscle soreness suggests that these substances may have been released. Electrical stimulation can cause minor tissue injury because of the abnormal muscle contractions and force development associated with this mode of activation. The role of kinins and prostaglandins during *voluntary* contractions is not clear (see Rowell and O'Leary, 1990).

It is important to keep in mind for the discussion of dynamic exercise (below) that release of vasoactive metabolites is most readily observed under conditions of *restricted blood flow*, that is, such as during isometric contractions rather than during the free-flow conditions of dynamic exercise. A reduction in muscle blood flow not only increases concentrations of metabolites in muscle venous blood, but often augments their production and their effects, especially for substances that might be diffusion-limited in normal free-flow conditions (i.e., the lower flow and longer transit time increases time for diffusion out of the muscle).

REFLEX RESPONSES TO VOLUNTARY ISOMETRIC CONTRACTIONS

As soon as isometric contractions become voluntary, there are the combined effects of central command and muscle reflexes to consider. As a beginning we assume that central command causes the initial increase in arterial pressure by rapidly increasing cardiac output through its sudden withdrawal of vagal activity. What then sustains and further increases the rise in arterial pressure?

An outgrowth of Alam and Smirk's (1937) original studies (see Figure 11-1) was the concept that the marked pressor responses to normal isometric contractions are also reflexly initiated by muscle ischemia. In this case the ischemia is presumed to be caused by mechanical compression of blood vessels and the consequent curtailment of blood flow during the contraction. With this hypothesis in mind isometric contraction, along with postexercise muscle ischemia, became the basic tools for the study of muscle chemoreflexes in humans, as well as in other species. The following sections review the findings that support the hypothesis.

What Stimuli Elicit the Pressor Response to Voluntary Isometric Contractions?

Depending on the type of muscle and the relative force development (percent of maximal voluntary contraction), isometric contractions impair muscle blood flow (see Chapter 8) and, as a consequence, lactic acid and other substances accumulate. Ischemia may exist only in portions of the muscle that are underperfused because of localized regions of high intramuscular pressure (Saltin et al., 1981). The examination of isometrically contracting forearm muscles with phosphorus 31 nuclear magnetic resonance spectroscopy indicates that activation of the muscle chemoreflex is closely associated with increments in intramuscular hydrogen ion activity, presumably associated with lactic acid formation (Victor et al., 1988). The onset of the reflex was identified by the sudden rise in muscle sympathetic nerve activity determined in a resting muscle by microneurography (see

Chapter 3). Increments in muscle sympathetic nerve activity (MSNA) (Victor et al., 1988) and in calf vascular resistance (Sinoway et al., 1989) were not significantly correlated with intramuscular concentrations of inorganic phosphate (Pi) and phosphocreatine (PCr) nor with their ratio, PCr/Pi (Pryor et al., 1990). During the pressor response to postexercise circulatory occlusion, all variables (except heart rate, which recovered) remained at levels near those observed at the final minute of contraction. Finally, MSNA did not rise during static contractions in patients with myophosphorylase deficiency (McArdle's disease) (Pryor et al., 1990). These patients are unable to break down muscle glycogen. Without glycolysis there is no lactic acid production. Together, all of these findings suggest that an event associated with muscle glycolysis and lactic acid production is required for reflex activation of MSNA during isometric contractions.

Sympathetic Nervous System, the Efferent Arm of Muscle Chemoreflexes and Mechanoreflexes

The current thinking is summarized in Figure 10-4, which attributes the initial increase in arterial pressure to central command and possibly a muscle mechanoreflex contributes as well. This scheme shows a delayed contribution from the muscle chemoreflex during the contraction and finally, it indicates that the persistent elevation in arterial pressure during the occlusion following contraction is caused exclusively by the muscle chemoreflex. Note also that this figure attributes none of the rise in heart rate to the muscle chemoreflex. Again, the reason for this idea is that heart rate recovers normally during postcontraction ischemia, meaning that arterial pressure must be kept elevated by sympathetic vasoconstriction rather than elevated cardiac output. This scheme is supported by the direct recordings of sympathetic nerve activity to resting muscles (MSNA) during an isometric contraction of other muscles.

Muscle Sympathetic Nerve Activity During Isometric Contractions

The rise in MSNA is delayed for approximately 0.5 to 2 minutes of an isometric contraction, depending on its severity (Mark et al., 1985; Saito et al., 1986; Seals et al., 1988a, 1988b; Seals, 1989a; Seals and Enoka, 1989; Victor and Seals, 1989) (Figure 11-3). This delay has been attributed to the time required for the accumulation of metabolites in the active muscle to a concentration needed to activate the muscle chemoreflex, which increases MSNA in the resting muscles (Mark et al., 1985). This assumption (there is no direct evidence) is supported by the finding that MSNA remains elevated *after* a contraction for as long as metabolites are entrapped within the muscle by vascular occlusion, as illustrated in Figure 11-3 (Mark et al., 1985; Seals et al., 1988a; Wallin et al., 1989). Seals (1989b) observed that the increases in arterial pressure and in MSNA are both roughly proportional to the mass of active muscle during the

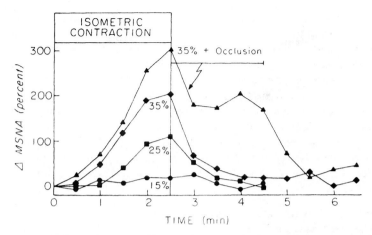

Figure 11-3 Average increases in muscle sympathetic nerve activity (ΔMSNA), expressed as percentage increase in total activity (burst frequency times amplitude), during and after 2.5 min of isometric contraction at 15, 25, and 35 percent of maximal voluntary contraction in eight subjects. Note that the muscle ischemia induced by postexercise occlusion prevents recovery of MSNA: this is a muscle chemoreflex. (Adapted from Seals et al., 1988a.)

contraction and also to the mass of muscle made ischemic by postexercise occlusion (Rowell et al., 1981). In general, these observations are all consistent with the assumption that MSNA is increased by muscle chemoreflexes. If mechanoreflexes rather than chemoreflexes were activated, one would expect an immediate rise in MSNA followed by rapid recovery at the end of contraction (Kaufman et al., 1983, 1988).

There is another way to interpret these results. The rise in MSNA is not only associated with rising hydrogen ion activity; it is also associated with increasing *fatigue* (Saito et al., 1989; Seals and Enoka, 1989). Thus the rise in MSNA might be related to increasing motor unit recruitment. This would suggest a possible role for central command in raising MSNA, an idea that has so far been discounted (see Victor et al., 1989). Nonfatiguing forearm contractions at 15 percent of maximum voluntary contraction force (MVC) are not accompanied by any rise in MSNA. With fatiguing contractions at 25 and 35 percent of MVC, MSNA (after a 1- to 2-minute delay), muscle electromyographic (EMG) activity, and arterial pressure all rise in parallel, as shown previously in Figure 8-9 (Seals and Enoka, 1989). Figure 8-9 also shows that with each successively more fatiguing contraction at 30 percent MVC, the rates of rise of MSNA, EMG activity, and arterial pressure increase so that peak values are reached at shorter contraction times (Saito et al., 1986; Seals and Enoka, 1989). The explanation by Seals and Enoka (1989) for the progressive rise in these variables was that the ischemia and resultant lactic acid production (not measured) induced by contraction would be expected to activate progressively chemosensitive muscle afferents during prolonged fatiguing contractions. Also, bear in mind that a fall in muscle pH impairs force development and requires greater motor unit recruitment which can be reflected by increased EMG activity (Hobbs, 1982; Hobbs and McCloskey, 1987). The findings could also be explained by the hypothesis of Hobbs (1982) (see Chapter 10) that activation of the cardiovascular system by central command is proportional to motor unit recruitment, which is augmented by fatigue and reflected in increased EMG activity.

We are left with a question. Is the fatigue-induced rise in arterial pressure due (wholly or in part) to augmented central command, or is the accelerated rise in MSNA attending fatigue related only to a crescendo of chemoreflex activity?

What Does the Increased Sympathetic Nerve Activity During Isometric Contractions Accomplish?

Earlier thinking held that the rise in sympathetic nerve activity during isometric contractions would cause vasoconstriction so that along with a rise in cardiac output, the fall in total vascular conductance would raise arterial pressure markedly. The rise in pressure was seen as a way of partially overcoming the mechanical restriction of muscle blood flow.

The question of what organs receive and respond to increased sympathetic nervous outflow during isometric contractions was discussed in Chapter 8. Arterial pressure during such contractions is increased by raising cardiac output; usually there is no significant change in total vascular conductance. There has been no discernable vasoconstriction in any of the organs investigated so far with the possible exception of the active muscle itself. Clearly, active muscle would be the least desirable target for the increased sympathetic vasoconstrictor activity. The muscle chemoreflex would, by vasoconstricting active muscle, set up a positive feedback condition that increases the accumulation of metabolites within the muscles and thereby worsens rather than improves metabolic conditions.

The muscle chemoreflex allegedly has as its primary function the improvement of the perfusion of active muscles. Conversely, if the reflex reduces muscle perfusion, perhaps we need to view it as a flow-sensitive, pressure-raising reflex rather than the flow-sensitive, flow-raising reflex that it was thought to be. The most important question to answer will be if the chemoreflex can raise muscle blood flow in dynamic exercise during which muscle perfusion and total vascular conductance normally increase.

Mechanoreflexes and Heart Rate: "The Muscle-Heart Reflex"

The current view is that heart rate is increased mainly by central command through its withdrawal of tonic vagal activity at the onset of exercise. Another view is that heart rate is also increased by the activation of muscle mechanoreflexes during the initial contractions at the onset of exercise. Some findings suggest that muscle mechanoreflexes mediated by group III afferents might initiate the rise in heart rate and some fraction of the rise in blood pressure during exercise. Hollander and Bouman (1975) offered evidence in support of a "muscle-heart reflex" in humans. Within 550 msec after the onset of either a voluntary or an electrically induced contraction (i.e., no central command), heart rate was suddenly increased by vagal withdrawal.

The entire increase in heart rate at the onset of exercise, or even a large portion of it, is probably not due to this mechanoreflex. For example, the sudden rise in heart rate in response to exercise is maintained in the face of sensory neuropathy or anesthetic blockade of sensory nerves (Freund et al., 1979; Duncan et al., 1981). One could, of course, argue the unlikely case that enough group III afferent activity was preserved in the patients with sensory loss and normal subjects with epidural anesthesia to explain their normal heart rate response. A more important point appears to be that there is more than one way to raise heart rate suddenly at the onset of exercise, that is, there is redundancy.

Role of Muscle Chemoreflexes in the Cardiovascular Responses to Isometric Contractions: A Summary

Figure 10-4 summarizes the idealized response to a strong isometric contraction. The immediate rise in arterial pressure is attributable to central command and its sudden withdrawal of tonic vagal outflow to the heart. The rise in blood pressure is proportional to the rise in cardiac output during the first seconds of contraction. Then, after a delay ranging from 30 seconds to 2 minutes, depending on the force of contraction, sympathetic activity to the heart and blood vessels of inactive muscles (MSNA) begins to increase. The rise in MSNA is attributed to the onset of a muscle chemoreflex initiated by the accumulation of metabolites within the contracting muscle. Metabolites accumulate because the muscle contractions mechanically impede its own blood flow (Chapter 8).

If muscle blood flow is arrested by vascular occlusion at the end of a contraction, the increase in MSNA measured during the contraction is maintained or may even increase despite the fall in arterial pressure to about one-half of its peak value during the contraction. The explanation for this persistent elevation in MSNA and arterial pressure is that the muscle chemoreflex is kept active by the continued accumulation of metabolites within the inactive muscle. The hypothetical explanation for the fall in arterial pressure below what it was during the contraction is that approximately one-half of the pressor response during contraction was induced by increased central command and the effects of vagal withdrawal on cardiac output. Thus the other half of the pressor response during contraction was attributed to the chemoreflex.

A generalization has emerged that the response to isometric contraction is governed by two separate mechanisms: one acts via the vagus nerve on heart rate and cardiac output, and the other acts via the sympathetic nervous system on the blood vessels. The increase in cardiac output is initiated by central command; the increase in sympathetic nervous activity is initiated by the muscle chemoreflex. Thus, the two components of the response exert their effects on the two separate arms of the autonomic nervous system. The notion that heart rate and arterial pressure are controlled by different mechanisms during and after isometric contraction came from the observation that heart rate fully recovers during postexercise occlusion when only the muscle chemoreflex is active, whereas arterial pressure is kept elevated by this chemoreflex (Lind, 1983; Mitchell and Schmidt, 1983; Rowell, 1986). Recall, however (Chapter 10), that Martin and colleagues (1974) and Maciel and colleagues (1987) saw a delayed but significant contribution of increased sympathetic activity to the rise in heart rate during isometric contraction; that is, part of the heart rate response was eliminated by the β-blocker propranolol. Thus the concept of separate control of the heart and vasculature may not be valid (see below).

IMPORTANCE OF THE MUSCLE CHEMOREFLEX DURING DYNAMIC EXERCISE

The shift from an analysis of control during isometric contraction of small muscle groups to control during dynamic exercise with large muscle groups is a large one. We direct our thinking away from a form of exertion characterized by an inability to secure adequate blood flow for contracting muscle. Cardiac output during isometric contraction is driven upward by central command and muscle reflexes without proportionate increases in total vascular conductance so that arterial pressure rises markedly. At moderate contraction forces the mechanical resistance to muscle blood flow overcomes this rising arterial pressure so that there is little or no increase in muscle blood flow. The perfusion of active muscle falls with greater force development. Therefore, isometric contractions provide conditions for initiating a muscle chemoreflex that are ideal.

Isometric contractions also provide experimental conditions that are comparable to those in so-called "open-loop" experiments. The receptors in the muscle can be virtually isolated from the influence of their efferent neural output on the cardiovascular system; that is, the muscles are deprived of the increased perfusion that counteracts the stimulus and tends to correct the error signal. This is not unlike investigating the systemic arterial pressor responses to changing pressure in the isolated carotid sinus. Carotid sinus pressure is not corrected by the change in systemic arterial pressure. In Chapter 6, the Cushing reflex was offered as one of the best-known examples of a similar condition. Such reflexes are commonly referred to as "positive feedback reflexes" because the responses to the error signal can increase the error. If the gain of the positive feedback is high, as it is the Cushing reflex (Chapter 6), then conditions will deteriorate rapidly.

Now, in contrast, consider *dynamic exercise,* for which response patterns are opposite to those during isometric contraction; there are large increases in total vascular conductance and only small increases in arterial pressure. The regulatory challenge is no longer to drive arterial pressure high enough to perfuse mechanically restricted muscle, but rather it is to drive cardiac output high enough to keep arterial pressure from falling. Thus the regulatory problems attending dynamic exercise are completely different from those associated with brief isometric contractions. A key question is whether the cardiovascular system can provide a high enough cardiac output during dynamic exercise to prevent the accumulation of metabolites within the muscle and the initiation of a muscle chemoreflex. The most important question is if there is a level of dynamic exercise at which the muscle chemoreflex becomes a tonically active controller of the cardiovascular system.

Importance of Muscle Mass in Dynamic Exercise

The preceding introduction pinpoints the regulatory challenge of dynamic exercise, which is to provide enough cardiac output to maintain arterial pressure. The discussion, therefore, is focused on dynamic exercise employing large masses of active muscle. Control may differ when the mass of active muscle is small.

Blomqvist and colleagues (1981) argued that there was little difference between the cardiovascular responses to isometric contractions and to dynamic exercise with small muscle groups. Clearly, at any given *absolute* oxygen uptake the smaller the muscle mass, the greater the demands for blood flow and oxidative capacity per 100 g of muscle. If the mass of dynamically active muscle is small, the drive to increase cardiac output will not be compensated by a large enough increase in total vascular conductance to prevent a rise in arterial pressure. It is an old observation that dynamic exercise with small muscle groups elicits cardiovascular responses that are exaggerated relative to the responses to exercise with large muscle groups at a given absolute oxygen uptake (see Bevegård et al., 1966, Freyschuss and Strandell, 1968). Thus the changes in MSNA attending rhythmic exercise with small muscle groups may not be representative of the changes in MSNA that might attend dynamic exercise with large muscles.

Characteristic Responses of Muscle Sympathetic Nerve Activity in Dynamic Exercise with Small Muscles

Rhythmic contractions with *small muscle groups* have the same effects on MSNA as characterized above for isometric contractions (Victor et al.,

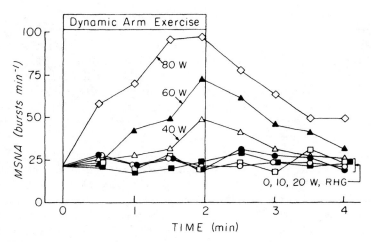

Figure 11-4 Muscle sympathetic nervous activity is increased in proportion to intensity of dynamic arm exercise (cycling). All data are unpublished observations from one of the investigators (D.R. Seals) in a study by Victor et al. (1987). This subject could reach 80 watts before body motion made microneurographic measurements from the peroneal nerve impossible. Two outstanding features: (1) Muscle sympathetic nerve activity (MSNA) did not rise until exercise level reached 40 watts (this threshold also existed for all six subjects). (2) The delay of the onset of increased MSNA was reduced at the highest level (80 watts). It rose high enough in 30 seconds to suggest the possibility that in heavier exercise, MSNA may increase immediately. (Data kindly provided by D.R. Seals.)

1987; Seals et al., 1988b; Victor and Seals, 1989), as shown in Figure 11-4. The exercise was with small muscle groups (i.e., dynamic arm exercise) because body motion attending exercise with larger muscles tended to disrupt microneurographic recordings. The main findings were as follows:

1. For rhythmic dynamic contractions the threshold for developed force is 33 percent of maximum before a rise in MSNA occurs. In relative terms, the exercise severity required to increase MSNA is greater for dynamic exercise than for isometric contractions. Once the increase in MSNA has occurred, it is proportional to the severity of exercise.
2. MSNA rises only after a delay of approximately 1 to 2 minutes depending on the force of contraction. It is important to remember that this delay is presumed to signify a chemoreflex origin and that this delay decreases with increasing severity of exercise (see Figure 11-4).
3. MSNA remains elevated during postexercise ischemia (muscle chemoreflex) and the rise is proportional to muscle mass.

There is one important addition: during rhythmic (dynamic) handgrip or two-arm cycling exercise, as exercise intensity is gradually increased and heart rate approaches 100 beats min^{-1}, MSNA begins to rise (also, spill-over of norepinephrine into plasma starts to increase) (Victor et al., 1987, 1989; Seals et al., 1988b) (Figure 11-5). At this heart rate in humans, nearly all vagal activity is withdrawn so that further *increases in heart rate require the activation of the more slowly responding sympathetic nervous system.*

As a first approximation it appears that during mild dynamic exercise at heart rates below 100 beats min^{-1} and before the sympathetic nervous system becomes active (see Figure 5-4), that control of the circulation could be dominated by central command signals, the actions of which are primarily on the parasympathetic nervous sytem. That is, the primary response is the withdrawal of vagal outflow to the heart and a rapid rise in its rate and output; initially, there are no sympathetically mediated events. This proposal for dynamic exercise is a logical outgrowth of what was said about circulatory control during isometric contractions.

Characteristic Responses of Overall Sympathetic Activity in Dynamic Exercise with Large Muscle Groups

Unfortunately we cannot compare the magnitude and time course of MSNA during dynamic exercise with small muscle groups to MSNA responses during exercise with large muscles, again because of the sensitivity of the microneurographic technique to the body motion. Figure 11-6 summarizes the known human sympathetic responses to "whole-body" dynamic exercise and continues the discussion that left off in Chapters 6 and 7. The data in Figure 11-6 were compiled from results and figures presented in those two chapters.

The important points in Figure 11-6 are as follows. *First:* Based on measurements of splanchnic and renal blood flows (along with arterial pressure and calculated vascular conductance) plus measurements of plasma norepinephrine concentration and renin activity, sympathetic nervous activity does not begin to rise in humans during dynamic exercise until heart rate approaches 100 beats min^{-1}. *Second:* At lower heart rates,

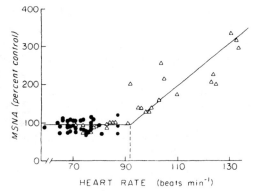

Figure 11-5 Relationship between heart rate and muscle sympathetic nerve activity during rhythmic hand-grip *(solid circles,* 10 to 50 percent of maximal voluntary contraction [MVC]) at 0 to 80 watts. When heart rate approached 100 beats min^{-1}, the progressive increase in muscle sympathetic nerve activity (MSNA) began. Compare with Figure 11-14. (Adapted from Victor et al., 1987.)

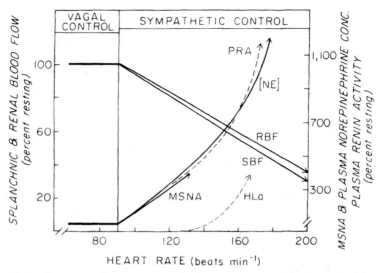

Figure 11-6 Summary of human sympathetic responses to mild-to-maximal dynamic exercise. Sympathetic nervous activity begins to rise when vagal withdrawal is nearly complete and heart rate approaches 100 beats min^{-1}. The indices of increased sympathetic control are splanchnic and renal vasoconstriction (decline in RBF and SBF), increased plasma norepinephrine (NE) concentration, and plasma renin activity (PRA). Skin and coronary arteries also vasoconstrict, suggesting a diffuse sympathetic outflow. The rise in MSNA (see Figure 11-5) was measured during arm cycling (small muscle mass), so its rate of rise versus heart rate may be different than for whole-body exercise. Lactic acid (HLa) does not rise until heart rate reaches 130 to 140 beats min^{-1} (50 to 60 percent $\dot{V}O_2$max). (Adapted from Rowell and O'Leary, 1990.)

the heart is predominantly under parasympathetic control. MSNA is also shown in Figure 11-6 because, as noted earlier, it also begins to increase during dynamic exercise (but with smaller muscle groups) when heart rate approaches 100 beats min^{-1}. Keep in mind, however, that MSNA has not been measured under the same conditions of dynamic exercise that apply to the other variables shown in Figure 11-6.

Some other features of sympathetic control in dynamic exercise (not shown in Figure 11-6) are the immediate constriction of cutaneous arteries and veins (Chapter 6) and even the constriction of coronary arteries and *active* skeletal muscle (the major source of norepinephrine spillover) as well as the inactive muscle (Chapter 7). Although the evidence is solid that there can be nonuniformity of sympathetic outflow with its sometimes discrete activation of some organs and not others (Simon and Riedel, 1975), it almost seems as though dynamic exercise is a condition under which sympathetic outflow is diffusely distributed. In fact, Figure 11-7 shows that virtually every organ examined by Hohimer and coworkers

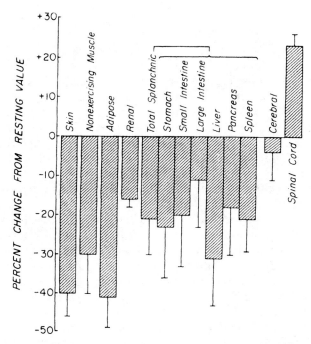

Figure 11-7 Humanlike redistribution of blood flow during mild dynamic exercise (cycling) in conscious baboons as measured from the distribution of radioactive microspheres. The spinal cord was the only inactive region in which blood flow rose during the 4-minute period of exercise in which oxygen uptake rose from 6.7 to 17.2 ml kg^{-1} min^{-1}; cardiac output from 2.75 to 4.14 L min^{-1}; heart rate from 118 to 157 beats min^{-1}; and arterial pressure from 106 to 117 mmHg. (From Rowell et al., 1986, with permission from Oxford University Press.)

(1983) in cycling, conscious baboons was vasoconstricted (as determined by distribution of labeled microspheres). Bear in mind that, although MSNA is by necessity measured in inactive muscles, any assumption that MSNA is not also increased in the *active* muscles as well is unsupported.

Is this uniform and highly reproducible pattern of sympathetic nervous activity the signature of an active muscle chemoreflex, or does something else cause this widespread increase in sympathetic activity?

Role of the Muscle Chemoreflex During Mild Dynamic Exercise

Is the muscle chemoreflex activated during mild dynamic exercise when muscle blood flow is unrestricted? Alternatively, is the muscle chemoreflex elicited only when muscle blood flow—or its oxygen delivery—falls below some critical level?

The Muscle Chemoreflex During Total Vascular Occlusion

When the muscle circulation is arrested immediately after *free-flow* dynamic exercise, the rise in arterial pressure seen during exercise persists as long as blood flow is arrested, as though the chemoreflex had raised pressure during exercise (Alam and Smirk, 1937; Rowell et al., 1976) (Figure 11-8). This blood pressure-raising reflex is augmented in proportion to the degree of oxygen deficiency in the muscle; oxygen deficiency was progressively increase by first beginning complete circulatory occlusion of both legs immediately at the end of exercise and then in subsequent bouts of exercise at 10, 20, and 30 seconds before exercise stopped in order to increase the quantity of metabolites trapped in the muscles when cycling stopped.

Note that the subject in Figure 11-8 showed a progressive tachycardia with increasing postexercise ischemia. In some subjects muscle ischemia had no effect on heart rate recovery, whereas one individual showed a progressive bradycardia with each increase in postexercise ischemia and arterial pressure. As is the case during isometric contractions, the cardiovascular system always finds a strategy for raising arterial pressure during muscle ischemia.

The recovery of ventilation was unaffected by muscle chemoreflexes (it actually falls faster during ischemia because oxygen consumption is lower). This was observed previously by Dejours and colleagues (1959). The point is that there seems to be no significant drive for muscle chemoreflexes to increase ventilation.

In a subsequent study with the same protocol as in Figure 11-8 (different subjects), the rise in arterial pressure was attributable to the maintenance of an elevated heart rate and cardiac output despite the large reduction in total vascular conductance caused by occluding both legs (Bonde-Petersen et al., 1978). The rise in heart rate during postexercise occlusion, in contrast to the rapid recovery during occlusion after an isometric contraction, argued that there is a heart rate component for the muscle chemoreflex.

Are Arterial Pressure and Heart Rate Controlled by Different Mechanisms During Exercise and Postexercise Ischemia?

During postexercise occlusion and muscle ischemia, the influences of central command and the mechanoreflex disappear and arterial pressure is kept elevated by the muscle chemoreflex. Despite the persistent chemoreflex, heart rate recovers fully during occlusion after an isometric contraction. Again, this has led to the idea that heart rate and sympathetic vasomotor outflow are controlled differently during and after isometric contractions (e.g., Lind, 1983; Mitchell and Schmidt, 1983; Rowell, 1986). Conversely, the rise in heart rate during ischemia after dynamic exercise would argue against the idea.

O'Leary (1991) studied the mechanism of heart rate control both during and after dynamic exercise with ischemia induced by vascular occlusion.

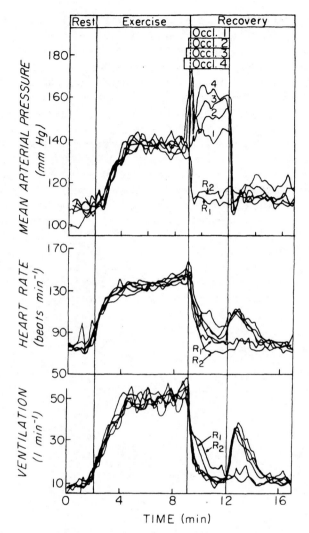

Figure 11-8 Circulatory and ventilatory responses from one subject during rest, leg exercise (cycling) at 150 watts with no occlusion, and then with total circulatory occlusion (Occl.) of both legs beginning immediately at the end of exercise, Occl. 1 (protocol for occlusions is at top), and 10, 20, and 30 seconds before the end of exercise (Occl. 2, 3, and 4, respectively). All occlusions persisted throughout the first 3 minutes of recovery (9-12 minutes). R_1 and R_2 denote normal recoveries from exercise without occlusion. Pressor responses during the 3-minute postexercise ischemia were graded in relation to duration of occlusion during exercise, that is, pressor responses 1 to 4 correspond to occlusions 1 to 4. Heart rate rose during postexercise occlusion in proportion to the rise in arterial pressure (not all subjects raised heart rate and one lowered it with each successive occlusion—owing to baroreflex influences; see Chapter 12). Postexercise ischemia of the muscle chemoreflex had no effect on ventilation which was lower during occlusion because oxygen uptake was lower. (Adapted from Rowell et al., 1976.)

The postexercise results are illustrated in Figure 11-9. The responses to exercise and postexercise occlusion are equivalent to those for isometric contractions in Figure 10-4 (the exception is that blood pressure remains at exercise levels during occlusion immediately after dynamic exercise). After parasympathetic blockade with atropine, both arterial pressure and heart rate remained elevated during postexercise ischemia (Figure 11-9). This means that sympathetic activity to the heart as well as to the blood vessels is sustained and that *heart rate as well as arterial pressure is under control of the muscle chemoreflexes* during postexercise ischemia. Normally, however, this sympathetic activation of the heart by the chemoreflex is overpowered by the dominance of parasympathetic control of cardiac pacemaker activity (Levy and Zieske, 1969). When exercise stops and both central command and vagal withdrawal end, the sudden restoration of vagal activity causes bradycardia and obscures the fact that heart rate is also under sympathetic control initiated by the muscle chemoreflex during dynamic exercise, isometric contractions, and postexercise ischemia (O'Leary, 1991). O'Leary's observation simplifies the discussion of dynamic exercise because, without a heart rate and cardiac output component, the muscle chemoreflex would not be able to raise muscle blood flow by increasing cardiac output.

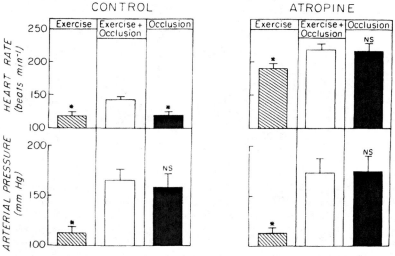

Figure 11-9 Evidence that heart rate is controlled both by central command and muscle chemoreflexes during both exercise with partial occlusion and postexercise ischemia. Atropine did not affect the increases in arterial pressure, but prevented the fall in heart rate during postexercise occlusion. Normally when exercise ends and occlusion continues, heart rate falls abruptly because both central command and inhibition of vagal activity end; sympathetic activation of the heart by the chemoreflex is normally overpowered by the reintroduction of vagal activity during postexercise ischemia, but atropine prevents this. (Adapted from O'Leary, 1991.)

Circulatory Responses After Elimination of the Muscle Chemoreflex by Sensory Blockade

None of the preceding experiments reveals whether the pressure-raising chemoreflex from ischemic muscle is actually part of a normal tonically *active* feedback to cardiovascular centers *during* dynamic exercise. Complete occlusion is an extreme stress, and the function of the pressor response to muscle ischemia might be to raise arterial pressure during crises such as intermittent claudication, when blood pressure falls to a critical level at which oxygen delivery is no longer adequate. Parenthetically, a pressor response does occur in such patients during claudication (Lorentsen, 1972).

Freund and colleagues (1979), blocked the muscle afferents by peridural anesthesia with the objective of seeing if cardiovascular responses to exercise were changed in the absence of the muscle chemoreflex. The sensory blockade abolished the pressor responses to postexercise ischemia, meaning that they had successfully blocked the afferent fibers for the muscle chemoreflex (see below). Figure 11-10 shows how the initial motor weakness exaggerated cardiovascular responses, but Figure 11-11 shows the responses to a later period of exercise during which sensory blockade of small fibers was still "complete" (as judged by the continued absence of a pressor response to postexercise ischemia), but much of the motor and proprioceptive functions had recovered. Although the muscle chemoreflex was still blocked, cardiovascular responses to mild dynamic exercise had returned to normal (i.e., preblockade). This suggests that the sensory fibers that mediate the pressor response to muscle ischemia are not essential for the normal matching between cardiovascular and metabolic responses during mild dynamic exercise.

The results of experiments employing differential anesthetic blockade have been difficult to interpret because the goal of leaving the large motor fibers intact while at the same time effecting a complete sensory loss has not been achieved (see Freund et al., 1979; Lassen et al., 1989; Mitchell et al., 1989; Fernandes et al., 1990). The critical problem is that it has not been possible to *abolish the pressor response to postexercise muscle ischemia without causing profound motor weakness.* Freund and colleagues (1979) argued that the persistance of any pressor response during postexercise occlusion meant that at least part of the muscle chemoreflex was intact and therefore responses could be due to both this reflex and central command. In the efforts of Fernandes and coworkers (1990), for example, to preserve motor strength, the muscle chemoreflex was not blocked (e.g., see Figures 12 and 13 in Mitchell, 1990). Their subjects were able to carry out moderate to heavy exercise, in contrast to those subjects of Freund and coworkers (1979), who had complete blockade of the muscle chemoreflex, but unfortunately they also had profound motor weakness and therefore could only perform mild exercise. This meant that the motor weakness may require that force be developed with the aid of additional

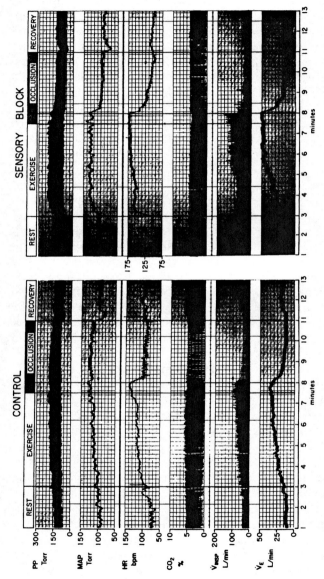

Figure 11-10 Abolishment of the pressor response to muscle ischemia by sensory block (peridural anesthesia). From top to bottom, variables are radial arterial pulse pressure (PP) in mmHg or torr, mean arterial pressure (MAP), heart rate (HR), end-tidal CO_2 concentration, inspiratory flow velocity (Vinsp), and ventilation (V_E). Left panel (control) shows normal responses to mild dynamic leg exercise (50 watts), 30-second occlusion during exercise, and 3 minutes of postexercise occlusion (as in Figure 11-8). Right panel shows responses from the same subject after sensory nerve block when motor weakness and proprioceptive loss was profound. Note the exaggerated cardiovascular responses and the loss of the postexercise pressor response during postexercise occlusion after sensory block. (From Freund et al., 1979, with permission from the American Physiological Society.)

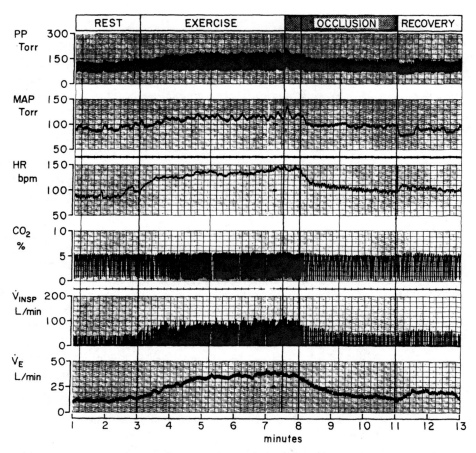

Figure 11-11 Responses to the second period of exercise after sensory blockade by peridural anesthesia (symbols as for Figure 11-10). Same subject as in Figure 11-10, but after much of motor and proprioceptive functions had recovered, and sensory nerve block and blockade of the muscle pressor responses persisted. Note the return of heart rate (and ventilation) toward the control levels shown in Figure 11-10. (From Freund et al., 1979, with permission from the American Physiological Society.)

muscle groups as validly argued by Lassen and coworkers (1989) and Fernandes and coworkers (1990).

The conclusion of Freund and colleagues (1979) that reflexes from active muscles are not tonically active during mild dynamic exercise was supported by experiments made in dogs with selective lesions in the lateral funiculus of the lumbar spinal cord. These lesions avoided most of the descending sympathetic and somatomotor pathways (Kozelka et al., 1987). The lesions selectively severed the ascending spinal pathways carrying afferent nerve traffic from the exercising hindlimbs (the dogs were trained to run on a treadmill on their hind legs only). The lesions markedly reduced

the increase in heart rate and arterial pressure in response to hindlimb
ischemia caused by occlusion of the left external iliac artery. However,
these lesions did not significantly affect the cardiovascular responses to
three levels of exercise without occlusion. The experiments of Kozelka
and colleagues (1987) make a second important point. The rise in arterial
pressure during exercise with muscle ischemia cannot be ascribed to an
increase in central command caused by the motor weakness; otherwise,
the pressor response to ischemia would not have been blocked, that is,
the pressor response is, as assumed, due to a muscle reflex.

Role of Muscle Chemoreflex in Maintaining Muscle Blood Flow During Mild Dynamic Exercise with Partial Occlusion of the Circulation to Active Muscle

A straightforward functional test of the chemoreflex hypothesis is made
by reducing blood flow to active muscle and observing the extent to which
the reflex restores blood flow. If the reflex restored blood flow two-thirds
of the way back to control blood flow before partial occlusion, the reflex
would have a sensitivity or open-loop gain of two, which is not unlike the
gain of the powerful arterial baroreflex (Chapter 12) (see Chapter 6, "Open-
Loop Experiments"). In short, if the reflex partially restores muscle blood
flow back to what it was before flow was reduced, it works; if it only raises
arterial pressure without partially restoring muscle blood flow, it does not
work purposefully. It was suggested earlier in this chapter that if a target
of chemoreflex-induced vasoconstriction is the contracting muscle from
which it originates, the reflex simply raises arterial pressure and overper-
fuses other organs without increasing active muscle blood flow enough to
wash out metabolites and reduce the metabolic error signal. That is, it
would be a *pressure-raising reflex with positive feedback and not a flow-
raising reflex with negative feedback.*

The extent of error correction by the chemoreflex would depend on its
gain or sensitivity and also the extent to which it is opposed by arterial
baroreflexes, if a rise in arterial pressure is involved; it also depends on
the extent to which active muscle is vasoconstricted. As the severity of
exercise increases, the margin for any "flow error" might decrease and
become extremely small, or even disappear, so that a persistent metabolic
error signal could maintain a tonically active muscle chemoreflex. This
would mean that the adequacy of muscle perfusion could be tonically
monitored during exercise. The goal of the experiments described below
is to provide information concerning the gain or sensitivity of the reflex
and to discover if it becomes tonically active during heavier exercise.

A Critical Test of the Chemoreflex Hypothesis

Figure 11-12 illustrates schematically a critial test of the muscle chemoreflex hypothesis. Figure 11-12A,D shows the basic experimental design
employed in the characterization of the muscle chemoreflex in voluntarily

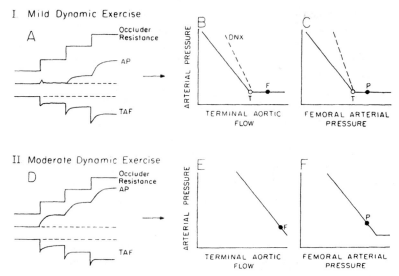

Figure 11-12   Schematic illustration of responses to the muscle chemoreflex during mild and moderate dynamic exercise. I. *Mild exercise.* (**A**) Graded increments in resistance across an occluder on the terminal aorta of an exercising dog will generate graded decrements in terminal aortic flow (TAF), but arterial pressure (AP) will not rise and TAF will not be partially restored until the chemoreflex becomes active, which happens at the second and third occlusions. The rise in AP causes a 50 percent recovery of TAF. (**B and C**) Stimulus-response curves for the chemoreflex show that the reflex has a threshold (T). "Prevailing" TAF (F, in Figure **B**) and femoral arterial pressure (P, in Figure **C**) represent their normal operating levels in exercise, which are on the flat (low-gain) parts of the curves. Therefore the chemoreflex is not tonically active and AP does not rise until TAF and/or femoral arterial pressure fall below some critical level. II. *Moderate dynamic exercise.* (**D**) Characteristic responses of a tonically active muscle chemoreflex. (**E and F**) Prevailing TAF and P are on the steep (high-gain) portion of the stimulus-response curves and there is no threshold. The dashed line (DNX) shows the effect of arterial baroreceptor denervation on the gain of the chemoreflex (see Chapter 12). (Adapted from Rowell and Sheriff, 1988, and Rowell and O'Leary, 1990.)

exercising dogs by Wyss and colleagues (1983) and Sheriff and colleagues (1987, 1990). They applied stepwise partial occlusions of the terminal aorta in dogs running at different speeds and grades on a motor-driven treadmill. If it is so that the muscle chemoreflex is *not* tonically active during mild dynamic exercise, but functions only when muscle blood flow is reduced below some critical level, responses would appear as they are shown in Panel A. The initial partial occlusion had no effect on arterial pressure (BP) and there was no restoration of terminal aortic flow (TAF) back toward preocclusion values; that is, there was neither a flow-raising nor a pressure-raising reflex. Figure 11-12B,C shows the stimulus-response curves relating systemic arterial pressure to the decrements in terminal aortic flow and in femoral arterial pressure below the terminal aortic occluder, that is muscle perfusion pressure. These two depictions of the muscle chemoreflex show it to have a disinct *threshold* (T) or break point for blood flow and femoral arterial pressure above which the gain is zero (or too small to be functionally significant) once the slope of the stimulus-response line is corrected for the mechanical effects of partial occlusion (this correction is not shown in Figure 11-12; see Wyss and colleagues, 1983). Above the threshold, the rise in systemic arterial pressure was four times greater than that attributed to the mechanical effect of occlusion. Inasmuch as large reductions in terminal aortic flow and in femoral pressure were required to reach this threshold, the margin for any "flow error" was large; therefore, the reflex must not be tonically active. Once the threshold was past and the reflex became active, its sensitivity or "open-loop gain" was calculated as the rise in systemic arterial pressure (again corrected for the mechanical effects of occlusion) divided by the fall in femoral arterial pressure below the occluder. Calculated gains for the reflex range from -2 to -3 (Sheriff et al., 1987, 1990), meaning that the "closed-loop gain" of the reflex was -0.67 to -0.75, based on the equation

$$G_{CL} = \frac{G_{OL}}{1 - G_{OL}}, \qquad (11\text{-}1)$$

where G_{CL} and G_{OL} are closed-loop and open-loop gains. Accordingly, beyond its threshold, the reflex can correct by 67 to 75 percent any deficit in muscle perfusion *pressure* when active muscle blood flow is restricted.

In agreement with Wyss and colleagues (1983) and Sheriff and colleagues (1987, 1990), Joyner (1991) found a distinct threshold for the pressor response in response to graded partial obstructions of muscle bloodflow during graded dynamic forearm exercise (rhythmic handgrip). Joyner (1991) reduced forearm blood flow by making stepwise increments in the pressure within a box surrounding the active arm. Analogous experiments carried out by Victor and Seals (1989) on human forearms with blood flow reduced by cuff inflations to subsystolic pressures (but with venous congestion) did not elicit increases in leg MSNA during mild arm cycling. Rather, complete vascular occlusion was required to increase MSNA; therefore, this reflex has a threshold during mild dynamic exercise.

Although the manner of calculating gain, described above, is the same one used to calculate the gain of the carotid sinus baroreflex, the muscle chemoreflex is supposed to be a flow-raising reflex, *not* a pressure-raising reflex. We have seen during isometric contractions that the reflex could raise arterial pressure without raising muscle blood flow; thus, these gain calculations could give a misleading impression of what the reflex is accomplishing if the rise in pressure does not raise blood flow and decrease the metabolic error signal.

Does the Muscle Chemoreflex Correct Blood Flow Errors?

Joyner (1991) saw no improvement in estimated forearm blood flow during rhythmic handgrip exercise when muscle ischemia and a rise in arterial pressure were elicited by partial occlusion, as shown in Figure 11-13. The pressure in the box used to lower muscle blood flow (50 mmHg; Figure 11-13) reduced calculated forearm blood flow by 20 to 25 percent, based on reductions in venous oxygen saturation. However, the approximately 20-mmHg rise in arterial pressure did not restore venous oxygen saturation—nor, by implication, muscle blood flow (the assumption is that forearm oxygen uptake did not change). Joyner (1991) concluded that the rise in sympathetic activity elicited by the chemoreflex vasoconstricted the active muscles and prevented the rise in muscle blood flow. Thus there was no correction of the metabolic "error signal."

The schematic representation of responses showing approximately 50 percent recovery of terminal aortic flow in Figure 11-12A,D is typical of the magnitude of blood flow correction measured by Sheriff and colleagues (1987, 1990). This response differs fundamentally from that described by Joyner (1991). Representative data from an animal during one of a sequence of partial occlusions are shown in Figure 11-14. Once the threshold

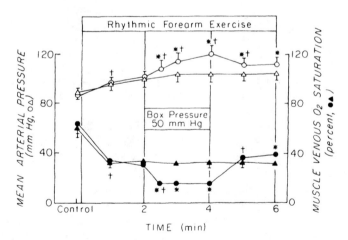

Figure 11-13 Apparent failure of the muscle chemoreflex to raise blood flow to ischemic forearm muscle during heavy rhythmic forearm exercise. Vasculature of active muscle was partially occluded by raising air pressure in a box surrounding the arm to 50 mmHg. Despite a rise in arterial pressure of 20 mmHg, deep forearm venous oxygen saturation did not increase, suggesting no increase in muscle perfusion, but rather an increase in its vascular resistance. Triangles show responses to control trial with no change in box pressure. Circles show responses to tests during which box pressure was raised. Asterisks and crosses denote significant changes with respect to control (*) or the previous minute of the same test (crosses). (Adapted from Joyner, 1991.)

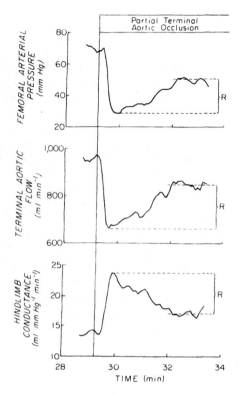

Figure 11-14 Successful action of the muscle chemoreflex in raising blood flow to ischemic exercising hindlimbs during partial terminal aortic occlusion. During moderate treadmill exercise graded partial occlusions were applied in the manner illustrated in Figure 11-12D. The occlusion shown here was midway through a sequence of graded occlusion. With each occlusion, terminal aortic flow was restored by approximately 50 percent by a rise in cardiac output and systemic arterial pressure (not shown). Vasodilation of the active muscle played a minor role as revealed by the fall in conductance during occlusion. (Data are from Sheriff et al., 1990.)

for the muscle chemoreflex is reached, this was the magnitude of recovery that was commonly observed at levels of partial occlusion that were both below and above the one shown.

The above findings are at odds with those of Joyner (1991), but not those of Rowell and colleagues (1991). Partial terminal aortic occlusion can be simulated in humans by lower body positive pressure. Subjects were sealed at the iliac crest into a large box containing a small cycle ergometer. Pressure in the box was increased in steps, just as was done in the box surrounding the forearm in Joyner's experiments. The reductions in leg blood flow were calculated from the increments in arterial-femoral venous oxygen difference (total oxygen uptake, at the mouth, remained constant). Figure 11-15 shows the effects of graded increments in box pressure at three levels of exercise requiring 1, 1.5, and 2 L O_2 min^{-1}. There was not, in contrast to other studies cited above, an obvious threshold for the pressure rise. Possibly the lowest work rate was above this threshold. Another point is that exercise was in the supine posture so that effective driving pressure for muscle blood flow is lower than in the upright position.

Rowell and colleagues (1991) concluded that opposition to the reduction in muscle blood flow by the chemoreflex must have been substantial

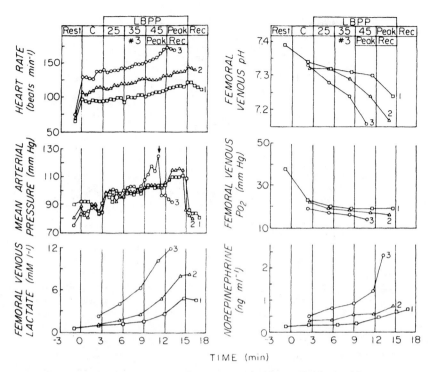

Figure 11-15 Responses of one subject to graded lower body positive pressure at 25, 35, 45, and 55 to 60 (peak) mmHg during mild to moderate supine cycling (oxygen uptake was ~1, 1.5, and 2.0 L min^{-1} at exercise levels 1, 2, and 3 [squares, triangles, and circles respectively]). There was no apparent threshold for the muscle chemoreflex, possibly because the load was not low enough or because supine exercise reduced effective muscle perfusion. The increments in mean arterial pressure were highly correlated with femoral venous lactate, pH, and Po$_2$. The rise in femoral venous norepinephrine signified marked increases in sympathetic activity at the highest exercise level (3). (Adapted from Rowell et al., 1991.)

inasmuch as the percentage decrements in leg vascular conductance during occlusion exceeded the reductions in muscle blood flow by twofold (Figure 11-16). Approximately 50 percent of the correction of muscle blood flow back toward control could be explained by the rise in heart rate (and thus in cardiac output assuming that stroke volume did not fall; see Bonde-Petersen and colleagues [1978]). Wyss and colleagues (1983) had come to the same conclusion when they measured cardiac output and determined the changes in vascular conductance for the entire animal and the hindlimb during partial occlusion of the terminal aorta. Part of the restoration in muscle perfusion indicated in Figure 11-16 could be explained by vasoconstriction as suggested by the high norepinephrine levels and also by the purely passive mechanical effects of partially occluding such a large mus-

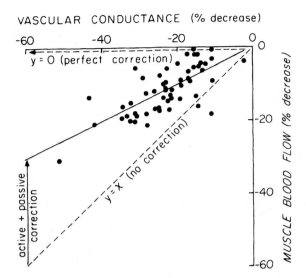

Figure 11-16   Indirect evidence for partial correction of muscle blood flow in exercising humans during partial occlusion of leg blood flow during supine exercise by lower body postitive pressure. See Figure 11-15 for protocol and representative data. Dashed line of identity ($y = x$) shows relationship of percent decrease in vascular conductance and muscle blood flow if there were no correction of muscle blood flow by increased arterial pressure (pressure constant). The horizontal dashed line ($y = 0$) shows what responses would be if there were perfect correction of muscle blood flow by increased arterial pressure. Solid regression line and filled circles suggest a *50 percent correction* of muscle blood flow; this could be accounted for partly by the calculated increase in cardiac output. Part of the correction was probably attributable to vasoconstriction and part to purely passive mechanical effects of partial occlusion, which could not be computed (see text). (From Rowell et al., 1991, with permission of the American Physiological Society.)

cle mass. Parenthetically, the effect of occlusion on mean arterial pressure cannot be calculated from the difference between intra-arterial pressure (unaffected by box pressure) and tissue pressure (or box pressure) for reasons discussed by Rowell and colleagues (1991).

What Causes the Threshold for the Muscle Chemoreflex?

In an earlier section of this chapter, evidence was presented that the rise in leg MSNA accompanying an isometric forearm contraction exceeding 15 percent of MVC is closely associated with the production of lactic acid in the muscle. Sheriff and colleagues (1987) proposed two models that might explain the accumulation of some "pressor substance" in the active muscle. In the first model the release of the pressor substance from the muscle simply depends on muscle blood flow, on the muscle's rate of work, and on the rate of washout of the substance from muscle interstitial space. During partial occlusion, this substance accumulates simply because the rate of washout from the muscle is reduced. In the second model, washout from muscle is also blood flow-dependent, but the substance's rate of production and release from muscle are governed by the adequacy of oxygen delivery; lactate provides an example of their second model.

Sheriff and colleagues (1987) found that the pressor response was initiated when oxygen delivery appeared to fall below the critical level. Figure 11-17 shows that when arterial oxygen content was lowered (this caused higher muscle blood flow), the pressor responses to partial terminal aortic occlusion occurred at higher blood flows (higher washout); but the *rate of oxygen delivery was the same* as when oxygen content and blood flow were normal. The pressor responses were most closely related to the

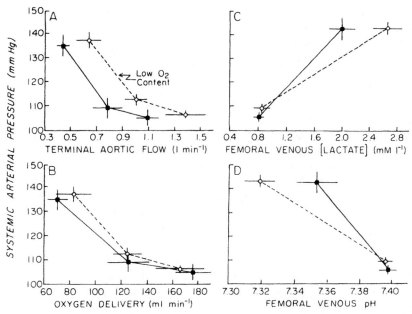

Figure 11-17 An experimental test of the hypothesis that muscle chemoreflexes are activated by a critical reduction in oxygen delivery rather than simply insufficient washout of metabolites. Average pressor responses (regression lines from multiple measurements on three dogs) to graded, partial terminal aortic occlusion are shown before (*solid lines*, normal response) and after blood flow was increased by reducing arterial oxygen content (dashed lines). (**A**) Reduced arterial oxygen content shifted the relationship between arterial pressure and terminal aortic flow, and the *threshold* for the pressor reflex to the right. (**B**) Relationship between arterial pressure and oxygen delivery was unaffected by lower oxygen content and higher blood flow. (**C**) and (**D**) Pressor responses were most closely related to femoral venous lactate concentration and pH, neither of which changed until after the threshold for the chemoreflex was reached. (From Rowell and Sheriff, 1988, with permission from the American Physiological Society.)

increments in femoral venous lactate (Figure 11-17C) and to decrements in pH (Figure 11-17D) at all levels of exercise. In agreement with these findings, Rowell and colleagues (1991) found during partial occlusion of the working legs by lower body positive pressure (Figure 11-15) that the rise in mean arterial pressure was well correlated with femoral venous pH and lactate concentration, and also Po_2, and O_2 content.

Thus the initiation of a muscle chemoreflex during dynamic exercise as well as during isometric contractions appears closely linked to a metabolic event that initiates production and accumulation of lactic acid in the muscle. Sheriff and colleagues (1987) found that the pressor response to ischemia was unrelated to the femoral venous concentration of potassium.

Summary. In summary, the studies employing partial occlusions of the circulation to active muscle during mild dynamic exercise usually show an approximately 50 percent recovery of muscle blood flow when the reflex is activated. About one-half of this 50 percent restoration of muscle blood flow is provided by the rise in heart rate and cardiac output. An increase in sympathetic vasoconstrictor outflow is also indicated by marked increases in neuronal leakage of norepinephrine into circulating plasma. In only one case has a partial correction of the fall in muscle blood flow during partial occlusion *not* been observed. The muscle chemoreflex has a distinct threshold and is clearly not tonically active during mild dynamic exercise. For simplicity, "open-loop" gain of the muscle chemoreflex has been calculated from the rise in systemic arterial pressure caused by the fall in femoral arterial pressure (below the vascular occluder). Calculated in this way, the open-loop gain of the reflex is -2 to -3. This assumes the rise in arterial pressure partially corrects the metabolic error signal by raising blood flow to the ischemic muscles. The closed-loop gain of the reflex is better estimated (but with more difficulty) from the percentage by which blood flow is restored; this is commonly about 50 percent, meaning the closed-loop gain expressed this way is 0.5 and the open-loop gain would be 1.0 (Equation 11-1). The threshold for the chemoreflex appears to be caused by a reduction in oxygen delivery rather than simply a fall in blood flow per se. Oxygen delivery falls below a critical level, causing increased tissue levels of lactic acid.

Role of the Muscle Chemoreflex in Maintaining Muscle Blood Flow During Moderate to Heavy Dynamic Exercise

The preceding section reveals that the adequacy of muscle perfusion appears not to be tonically monitored during mild dynamic exercise. It is possible in dogs, for example, to cause large reductions in muscle blood flow without increasing the "metabolic error signal" which is directly or indirectly linked to the production and release of lactic acid from the muscle. We come now to a crucial question raised previously: As exercise becomes more severe, does the margin for "blood flow error" become so small that a persistent metabolic error signal could maintain a tonically active muscle chemoreflex? This question is vital in establishing if the chemoreflex is involved in normal exercise responses or conversely, is only active when blood flow is artifically restricted or reduced to subnormal levels by vascular disease; that is, is this chemoreflex only for "emergencies"?

Figure 11-12D,E, and F schematically illustrate the results of experiments by Wyss and colleagues (1983) and Sheriff and colleagues (1987, 1990), this time with partial terminal aortic occlusion applied in steps during *moderate* exercise. These results are what would be expected if the muscle chemoreflex were *tonically active*. Each stepwise occlusion caused an immediate rise in arterial pressure that exceeded, by a factor of 4, the rise owing to the passive mechanical effect of increased hindlimb vascular resistance (Wyss et al., 1983). *The reflex had no apparent threshold.* Figure 11-12D shows that, during each partial occlusion, the muscle chemoreflex restored the muscle blood flow halfway back to the preocclusion level, that is, 50 percent recovery. Figure 11-12E,F show that the prevailing terminal aortic blood flow (point *F*) and the prevailing arterial pressure (point *P*) are moved by heavier exercise from the flat—zero gain—portion of the stimulus-response curve (as for mild exercise in Figure 11-12B,C) to the steep portion of the curve, reflecting possible tonic activity of the reflex. This activity is qualified as "possibly" tonic because it is not established whether the operating point of the reflex is just at the threshold and therefore not active until there is a slight decrease in blood flow. Alternatively, the reflex could be operating well up on its stimulus-response curve so that it is constantly responding to any small increase or decrease in blood flow.

Again, the estimates of gains based on the rise in arterial pressure versus those based on restoration of blood flow were not the same. Based on the corrected (for passive resistance effects) slope of the relationship between systemic arterial and femoral arterial pressure, open-loop gain of the reflex averaged -2 to -3 or 0.67 to 0.75 for closed-loop gain (Sheriff et al., 1987, 1990). The estimated open-loop gain based on a 50 percent correction of blood flow would, of course, be -1. These numbers are the same as those obtained after the reflex was activated during mild exercise. Although there has been no indication that the gain of the chemoreflex becomes greater with increases in exercise intensity, an increase in gain would be expected were the mass of active muscle to increase along with work intensity. The pressor response to the muscle chemoreflex increases in proportion to muscle mass (Freund et al., 1978).

The gain of the muscle reflex could not be reliably computed in exercising humans because it was not possible to correct for the mechanical effects of positive air pressure surrounding the legs on local and systemic vascular resistance (Rowell et al., 1991). Again, the veins were fully collapsed at low box pressures. The low gain of -0.35 to -0.39 for the chemoreflex in forearm muscle, calculated by Joyner (1991), was in part due to the small muscle mass and partly to the method of computing gain. In Joyner's study gain for the correction of muscle blood flow was zero, that is, there was no correction. A muscle chemoreflex elicited by a fall in total muscle blood flow during severe whole-body exercise might have an open-loop gain possibly as high as -4 or -5, again because the gain probably increases in proportion to muscle mass. So far we lack quantitative data on this point.

Bear in mind that all of these gain calculations have been made without any consideration of the arterial baroreflex (see Chapter 12). If this reflex is active and has an open-loop gain of 2 to 3, then presumably it would oppose the rise in arterial pressure attributable to the chemoreflex and reduce it by at least one-half. This would mean that the true open-loop gain of the chemoreflex pressor response would be in the order of -4 to -6 and not -2 to -3. The complex interplay between these two powerful and competing reflexes is dealt with in Chapter 12.

Can Muscle Chemoreflexes Explain the Rise in Sympathetic Nervous Activity During Moderate to Heavy Dynamic Exercise?

If it is true that central command determines parasympathetic outflow, whereas muscle chemoreflexes determine sympathetic nervous outflow (i.e., this is the model discussed previously for isometric contractions) then the events described in Figure 11-6 for moderate to heavy dynamic exercise could be explained by activation of this chemoreflex. Against this idea is the fact that the release of lactic acid from active muscle does not begin in dynamically exercising humans until rates of work far exceed those at which sympathetic nervous activity increases significantly. In physically unconditioned subjects plasma lactic acid concentration does not increase until exercise requires approximately 50 to 60 percent of $\dot{V}o_2max$, and not before heart rate reaches 130 to 140 beats min^{-1}. In physically well-conditioned individuals, lactate release may not begin until exercise requires 80 percent or more of $\dot{V}o_2max$. Yet the increase in sympathetic nervous activity with exercise follows the same relation to heart rate portrayed in Figure 11-6, irrespective of the point at which lactate concentration first increases, and irrespective of the magnitude of $\dot{V}o_2max$ (Rowell, 1974).

If we agree that the onset of the muscle chemoreflex in dogs and humans parallels the rise in muscle venous lactic acid concentration, how can we explain the steady increase in sympathetic nervous activity and reflex vasoconstriction that occurs in humans when heart rate rises above 100 beats min^{-1}, that is, long before production of lactic acid begins?

There is another problem. Canine muscle has high oxidative capacity and its release of lactate probably does indicate a reduction in oxygen delivery below a critical level. The same could be true as well in humans when muscle blood flow is actively reduced, for example, by intermittent claudication. However, the problem is that when lactate release begins in dynamically exercising humans under normal, free-flow conditions, it does not normally reflect inadequate delivery of oxygen to the active muscle. It is well known that oxidative capacity of human muscle is far below that of dogs. In humans lactate is released as soon as muscle glycolysis and oxidation of glucose become a significant part of total oxidative metabolism. This occurs when β-oxidation of free-fatty acids can no longer provide the active acetate needed for oxidative reactions of the tricarboxylic acid cycle. Because of the increased utilization of glucose, more pyruvate is produced than can be utilized in the tricarboxylic acid cycle (Gollnick et al., 1985). Thus, the appearance of lactate reflects our limited ability to utilize pyruvate—not inadequate oxygen delivery, or an "anaerobic threshold," as this substrate transition has been inappropriately labeled. In short, there is no reason to propose that the appearance of lactic acid during normal (free-flow) dynamic exercise would be associated with the initiation of a muscle chemoreflex. Therefore, some other stimulus must be responsible for the increase in sympathetic nervous activity once heart rate exeeds 100 beats min^{-1} (Chapter 12).

Does Muscle Sympathetic Nerve Activity Reflect the Overall Rise in Sympathetic Nervous Activity During Moderate to Heavy Dynamic Exercise?

The evidence indicating that the rise in MSNA during isometric contractions is related to the initiation of a muscle chemoreflex appears to be solid. In isometric contractions the setting is ideal; blood flow and oxygen delivery *decreases* with *increases* in both contraction force and oxygen demand. Regrettably, however, the reflex appears not to improve muscle blood flow.

Moderate dynamic exercise with relatively *small* muscle groups (e.g., arms) increases MSNA when heart rate approaches 100 beats min^{-1} (Figure 11-5). As pointed out by Blomqvist and colleagues (1981), Bevegård and colleagues (1966), and Freyschuss and Strandell (1968), cardiovascular responses and lactate release are much greater at a given absolute oxygen uptake during exercise with the arms than with the legs. As with isometric contractions, the increase in MSNA during arm exercise is delayed, so it is assumed here as well that this rise is attributable to the initiation of a muscle chemoreflex. Inasmuch as the absolute demands for blood flow and oxygen can be high relative to the small mass of active muscle during arm exercise, the chemoreflex hypothesis may be valid here as well.

The critical question is: Does MSNA rise along with sympathetic vasomotor outflow to the splanchnic organs, kidneys, skin and so on during dynamic exercise with large muscles? The question, which cannot now be answered, is raised to direct attention to the inclusion of MSNA along with other sympathetically mediated variables in Figure 11-6. If MSNA were to rise, as it is shown in Figure 11-6, we would have to conclude that the stimulus is not the muscle chemoreflex because the rise precedes that of lactic acid.

There is one clue from some unpublished results kindly provided by Dr. Douglas Seals and shown in Figure 11-4. It shows the responses to dynamic arm exercise, including data from one investigator (Dr. Seals), at a level as high as 80 watts. Ths most important point in this figure is that the delay in the onset of MSNA shrinks as work rate increases. It suggests that with heavy dynamic exercise, MSNA may rise as quickly (10 to 20 seconds) as sympathetic nervous outflow to other regions. This might again suggest that something other than the muscle chemoreflex turns on MSNA during heavy dynamic exercise. One would not expect an immediate accumulation of metabolites with the high rates of blood flow, despite the high metabolic rate, during heavy dynamic exercise.

We need answers to the following questions (see Rowell and O'Leary, 1990):

1. Is the time delay in the onset of MSNA inversely proportional to active muscle mass and to the rate of work?
2. Does MSNA parallel the sympathetic vasomotor outflow to other regions such as splanchnic and kidneys; that is, does it increase within a few seconds after the onset of dynamic exercise with large muscles when heart rates exceeds 100 beats min^{-1}, as implied by its inclusion in Figure 11-6? Cutaneous vasoconstriction (Taylor et al., 1988) and probably splanchnic vasoconstriction (Clausen and Trap-Jensen, 1974) may occur within 10 to 15 seconds, so why would MSNA rise later?
3. Alternatively, does MSNA rise only when lactic acid appears in blood? This would be consistent with the idea that MSNA is increased by the muscle chemoreflex.

Possibly a separate neuron pool directs the rapid rise in sympathetic activity to skin and visceral organs, this rise being elicited by a reflex other than the muscle chemoreflex. Clearly, overall sympathetic activity to several regions, but perhaps not MSNA, rises well before any known metabolic error signal exists.

Is the Muscle Chemoreflex Functionally Important During Severe Whole-Body Exercise?

We come to an extremely difficult problem in dealing with how the chemoreflex could function effectively during a condition under which there is little reserve in cardiac output or regional vascular conductance. The condition is severe whole-body exercise; cardiac output approaches its maximum; active muscle comprises 85 percent or more of total vascular conductance; and finally, vascular conductance of inactive regions is minimum owing to their marked sympathetically mediated vasoconstriction. The point is that the activation of the muscle chemoreflex in that setting would require that any rise in arterial pressure be achieved by vasoconstriction of active muscle—there is no other way to raise blood pressure.

Again, this is positive feedback as the rise in arterial pressure by the *chemoreflex cannot restore or raise muscle blood flow*.

If we look back for a moment and consider moderate exercise, a deficit in muscle blood flow created by partial occlusion can be corrected by approximately 50 percent. This is accomplished by a rise in cardiac output and also by some vasoconstriction in inactive regions. The partial restoration in muscle blood flow is accomplished by raising arterial pressure and by little additional vasodilation in the muscle, as shown in Figure 11-14. It is clear from Figure 11-6 that there is already significant regional vasoconstriction during moderate exercise, say, for example, at a heart rate of 150 beats min^{-1}. Evidence presented in Chapter 7 indicates that the active skeletal muscles are an important source of the norepinephrine spilled over into plasma from sympathetic vesicles during exercise. Thus active muscle appears to be as much a target for vasoconstriction during moderate exercise as other organs. At a heart rate of 150 beats min^{-1}, plasma lactate concentration increases, and this could signal activation of the muscle chemoreflex, which at this level of exercise may not be able to raise muscle blood flow. We return to the recurrent question of whether the progressive rise in sympathetic activity and vasoconstriction revealed in Figure 11-6 could be initiated by the muscle chemoreflex, which becomes increasingly stronger as exercise becomes more severe.

Another point to keep in mind is that in humans the demands of muscle for blood flow can exceed cardiac pumping capacity (see Chapter 7). We do not know yet the level of whole-body exercise at which any potential imbalance between cardiac output and muscle vasodilation might occur. At some point during whole-body exercise of increasing severity, vasoconstriction in active muscle must become important if a fall in arterial pressure is to be prevented. The marked rise in sympathetic nervous activity that attends severe exercise probably reveals the activity of a reflex that prevents vasodilation from outstripping cardiac output. Would one assign this function to a chemoreflex or to a baroreflex?

The discussion that follows temporarily sets aside the view that the simplest way to correct a mismatch between blood flow and vascular conductance (i.e., a pressure error) would be by a baroreflex, not by a chemoreflex. We ask instead what role the muscle chemoreflex might play in the mismatch that is thought to occur between muscle vascular conductance and cardiac output during severe whole body exercise. What follows is speculation, which postulates a role for a chemosensitive *pressure-raising reflex* in a setting in which the chemoreflex cannot increase total muscle blood flow. Skeletal muscle is on both the afferent and efferent arms of a positive-feedback reflex that would serve the body only by limiting reductions in arterial pressure rather than by preserving muscle blood flow.

Rowell and Sheriff (1988) chose, as an example of a mismatch between blood flow and metabolism, the condition of near-maximal leg exercise during which heavy exercise with the arms is suddenly added. Total demands for muscle blood flow now exceed cardiac pumping capacity and the only way to prevent a fall in arterial pressure is to vasoconstrict active muscle. Both cardiac output and total muscle blood flow remain constant at their maxima, but arterial pressure and blood flow per kg of active muscle must decline because there are more kilograms of active muscle that must receive the same total blood flow. The decrease in muscle blood flow per kilogram of muscle activates (or further activates) the muscle chemoreflex which in turn causes active muscle to vasoconstrict more. With its closed-loop gain of -0.67 to -0.75, the chemoreflex will restore blood pressure (not blood flow) two-thirds or three-fourths of the way back to where it was before the additional vasodilation caused pressure to fall. The persistent metabolic error signal could force the system through several cycles of adjustment with each one becoming increasingly smaller until stability is finally achieved. At this new steady state, there would be somewhat lower muscle vascular conductance and higher arterial pressure. Total muscle blood flow would remain the same but would now perfuse a larger muscle mass.

The preceding scheme has obvious pitfalls, not the least of which is the need to direct the greatest vasoconstriction to the least active muscles so that the most active muscles receive the bulk of the unchanged total blood flow. This could work if the effectiveness of sympathetic vasoconstriction were to decrease in inverse proportion to the metabolic rate of the muscle (i.e., "sympatholysis"). That is, the most active muscles would vasoconstrict the least and the least active muscles would vasoconstrict the most. The inhibitory effects of local metabolites on the effectiveness of vasoconstriction are small (see Chapter 7), and as yet we know of no way to redistribute actively (by reflex) muscle blood flow in accordance with local needs. In short, there is no way for the muscle chemoreflex to raise total blood flow to active muscles in severe exercise, but the distribution of blood flow among active muscles could be improved, were the least active muscle to be vasoconstricted significantly more than the most active muscle.

SUMMARY

In summary, the muscle chemoreflex does little to correct a "metabolic error signal" in isometrically contracting muscle; it may actually increase the error and contribute to the continuous rise in arterial pressure. The chemoreflex does help to restore muscle blood flow during mild dynamic exercise whenever oxygen delivery to the muscle falls below a critical level needed to maintain oxidative metabolism. That is, the reflex has a threshold and thus appears not to be part of a tonically active feedback control system serving to govern cardiovascular responses to mild exercise. As the severity of exercise increases to moderate, the margin for any blood flow error decreases and the reflex could be tonically active, but it has less reserve of cardiac output and regional vasoconstriction from which to raise muscle blood flow. As exercise becomes more severe the blood flow reserve (from either cardiac output or vasoconstriction) becomes less and less significant. The chemoreflex, if activated in this setting, can serve only to raise arterial blood pressure by vasoconstricting the active muscle to which most of the cardiac output is directed. In short, the chemoreflex becomes a pressure-raising rather than a flow-raising reflex, and would tend to increase rather than reduce a metabolic error signal. Its most important function in severe exercise may be to supplement other reflexes which prevent a fall in arterial pressure. Finally, it is also possible that the chemoreflex-induced vasoconstriction in the active muscle might, through local modulation of vasoconstriction, redirect muscle blood flow to the most active and away from the least active muscles without significantly reducing total muscle blood flow. There is no evidence to support this speculation. At this time it is not possible to say whether the muscle chemoreflex is normally one of the controllers of the circulation during dynamic exercise, or if it functions only in crises in which blood flow to muscle falls below a level needed to maintain oxygen delivery.

REFERENCES

Alam, M., and F.H. Smirk (1937). Observations in man upon a blood pressure raising reflex arising from the voluntary muscles. *J. Physiol. (Lond.) 89,* 372–383.

Bevegård, S., U. Freyschuss, and T. Strandell (1966). Circulatory adaptation to arm and leg exercise in supine and sitting position. *J. Appl. Physiol. 21,* 37–46.

Blomqvist, C.G., S.F. Lewis, W.F. Taylor, and R.M. Graham (1981). Similarity of the hemodynamic responses to static and dynamic exercise of small muscle groups. *Circ. Res. 48 (Suppl. 1),* 87–92.

Bonde-Petersen, F., L.B. Rowell, R.G. Murray, C.G. Blomqvist, R. White, E. Karlsson, W. Campbell, and J.H. Mitchell (1978). Role of cardiac output in the pressor responses to graded muscle ischemia in man. *J. Appl. Physiol. (Respir. Environ. Exerc. Physiol.) 45,* 574–589.

Clausen, J.-P., and J. Trap-Jensen (1974). Arteriohepatic venous oxygen difference and heart rate during initial phases of exercise. *J. Appl. Physiol. 37,* 716–719.

Coote, J.H., S.M. Hilton, and J.F. Perez-Gonzalez (1971). The reflex nature of the pressor response to muscular exercise. *J. Physiol. (Lond.) 215,* 789–804.

Dejours, P., J.C. Mithoefer, and J. Raynaud (1959). Evidence against the existence of specific ventilatory chemoreceptors in the legs. *J. Appl. Physiol. 10,* 367–371.

Duncan, G., R.H. Johnson, and D.G. Lambie (1981). Role of sensory nerves in the cardiovascular and respiratory changes with isometric forearm exercise in man. *Clin. Sci. Lond. 60,* 145–155.

Fernandes, A., H. Galbo, M. Kjaer, J.H. Mitchell, N.H. Secher, and S.N. Thomas

(1990). Cardiovascular and ventilatory responses to dynamic exercise during epidural anesthesia in man. *J. Physiol. (Lond.) 420*, 281–293.

Freund, P.R., S.F. Hobbs, and L.B. Rowell (1978). Cardiovascular responses to muscle ischemia in man: dependency on muscle mass. *J. Appl. Physiol. (Respir. Environ. Exerc. Physiol.) 45*, 762–767.

Freund, P.R., L.B. Rowell, T.M. Murphy, S.F. Hobbs, and S.H. Butler (1979). Blockade of the pressor response to muscle ischemia by sensory nerve block in man. *Am. J. Physiol. 236 (Heart Circ. Physiol. 6)*, H433–H439.

Freyschuss, U., and T. Strandell (1968). Circulatory adaptation to one- and two-leg exercise in supine position. *J. Appl. Physiol. 25*, 511–515.

Gollnick, P.D., M. Riedy, J.J. Quintinskie, and L.A. Bertocci (1985). Differences in metabolic potential of skeletal muscle fibres and its significance for metabolic control. *J. Exp. Biol. 115*, 191–199.

Hobbs, S.F. (1982). Central command during exercise: parallel activation of the cardiovascular and motor systems by descending command signals. In O.A. Smith, R.A. Galosy, and S.M. Weiss, eds. *Circulation, Neurobiology and Behavior*, pp. 217–231. Elsevier, New York.

Hobbs, S.F., and D.I. McCloskey (1987). Effects of blood pressure on force production in cat and human muscle. *J. Appl. Physiol. 63*, 834–839.

Hohimer, A.R., J.R.S. Hales, L.B. Rowell, and O.A. Smith (1983). Regional distribution of blood flow during mild dynamic leg exercise in the baboon. *J. Appl. Physiol. (Respir. Environ. Exerc. Physiol.) 55*, 1173–1177.

Hollander, A.P., and L.N. Bouman (1975). Cardiac acceleration in man elicited by a muscle-heart reflex. *J. Appl. Physiol. 38*, 272–278.

Joyner, M.J. (1991). Does the pressor response to ischemic exercise improve blood flow to contracting muscles in humans? *J. Appl. Physiol. 71*, 1496–1501.

Kalia, M., S.S. Mei, and F.F. Kao (1981). Central projections from ergoreceptors (C fibers) in muscle involved in cardiopulmonary responses to static exercise. *Circ. Res. 48 (Suppl. 1)*, 48–62.

Kaufman, M.P., J.C. Longhurst, K.J. Rybicki, J.H. Wallach, and J.H. Mitchell (1983). Effects of static muscular contraction on impulse activity of groups III and IV afferents in cats. *J. Appl. Physiol. (Respir. Environ. Excerc. Physiol.) 55*, 105–112.

Kaufman, M.P., D.M. Rotto, and K.J. Rybicki (1988). Pressor reflex response to static muscular contraction: its afferent arm and possible neurotransmitters. *Am. J. Cardiol. 62*, 58E–62E.

Kaufman, M.P., and K.J. Rybicki (1987). Discharge properties of group III and IV muscle afferents: their responses to mechanical and metabolic stimuli. *Circ. Res. 61 (Suppl. 1)*, 60–65.

Kaufman, M.P., K.J. Rybicki, T.G. Waldrop, and G.A. Ordway (1984). Effect of ischemia on responses of group III and IV afferents to contraction. *J. Appl. Physiol. (Respir. Environ. Exerc. Physiol.) 57*, 644–650.

Kniffki, K.-D., S. Mense, and R.F. Schmidt (1981). Muscle receptors with fine afferent fibers which may evoke circulatory reflexes. *Circ. Res. 48 (Suppl. 1)*, 25–31.

Kozelka, J.W., G.W. Christy, and R.D. Wurster (1987). Ascending pathways mediating somatoautonomic reflexes in exercising dogs. *J. Appl. Physiol. 62*, 1186–1191.

Lassen, A., J.H. Mitchell, D.R. Reeves, Jr., H.B. Rogers, and N.H. Secher (1989).

Cardiovascular responses to brief static contractions in man with topical nervous blockade. *J. Physiol. (Lond.) 409*, 333–341.

Levy, M.N., and H. Zieske (1969). Autonomic control of cardiac pacemaker activity and atrioventricular transmission. *J. Appl. Physiol. 27*, 465–470.

Lind, A.R. (1983). Cardiovascular adjustments to isometric contractions: static effort. In J.T. Shepherd, F.M. Abboud, and S.R. Geiger, eds. *Handbook of Physiology. The Cardiovascular System: Peripheral Circulation and Organ Blood Flow*, sect. 2, vol. III, pp. 947–966. American Physiological Society, Bethesda, MD.

Lorentsen, E. (1972). Systemic arterial blood pressure during exercise in patients with atherosclerosis obliterans of the lower limbs. *Circulation 46*, 257–263.

Maciel, B.C., L. Gallo, Jr., J.A. Marin Neto, and L.E.B. Martins (1987). Autonomic nervous control of the heart rate during isometric exercise in normal man. *Pflugers Arch. 408*, 173–177.

Mark, A.L., R.G. Victor, C. Nerhed, and B.G. Wallin (1985). Microneurographic studies of the mechanisms of sympathetic nerve responses to static exercise in humans. *Circ. Res. 57*, 461–469.

Martin, C.E., J.A. Shaver, D.F. Leon, M.E. Thompson, P.S. Reddy, and J. J. Leonard (1974). Autonomic mechanisms in hemodynamic responses to isometric exercise. *J. Clin. Invest. 54*, 104–115.

McCloskey, D.I., P.B.C. Matthews, and J.H. Mitchell (1972). Absence of appreciable cardiovascular and respiratory responses to muscle vibration. *J. Appl. Physiol. 33*, 623–626.

McCloskey, D.I., and J.H. Mitchell (1972). Reflex cardiovascular and respiratory responses originating in exercising muscle. *J. Physiol. (Lond.) 224*, 173–186.

Mense, S. (1978). Effects of temperature on the discharges of muscle spindles and tendon organs. *Pflugers Arch. 374*, 159–166.

Mitchell, J.H. (1990). Neural control of the circulation during exercise. *Med. Sci. Sports Exerc. 22*, 141–154.

Mitchell, J.H., D.R. Reeves, Jr., H.B. Rogers, and N.H. Secher (1989). Epidural anaesthesia and cardiovascular responses to static exercise in man. *J. Physiol. (Lond.) 417*, 13–24.

Mitchell, J.H., B. Schibye, F.C. Payne III, and B. Saltin (1981). Response of arterial blood pressure to static exercise in relation to muscle mass, force development, and electromyographic activity. *Circ. Res. 48 (Suppl. 1)*, 70–75.

Mitchell, J.H., and R.F. Schmidt (1983). Cardiovascular reflex control by afferent fibers from skeletal muscle receptors. In J.T. Shepherd, F.M. Abboud, and S.R. Geiger, eds. *Handbook of Physiology. The Cardiovascular System: Peripheral Circulation and Organ Blood Flow*, sect. 2, vol. III, pp. 623–658. American Physiological Society, Bethesda, MD.

O'Leary, D.S. (1991). Autonomic mechanisms of muscle metaboreflex control of heart rate during post-exercise muscle ischemia in conscious dogs. *The Physiologist 34*, 239, 1991.

Pryor, S.L., S.F. Lewis, R.G. Haller, L.A. Bertocci, and R.G. Victor (1990). Impairment of sympathetic activation during static exercise in patients with muscle phosphorylase deficiency (McArdle's disease). *J. Clin. Invest 85*, 1444–1449.

Rotto, D.M., and M.P. Kaufman (1988). Effect of metabolic products of muscular contraction on discharge of group III and IV afferents. *J. Appl. Physiol. 64*, 2306–2313.

Rotto, D.M., K.D. Massey, K.P. Burton, and M.P. Kaufman (1989a). Static contraction increases arachidonic acid levels in gastrocnemius muscles of cat. *J. Appl. Physiol. 66*, 2721–2724.

Rotto, D.M., H.D. Schultz, J.C. Longhurst, and M.P. Kaufman (1990). Sensitization of group III muscle afferents to static contraction by arachidonic acid. *J. Appl. Physiol. 68*, 861–867.

Rotto, D.M., C.L. Stebbins, and M.P. Kaufman (1989b). Reflex cardiovascular and ventilatory responses to increasing H^+ activity in cat hindlimb muscle. *J. Appl. Physiol. 67*, 256–263.

Rowell, L.B. (1974). Human cardiovascular adjustments to exercise and thermal stress. *Physiol. Rev. 54*, 75–159.

Rowell, L.B. (1980). What signals govern the cardiovascular responses to exercise? *Med. Sci. Sports 12*, 307–315.

Rowell, L.B. (1986). *Human Circulation: Regulation During Physical Stress*. Oxford University Press, New York.

Rowell, L.B., P.R. Freund, and S.F. Hobbs (1981). Cardiovascular responses to muscle ischemia in humans. *Circ. Res. 48 (Suppl. 1)*, 37–47.

Rowell, L.B., L. Hermansen, and J.R. Blackman (1976). Human cardiovascular and respiratory responses to graded muscle ischemia. *J. Appl. Physiol. 41*, 693–701.

Rowell, L.B., and D.S. O'Leary (1990). Reflex control of the circulation during exercise: chemoreflexes and mechanoreflexes. *J. Appl. Physiol. 69*, 407–418.

Rowell, L.B., M.V. Savage, J. Chambers, and J.R. Blackmon (1991). Cardiovascular responses to graded reductions in leg perfusion in exercising humans. *Am. J. Physiol. 261 (Heart Circ. Physiol. 30)*, H1545–H1553.

Rowell, L.B., and D.D. Sheriff (1988). Are muscle "chemoreflexes" functionally important? *News Physiol. Sci. 3*, 250–253.

Rybicki, K.J., T.G. Waldrop, and M.P. Kaufman (1985). Increasing gracilis muscle interstitial potassium concentrations stimulate group III and IV afferents. *J. Appl. Physiol. 58*, 936–941.

Saltin, B., G. Sjøgaard, F.A. Gaffney, and L.B. Rowell (1981). Potassium, lactate, and water fluxes in human quadriceps muscle during static contractions. *Circ. Res. 48 (Suppl. I)*. 18–24.

Saito, M., T. Mano, H. Abe, and S. Iwase (1986). Responses in muscle sympathetic nerve activity to sustained hand-grips of different tensions in humans. *Eur. J. Appl. Physiol. Occup. Physiol. 55*, 493–498.

Saito, M., T. Mano, and S. Iwase (1989). Sympathetic nerve activity related to local fatigue sensation during static contraction. *J. Appl. Physiol. 67*, 980–984.

Sato, A., and R.F. Schmidt (1973). Somatosympathetic reflexes: afferent fibers, central pathways, discharge characteristics. *Physiol. Rev. 53*, 916–947.

Seals, D.R. (1989a). Sympathetic neural discharge and vascular resistance during exercise in humans. *J. Appl. Physiol. 66*, 2472–2478.

Seals, D.R. (1989b). Influence of muscle mass on sympathetic neural activation during isometric exercise. *J. Appl. Physiol. 67*, 1801–1806.

Seals, D.R., P.B., Chase, and J.A. Taylor (1988a). Autonomic mediation of the pressor responses to isometric exercise in humans. *J. Appl. Physiol. 64,* 2190–2196.

Seals, D.R., and R.M. Enoka (1989). Sympathetic activation is associated with increases in EMG during fatiguing exercise. *J. Appl. Physiol. 66,* 88–95.

Seals, D.R., R.G. Victor, and A.L. Mark (1988b). Plasma norepinephrine and muscle sympathetic discharge during rhythmic exercise in humans. *J. Appl. Physiol. 65,* 940–944.

Shepherd, J.T., C.G. Blomqvist, A.R. Lind, J.H. Mitchell, and B. Saltin (1981). Static (isometric) exercise: retrospection and introspection. *Circ. Res. 48, Suppl. 1,* 179–188.

Sheriff, D.D., D.S. O'Leary, A.M. Scher, and L.B. Rowell (1990). Baroreflex attenuates pressor response to graded muscle ischemia in exercising dogs. *Am. J. Physiol. 258 (Heart Circ. Physiol. 27),* H305–H310.

Sheriff, D.D., C.R. Wyss, L.B. Rowell, and A.M. Scher (1987). Does inadequate O_2 delivery trigger the pressor response to muscle hypoperfusion during exercise? *Am. J. Physiol. 253 (Heart Circ. Physiol. 22),* H1199–H1207.

Simon, E., and W. Riedel (1975). Diversity of regional sympathetic outflow in integrative cardiovascular control: patterns and mechanisms. *Brain Res. 87,* 323–333.

Sinoway, L., S. Prophet, I. Gorman, T. Mosher, J. Shenberger, M. Dolecki, R. Briggs, and R. Zelis (1989). Muscle acidosis during static exercise is associated with calf vasoconstriction. *J. Appl. Physiol. 66,* 429–436.

Stebbins, C.L., B. Brown, D. Levin, and J.C. Longhurst (1988). Reflex effect of skeletal muscle mechanoreceptor stimulation on the cardiovascular system. *J. Appl. Physiol. 65,* 1539–1547.

Stebbins, C.L., and J.C. Longhurst (1985). Bradykinin-induced chemoreflexes from skeletal muscle: implications for the exercise reflex. *J. Appl. Physiol. 59,* 56–63.

Stebbins, C.L., and J.C. Longhurst (1986). Bradykinin in reflex cardiovascular responses to static muscular contraction. *J. Appl. Physiol. 61,* 271–279.

Stebbins, C.L., and J.C. Longhurst (1989). Potentiation of the exercise pressor reflex by muscle ischemia. *J. Appl. Physiol. 66,* 1046–1053.

Taylor, W.F., J.M. Johnson, W.A. Kosiba, and C.M. Kwan (1988). Graded cutaneous vascular responses to dynamic leg exercise. *J. Appl. Physiol. 64,* 1803–1809.

Thimm, F., M. Carvalho, M. Babka, and E. Meier zu Verl (1984). Reflex increases in heart-rate induced by perfusing the hind leg of the rat with solutions containing lactic acid. *Pflugers Arch. 400,* 286–293.

Victor, R.G., L.A. Bertocci, S.L. Pryor, and R.L. Nunnally (1988). Sympathetic nerve discharge is coupled to muscle cell pH during exercise in humans. *J. Clin. Invest. 82,* 1301–1305.

Victor, R.G., S.L. Pryor, N.H. Secher, and J.H. Mitchell (1989). Effects of partial neuromuscular blockade on sympathetic nerve responses to static exercise in humans. *Circ. Res. 65,* 468–476.

Victor, R.G., and D.R. Seals (1989). Reflex stimulation of sympathetic outflow during rhythmic exercise in humans. *Am. J. Physiol. 257 (Heart Circ. Physiol. 26),* H2017–H2024.

Victor, R.G., D.R. Seals, and A.L. Mark (1987). Differential control of heart rate and sympathetic nerve activity during dynamic exercise. *J. Clin. Invest. 79,* 508–516.

Wallin, B.G., R.G. Victor, and A.L. Mark (1989). Sympathetic outflow to resting muscles during static handgrip and postcontraction muscle ischemia. *Am. J. Physiol. 256 (Heart Circ. Physiol. 25)*, H105–H110.

Wyss, C.R., J.L. Ardell, A.M. Scher, and L.B. Rowell (1983). Cardiovascular responses to graded reductions in hindlimb perfusion in exercising dogs. *Am. J. Physiol. 245 (Heart Circ. Physiol. 14)*, H481–H486.

Zuntz, N., and J. Geppert (1886). Über die Natur der normalen Atemreize und den ort ihrer Wirkung. *Pflugers Arch. 38*, 337–338.

12

Arterial Baroreflexes, Central Command, and Muscle Chemoreflexes: A Synthesis

The evidence presented in preceding chapters supports the idea that central command sets the basic patterns of effector activity at the beginning of exercise, as summarized in Figure 12-1. However, we still have the unsolved mystery regarding the causes of the rise in sympathetic nervous activity when heart rate approaches 100 beats min^{-1} during dynamic exercise, as illustrated in Figure 11-6. Recall from Chapters 10 and 11 that central command appears to raise cardiac output by withdrawal of vagal activity; it has minimal effect on the sympathetic nervous system. Based on the delayed onset of increased muscle sympathetic nerve activity (MSNA) and the rise in blood lactate levels during *isometric* contractions, the sympathetic nervous system could, in those settings, be activated by muscle chemoreflex, but there is no evidence yet to support the action of this chemoreflex during mild to moderately heavy dynamic exercise under normal, free-flow conditions.

The primary question raised in this chapter is: What causes overall sympathetic nervous activity to increase with such remarkable consistency when heart rate approaches 100 beats min^{-1} during *whole-body dynamic exercise?* Dynamic exercise at this low heart rate is mild, and there are ample reserves to correct any mismatch between blood flow and metabolism. Blood lactate levels do not rise until heart rate approaches 130 to 140 beats min^{-1} in sedentary individuals and not until much higher heart rates (and percentages of $\dot{V}O_2max$) are reached in athletes. Thus there is no hint of any mismatch between blood flow and metabolism, and therefore no discernable metabolic error signal. If neither central command nor the muscle chemoreflex initiates the activation of the sympathetic nervous system in humans, then we are left with muscle mechanoreflexes and the arterial baroreflex. Muscle mechanoreflexes appear to be only transiently active at the onset of isometric contractions, but during dynamic exercise they may be activated with each contraction. There is no way at this time to rule in or out mechanoreflexes as potentially significant activators of the sympathetic nervous system during steady-state dynamic exercise.

Arterial mean pressure is well maintained over a wide range of dynamic exercise intensities; it increases by a few millimeters of mercury from mild

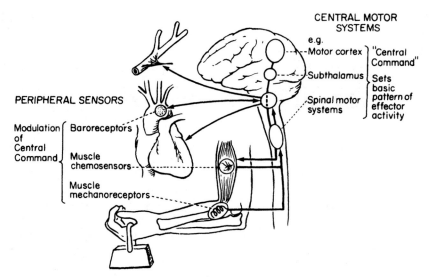

Figure 12-1 Proposed scheme for initiating of the cardiovascular responses to exercise in which "central command" initiates the effector activity that is in turn modulated by arterial baroreceptors and muscle chemo- and mechanosensors as appropriate error signals develop. (From Rowell, 1982, with permission from Elsevier.)

exercise up to levels requiring the $\dot{V}o_2$max (see Figure 5-11). Many would argue, validly, that simply because arterial pressure remains relatively constant during exercise does not mean that pressure is the variable being regulated; the variable could, for example, be cardiac output. In fact, some have even maintained that the arterial baroreflex is so insensitive during exercise that it is in essence inoperative.

One could also argue that despite the constancy of arterial pressure, a pressure error could still be perceived by the central nervous system. For example, the prevailing pressure might simply be below the operating point, or so-called "set point," for a baroreflex that had been reset to a higher pressure by the central nervous system. In other words, if arterial pressure were reset upward, for example, by central command, at the onset of exercise and arterial pressure failed to rise to the new operating point, the central nervous system would perceive "hypotension" and make the appropriate corrections.

Any speculation that "resetting" of the baroreflex can explain blood pressure control during exercise has often been viewed with skepticism because the origin of the stimulus that resets the baroreflex is not defined. Clearly, if the arterial baroreflex were "reset" to higher operating points in proportion to exercise intensity, all cardiovascular responses to exercise could easily be explained on the basis of a need to correct centrally perceived "pressure errors." The argument that arterial baroreflexes could not be controllers of the circulation during exercise because arterial pressure does not fall would disappear simply because a fall cannot be perceived if the new reset operating point is not defined. The fact that the putative new operating point is never identified is an obvious weakness. This concept of "resetting" means that the arterial baroreflex would actually cause the rise in arterial pressure during exercise, rather than opposing it, as it is commonly assumed to do.

To begin, three questions must be answered:

1. Is the baroreflex operative and effectively so during exercise?
2. Is the operating point of the baroreflex shifted upward to a higher pressure during exercise?
3. What might shift the operating point of the baroreflex?

Keep in mind the *focus of this chapter is on dynamic exercise with large muscle groups,* often called "whole-body exercise."

OVERALL ASSESSMENT OF BAROREFLEX REGULATION OF ARTERIAL PRESSURE DURING EXERCISE

Although arterial pressure during exercise could simply be the resultant of regulation of cardiac output and total vascular conductance by other reflexes, this solution seems untenable based on the evidence discussed in Chapters 10 and 11. Central command or reflexes originating in skeletal muscle would appear not to explain the increase in sympathetic nervous outflow. The arterial baroreflex is another possible controller of the circulation, but there has been a long-standing argument about the significance of this reflex during exercise (for reviews, see Ludbrook, 1983; Rowell, 1986; Rowell and O'Leary, 1990; Walgenbach-Telford, 1991). Debate has centered on several issues, one of the oldest of which concerns the changes in arterial pressure at the onset of exercise.

Does Arterial Pressure Fall at the Onset of Dynamic Exercise with Large Muscle Groups?

The original thinking on this question was that muscle vasodilated faster than cardiac output could increase so that arterial pressure fell at the onset of exercise. This provided the initial stimulus to increase heart rate and arterial pressure. Surprisingly, there is still significant debate about the initial change in arterial pressure at the onset of exercise. The history of earlier observations was reviewed by Holmgren (1956), whose own findings concerning the *initial* pressure response during the transition from seated upright rest to upright exercise are summarized in Figure 12-2. This figure shows the changes in arterial pressure beginning with a brief small rise and then a longer but still brief fall followed by a steady-state level not much different from rest. Rowell and colleagues (1968) observed the same transients in simultaneous recordings from the aortic arch and the radial artery (especially during severe exercise) and also observed (as have others; see Holmgren, 1956) many cases during which arterial pressure

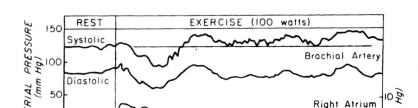

Figure 12-2   Oscillations in blood pressure at the onset of upright (seated) cycling such as illustrated here were often observed in the transition from upright rest to cycling, but usually disappeared on repeated trials. (Redrawn from Holmgren, 1956.)

did not dip slightly at the onset of submaximal exercise. In fact, Holmgren (1956) saw that in repeated starts from seated rest to exercise, the transient decline in arterial pressure progressively disappeared. He also saw that a sudden transition from one level to a heavier one was attended by an immediate rise in arterial pressure without any transient dip; that is, a fall in pressure was not the stimulus to raise cardiac output.

Sprangers (1991) observed that both arterial and right atrial pressures rose during a *3-second* burst of upright cycle exercise; arterial pressure fell suddenly when exercise was terminated. Local vasodilation probably explains the fall in pressure immediately after muscle pumping had suddenly stopped. However, Sprangers' interpretation was that the sudden forceful contraction of leg and abdominal muscles forced blood from the peripheral vasculature to intrathoracic vessels; the subsequent increase in cardiac filling pressure stimulated cardiopulmonary baroreceptors, causing a release of vasoconstriction and the secondary fall in arterial pressure. Sprangers saw this as the cause of the transient dip in pressure shown in Figure 12-2. This interpretation is difficult to accept because these events occur within seconds and the time constant of the sympathetic nervous response is much longer (see Figure 5-5).

The main point of this discussion is that the occurrence of a transient dip in arterial pressure is probably not an important signal for the overall cardiovascular response to exercise; the dip is transient and does not occur when work intensity increases suddenly from one level to another, and therefore it is not useful in any straightforward analysis of the steady-state response.

Is Baroreflex Sensitivity or Gain Reduced During Exercise?
What is Meant by Baroreflex Sensitivity?

Sensitivity refers to the change in systemic arterial pressure caused by a given change in pressure at the arterial baroreceptors (most commonly the isolated carotid sinus). It also refers to the slope of the relationship between systemic arterial pressure and carotid sinus pressure, as shown in Figure 12-3; this slope is commonly called *gain*.

Figure 12-3 shows some hypothetical stimulus-response curves for the carotid sinus baroreflex, and provides some definitions for subsequent discussion. Figure 12-3A shows a characteristic stimulus-response curve for the reflex with a threshold at the upper limit and saturation (arrow with S) at the lower limit. The *operating point* for the reflex is the carotid sinus pressure at which the slope of the stimulus-response curve, or the gain, is maximum (cf. Sagawa, 1983). Figure 12-3B illustrates a reduction in baroreflex sensitivity (i.e., reduced maximal slope) going from curve 1 to 2 (ignore for now the small shift in operating point which need not occur with a change in sensitivity). This reduction in the sensitivity of the reflex, shown in Figure 12-3B, means that any baroreflex opposition to an increase in arterial pressure would be lessened. An acute alteration in sensitivity of the baroreflex is normally initiated centrally by a perturbation that acts on the central motor neuron pool involved in baroreflexes. For example, baroreflex sensitivity could be reduced or raised by central command signals.

The ideal method for assessing the sensitivity of the baroreflex is to determine the maximal slope of the stimulus-response curve as illustrated in Figure 12-3A. Although this can be done in humans by applying a range of positive or negative pressures to the neck over the carotid sinus (as discussed in Chapter 2), the responses are opposed by the aortic baroreflex. That is, when carotid sinus transmural pressure is increased, the

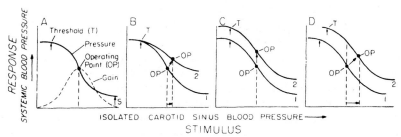

Figure 12-3 Hypothetical stimulus-response curves for the carotid sinus baroreflex (or baroreflex function curves). The most important landmarks on the curves are defined in Figure A (*S* marks the point of saturation). **(A)** The dashed line shows the gain or sensitivity of the reflex over the slope of the curve. By definition, the point of maximum gain is the baroreflex operating point. **(B)** A change in the baroreflex in which operating point (OP) and systemic pressure are shifted upward with a decrease in gain and no change in threshold. **(C)** An upward shift in response (systemic pressure) with no change in threshold, gain, OP, or the baroreflex. **(D)** A shift in threshold and OP to a higher carotid sinus and systemic pressure. This is the classical picture of so-called baroreceptor "resetting." (Adapted from Korner, 1979, and Rowell, 1986.)

hypotensive response is opposed and diminished by the aortic barorecep-tors. Another problem with this approach is that the stimulus-response curve for the carotid sinus reflex is often obtained by applying each pres-sure to the sinus for only a few seconds. Inasmuch as full activation of the sympathetic nervous system may take 10 to 15 seconds or longer, these stimulus-response curves are dominated by vagal activation or inhibition of heart rate with some mix of lagging sympathetic vasoconstriction. In animals, carotid sinus stimulus-response curves can be constructed after a surgical denervation of the aortic receptors plus an isolation of the sinus and direct measurement of their transmural pressure (described later).

Evidence Suggesting Inoperative Arterial Baroreflex or Reduced Baroreflex Sensitivity During Exercise

Complete and chronic denervation of the carotid sinus and aortic barore-ceptors in chronically instrumented dogs caused no obvious deficit in either the level to which blood pressure rose or in its stability once that level was reached during *moderate* exercise (Vanhoutte et al., 1966; McRitchie et al., 1976). These observations imply either that the baroreflex is totally insensitive or inoperative during exercise or that control is achieved by some other *redundant* mechanism. Although Krasney and coworkers (1974) saw only a small reduction in heart rate and cardiac output during the steady state of exercise, they also noted a sluggish increase in heart rate and cardiac output at the onset of exercise in their denervated dogs.

A few studies on humans have also suggested to some that baroreflex sensitivity is depressed by exercise. Unfortunately this conclusion was based on an assessment of "sensitivity" by observing the changes in the R-R interval of the electrocardiogram in response to increments in arterial pressure induced by bolus injections of the powerful vasoconstrictor, phenylephrine. The sudden rise in arterial pressure caused baroreflex-induced bardycardia. The change in the slope of the line relating the time between heart beats (R-R interval) to the increase in arterial pressure was taken as a measure of the sensitivity of the entire baroreflex. The smaller the increase in R-R interval per unit increase in arterial pressure, the lower the baroreflex sensitivity was assumed to be (e.g., Bristow et al., 1971; Cunningham et al., 1972). Actually under the conditions of exercise it was a measure of neither the sensitivity of the heart rate nor of vascular resistance components of the baroreflex. One problem with this technique, outlined earlier (see Chapter 4 and Figure 4-6), is that for any increase in heart rate, the corresponding change in R-R interval becomes less and less as the initial or baseline heart rate becomes higher. A second problem is that the sensitivity of the arterial baroreflex is determined by the combined sensitivities of the cardiac output response and the vasomotor response. The substitution of heart rate for cardiac output assumes constant stroke volume; the gains do not simply add when cardiac output does not change in proportion to heart rate (see Ludbrook, 1984).

baroreflex gain $\propto$ heart rate gain + total vascular resistance gain.

Sudden increases in blood pressure with phenylephrine injections stem from rapid changes in cardiac output (i.e., within one beat owing to the speed of vagal action on the sinus node [approximately 0.5 seconds]) (Figure 5-5). The slower sympathetic vasomotor component of the reflex is abolished by the drug. The main point is that normally, changes in either heart rate (i.e., cardiac output) or in vascular resistance, or both, can dominate the response to a baroreflex during exercise; the response will depend on the duration of the stimulus, the intensity of exercise, and any other factors that affect differentially one of the two adjustments.

Evidence Suggesting That Baroreflex Sensitivity Is Not Reduced by Exercise

Historically, those who have evaluated baroreflex sensitivity during exercise in humans by examining the relationship between heart rate (rather than R-R interval) and arterial pressure have concluded that this index of baroreflex sensitivity was unaffected by exercise because the slope of this relationship was unchanged (Bevegård and Shepherd, 1966; Robinson et al., 1966). Ironically, virtually the same results (i.e., for heart rate) were obtained by those who concluded that exercise reduced sensitivity, but based on the relationship of R-R interval rather than heart rate to changes in arterial pressure.

If one uses instead of heart rate the change in systemic blood pressure in response to a change in distending pressure at the baroreceptors, then the response to a change in arterial pressure combines the cardiac and vasomotor components of the reflex; it looks at the reflex in its entirety. That is,

Blood pressure = [cardiac output] × [total vascular resistance].

For example, application of negative pressure to the neck over the carotid sinus reflexly lowers arterial pressure (Ludbrook, 1983; Ebert, 1986) via its combined effects on cardiac output and vascular resistance (Bevegård and Shepherd, 1966). In animals, partial occlusion of the common carotid artery achieves the same goal. The sensitivity of the carotid sinus reflex, based on the changes in arterial pressure for a given change in carotid sinus transmural pressure is *unaffected by mild to heavy dynamic exercise* in humans and other species (Bevegård and Shepherd, 1966; Melcher and Donald, 1981; Ludbrook, 1983; Walgenbach-Telford, 1991) even during isometric contractions (Ludbrook, 1983; Ebert, 1986).

One problem inherent in these studies is that the decline in arterial pressure in response to the carotid sinus baroreflex is partially counteracted by the intact aortic baroreflex. The assumption is that the gains of the aortic baroreflex and the carotid sinus reflex remain similar over the range of arterial pressures occurring from rest through increasing intensities of exercise. Angell-James and Daly (1971) found in dogs the same operating points for carotid sinus and aortic baroreflexes over a wide range of pressures when they applied the pressures to the receptors in pulsatile fashion. This suggests that there is more or less uniform opposition of the carotid sinus baroreflex by the aortic baroreflex over a normal range of arterial pressures.

Strange and coworkers (1990) observed similar declines in arterial pressure in response to pulsatile neck suction during rest and moderate upright exercise (40 percent of $\dot{V}O_2max$). A negative pressure of -50 mmHg was applied pulsatilely to the carotid sinus at each electrocardiographic R-wave for 250 to 400 ms, depending on heart rate (see Figure 12-4). The fall in systemic arterial pressure was sustained only when the negative pressure was applied to the sinus in a pulsatile rather than a steady manner (see Figure 12-5). At the two higher work rates (averages 69 percent and 88 percent of $\dot{V}O_2max$), the decrements in systemic arterial pressure were smaller than those at the lowest work intensity (Figure 12-6A). Also, the fall in heart rate with neck suction decreased with increasing work rate as did the rise in vascular conductance of the exercising legs (Figure 12-6C). In general, the findings of Strange and co-workers (1990) suggest that sensitivity of the carotid sinus baroreflex may decrease slightly during *severe* exercise or alternatively, other reflexes may compete with it, as is discussed later in this chapter.

Vatner and coworkers (1970) observed that electrical stimulation of the carotid sinus nerve in voluntarily exercising dogs causes a similar drop in arterial blood pressure during rest and exercise. This fall in pressure was caused by increases in mesenteric, renal, and iliac vascular conductance. The baroreflexes appear equally effective during rest and exercise. However, the finding of a tonic vasoconstriction that could be withdrawn from active muscles of dogs did not fit with Donald and colleagues' (1970) earlier observation that active hindlimbs received no tonic sympathetic

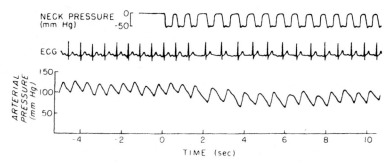

Figure 12-4 Experimental technique for studying carotid sinus reflex during exercise. Pulsatile neck suction was triggered by computer on the R-wave. Duration of the stimulus was varied between 400 and 200 ms, depending on heart rate. Neck-chamber pressure fell 50 mmHg in 70 ms. Note the increase in R-R interval and the fall in electronically damped femoral arterial pressure during neck suction. (Adapted from Strange et al., 1990.)

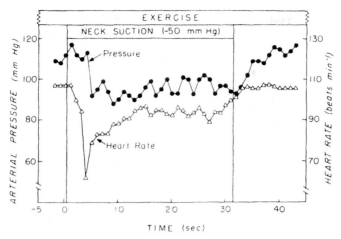

Figure 12-5 Effect of pulsatile neck suction on femoral arterial pressure and heart rate during moderate exercise. Each period of suction was maintained for 35 sec to allow time from measurements of blood flow. Decline in arterial pressure was better maintained when suction was pulsatile. (Adapted from Strange et al., 1990.)

vasoconstriction. The cause for this discrepancy is unknown. Vatner and colleagues' (1970) results do, however, fit with those of Strange and colleagues (1990).

FUNCTIONAL CHARACTERISTICS OF THE CAROTID SINUS REFLEX DURING EXERCISE

Two important series of studies carried out during the 1980s by Donald and his coworkers in the United States and Ludbrook and his colleagues in Australia provided our first detailed look at the functional characteristics of the arterial baroreflex, and particularly the carotid sinus reflex in exercising animals. These studies have been reviewed by Ludbrook (1983), Walgenbach and Shepherd (1984), Walgenbach-Telford (1991), and Rowell and O'Leary (1990). The studies are characterized by their skillful design and great complexity. Their complexity makes them difficult to discuss succinctly, but their importance warrants the effort.

   The vascular isolation of the carotid sinus, either in conscious dogs or rabbits, provided a means of controlling pressures within the carotid sinus separately from the pressures existing at other receptor sites. This gave us the first detailed information on the effects of exercise on baroreflex stimulus-response curves. These techniques provided information about their maximal sensitivity, their operating points, and how these variables change in response to exercise. These studies also allow us to address the most important question of all: Is the arterial baroreflex "reset" or shifted to a higher operating point in response to exercise?

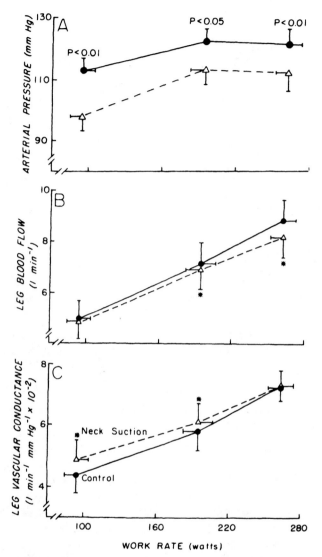

Figure 12-6 **(A)** Average arterial pressure during three levels of exercise requiring 40, 69, and 88 percent of V̇O₂max. The higher pressures (*solid circles*) are controls and the lower pressure (*open triangles*) were those decreased by neck suction during the same bouts of exercise. Responses to carotid sinus hypertension were greatest at 40 percent of V̇O₂max and less but equal at 69 and 88 percent of V̇O₂max, suggesting lower baroreflex sensitivity at the two higher levels of exercise. **(B)** Blood flow by femoral venous thermodilution in one leg during two-legged cycling at 40, 69, and 88 percent of V̇O₂max. Pulsatile neck suction (see Figure 12-4) significantly reduced leg blood flow at 69 and 88 percent of V̇O₂max. **(C)** At 40 and 69 percent of V̇O₂max carotid sinus hypertension increased leg vascular conductance by reducing sympathetic vasoconstriction in the active muscle. Leg vascular conductance was unaffected by neck suction at 88 percent V̇O₂max. (Redrawn from Strange et al., 1990.)

Initial Studies on the Vascularly Isolated Carotid Sinus

Complete baroreflex stimulus-response curves (systemic arterial versus carotid sinus pressure) for the vascularly isolated carotid sinus in dogs with intact aortic baroreflexes during rest and exercise revealed that mild to heavy exercise caused no changes in the threshold, slope (or gain), or saturation level of the curves; that is, the operating point of the reflex is unchanged (Melcher and Donald, 1981). However, this baroreflex function curve was displaced vertically to higher systemic arterial pressure. This response is typified in Figure 12-3C. In these experiments the effects on the curves were unlike those described for Figure 12-3B or D, in which some stimulus acts on the central neurons involved in the baroreflex and causes "resetting" of the reflex to a higher operating point, shown by a rightward shift in the curve. Conversely, the vertical shift in the stimulus-response curve (illustrated in Figure 12-3C) is attributable to an elevation in systemic arterial pressure caused by a rise in either cardiac output or by sympathetic vasoconstriction, or both, and not to any change in the functional characteristics of the carotid sinus baroreflex (Korner, 1979).

Two disadvantages of the isolated carotid sinus preparation have been the use of nonpulsatile pressures and the presence of intact aortic baroreflexes that buffer or oppose the carotid sinus reflex. Therefore the aortic baroreflex could mask any resetting of the carotid sinus. For example, in resting dogs interruption of the aortic baroreflex markedly altered the shape and position of the isolated carotid sinus stimulus-response curve so that its overall sensitivity was much greater and point of maximal gain ("operating point") was at a higher intrasinus pressure. A reduction in sinus pressure without intact aortic baroreceptors caused marked hypertension and the range as well as gain of the reflex was increased (Walgenbach and Donald, 1983b). A rise in carotid sinus pressure in exercising dogs without functioning aortic baroreceptors caused such instability in systemic arterial pressure that stimulus-response curves could not be constructed. These experiments reveal that the sensitivity of the carotid sinus baroreflex is well maintained during exercise and this sensitivity is increased by elimination of aortic baroreceptors. Therefore, the question is no longer if the baroreflex maintains its sensitivity during exercise, but rather what happens to its operating point and why.

Role of Arterial Baroreflexes at the Onset of Exercise

As shown in Figure 12-7, arterial pressure falls abruptly and markedly at the onset of exercise when all arterial and cardiopulmonary baroreceptors are denervated, and the central nervous system receives no neural feedback from them. If exercise is mild, arterial pressure falls less but remains depressed throughout the exercise, whereas in moderate to heavy exercise, arterial pressure falls more but then rises to preexercise levels, after a delay of 1 to 2 minutes (a similar delay in the onset of MSNA was

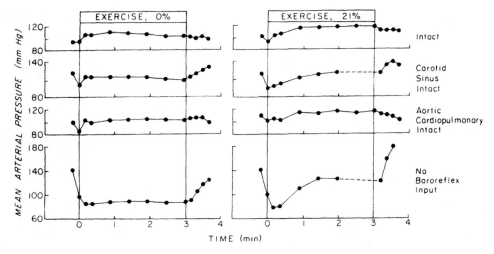

Figure 12-7   Effects of losses of arterial and cardiopulmonary baroreceptors on the responses of arterial pressure to mild treadmill exercise at 0 percent grade, 5.5 km h^{-1} and heavy exercise at 21 percent grade, 5.5 km h^{-1}. Top panel shows normal responses with all baroreceptors intact. Next panel shows responses with only carotid sinus baroreflex intact. Next panel shows responses with intact aortic and cardiopulmonary baroreflexes with carotid sinus isolated. Finally, all baroreflex input is lost. (Redrawn from Melcher and Donald, 1981.)

described in Chapter 11; see below). Recall that in some studies, sinoaortic denervation appeared to have no effect on the cardiovascular responses to exercise in the steady state (Vanhoutte et al., 1966; Krasney et al., 1974; McRitchie et al., 1976). However, Krasney and colleagues (1974) observed the transient hypotensive responses typified in Figure 12-7. In subsequent studies, others also saw that total baroreceptor denervation caused a sudden drop in arterial pressure at the onset of exercise (Ardell et al., 1980; Melcher and Donald, 1981, and Walgenbach and Donald, 1983b; Hales and Ludbrook, 1988). Of particular interest is the fact that during mild exercise, arterial pressure remained depressed, whereas in heavier exercise, the drop was transient and arterial pressure recovered to the pre-exercise level after 2 to 3 min despite the absence of the baroreflex (Figure 12-7). This recovery is caused by reflexes from hypoperfused muscles (due to low pressure, as discussed later) and has no bearing on baroreflexes.

One problem with sinoaortic denervation is that the period of recovery between denervation and the first experiments, which has varied in different studies, can provide the potential for the animal to adapt to the loss of baroreceptors. Effects of denervation change with time over days (Ludbrook et al., 1986). This could account for some of the different responses in the studies just cited. Thus responses may reveal more about the adaptation to the loss than about the acute effects of interrupting the feedback from the baroreceptors.

The solution to the dilemma caused by adaptation came with the technique allowing reversible isolation of the carotid sinus from the remainder of the circulation. In contrast to animals with baroreceptor denervation, *the central nervous system is not deprived of the neural feedback from these baroreceptors;* for unknown reasons (there are many ideas) this feedback profoundly alters the responses. Pressure within the isolated sinus could be changed back and forth between preset static pressures at different levels or open to normal systemic pressure (free-running) (Melcher and Donald, 1981; Walgenbach and Donald, 1983b; Ludbrook et al., 1986). Melcher and Donald (1981) and Walgenbach and Donald (1983b) interrupted the carotid sinus reflex by holding intra-sinus pressure below the threshold level of receptor firing. Figure 12-7 shows a typical sequence in which Melcher and Donald (1981) studied the responses to exercise at various stages of baroreceptor denervation. They found that a normal initial arterial pressure response to exercise required either an intact carotid sinus or the combination of intact aortic and cardiopulmonary baroreflexes (the cardiopulmonary receptors proved in later studies to be unimportant). When all three of these baroreceptor groupings were eliminated, the normal rise in arterial pressure after the brief initial dip was abolished. *In short, the rise in arterial pressure in response to exercise requires the active participation of the arterial baroreflexes.*

Why Did Baroreceptor Denervation Cause Hypotension at the Onset of Exercise?

Walgenbach and Donald (1983b) investigated the cause of the transient drop in pressure at the onset of exercise in dogs with aortic baroreceptors denervated, carotid sinuses isolated and held at a constant static pressure, and with the carotid sinuses exposed to normal arterial pulsatile pressure. Cardiac output rose normally in proportion to the intensity of exercise in all cases. This means that the sudden fall in arterial pressure occurred because there was a much greater rise in total vascular conductance in dogs acutely deprived of arterial baroreflexes. Again, this points strongly to the idea that arterial baroreflexes support the rise in arterial pressure at the onset of exercise by causing vasoconstriction and decreasing vascular conductance. For example, a sudden and large (414 percent) rise in renal sympathetic nerve activity in response to exercise in rabbits was abolished by sinoaortic denervation (DiCarlo and Bishop, 1992). The findings suggest that the rise in cardiac output at the onset of exercise may be "too slow" so that the baroreflex had to correct a mismatch between cardiac output and vascular conductance by eliciting vasoconstriction.

Inasmuch as the acute interruption of arterial baroreflexes can alter arterial pressure during exercise without affecting heart rate or cardiac output, Walgenbach and Shepherd (1984) concluded: "Thus the role of arterial baroreflexes is to govern the total systemic vascular resistance during and after exercise. Heart rate and cardiac output are regulated by different mechanisms" (i.e., different from those regulating systemic vascular resistance). This has the familiar sound of an argument stated repeatedly in previous chapters; namely, in response to exercise, heart rate and cardiac output are increased by central command, whereas afferent feedback arising from other reflexes—muscle chemoreflexes (?), or arterial baroreflexes (?), or both—may regulate vascular conductance. Some findings, discussed later, argue against this generalization—at least for dynamic exercise.

Ludbrook and his colleagues (1986) looked at the importance of arterial baroreflexes in the response to the onset of dynamic exercise in rabbits trained to hop while on a motor-driven treadmill. After sinoaortic denervation the rabbits' arterial pressure fell at the onset of exercise, just as in dogs (i.e., Melcher and Donald, 1981). Ludbrook and his colleagues directed attention to the first 10 seconds of mild exercise in order to explain the mechanism of hypotension in their baroreceptor-denervated rabbits (Ludbrook and Graham, 1985; Ludbrook et al., 1986; Hales and Ludbrook, 1988). Ludbrook and Graham (1985) concluded that at the onset of exercise in normal rabbits the arterial baroreflex immediately ceases to exert most of its tonic inhibitory effects on heart rate and systemic vascular resistance, and, as a consequence, heart rate and systemic vascular resistance rise suddenly *causing arterial pressure to rise.* When Ludbrook and his colleagues (1986) inflated a cuff on the carotid artery to unload the carotid sinus baroreceptor at the onset of exercise (all of the other baroreceptors were denervated), the increases in heart rate, systemic vascular resistance, and arterial pressure were suppressed, that is, as though the baroreflex was essential for the normal (i.e., opposite) responses. After sinoaortic denervation, a fall in mean arterial pressure with the onset of exercise coincided with a much greater fall in systemic vascular resistance and little (Ludbrook and Graham, 1985) or no (Hales and Ludbrook, 1988) effect on cardiac output.

Hales and Ludbrook (1988) concluded that approximately 40 percent of the initial rise in muscle blood flow during the first 20 seconds of exercise in their rabbits was contributed by regional vasoconstriction and diversion of blood flow from inactive regions (splanchnic organs, kidneys, and skin) to active skeletal muscle (recall that exercise was very mild and that rabbits have small hearts with small output). Presumably the regional vasoconstriction is a necessary consequence of the long time (approximately 40 seconds) required for cardiac output to rise to a steady level in rabbits. Again this creates a mismatch between cardiac output and total vascular conductance or a "pressure error." This diversion of blood flow to active muscle was lost after arterial baroreceptor denervation and, as a consequence, arterial pressure fell markedly at the onset of exercise. Again, this initial vasoconstrictor response has been interpreted as a loss of tonic baroreceptor restraint on sympathetic vasoconstriction. That is, arterial baroreflexes were presumed to be momentarily "shut off," or insensitive, at the onset of exercise (Hales and Ludbrook, 1988).

Another interpretation of the preceding results, and one supported by other studies, is that the baroreflex is immediately shifted upward to a higher operating point at the onset of exercise, and it is the baroreflex that becomes the stimulus to increase vasoconstrictor outflow to inactive regions whereby aiding the rapid rise in blood pressure. The hypothesis is that the baroreflex is not actually suppressed at the onset of exercise (although the effect is the same); rather, the reflex is immediately shifted rightward to a higher operating point, as illustrated in Figure 12-8A. Figure 12-8A also shows (vertical arrow from OP$_1$) that the new rightward-shifted stimulus-response curve is insensitive to the prevailing arterial pressure at OP$_1$ before this pressure has time to rise to OP$_2$. This is theory.

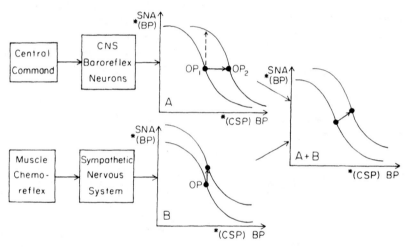

Figure 12-8 Hypothetical baroreflex-function curves to illustrate the contrasting effects of central command and muscle chemoreflexes on curve position and operating points (OP). Function curves can be expressed as the relationship between systemic arterial pressure (BP) and sympathetic nervous activity (SNA) or, as often done experimentally, as carotid sinus pressure *(CSP) substituted for SNA on the x-axis versus systemic arterial pressure *(BP), substituted for SNA on the y-axis. **(A)** In theory, central command "resets" the baroreflex to OP$_2$ by acting on the neuron pool receiving baroreceptor afferents. The vertical dashed arrow from OP$_1$ (initial operating point) to the reset curve shows that any perturbation of pressure around the original OP is poorly corrected because this pressure falls on the insensitive region of the new curve (i.e., the baroreflex is momentarily insensitive at the onset of exercise). **(B)** A vertical shift in the baroreflex function curve signifies that the muscle chemoreflex raises BP or SNA without changing OP because the stimulus acts only on the efferent arm of the reflex and not the central neurons controlling the reflex. A + B illustrates the combined predicted effects of both stimuli on the baroreflex function curve during exercise. (Modified from Rowell and O'Leary, 1990.)

One important difference between the studies by Ludbrook and colleagues and those by Donald's group was that the former studies focused on the changes in the baroreflex during the first 10 seconds of exercise, whereas Donald and colleagues investigated the characteristics of the baroreflex during a steady state of exercise after initial shifts in the baroreflex function curves had occurred. Once the steady-state and normal sensitivity of the baroreflex is achieved during mild exercise, the reflex serves to stabilize arterial pressure. Note in Figure 12-9 the instability of blood pressure during mild exercise in dogs deprived of all baroreceptors. This stability improves as the intensity of exercise increases as shown in this figure.

Summary.   In summary, arterial pressure does not rise in response to exercise or in proportion to work intensity if animals are without any feedback from the baroreceptors due either to their denervation or, alternatively, to keeping transmural pressure of the isolated intact baroreceptors below a threshold level. If baroreceptor transmural pressure is held at resting levels, then the central nervous system continues to receive information from the baroreceptors and the central neurons activate the sympathetic nervous system causing extreme vasoconstriction, as will be shown in the next section.

What is the Evidence for "Resetting" of the Arterial Baroreflex to Higher Pressures?

The term *resetting* has been borrowed from the field of engineering to describe a rather restricted scheme that describes the shifts in one definite, preset or control value for arterial pressure (a "set point"). Although the

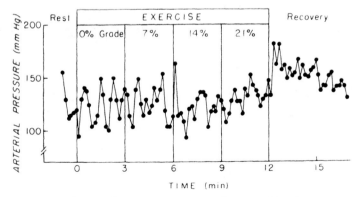

Figure 12-9   Typical arterial pressure responses during mild to heavy exercise in a dog without arterial or cardiopulmonary baroreflexes. Note the marked instability of pressure during mild exercise as opposed to greater stability during heavy exercise. (Redrawn from Walgenbach and Donald, 1983b.)

reviews of Korner (1979) and Sagawa (1983) point out that instead of a single "set point," there are what they prefer to call *operating points* of reflexes that can be continuously variable over a range of pressures. That is, there is no firmly fixed "set point." For simplicity, the operating point of the reflex will be treated as illustrated in Figure 12-3A. It shows the operating point of the baroreflex to be the point of maximum slope or highest gain of the stimulus-response curve. A rightward shift in the baroreflex stimulus-response curve (or function curve), regardless of definitions, conveys the essential idea that the reflex has been "reset" and that the operating point (or "set-point" if you prefer) has shifted to a higher pressure.

The basic question we face here is whether the stimulus-response curve for the entire baroreflex (receptors, central neuron pool, and effectors) is altered during exercise so that pressure that is regulated by the reflex is higher than the prevailing pressure at rest. If one assumes that the stimulus-response curve of the human arterial baroreflex has the same sigmoid shape observed in other species (see Sagawa, 1983), then we can describe the changes that might occur at the onset of exercise as in Figure 12-8. This figure shows hypothetical stimulus-response curves for the arterial baroreflex expressed as the relationship between sympathetic nervous activity (SNA) and systemic arterial pressure (BP). The y-axis is also labeled *(BP) and the x-axis is labeled *(CSP) simply to show also that the arterial baroreflex is often described as the relationship between the isolated carotid sinus pressure *(CSP) and systemic arterial pressure *(BP) (e.g., as in Figure 12-3).

The carotid sinus stimulus-response curves described by Melcher and Donald (1981) had the form shown in Figure 12-8B. This *vertical shift* in the carotid sinus stimulus-response curve is described in Figure 12-3C and is unrelated to the rightward shift in the curve that signifies "resetting." In general, a vertical shift in the baroreflex curve presumably stems from a disturbance that activates only the efferent arm of the reflex (i.e., the sympathetic nervous system) and raises systemic arterial pressure without affecting the carotid sinus threshold or operating point. Inasmuch as the operating point for the reflex is unchanged, the reflex is not "reset."

The findings of Melcher and Donald (1981) are not an argument against resetting of the baroreflex because the aortic baroreceptors were intact, and Walgenbach and Donald (1983b) showed that their removal unmasked large effects of exercise on the gain and position (on its pressure axis) of the carotid sinus stimulus-response curve.

Figure 12-8A (also Figure 12-3D) shows the lateral shifts in the stimulus-response curve that typify resetting and again which are, in theory, caused by disturbances acting on the central neuron pool that integrates the entire reflex (Korner, 1979; Sagawa, 1983). Central command could act on the central neurons involved in the baroreflex and elicit such a lateral shift in the baroreflex function curve (see Korner, 1979). In contrast, the muscle chemoreflex, for example, might be expected to cause the vertical shift in the curve because it presumably activates neurons that directly control the sympathetic nervous system without affecting the entire baroreflex.

It is now clear that the arterial baroreceptors themselves are not simply adapting to a higher pressure caused by a higher cardiac output in exercise (O'Leary et al., 1989). As discussed in Chapter 2, any mechanoreceptors, such as baroreceptors, adapt rapidly to a higher *static* pressure, but they do not adapt similarly to pulsatile pressures (Mendelowitz and Scher, 1988). In short, it is the entire reflex and not just the receptors that are reset.

The first line of evidence in support of resetting of the arterial baroreflex during exercise comes from the demonstration that arterial pressure does not rise at the onset of exercise in dogs after sinoaortic denervation; rather, pressure falls (Krasney et al., 1974; Ardell et al., 1980; Melcher and Donald, 1981; Walgenbach and Donald, 1983b; Ludbrook and Graham, 1985; Ludbrook et al., 1986; Hales and Ludbrook, 1988). Inasmuch as the *arterial baroreflex is essential for the normal rise in arterial pressure at the onset of exercise,* it is assumed that the baroreflex must have been reset to a higher pressure. This is further indicated by the fact that the baroreflex will continue to oppose any extreme rise in arterial pressure (e.g., Strange et al., 1990). That is, above the operating point the reflex still functions in its "usual" manner by opposing hypertension.

One of the most convincing albeit indirect demonstrations of resetting of the arterial baroreflex occurred when Walgenbach and Donald (1983b) held blood pressure within the isolated carotid sinuses of exercising dogs at a level equivalent to resting arterial pressure (i.e., a static pressure of 140 mmHg was required to maintain normal resting systemic arterial pressure). The remaining baroreceptors in these dogs had been surgically eliminated. Figure 12-10 shows the changes in arterial pressure, heart rate, and cardiac output in these dogs when they were intact and then after sinoaortic denervation and surgical isolation of their carotid sinuses, again with sinus pressure maintained at constant "resting" level. The increases in cardiac output were essentially the same in these dogs before and after their surgery, but after an initial transient fall, the increments in arterial pressure were extreme when the sinuses were isolated. After an initial rise in total vascular conductance between rest and exercise at 0 percent grade, conductance increased no further. This means that a powerful vasoconstrictor outflow successfully opposed any further vasodilation in active muscle; other regions had to be maximally vasoconstricted as well to explain the rise in arterial pressure. *"Resting" carotid sinus pressure must have been interpreted by the central nervous system as a progressively increasing hypotensive stimulus* with increasing severity of exercise. This would be the expected result of a step-wise resetting of the arterial baroreflex in proportion to increasing work rate. At each resetting, isolated carotid sinus pressure failed to increase so that a maximal vasoconstrictor stimulus was directed by the central nervous system to all vasculature

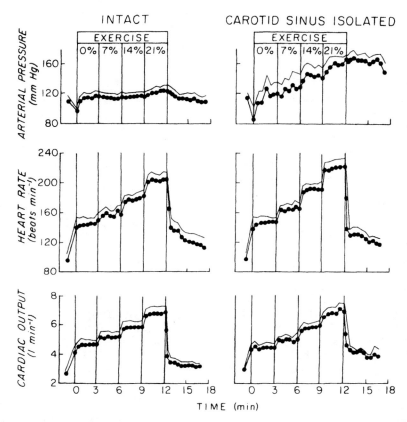

Figure 12-10   Evidence for upward resetting of the arterial baroreflex in proportion to intensity of exercise. Data are from dogs with intact baroreflex (*left*) and after denervation of aortic baroreceptors and surgical isolation of carotid sinuses (*right*) with sinus pressure kept at constant static level to reproduce resting baroreceptor afferent activity. In dogs with isolated carotid sinuses, cardiac output rose normally, heart rate was augmented, but elevations in arterial pressure were extreme owing to intense vasoconstriction—even in active muscles. "Resting" carotid sinus pressure must have been interpreted centrally as a progressively increasing hypotensive stimulus with each workload-dependent resetting of the baroreflex. (Redrawn from Walgenbach and Donald, 1983b.)

with such power that even active muscle did not vasodilate at the higher intensities of exercise. In short, the central nervous system did everything possible to raise carotid sinus pressure to the elevated level it was seeking but could never attain.

DiCarlo and Bishop (1992) also tested the hypothesis that the rise in arterial pressure and sympathetic nerve activity during exercise depends on a sudden resetting of the arterial baroreflex. When they prevented the normal rise in arterial pressure attending exercise in rabbits by infusing the vasodilator nitroglycerin, as shown in Figure 12-11, exercise was

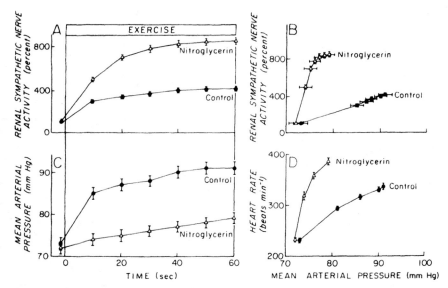

Figure 12-11   Further evidence that onset of exercise shifts arterial baroreflex operating point to higher pressures. Delaying the rise in arterial pressure (in rabbits) during exercise by infusing nitroglycerin (panel C) caused marked increase in renal sympathetic nerve activity (panel A) and also heart rate. Panels B and D show the exaggerated increases in sympathetic outflow and heart rate at any given arterial pressure when the rise in pressure was delayed by nitroglycerin. (Redrawn from DiCarlo and Bishop, 1992.)

accompanied by an abnormally large (848 percent) increase in renal sympathetic nerve activity and also a greater-than-normal rise in heart rate. Figure 12-11B,D show a marked upward shift in the relationship between renal sympathetic nerve activity and heart rate at any given arterial pressure when the rise in pressure was suppressed by nitroglycerin infusion. Again, these responses appear to reflect an attempt by the central nervous system and the arterial baroreflex to raise arterial pressure to a reset operating point.

Summary.   In summary, arterial blood pressure does not rise at the onset of exercise or in proportion to work intensity if animals are without any feedback from the baroreceptors due either to their denervation or to keeping their transmural pressure below threshold level (a subsequent rise in pressure during heavier exercise is caused by the muscle reflex described in Chapter 11). If the transmural pressure of intact baroreceptors is held at resting levels while animals exercise, then the central nervous system receives feedback from the baroreceptors and activates the sympathetic nervous system so that extreme increases in nerve traffic are directed to kidneys, for example, and to active skeletal muscle to the extent that its vasodilation during even severe exercise is prevented. Although these experimental results do not prove that at the onset of exercise the arterial baroreflex was rapidly shifted upward to a new operating point; they do reflect what would occur had the reflex been so altered.

Experiments by Ebert (1986) and by Scherrer and colleagues (1990) may come the closest to revealing an upward resetting of the carotid sinus baroreflex in humans (both used isometric contractions, but the point can still be made). Ebert applied a sequence of positive and negative pressures to the neck over the carotid sinus during (1) supine rest (control), (2) during the period of anticipation just before an isometric contraction began, and (3) during an isometric contraction at 20 percent of MVC. The stimulus-response curve for the carotid sinus reflex during rest and isometric contraction is shown in Figure 12-12. Isometric contraction caused a rightward shift in the line relating carotid sinus distending pressure to radial intra-arterial pressure, suggesting a rightward shift in the operating point of the reflex with the unchanged slope of the line indicating an unaltered baroreflex sensitivity. Inasmuch as neck pressure was changed every 5 seconds, the stimulus-response curves in Figure 12-12 represent the mixed results of the rapid changes in heart rate, which is probably the dominant factor along with cardiac output, and a slow (10- to 15-second) sympathetic vasoconstriction which lags behind heart rate by two or three periods of neck pressure.

Of particular interest in this study was the finding that immediately before contraction, anticipation of the task blunted the responses of heart rate and arterial pressure to altered carotid sinus transmural pressure. It

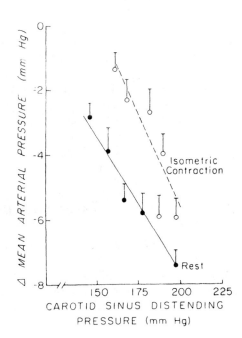

Figure 12-12 Evidence from humans that isometric forearm contraction shifts the operating point of the arterial baroreflex to higher pressures. Carotid sinus distending pressure was increased by application of negative pressure to the neck over the sinuses in 5-second steps. The rightward shift of the slope indicated resetting without a change in gain or sensitivity (i.e., no significant change in slope with contraction). *Anticipation* of a contraction also caused a rightward shift in the curve for "contraction." (Redrawn from Ebert, 1986.)

appears that resetting of the baroreflex to a higher operating point may have commenced just before the contraction began.

When Scherrer and coworkers (1990) pharmacologically suppressed the rise in arterial pressure in response to an isometric forearm contraction, increases in heart rate and especially MSNA were greatly increased above those observed during normal contraction. Their results are interpreted here (not by the authors) as evidence for resetting of the arterial baroreflex.

Why Does Central Command Not Raise Arterial Pressure at the Onset of Exercise If Baroreflexes Are Absent?

It has been proposed often that it is central command that rapidly raises arterial pressure by raising heart rate and cardiac output at the onset of exercise. Why then does arterial pressure drop at the onset of exercise in animals with sinoaortic denervation if central command is still operating? One answer is that central command could exert its effects on arterial pressure by resetting the arterial baroreflex (Rowell, 1986; Houk, 1988; Rowell and O'Leary, 1990). Presumably central command cannot reset the baroreflex if there is no baroreflex to reset. That is, the central nervous system does not raise arterial pressure without some afferent nerve traffic being fed back, which can be centrally modulated. In this scheme, at the onset of exercise when the arterial baroreflex is immediately reset rightward to a higher pressure by central command, as in Figure 12-8, the system would then perceive hypotension relative to its new operating point. Therefore, heart rate and sympathetic vasoconstrictor activity must increase immediately to raise arterial pressure to the new operating point (Ludbrook and Graham, 1985; Ludbrook et al., 1986); otherwise pressure would fall because of uncompensated vasodilation in the active muscles (as in Hales and Ludbrook, 1988).

We have seen that an intact arterial baroreflex appears to be essential for the sudden rise in arterial pressure at the onset of exercise. At this moment, central command could cause a virtually instantaneous resetting of the arterial baroreflex so that its operating point is immediately shifted to a higher pressure; however, a finite period of time is required for arterial pressure to rise and reach its new operating point. Presumably it is this error signal derived from the elevated operating point and the lagging rise in arterial pressure (i.e., a pressure error) that causes the vasoconstriction.

Does Central Command Affect Sympathetic Activity and Heart Rate Directly or as a Secondary Effect of Resetting the Arterial Baroreflex?

It appears that with initiation of central command, arterial baroreflex control of renal sympathetic nerve activity is reset (DiCarlo and Bishop, 1992). The vagal withdrawal attributed to increased central command appears to be independent of the arterial baroreflex (Daskalopoulos et al., 1984), but the rise in heart rate attributable to increased cardiac sympathetic nerve activity appears to depend on an intact baroreflex (DiCarlo

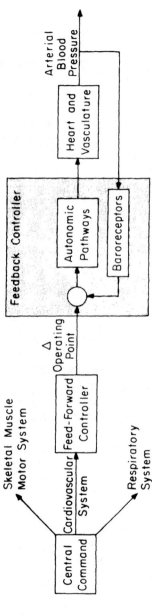

Figure 12-13 A scheme for coordination of feed-forward and feedback control of the cardiovascular system during exercise. Motor system signals used to initiate locomotion initiate feed-forward actions (central command) on the cardiovascular system. Coordination with feedback control (the arterial baroreflex) is accomplished by sending the feed-forward command to the feedback controller which resets the operating point for arterial pressure regulation during exercise. (Adapted from Houk, 1988.)

and Bishop, 1992). Therefore the increase in sympathetic outflow to the heart and kidneys at the onset of exercise appears to be secondary to the resetting of the arterial baroreflex, presumably by central command.

The proposal that a feed-forward controller such as central command could work by resetting the arterial baroreflex is not a new idea (e.g., Rowell, 1986; Houk, 1988). This is another way of saying that central command as a feed-forward controller also works in combination with a feedback controller, that is, the arterial reflex. Houk's scheme, illustrated in Figure 12-13, is that the feedback controller of the circulation in exercise is the arterial baroreflex which sends its forcing functions (output) to a controlled system, the heart and vasculature, in order to regulate arterial pressure. The coordination of feedback control with feed-forward control is accomplished by directing feed-forward command to the feedback controller where it resets the operating point of the arterial baroreflex (Houk, 1988).

ROLE OF CARDIOPULMONARY BARORECEPTORS IN DYNAMIC EXERCISE

The filling pressure of the heart during dynamic exercise is determined mainly by the effectiveness of the muscle pump and also by the redistribution of cardiac output between active muscle and the inactive organs whose blood flow must be curtailed by sympathetic vasoconstriction if central venous pressure is to be maintained (Chapter 5, Figures 5-14 and 6-8). The maintenance of ventricular filling pressure during exercise requires a balance between the purely mechanical effects of the muscle pump and the sympathetic control of the blood vessels. The increased muscle pumping activity and the high percent of cardiac output passing through active muscle during severe exercise increases ventricular filling pressure (Figure 5-7), which could be opposed by cardiopulmonary baroreflexes as suggested by Sprangers (1991). The point of this brief review of Chapter 5 is to emphasize that if the cardiopulmonary mechanoreflexes responded to the rise in filling pressure during exercise by releasing vasoconstriction, cardiac filling pressure and stroke volume would fall. There is no evidence to suggest that the cardiopulmonary baroreflex opposes the *rise* in central venous pressure during exercise. There is indirect evidence from humans that the cardiopulmonary baroreflexes may counteract the *fall* in central venous pressure and stroke volume accompanying vasodilation of skin during exercise and heat stress (Mack et al., 1988). The uncertainty is due to the possibility that small changes in aortic pulse pressure rather than the fall in central venous pressure could initiate the vasoconstriction through an arterial baroreflex.

Inasmuch as the cardiopulmonary receptors are hydraulically separated from the arterial side of the circulation and cannot "sense" arterial pressure, they cannot be involved in its traditional feedback regulation. A number of experiments discount any significant role of cardiopulmonary baroreceptors in cardiovascular control during dynamic exercise (the same conclusion was made for isometric contractions; e.g., Seals, 1988). For example, when Melcher and Donald (1981) interrupted the cardiopulmonary baroreceptors in dogs by bilateral vagotomy, there were no significant effects on arterial pressure during mild to heavy exercise as long as the carotid baroreflex was intact. Walgenbach and Donald (1983a) made progressive interruptions of the baroreflexes and found that interruption of cardiopulmonary baroreflexes caused no further disruption of the cardiovascular response.

CENTRAL COMMAND, MUSCLE CHEMOREFLEXES AND ARTERIAL BAROREFLEXES: HOW DO THEY OPERATE TOGETHER?

General Hypothesis

Based on the findings discussed so far, in this and in previous chapters, the following general hypothesis about cardiovascular control during exercise seems reasonable: In the response to dynamic exercise after central command "resets" the arterial baroreflex to a higher operating pressure and raises cardiac output by vagal withdrawal; the initial error corrected by the sympathetic nervous system is an "arterial pressure error." That is, the prevailing level of arterial pressure at the onset of exercise is perceived by the central nervous system to be hypotensive relative to the new baroreflex operating point. Hence a sustained increase in sympathetic outflow is needed to reduce vascular conductance and raise cardiac output in order to reduce the perceived "arterial pressure error."

If we reexamine Figure 11-6, the preceding hypothesis suggests that for some reason the rise in cardiac output before heart rate reaches 100 beats min^{-1} is sufficient to prevent any mismatch between vascular conductance and cardiac output; that is, there is no arterial pressure error that has to be corrected by an increase in sympathetic vasoconstrictor activity. The muscle chemoreflex can apparently be ruled out as a mechanism for the instantaneous resetting of the arterial baroreflex and the sudden rise in cardiac output and blood pressure at the onset of exercise. *First*, if the response time of the chemoreflex were actually 1 to 2 minutes (owing to the time needed to accumulate metabolites in muscle; see Chapter 11), it would be much too slow to have such a rapid effect. *Second*, the chemoreflex is reputed to act only on the sympathetic nervous system, which is too slow to generate the rapid increases in heart rate seen when the rate is below 100 beats min^{-1}. A role for muscle mechanoreflexes cannot be ruled out; not enough is known to comment.

Above a heart rate of 100 beats min^{-1}, when most tonic vagal activity is withdrawn, sympathetic vasoconstrictor activity increases steeply with increasing oxygen uptake and cardiac output, suggesting that a "pressure error'' or some other error signal begins to develop above this heart rate. Whatever the error might be, its correction requires parallel increases in sympathetic outflow to the heart to increase heart rate, to the blood vessels to reduce blood flow, and to the kidneys to increase renin release (Figure 11-6). A probable stimulus to sympathetic outflow is the muscle chemoreflex; any sudden contribution from muscle mechanoreflexes at that time seems unlikely. In fact, the muscle chemoreflex would be an excellent candidate for the stimulus if a mismatch between muscle blood flow and metabolism develops when heart rate reaches 100 beats min^{-1}. Vasoconstriction would divert blood flow away from inactive regions and thereby improve its perfusion of active muscle and reduce the metabolic error signal. However, there is no evidence that the chemoreflex is normally active at these low levels of exercise unless there is some impedance to blood flow. In fact, even when heart rate is well in excess of 100 beats min^{-1}, without partial obstruction of muscle blood flow (i.e., free-flow conditions), none of the metabolites currently associated with the muscle chemoreflex are evident in blood draining the active muscles. Muscle blood flow appears to be well above the threshold for the chemoreflex. Also keep in mind that active muscle also receives the increase in sympathetic activity as well as the inactive regions (Chapter 7).

Eventually, at heart rates of 130 to 140 beats min^{-1} (or higher in well-conditioned individuals), blood lactate concentration begins to rise, but this still may not signal the activation of the chemoreflex. Even this rise in lactate may not represent a true metabolic error signal. Although accumulation of lactate is closely associated with the onset of increased MSNA and may reflect a critical reduction in oxygen delivery during isometric contraction, this appears not to be the case during dynamic exercise when lactate is released long before a mismatch between blood flow and metabolism or any real deficiency in oxygen delivery exists. This overflow of lactate owing to the accelerated breakdown of muscle glycogen occurs readily in human muscle (in comparison to dog muscle, for example) because of its low oxidative capacity; lactate accumulates by simple mass action because of our limited ability to metabolize pyruvate. It is not known if such an increase in lactate release from muscle is a stimulus for the chemoreflex during dynamic exercise.

In the hypothetical scheme to be developed in this chapter, it is proposed that the correction of metabolic errors is secondary to the correction of arterial pressure errors. Aside from conditions that mechanically restrict muscle blood flow and cause it to fall below a critical level, the chemoreflex may not be tonically active until the severity of exercise becomes so great that the heart can no longer provide the active muscles with the blood flow they require.

This last condition provides us with the most difficult problem of all to solve, because the only way to prevent a fall in arterial pressure when cardiac output approaches its maximum, and 85 percent of the total blood flow goes to active muscle, is to vasoconstrict active muscle.

When Are Arterial Baroreflexes and Muscle Chemoreflexes Activated During Dynamic Exercise?

The exceedingly complex story unraveling the significance of arterial baroreflexes in cardiovascular control during exercise can be summarized in five main points. Some of these points have already been developed in this chapter. They are as follows:

1. The sensitivity or gain of the arterial baroreflex is similar during rest and steady-state exercise.
2. The arterial baroreflex is essential for the rise in arterial pressure at the onset of dynamic exercise as a consequence of the immediate shift of its operating point to a higher arterial pressure.
3. The arterial baroreflex is essential to the maintenance of a stable arterial pressure during mild exercise—but not during heavy exercise.
4. The gain of the arterial baroreflex is less than that of the muscle chemoreflex when the latter is also treated as a (flow-sensitive) pressure-raising reflex. The two reflexes buffer or oppose one another.
5. The arterial baroreflex and/or the muscle chemoreflex must counteract mismatches between vascular conductance and cardiac output by vasoconstricting active muscle to maintain blood pressure during severe dynamic exercise.

Hypothesis 1: Mild Exercise

The arterial baroreflex will not elicit an increase in sympathetic nervous activity at the onset of mild dynamic exercise when the rise in cardiac output is rapid enough to raise arterial pressure to its new and immediately elevated operating point. This hypothesis has two parts which are based on what has been described previously in this chapter (see also Rowell and O'Leary, 1990). *First,* central command immediately shifts the operating point of the arterial baroreflex to a higher pressure and withdraws vagal outflow to the heart at the onset of exercise. *Second,* if the consequent rise in cardiac output is fast enough and large enough to raise arterial pressure to the new baroreflex operating point without significant delay, then there is no arterial pressure error and no increase in sympathetic nervous activity.

The following observations, described earlier in this chapter, are consistent with hypothesis 1. First, arterial baroreceptor denervation will, by depriving the central nervous system of any feedback from the baroreceptors, prevent the rise in arterial pressure at the onset of exercise (see Figure 12-7). Second, baroreceptor denervation also prevents the regulation of cardiac output and arterial pressure during exercise after initial responses are over. Figure 12-9 shows that during mild exercise, arterial pressure never rises to a stable level and it fluctuates markedly and randomly.

Without the arterial baroreflex, arterial pressure remains depressed and is highly unstable because all extraneous influences on pressure such as noise, mild excitement, and so on are unbuffered.

Hypothesis 2: Moderate Exercise

If the fast vagal component of the rise in cardiac output at the onset of moderate exercise is not sufficient to raise arterial pressure close to its new operating point, then the sympathetic nervous system must increase its activity in order to complete the rise in arterial pressure and minimize the "pressure error." The key to this hypothesis is the speed of the increases in heart rate and cardiac output. The specific hypothesis is that during moderate exercise, when heart rate exceeds 100 beats min^{-1}, the activation of vagal withdrawal by central command still increases cardiac output, but not enough. The *rapid* rise in heart rate does not raise cardiac output to a level that is sufficient to compensate fully for the sudden vasodilation in active muscle; as a consequence, arterial pressure cannot be increased *immediately* to its new, reset (i.e., reset in proportion to exercise intensity) operating point so there is a "pressure error." As a consequence of this error, sympathetic nervous activity to both the heart and to the resistance vessels increases. The sympathetically mediated increase in heart rate and cardiac output is much slower (by 15- to 20-fold) than the parasympathetically mediated rise. Thus vasoconstriction in splanchnic, renal, and cutaneous regions and skeletal muscle, both resting and active, becomes a necessary adjunct to increased cardiac output in order to raise arterial pressure as quickly as possible to minimize the pressure error.

The basic scheme is therefore the same as that put forward for hypothesis 1 except that here, the arterial baroreflex must activate the sympathetic nervous system in order to complete the rise in arterial pressure to its new operating point. This hypothetical scheme is illustrated schematically in Figure 12-14.

Is the Muscle Chemoreflex Involved in the Activation of Sympathetic Nervous Activity?

When the level of exercise is too low to activate the muscle chemoreflex, the arterial baroreflex must be essential to modulate cardiac output and sympathetic activity in order to maintain a stable arterial pressure. Figures 12-7 and 12-9 show that denervation of arterial baroreceptors disrupts arterial pressure regulation during mild exercise. Pressure falls markedly and remains depressed and is also unstable because all extraneous influences on pressure remain unbuffered (Walgenbach and Shepherd, 1984). This instability may also originate from the fact that the level of exercise was too mild to elicit a chemoreflex during the period when pressure was low. Note in Figure 12-9 that arterial pressure is more stable at the higher work rates when the muscle chemoreflex is presumably active. These results show that *when there is neither a functional arterial baroreflex nor*

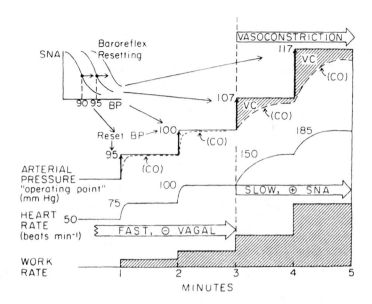

Figure 12-14   Schematic illustration of hypotheses 1 and 2, which propose that errors in arterial pressure regulation occur whenever the rise in cardiac output (CO) at the onset of exercise (or sudden increase in work intensity) is not rapid enough to raise arterial pressure immediately to its new (reset) operating point. At each onset of exercise and first increment in work rate, heart rate increases *rapidly* from 50 to 75 and then to 100 beats min^{-1} by fast vagal withdrawal so that blood pressure rises rapidly to its reset value, that is, to 95 and 100 mmHg by a sudden increase in cardiac output shown as (CO) and dashed line. At each additional increment in work rate with heart rate rising from 100 to 150 to 185 beats min^{-1}, the rate of rise in heart rate and CO is slow because the response to increased sympathetic nervous activity (+SNA) is 10 to 15 times slower than parasympathetic responses. Thus the rise in arterial pressure from 100 to 107 to 117 mmHg is delayed and the gap between these reset pressures and CO must be corrected by *vasoconstriction* (VC in shaded regions). Therefore, sympathetic nervous activity and vasoconstriction begin after heart rate reaches 100 beats min^{-1} (Figure 11-6) because of the transient mismatch between CO and total vascular conductance caused by (1) the sudden shift of baroreflex operating point to a higher pressure with each increase in work rate (baroreflex resetting shown by baroreflex-function curves in the inset), and (2) the slow rise in cardiac output attributable to slow sympathetically mediated responses (Rowell and O'Leary, 1990). (Modified from Rowell, 1991.)

an active muscle chemoreflex, regulation of heart rate, cardiac output, and arterial pressure are lost during mild exercise.

At the onset of moderate to heavy exercise, arterial pressure falls in dogs with sinoaortic denervation, but within 1 or 2 minutes pressure returns to the control level (Figure 12-7) and remains stable thereafter. It is presumed that the fall in arterial pressure caused muscle blood flow to fall beyond the threshold for activation of the muscle chemoreflex (Figure

11-12) so that the chemoreflex caused the return of arterial pressure to normal. Any further fluctuations in arterial pressure caused by changing muscle blood flow would be modulated by the tonically active chemoreflex. In this setting the chemoreflex serves as a secondary or backup "regulator" of arterial pressure; but this regulation is achieved primarily by controlling muscle blood flow by changes in cardiac output and regional vasoconstriction (exercise is moderate so that corrections in muscle blood flow are possible).

Another putative cause for this recovery of pressure in the sinoaortic-denervated dog is that the hypotension and fall in muscle blood flow so weakens the muscle (Hobbs and McCloskey, 1987) that central command raises arterial pressure (see Seals and Enoka's findings of the close relationship between muscle fatigue, increased electromyographic activity and muscle sympathetic nerve activity in Figure 8-9). This idea is countered first by the finding of Kozelka and colleagues (1987) that when spinal cord lesions block traffic from muscle afferents, muscle ischemia will not raise arterial pressure; that is, central command was not the mechanism for the rise in pressure in these voluntarily exercising dogs. Second, central command appears not to influence sympathetic activity directly, but rather its effects are secondary to upward resetting of the arterial baroreflexes.

Importance of Species Differences in Ranges of Autonomic Control

In moderate exercise sympathetic nervous responses among different species will depend on their cardiac pumping capacity, and again on their ability to increase heart rate and cardiac output rapidly via parasympathetic control. At moderate levels of exercise, depending on the species, responses will vary from the marked sympathetic vasoconstriction observed in rabbits, to modest vasoconstriction in humans (Figure 11-6), to virtually no regional vasoconstriction in dogs (Donald et al., 1970; Vatner, 1975). In normal dogs, regional vasoconstriction appears not to occur until their heart rates exceed 160 to 180 beats min^{-1} when vagal activity has nearly all been withdrawn (Vatner, 1975; Rowell and O'Leary, 1990). In contrast, if the pumping capacity of the heart or the oxygen carrying capacity of the blood are experimentally compromised, regional vasoconstriction occurs at the onset of modest intensities of exercise in dogs (Vatner, 1975). Rowell and O'Leary (1990) postulated that one feature that may link the cardiovascular responses to exercise across the species could be the extent to which cardiac output and arterial pressure can be rapidly increased by central command and vagal withdrawal.

Influence of Stresses or Adaptations That Alter Autonomic Control of Heart Rate During Exercise

If hypotheses 1 and 2 (above) are correct, the *range of parasympathetic control of the heart would determine the level of exercise at which activation of sympathetic nervous system first occurs*. This is a fundamental point that was first raised in Chapter 5 and in Figure 5-2 and Table 5-3, which showed the small range of parasympathetic control in patients with low cardiac output and high resting heart rate as opposed to the extremely wide parasympathetic control in endurance athletes, whose high stroke volumes permit normal resting cardiac output with low heart rate. The point is remade here that in the patients, normally active subjects, and endurance athletes, sympathetic control of the cardiovascular system becomes obvious when heart rate reaches 100 beats min^{-1}; near this heart rate all three groups reveal the beginning of regional vasoconstriction and increased spillover of norepinephrine into plasma, increased plasma renin activity, and so on. In short, their responses are consistent with the hypotheses stated above. Another illustration of this point is seen in normal individuals in whom the relationship between heart rate and work rate or oxygen uptake is changed acutely by heat stress or changed over weeks by physical conditioning. These acute or chronic adjustments have no effect on the relationships among heart rate and any of the indexes of increased sympathetic nervous activity shown in Figure 11-6, even though the relationship between *heart rate* and variables such as cardiac output, oxygen uptake or work intensity are altered markedly. For example, during heat stress the higher heart rate at a given oxygen uptake simply means that regional vasoconstriction begins at a lower oxygen uptake, as shown previously (see Chapter 6 and Figure 6-3). In all of the examples, sympathetic nervous activity begins to increase whenever parasympathetic control of heart rate is no longer effective.

The Importance of Skeletal Muscle Vasoconstriction

Before moving into the most difficult part of this discussion, namely, how baroreflexes and chemoreflexes might interact during severe exercise when most of the cardiac ouput goes to active muscle, it is necessary to look briefly at the importance of skeletal muscle itself in the vasomotor adjustments to exercise. Things would be much simpler if all vasomotor adjustments required to correct any "pressure errors" or "blood flow errors" could be provided by inactive regions. Unfortunately this is not possible when their fraction of the total vascular conductance becomes only a few percent as the intensity of moderate exercise increases.

Evidence indicating that blood flow to active skeletal muscle is restricted by increased sympathetic nerve activity during dynamic exercise was discussed in Chapters 7 and 9. One point of view is that muscle blood flow must be curtailed by the sympathetic vasoconstriction during severe exercise in order to prevent muscle vasodilation from outstripping the pumping capacity of the heart. However, this thinking cannot explain the cause for the vasoconstriction of active muscle during submaximal exercise when cardiac pumping reserves are ample.

Why Active Muscle?   When the arterial baroreflex is rapidly reset to higher operating points that increase in proportion to the intensity of exercise, the prevailing arterial pressure will tend to remain on the most sensitive portion of the baroreflex-function curve. Thus the strength of the reflex will be undiminished as exercise becomes more and more severe as long as the slope of the curve does not decrease (e.g., Figure 12-3B). A potential obstacle to this scheme is the fact that at some level of exercise, active muscle must become the most important site for baroreflex-induced vasoconstriction. For example, in moderate exercise with large muscle groups, approximately 70 percent of the total vascular conductance is in the active muscle. If heart rate were 150 beats min^{-1}, it is evident from Figure 11-6 that blood flow to visceral organs is already reduced more than one-half by vasoconstriction. Thus, further vasoconstriction of these organs would not contribute much to a rise in arterial pressure. In short, as the intensity of exercise increases, the relative contribution of inactive regions to raising or maintaining arterial pressure decreases and the contribution of active muscle increases.

To What Extent Will the Active Muscles Vasoconstrict?   This question was discussed in some detail in Chapter 7, which concluded that the so-called "functional sympatholysis" virtually disappears when the vasoconstriction is expressed as a change in vascular conductance rather than in vascular resistance. Again this relates to the old problem of changing baselines (analogous to our discussion of R-R interval versus heart rate). In short, when muscle blood flow is high, vasoconstriction causes large changes in vascular conductance and blood pressure, but only small changes in resistance.

Figure 12-15 shows the vasoconstriction in the exercising dog hindlimb; about 87 percent of the total hindlimb blood flow (at rest; it will be more in exercise), is to skeletal muscle. The vasoconstriction is in response to carotid sinus occlusion which was, of course, opposed and diminished some by the intact aortic baroreflex (O'Leary et al., 1991). The responses cannot be explained by autoregulation (Koch et al., 1991). In these experiments, the reflex-induced reduction in terminal aortic vascular conductance also increased even though the stimulus appeared to be constant. This agrees with those who find that vasoconstriction, for example by norepinephrine infusion, can actually be increased by exercise (Rowlands and Donald, 1968). The idea is that the ability of the vascular smooth muscle to develop tension increases as its initial fiber length increases with metabolic vasodilation. Nevertheless, there are indications still that in severe exercise, the vasoconstrictor response to sympathetic activation may be slightly blunted but it is far from being abolished (see Donald et al., 1970, and Figure 7-5, also Koch et al., 1991; for review, see Britton and Metting, 1991).

At What Level of Exercise Does Active Skeletal Muscle Vasoconstrict in Humans?   Chapter 7 reviews a series of experiments indicating that vasoconstriction develops in active leg muscles when additional muscles

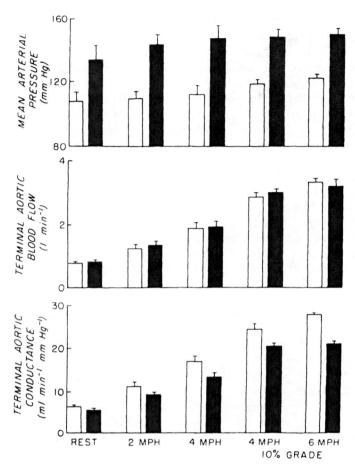

Figure 12-15   Maintained responsiveness of skeletal muscle vasculature to vasoconstriction elicited by the carotid sinus baroreflex during rest and mild to heavy exercise.
Carotid sinus pressure was reduced by 2-minute periods of carotid artery occlusion.
Each occlusion caused approximately the same rise in systemic arterial pressure. The
magnitude of reduction in terminal aortic conductance during carotid occlusion
increased in proportion to the level of terminal aortic flow just before occlusion
($r = 0.86$) so that the higher the muscle blood flow the greater the vasoconstriction
in response to this stimulus. (Redrawn from O'Leary et al., 1991.)

(e.g., arms) are activated during near-maximal exercise with the legs (e.g.,
Secher et al., 1977). The conclusion was that active muscle must vasoconstrict in order to reduce any mismatch between cardiac output and total
vascular conductance. Further, this idea was reinforced by experiments
(see Figure 7-13) showing that peak blood flow to active human quadriceps
muscle could be much higher than the heart could provide to 10 to 15 kg
of similarly active muscle with similar blood flow capacity.

A puzzle was the additional finding by Secher and coworkers (1977) that active legs also vasoconstricted when arm exercise was superimposed during *submaximal* as well as near-maximal cycling. There was no need for such vasoconstriction during submaximal exercise and the cause was unknown. There was no fall in arterial pressure and thus no reason at the time to think that the arterial baroreflex would elicit this vasoconstriction. The experiments of Strange and colleagues (1990) produced another surprising finding. When the application of pulsatile negative pressure on each heart beat over the carotid sinus (Figure 12-4) lowered arterial pressure (Figure 12-6A), it increased vascular conductance in the exercising legs (Figure 12-6C). Strange and colleagues (1990) calculated that at the lowest level of exercise, almost all of the *increase in total vascular conductance could be explained by the release of vasoconstrictor tone in the two exercising legs*. This can only mean that tonic sympathetic vasoconstrictor outflow to the active muscles had been withdrawn by carotid sinus hypertension. Figure 12-6C, shows that the largest effect of neck suction on leg vascular conductance was at the lowest intensity of exercise which required only 40 percent of $\dot{V}o_2$max. The realization that active skeletal muscle is tonically vasoconstricted at such relatively low rates of work first stimulated the ideas expressed in hypotheses 1 and 2 above.

What Causes Active Skeletal Muscle to Vasoconstrict During Moderate Submaximal Exercise?   The muscle chemoreflex appears not to be active at 40 percent of $\dot{V}o_2$max during large-muscle dynamic exercise (it is not known if muscle is vasoconstricted at lower levels of exercise). Nevertheless, based on hypotheses 1 and 2 (above), vasoconstriction of active muscle would be expected. If vasoconstriction is needed to raise arterial pressure to its operating point, then active muscle must eventually become the major site for a change in total vascular conductance; that is, conductance of other regions is too small a fraction of the total to account for a significant change in arterial pressure. Based on the reasoning in hypotheses 1 and 2, when Strange and colleagues (1990) raised carotid sinus transmural pressure, they presumably raised arterial pressure above its operating point for a particular level of exercise. Vasoconstriction in the active muscle would have to cease in order to restore arterial pressure downward toward its operating point. Furthermore, when Secher and coworkers (1977) added arm exercise to submaximal leg exercise, they increased both the total work rate and total vascular conductance and they presumably raised the baroreflex operating point. Vasoconstriction in the active muscles must have been required to increase arterial pressure to its new operating point—much the same as would have occurred had leg exercise simply been increased from one submaximal level to a higher one (all above heart rate 100 beats min^{-1}).

Although the experiments of Strange and his colleagues (1990) show that activation of the carotid sinus reflex can abolish tonic vasoconstrictor outflow to active muscle, these studies do *not* establish that the arterial baroreflex was what had caused the vasoconstriction in the first place. The findings are consistent with hypotheses 1 and 2, but they are not proof.

Do Arterial Baroreflexes and Muscle Chemoreflexes Oppose or Reinforce One Another During Severe Exercise?

If we are actually on the verge of arterial hypotension as we approach "maximal" whole-body exercise so that arterial pressure could only be maintained by vasoconstriction in active muscles (which, incidentally, would explain their extremely high oxygen extraction), then carotid sinus hypertension (neck suction) would be expected to cause systemic hypotension. Contrary to prediction, Strange and colleagues (1990) observed *less* effect of neck suction on arterial blood pressure at the highest levels of exercise (80 to 95 percent of $\dot{V}o_2$max) than at the lowest level (40 percent $\dot{V}o_2$max) (Figure 12-6). Possibly the high level of vasoconstrictor outflow to muscle in severe exercise does not originate from the arterial baroreflex if it cannot be reduced by carotid sinus hypertension.

Strange and colleagues suggested that another arterial pressure-raising reflex, for example, the muscle chemoreflex, may compete with the carotid sinus reflex during severe exercise and thereby prevent the anticipated fall in arterial pressure with carotid sinus hypertension. Figure 12-6C shows that carotid sinus stimulation had no effect on leg vascular conductance during severe exercise. The fall in arterial pressure was accompanied by a significant fall in leg blood flow and in leg oxygen uptake and a rise in lactate release from the legs; both are conditions needed for activation of the chemoreflex (Sheriff et al., 1987).

An implication of the findings in Figure 12-6 was that the muscle chemoreflex might compete successfully against the arterial baroreflex during severe exercise. In this case the tendency for carotid sinus hypertension to lower arterial pressure would be opposed by a chemoreflex which would vasoconstrict active muscle and raise blood pressure. The experiments of Sheriff and associates (1990) show the extent to which the two reflexes oppose one another. When both reflexes are intact, muscle chemoreflexes can correct approximately 67 percent (closed-loop gain = 0.67) of any deficit in muscle perfusion *pressure* (not flow) if exercise is severe. Melcher and Donald (1981) and Sheriff and colleagues (1990) observed similar closed-loop gains of the arterial baroreflex (the former group, -0.72 and the latter, -0.60). Sheriff and colleagues found the closed-loop gain for the chemoreflex was 0.74 when the arterial baroreflex was intact; in the same dogs after chronic sinoaortic denervation, the closed-loop gain of the chemoreflex increased to 0.86 (Figure 12-16). That is, the open-loop gains rose from -2.8 to -6.3, meaning that the *baroreflex is able to reduce by 60 percent the effect of the muscle chemoreflex on arterial pressure*. Stated differently, the strength of the muscle chemoreflex is increased nearly 2.5 times in sinoaortic-denervated dogs.

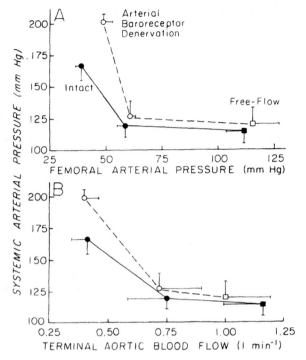

Figure 12-16 Effect of complete arterial baroreceptor denervation on the pressor response to muscle ischemia (muscle chemoreflex) caused by graded reduction in terminal aortic flow during mild dynamic exercise, 2 miles h^{-1}, 0 percent grade. **(A)** Femoral arterial pressure downstream from the terminal aortic occluder during free-flow (control) conditions; at the threshold of the pressor reflex; and at the peak of the rise in systemic arterial pressure caused by the pressor reflex. Baroreceptor denervation increased gain of the muscle chemoreflex (slope of the pressor response line) from -2.8 to -6.3. Note that the threshold for the chemoreflex was unaffected by baroreceptor denervation. **(B)** Baroreceptor denervation had no significant effect on terminal aortic blood flow during free-flow conditions and it did not significantly alter the blood flow at the threshold, but it did increase blood flow at the peak of the pressor response. (Redrawn from Sheriff et al., 1990.)

It must be emphasized that the gains of neither reflex during severe exercise are known. The chemoreflex could become much more powerful with increasing severity of exercise because a larger active muscle mass is involved. As pointed out in Chapter 11, the strength of the chemoreflex is a function of active muscle mass (Rowell et al., 1981). The current numbers for the gain of the muscle chemoreflex (i.e., as a pressure-raising reflex) are based on experiments in which only about one-third of the muscle mass was mildly to moderately active—and in dogs (Wyss et al., 1983; Sheriff et al., 1987, 1990).

In heavy to severe exercise the sensitivity of the baroreflex may be slightly lower as suggested by the smaller decreases in arterial pressure in response to carotid sinus hypertension, shown in Figure 12-6A. In order to understand how the muscle chemoreflex and baroreflex interact, we would need to know how far to the right the baroreflex function curve is shifted by exercise, and whether its maximal slope or sensitivity has been changed. We also need to know what has happened to the strength of the muscle chemoreflex under conditions in which it can only serve to raise arterial pressure but not (total) muscle blood flow.

The Importance of Cardiac Limitations

If our cardiac pumping limitation is such that total muscle vasodilation can outstrip cardiac pumping ability, then we are in danger of falling arterial pressure when whole-body exercise becomes severe. If the gain of the baroreflex were reduced, so would be its opposition to the chemoreflex if the gain of the latter were unaltered. It seems more likely that, as the large mass of active muscle approaches a blood-flow limited metabolic rate at $\dot{V}o_2$max, it will elicit a powerful muscle chemoreflex that could raise arterial pressure.

Possibly the arterial baroreflex and the muscle chemoreflex work in synergy with the chemoreflex serving to amplify any baroreflex vasoconstriction of active muscle. In Chapter 11, it was suggested that these two vasoconstrictor reflexes (i.e., in this setting) could optimize the distribution of blood flow between the most active and the least active muscles while at the same time keeping the same total muscle blood flow through all active muscle with maintained arterial pressure. Again, there is no evidence—this is speculation. One point that remains clear in all of this discussion is that no matter how much muscle we try to engage maximally during the most severe exercise, arterial pressure does not fall.

Vasoconstriction and Capillary Fluid Transfer

Finally, one other potentially important point about the importance of sympathetic vasoconstriction in active muscle has been made by Mellander and his colleagues (e.g., Maspers et al., 1990). In their view, sympathetic discharge to the active muscles might serve as an important protective mechanism directed against excessive transcapillary plasma fluid loss into exercising muscle. They have demonstrated that this vasoconstriction does lower muscle capillary pressures and reduces outward filtration in electrically stimulated cat hindlimb muscles. Might this vasoconstriction be an adjunct to the muscle pump that serves to foster fluid absorption between contractions? In so doing, would the effect be to lessen the interstitial volume only, or would it alter the interstitial *concentration* of substances that activate chemosensitive afferents? Could a benefit of this vasoconstriction be a reduction of the metabolic error signal, rather than an increase as presumed?

Given the effectiveness of the muscle pump, the scheme appears to provide no advantage. For example, if it is correct that negative venular pressures accompany relaxation of the muscle pump (Chapter 7), this would steepen the pressure drop across the capillaries and *lower* capillary pressure. Another argument is that during heavy exercise the vasoconstriction of active muscle appears to keep arterial pressure from falling. In this setting the vasoconstriction within the active muscles could prevent a fall in capillary pressures rather than protect them from a rise. A final point is that this vasoconstriction cannot prevent the enormous increases in muscle perfusion that accompany severe exercise. Also, when small muscle groups are active, this vasoconstriction is not evident, meaning that capillaries would be unprotected by vasoconstriction at a time when the highest peak flows for active muscles are attained. The critical question to be answered is whether the vasoconstriction of active muscles influences neural feedback from the muscle chemoreflex by raising or lowering the metabolic error signal.

SUMMARY

This chapter presented a hypothesis that central command could effect its control over the cardiovascular system during dynamic exercise by resetting the operating point of the arterial baroreflex to a higher pressure. It was concluded that the baroreflex operates effectively and with high enough gain to correct by 60 to 75 percent any blood pressure error. Arguments for resetting of the baroreflex at exercise are supported by the following observations:

1. Without a functioning arterial baroreflex, arterial presusre cannot rise during exercise, but rather remains depressed and is unstable during mild exercise below the threshold for the muscle chemoreflex. In heavier exercise, arterial pressure falls at the onset of exercise and after a 1- to 2-minute delay is restored presumably by the muscle chemoreflex.
2. When the rise in arterial pressure in response to exercise is prevented, the reaction is of that to severe arterial hypotension; increases in sympathetic outflow become extreme.

It is proposed that central command resets the arterial baroreflex and in turn raises cardiac output by sudden withdrawal of tonic vagal outflow to the heart. Cardiac output rises because the muscle pump is also engaged. The rise in cardiac output and arterial pressure are rapid so that pressure is raised immediately to the new operating point of the reflex. The central nervous system perceives no pressure error. Only when parasympathetic control is exhausted and control is shifted to the sympathetic nervous system do centrally perceived pressure errors develop (as heart rate approaches 100 beats min^{-1}). This "error" stems from the much slower action of the sympathetic nervous system on cardiac output and arterial pressure. Arterial pressure cannot be raised immediately to its new, reset operating point so that sympathetic nervous outflow to the heart and blood vessels increases so as to minimize this pressure error. It appears, therefore, that the range of parasympathetic control of the heart by central command determines the level of exercise at which activation of the sympathetic nervous system occurs. This is borne out by comparisons of responses of individuals in whom the relationship between heart rate and variables such as cardiac output or oxygen uptake, or work intensity are altered drastically by cardiac disease, physical conditioning, heat stress, and so on; in all cases the relationship between all indices of sympathetic nervous activity and heart rate is fixed. Sympathetic outflow increases only when the fast vagal component of cardiac control is no longer effective. The shift from predominantly cardiac control of arterial pressure to combined cardiac and vasomotor control inolves most major organ systems but as severity of exercise increases, active skeletal muscle beomes the most important target because only its vascular conductance is large enough to significantly alter arterial pressure. Vasoconstriction of active muscle begins at moderate exercise intensities, but there is no evidence that this vasoconstriction reduces muscle blood flow to levels that activate the muscle chemoreflex. A preponderance of evidence suggests that this reflex is only active during mild to moderately heavy exercise when muscle blood flow is reduced below a level at which its oxygen delivery is compromised.

We still lack any evidence that the muscle chemoreflex is a tonically active controller of the circulation during severe exercise when its only significant effect on blood pressure can be achieved by vasoconstricting active muscle. In short, the chemoreflex goes from a flow-sensitive, flow-raising reflex during mild dynamic exercise to a flow-sensitive, pressure-raising reflex if it is activated during severe exercise. In the latter setting, the chemoreflex could work in synergy with the arterial baroreflex even though the strength of the chemoreflex in raising arterial pressure may be reduced markedly by the opposition of the arterial baroreflex. The strength of neither reflex is known during severe exercise. Together, the two reflexes may maintain blood pressure when extreme vasodilation in active muscle is sufficient to outstrip the pumping capacity of the heart so as to threaten arterial pressure. An important question remains unanswered: Is the muscle chemoreflex ever a tonically active controller of the cardiovascular system during dynamic exercise when muscle blood flow is unrestricted?

REFERENCES

Angell-James, J.E., and M. De B. Daly (1971). Effects of graded pulsatile pressure on the reflex vasomotor responses elicited by changes of mean pressure in the perfused carotid sinus-aortic arch of the dog. *J. Physiol. (Lond.) 214,* 51–64.

Ardell, J.L., A.M. Scher, and L.B. Rowell (1980). Effects of baroreceptor denervation on the cardiovascular response to dynamic exercise. In P. Sleight, ed. *Arterial Baroreceptors and Hypertension,* p. 311–317. Oxford University Press, Oxford, UK.

Bevegård, B.S., and J.T. Shepherd (1966). Circulatory effects of stimulating the carotid arterial stretch receptors in man at rest and during exercise. *J. Clin. Invest. 45,* 132–142.

Bristow, J.D., E.B. Brown, Jr., D.J.C. Cunningham, M.G. Howson, E.S. Petersen, T.G. Pickering, and P. Sleight (1971). Effect of bicycling on the baroreflex regulation of pulse interval. *Circ. Res. 28,* 582–592.

Britton, S.L., and P.J. Metting (1991). Reflex regulation of skeletal muscle blood flow. In I.H. Zucker and J.P. Gilmore, eds. *Reflex Control of the Circulation,* pp. 737–764. CRC Press, Boca Raton, FL.

Cunningham, D.J.C., E. Strange Petersen, R. Peto, T.C. Pickering, and P. Sleight (1972). Comparison of the effect of different types of exercise on the baroreflex regulation of heart rate. *Acta Physiol. Scand. 86,* 444–455.

Daskalopoulos, D.A., J.T. Shepherd, and S.C. Walgenbach (1984). Cardiopulmonary reflexes and blood pressure in exercising sinoaortic-denervated dogs. *J. Appl. Physiol. 57,* 1417–1421.

DiCarlo, S.E., and V.S. Bishop (1992). Onset of exercise shifts operating point of arterial baroreflex to higher pressures. *Am. J. Physiol. 262 (Heart Circ. Physiol. 31),* H302–H307.

Donald, D.E., D.J. Rowlands, and D.A. Ferguson (1970). Similarity of blood flow in the normal and the sympathectomized dog hind limb during graded exercise. *Circ. Res. 26,* 185–199.

Ebert, T. (1986). Baroreflex responsiveness is maintained during isometric exercise in humans. *J. Appl. Physiol. 61,* 797–803.

Hales, J.R.S., and J. Ludbrook (1988). Baroreflex participation in redistribution of cardiac output at onset of exercise. *J. Appl. Physiol. 64,* 627–634.

Hobbs, S.F., and D.I. McCloskey (1987). Effects of blood pressure on force production in cat and human muscle. *J. Appl. Physiol. 63,* 834–839.

Holmgren, A. (1956). Circulatory changes during muscular work in man: with special reference to arterial and central venous pressures in the systemic circulation. *Scand. J. Clin. Lab. Invest. 8 (Suppl. 24),* 1–97.

Houk, J.C. (1988). Control strategies in physiological systems. *FASEB J. 2,* 97–107.

Koch, L.G., D.M. Strick, S.L. Britton, and P.J. Metting (1991). Reflex versus autoregulatory control of hindlimb blood flow during treadmill exercise in dogs. *Am. J. Physiol. 260 (Heart Circ. Physiol. 29),* H436–H444.

Korner, P.I. (1979). Central nervous control of autonomic cardiovascular function. In R.M. Berne, N. Sperelakis, and S.R. Geiger, eds. *Handbook of Physiology. The Cardiovascular System: The Heart,* vol. I, sect. 2, pp. 691–739. American Physiological Society, Bethesda, MD.

Kozelka, J.W., G.W. Christy, and R.D. Wurster (1987). Ascending pathways mediating somatoautonomic reflexes in exercising dogs. *J. Appl. Physiol. 62,* 1186–1191.

Krasney, J.A., M.G. Levitzky, and R.C. Koehler (1974). Sinoaortic contribution to the adjustment of systemic resistance in exercising dogs. *J. Appl. Physiol.* 36, 679–685.

Ludbrook, J. (1983). Reflex control of blood pressure during exercise. *Annu. Rev. Physiol.* 45, 155–168.

Ludbrook, J. (1984). Concern about gain: Is this the best measure of performance of cardiovascular reflexes? *Clin. Exp. Pharmacol. Physiol.* 11, 385–389.

Ludbrook, J. and W.F. Graham (1985). Circulatory responses to onset of exercise: role of arterial and cardiac baroreflexes. *Am. J. Physiol. 248 (Heart Circ. Physiol. 17),* H457–H467.

Ludbrook, J., W.F. Graham, and S.M. Potocnik (1986). Effects of acute versus chronic deletion of arterial baroreceptor input on the cardiovascular responses to exercise in the rabbit. *Clin. Exp. Pharmacol. Physiol.* 13, 25–37.

Mack, G.W., H. Nose, and E.R. Nadel (1988). Role of cardiopulmonary baroreflexes during dynamic exercise. *J. Appl. Physiol.* 65, 1827–1832.

Maspers, M., J. Bjornberg, and S. Mellander (1990). Relation between capillary pressure and vascular tone over the range from maximum dilatation to maximum constriction in cat skeletal muscle. *Acta Physiol. Scand. 140,* 73–83.

McRitchie, R.J., S.F. Vatner, D. Boettcher, G.R. Heyndrickx, T.A. Patrick, and E. Braunwald (1976). Role of arterial baroreceptors in mediating cardiovascular response to exercise. *Am. J. Physiol.* 230, 85–89.

Melcher, A., and D.E. Donald (1981). Maintained ability of carotid baroreflex to regulate arterial pressure during exercise. *Am. J. Physiol. 241 (Heart Circ. Physiol. 10),* H838–H849.

Mendelowitz, D., and A.M. Scher (1988). Pulsatile sinus pressure changes evoke sustained baroreflex responses in awake dogs. *Am. J. Physiol. 255 (Heart Circ. Physiol. 24),* H673–H678.

O'Leary, D.S. (1991). Regional vascular resistance vs. conductance: which index for baroreflex responses? *Am. J. Physiol. 260 (Heart Circ. Physiol 29),* H632–H637.

O'Leary, D.S., L.B. Rowell, and A.M. Scher (1991). Baroreflex-induced vasoconstriction in active skeletal muscle of conscious dogs. *Am. J. Physiol. 260 (Heart Circ. Physiol 29),* H37–H41.

O'Leary, D.S., A.M. Scher, and J.E. Bassett (1989). Effects of steps in cardiac output and arterial pressure in awake dogs with AV block. *Am. J. Physiol. 256 (Heart Circ. Physiol. 25),* H361–H367.

Robinson, B.F., S.E. Epstein, G.D. Beiser, and E. Braunwald (1966). Control of heart rate by the autonomic nervous system: studies in man on the interrelation between baroreceptor mechanisms and exercise. *Circ. Res.* 19, 400–411.

Rowell, L.B. (1981). Neural control of the circulation in exercise. In O.A. Smith, R. Galosy, and S. Weiss, eds. *Circulation, Neurobiology, and Behavior,* pp. 85–96. Elsevier North-Holland, New York.

Rowell, L.B. (1986). *Human Circulation. Regulation During Physical Stress.* Oxford University Press, New York.

Rowell, L.B. (1991). Control of regional circulations during dynamic exercise. In I.H. Zucker and J.P. Gilmore, eds. *Reflex Control of the Circulation,* pp. 795–828. CRC Press, Boca Raton, FL.

Rowell, L.B., G.L. Brengelmann, J.R. Blackmon, R.A. Bruce, and J.A. Murray

(1968). Disparities between aortic and peripheral pulse pressures induced by upright exercise and vasomotor changes in man. *Circulation 37*, 954–964.

Rowell, L.B., P.R. Freund, and S.F. Hobbs (1981). Cardiovascular responses to muscle ischemia in humans. *Circ. Res. 48, Suppl. I*, 37–47.

Rowell, L.B., and D.S. O'Leary (1990). Reflex control of the circulation during exercise: chemoreflexes and mechanoreflexes. *J. Appl. Physiol. 69*, 407–418.

Rowlands, D.J., and D.E. Donald (1968). Sympathetic vasoconstrictive responses during exercise- or drug-induced vasoconstriction. *Circ. Res. 23*, 45–60.

Sagawa, K. (1983). Baroreflex control of systemic arterial pressure and vascular bed. In J.T. Shepherd, F.M. Abboud, and S.R. Geiger, eds. *Handbook of Physiology. The Cardiovascular System: Peripheral Circulation and Organ Blood Flow*, vol. III, sect. 2, part 2, pp. 453–496. American Physiological Society, Bethesda, MD.

Scherrer, U., S.L. Pryor, L.A. Bertocci, and R.G. Victor (1990). Arterial baroreflex buffering of sympathetic activation during exercise-induced elevations in arterial pressure. *J. Clin. Invest. 86*, 1855–1861.

Seals, D.R. (1988). Cardiopulmonary baroreflexes do not modulate exercise-induced sympathoexcitation. *J. Appl. Physiol. 64*, 2197–2203.

Secher, N.H., J.P. Clausen, K. Klausen, I. Noer, and J. Trap-Jensen (1977). Central and regional circulatory effects of adding arm exercise to leg exercise. *Acta Physiol. Scand. 100*, 288–207.

Sheriff, D.D., D.S. O'Leary, A.M. Scher, and L.B. Rowell (1990). Baroreflex attenuates pressor response to graded muscle ischemia in exercising dogs. *Am. J. Physiol. 258 (Heart Circ. Physiol. 27)*, H305–H310.

Sheriff, D.D., C.R. Wyss, L.B. Rowell, and A.M. Scher (1987). Does inadequate O_2 delivery trigger the pressor response to muscle hypoperfusion during exercise? *Am. J. Physiol. 253 (Heart Circ. Physiol. 22)*, H1199–H1207.

Sprangers, R.L.H., K.H. Wesseling, A.L.T. Imholz, B.P.M. Imholz, and W. Wieling (1991). Initial blood pressure fall on stand up and exercise explained by changes in total peripheral resistance. *J. Appl. Physiol. 70*, 523–530.

Strange, S., L.B. Rowell, N.J. Christensen, and B. Saltin (1990). Cardiovascular responses to carotid sinus baroreceptor stimulation during moderate to severe exercise in man. *Acta Physiol. Scand. 138*, 145–153.

Vanhoutte, P.M., E. Lacroix, and I. Leusen (1966). The cardiovascular adaptation of the dog to muscular exercise: role of the arterial pressoreceptors. *Arch. Int. Physiol. Biochim. 74*, 201–222.

Vatner, S.F. (1975). Effects of exercise on distribution of regional blood flows and resistances. In R. Zelis, ed. *The Peripheral Circulations*, pp. 211–233. Grune & Stratton, New York.

Vatner, S.F., D. Franklin, R.L. Van Citters, and E. Braunwald (1970). Effects of carotid sinus nerve stimulation on blood flow distribution in conscious dogs at rest and during exercise. *Circ. Res. 27*, 495–503.

Walgenbach, S.C., and D.E. Donald (1983a). Cardiopulmonary reflexes and arterial pressure during rest and exercise in dogs. *Am. J. Physiol. 244 (Heart Circ. Physiol. 13)*, H362–H369.

Walgenbach, S.C., and D.E. Donald (1983b). Inhibition by carotid baroreflex of exercise-induced increases in arterial pressure. *Circ. Res. 52* 253–262.

Walgenbach, S.C., and J.T. Shepherd (1984). Role of arterial and cardiopulmonary mechanoreceptors in the regulation of arterial pressure during rest and exercise in conscious dogs. *Mayo Clin. Proc. 59,* 467–475.

Walgenbach-Telford, S. (1991). Arterial baroreflex and cardiopulmonary mechanoreflex function during exercise. In I.H. Zucker and J.P. Gilmore, eds. *Reflex Control of the Circulation,* pp. 765–793. CRC Press, Boca Raton, FL.

Wyss, C.R., J.L. Ardell, A.M. Scher, and L.B. Rowell (1983). Cardiovascular responses to graded reductions in hindlimb perfusion in exercising dogs. *Am. J. Physiol. 245 (Heart Circ. Physiol. 14),* H481–H486.

Index

aldosterone, 99, 100
alpha-adrenergic innervation
  cotransmitters, 82, 83
  distribution, 82
  density of, 83
  differential control of, 83, 84
  heterogeneity, 83
  tonic activity, 58, 82
alpha-receptors, 69, 70, 82–84, 223
  density of, 83
  heterogeneity, 83, 242
altitude and. *See* hypoxemia
"anaerobic threshold", 431
angiotensin I, 98, 100
  angiotensinogen, 98
  converting enzyme, 98, 100
  endothelium, 98
angiotensin II, 84, 98, 99, 100
  anephric patients, 100
  blockade of, 100
  central nervous action, 99
  potentiation of sympathetic activity,
    84, 99
  regional blood flow and, 100
  vasoconstrictor potency, 98, 99, 100
antidiuretic hormone (ADH). *See*
  vasopressin
aortic baroreceptors, 56
arginine vasopressin. *See* vasopressin
arterial baroreceptors, 56
  central hypervolemia and, 103–107,
    109–113
  operating point or "set point", 62–
    64
  pulsatile pressures and, 64
  resetting of, 62–64, 127
  vasopressin and. *See* arterial
    baroreflex
arterial baroreflex, 56–64, 94–96

aortic pulse pressure and, 54, 59
cardiopulmonary baroreflexes and,
  60, 61
importance of, 59, 60
operating point, 62–64
orthostasis and, 59–62
regional vasoconstriction and, 61,
  62
resetting, 62–64, 127
sensitivity (gain), 128, 129
"set point". *See* operating point
upright posture, 56–64
vagal versus sympathetic, 57, 58
vasopressin, 103–107, 109–113
arterial baroreflex, exercise, 441–479
  adaptation, autonomic control, 470
  adaptation, receptor, 458
  aortic baroreflex, 447, 448, 451
  cardiac pumping limitations and,
    477
  carotid sinus baroreflex, 447, 448,
    451
  central command and, 442, 457,
    462–464, 467, 468
  closed-loop and open-loop gains,
    475
  function curves, 445, 446, 455, 457
  muscle chemoreflex versus, 475–
    477
  muscle vascular conductance and,
    450
  neck suction and, 448, 461, 475
  operating point ("set-point"), 442,
    445, 448, 449, 455–457, 460,
    467
  pressure errors, 442, 454, 465, 467
  pulsatile versus steady forcing, 448,
    450, 451, 458
  renal sympathetic activity and, 459

arterial baroreflex, exercise
  (*continued*)
  "resetting", 442, 445, 448, 455–465
  responses to onset, 443, 453–456,
    462
  R-R interval and sensitivity, 446
  sensitivity (gain), 444–449, 475
  sinoaortic denervation, 55, 446,
    452, 458, 462, 475
  species differences, autonomic
    control, 470
  stimulus-response curves. *See* func-
    tion curves
  sympathetic vasoconstriction, 465,
    467–475
arterial blood pressure
  exercise, 182–185
  exercise and heat stress, 228, 230,
    231
  ischemia, cerebral, 245–248
  ischemia, muscle, 383, 397, 414–420
  isometric contractions and, 313–315
  orthostasis, 6–12
  wave amplification, 182
arterial compliance, 12, 13, 15
arterial oxygen saturation, exercise.
    See also limitations to oxygen
    uptake, respiration, 187, 188,
    331–335
arteriovenous oxygen difference,
    systemic in exercise, 166, 169,
    171, 187–190
  arterial oxygen content, determi-
    nants of, 187, 188, 331–335
  Bohr shift, 188–190
  capillary blood volume and, 190
  capillary diffusion distances and,
    190
  capillary mean transit time and, 190
  endurance athletes and, 166, 169
  hypoxemia and, 171
  maximal values, 169
  mitral stenosis and, 166, 170
  mixed venous oxygen content, 188–
    190
  muscle capillary recruitment, 189–
    190
  oxygen dissociation curve, 188, 189
  physical conditioning, 192, 289,
    350, 351, 359

atherosclerosis obliterans, 30
  muscle chemoreflex and, 465–470,
    475–479
  muscle pump and, 30
atrial natriuretic factor, 104, 110–112
atriopeptin. *See* atrial natriuretic
    factor
atriorenal reflexes. *See* cardiorenal
    reflexes
autacoids, 84
autonomic dysfunction. *See also*
    orthostatic intolerance, 153–
    158
  cerebral autoregulation, 154
  diabetic neuropathy, 156–158
  epinephrine, 154, 157
  myogenic response, 156
  norepinephrine, 154, 157
  paraplegia, quadriplegia (tetraple-
    gia), 154–156
  renal baroreflex, 156, 157
  renin activity, 154–158
  spinal cord injury, 153, 156
  spinal sympathetic reflexes, 154–
    156
  splanchnic circulation and, 156, 157
  sympathetic venoarteriolar reflexes,
    155–157
  tonic sympathetic activity, 154
  vasopressin, 156
autoregulation
  cerebral, 8, 10, 245
  renal, 237

Bainbridge reflex, 54, 55, 103, 106,
    107, 111, 112
baroreceptor "resetting", 62–64
basal tone, 84, 271
blood flow distribution. *See* regional
    circulations
blood pressure regulation. *See* arterial
    baroreflexes
blood volume distribution
  exercise, 195, 196, 213–215
  exercise and heat stress, 228–232
  heat stress, 121–123, 219
  orthostasis, 120–126

blood volume, physical conditioning and, 195, 196
body temperature, exercise, 224–228, 231, 233, 235
  brain and body cooling, 233
  skin blood flow and, 223–233
Bohr shift, 188–190
bradykinin, 220, 401, 402
breathing
  pericardectomy and, 42
  right versus left ventricular stroke volume and, 42, 43

capillary blood volume
  pulmonary, 345–347
  skeletal muscle, 294, 351, 360
cardiac depressor reflex, 130, 137–139
  beta$_1$-adrenergic mechanisms, 137, 138
  Bezold-Jarisch reflex, 137
  bradycardia, 137, 138
  ventricular c fibers, 137
  ventricular "receptors", 137
  ventricular volume, 139
cardiac dimensions. See heart volume
cardiac filling pressure. See ventricular filling pressure
cardiac output, 38, 40, 168
  cardiac index versus, 168
  effects of breathing on, 42, 43
  endurance athletes and, 166, 168, 170, 173
  exercise, 166, 168, 171
  heat stress and exercise, 223–235
  hypoxemia, 171
  isometric contractions and, 312, 315, 316
  maximal values, 168
  mitral stenosis and, 166, 168, 170, 173
  orthostasis, 40, 41
  physical conditioning, 192
  range, 166
  relationship to central venous pressure in orthostasis, 44, 45
  vagal versus sympathetic control, 42, 57, 58

cardiac output, distribution of. See regional circulations
cardiac performance. See ventricular function
cardiac reflexes. See cardiorenal reflexes and cardiac depressor reflex
cardiopulmonary baroreflexes, 53–56, 94–96, 97, 100, 101
  cardiac transplants and, 55, 56
  exercise and, 444, 451, 453, 464
  heat stress, exercise and, 464
  interaction with arterial baroreflexes, 60, 61
  orthostasis and, 53–56
  regional vasoconstriction and, 53–55
  sinoaortic denervation and, 55
  upright posture, importance in, 53
  ventricular filling pressure and, 464
  ventricular receptors and, 53
cardiorenal reflexes (Henry-Gauer reflex), 96, 97, 101–112
  free-water clearance, 102
  natriuresis, diuresis, 102
  quadrupeds versus bipeds, 97
  thoracic blood volume and, 101, 102
  vasopressin and, 103, 106, 107, 109, 110
  water immersion and, 102
cardiovascular control in exercise: central command versus chemoreflexes versus baroreflexes, 465–479
  general hypothesis, 465–467
  heart rate control, 470
  hypothesis 1: mild exercise, 467
  hypothesis 2: moderate exercise, 468
  muscle chemoreflex, sympathetic activity, 468–470
  regional vasoconstriction, 470–475
  skeletal muscle vasoconstriction and, 471–475
  species differences and, 470
"cardiovascular drift", 228, 230
cardiovascular dysfunction. See also orthostatic intolerance, 139–152

cardiovascular dysfunction
    (*continued*)
    cardiac transplants, 152
    congestive heart failure, 150–152
    epinephrine and, 134, 136–139, 142,
        143, 146, 148, 154, 157
    hypoxemia and, 139–149
    prejunctional inhibition, 141, 144,
        145
    splanchnic circulation, 140, 148
    valvular heart disease, 148
    vasomotor impairment, 140–144
carotid sinus baroreflex, 56, 58, 59
    neck suction and, 58, 59, 60, 61, 128
catecholamines. *See* epinephrine and
        norepinephrine
central blood volume, 60, 61, 101, 102
central circulatory adjustments, exer-
        cise, 162–199
    arterial blood pressure, 182, 183
    arteriovenous oxygen difference,
        169, 187–190
    cardiac output, 168
    heart rate, 168, 172–175
    stroke volume, 175–182
    total vascular conductance, 183–185
    ventricular filling pressure, 186,
        194–199
central circulatory adjustments, heat
        stress and prolonged exercise,
        228–232
central circulatory adjustments,
        orthostasis, 39–42, 44–51, 54,
        59
central circulatory adjustments, physi-
        cal conditioning, 190–199
central command, 371–393, 403, 404,
        407, 414, 430, 454, 468
    arterial baroreflex "resetting" and,
        457, 462–464, 468
    arterial pressure and, 405
    decorticate and decerebrate animals
        and, 381
    EMG activity and, 388, 389, 405
    feed-forward control, 373, 380, 386–
        392
    feed-forward plus feedback con-
        trol?, 386–392
    "fictive" locomotion, 381
    "fields of Forel", 379–381

    heart rate and, 384–386
    hypotheses, 371–373, 378
    involuntary contractions and, 376,
        379
    motor paralysis and, 373, 375
    motor unit recruitment, 386, 390,
        405, 406
    muscle mass and, 388
    muscle reflexes and, 375, 392
    muscle sympathetic nerve activity
        (MSNA), 383–386, 405
    neural organization, 378
    neuromuscular blockade and, 373,
        387, 388
    parasympathetic versus sympathetic
        activity by, 382–386, 392
    perception of effort and, 375, 376,
        388
    posterior hypothalamus, 379, 382,
        391
    sensory blockade and, 375, 377
    sensory neuropathies and, 374
    spinal cord, role of, 390
    subthalamic locomotor region, 379
    sympathetic activation and, 405,
        407, 408, 430, 441, 462–464
    vagal withdrawal and, 403, 407,
        430, 441, 462–464, 468
central hypervolemia, 101–113
central hypovolemia, 101, 102, 104,
        109, 110
central venous pressure. *See also*
        ventricular filling pressure, 38,
        67
    cardiac output and, 48–51, 67–69,
        186
    exercise and, 180–182, 186, 194–
        199
    flow dependency of, 46–51, 67–69,
        186, 187
    gravity and, 6–12, 41
    heat stress and, 228–232
    muscle pump and, 180–182, 186
    orthostasis, 7, 8, 12, 44
    vasoconstriction, vasodilation, and,
        46–50
    venous return and, 45, 46, 71, 72
cerebral circulation, 8, 51, 130, 241–
        249
    adenosine, 243

cerebral circulation (*continued*)
  alpha-receptors, 242
  autoregulation, 8, 10, 51, 130, 154, 245
  blood-brain barrier, 241, 245
  blood flow, 8, 10, 42, 51, 242
  carbon dioxide, 243, 244
  cerebrospinal fluid, 51, 243
  exercise, 248
  gravity, effects of, 8, 10, 51
  hormonal control, 245
  hypoxemia, effects of, 244
  measurement of, 241
  metabolic control, 241, 243–245
  neural control, 242, 243
  norepinephrine, 242
  oxygen, 243, 244
  vasovagal syncope and, 130
cerebral siphon effect, 19
  cerebral veins and, 19
  giraffe, 19
  venous collapse and, 19
cerebral spinal fluid pressure, 9, 10, 19, 22, 245, 247
cerebral veins, 8, 9, 10, 19
compliance
  arterial versus venous, 12
  definitions, 13
  distribution of, 12, 13
  interstitial, 26
  systemic, 13
  venous, 13, 68, 69
  volume-pressure relationship, 13–16
congestive heart failure. *See also* cardiovascular dysfunction, 150–152
  beta-adrenergic effects, 152
  cardiopulmonary baroreflex, 150
  epinephrine, 152, 154, 157
  norepinephrine spillover, 150
  paradoxical vasodilation, 150
  renin-angiotensin system, 152
  sympathetic venoarteriolar reflex, 151
  ventricular preload and afterload, 150
contractility. *See also* ventricular function, 176, 179, 193
coronary circulation, 256–265
  adenosine, 263

alpha-receptors, 264, 265
beta-receptors, 255
blood flow, range, 257–261
epicardial, endocardial blood flow, 262, 265
exercise, 412
"maximal" versus "peak" blood flow, 258, 260
measurement, 257
mechanical effects, 262
metabolic control, 263
neural control, 264, 265
norepinephrine spillover from, 86
oxygen uptake, determinants, 261
pressure-rate product, 262, 263
subendocardial, subepicardial flow ratios, 262, 265
time-tension index, 262
Cushing reflex, 245–248
  arterial blood pressure, 247
  cerebral spinal fluid pressure, 245, 247
  ischemia, 245, 247
cutaneous circulation, 219–235
  alpha-adrenoreceptors, 84, 226
  blood flow, 219, 220
  blood volume, 219, 220
  bradykinin hypothesis, 220–221
  cholinergic, 220, 221
  cutaneous veins, 222, 223
  exercise, 223–235, 412
  exercise and heat stress, 224–235
  heat stress, 219, 224, 225
  humoral control, 222
  isometric contractions and, 318, 319
  local control, 222
  measurement, 219
  neural control, 220, 221, 224, 226
  nonthermoregulatory control, 223–226
  norepinephrine spillover from, 86
  orthostasis and, 59, 60
  orthostatic reflexes and, 51, 52, 55, 56
  reflex control, 223–227
  sweating, 220, 221, 224–226
  sympathetic vasodilation, 220
  vasoactive intestinal polypeptide (VIP) and, 220, 221

cutaneous veins, 69, 222, 223
  alpha-adrenoreceptors, 70, 84, 223
  reflex control, 222
  temperature, 222, 223

delayed compliance, stress-relaxation,
  14–16
distribution of cardiac output. *See*
  regional circulations
diuresis, 102

edema, 4, 25–27, 30, 38, 39, 81
ejection fraction, 177, 179, 180, 193
end-diastolic and end-systolic volume.
  See ventricular function
endothelium, vascular, 272, 273, 401
  endothelial-derived relaxing factor
    (EDRF), 272
  nitric oxide, 272
epinephrine, 134, 136–139, 142, 143,
    146, 148, 154, 157
  beta$_1$-receptors, 137
  beta-$_2$-receptors, 136, 137
  cardiac depressor reflexes and,
    137–139
  cardiovascular effects, 134, 136
  hypoxemia and, 142, 146, 148, 149
  syncope and, 134–137
exercise, cardiovascular responses to
  dynamic, 162–199
  heat stress and, 223–235
  static, isometric, 302–323
exercise capacity. *See* work capacity

feedback control, 56
  redundancy, 82
  positive versus negative, 246, 322,
    406, 408, 420, 433
Fick Principle, 162, 205, 219, 236,
    241, 327
Fields of Forel, 379–381
force-velocity relationship, 176, 193
Frank-Starling relationship, 40, 43,
    175, 176, 193

free-water clearance, 102–104, 106,
    107
functional capacity, 162, 163

giraffe
  antigravity suit, 17, 26
  arterial pressure in, 17, 18, 26
  cerebral siphon effect, 19
  interstitial fluid pressure in, 17, 26
  transmural pressure in, 17, 26
  venous pressure in, 17, 18, 26
gravitational pooling, structural coun-
    teraction of, 20
gravity. *See* orthostasis

heart rate, 40, 44, 57, 58, 168–175
  beta$_1$-adrenoreceptors, 172
  maximal, 168, 169
  norepinephrine, relationship to, 175
  orthostasis, ineffectiveness in, 40,
    44
  pharmacological blockade and
    orthostasis, 44, 59
  regional blood flow, relationship to,
    88, 210–212, 411, 412
  regulation in exercise, 172–175
  sympathetic activity, relationship
    to, 88, 210–212, 411, 412
  vagal versus sympathetic control,
    40, 57, 58, 172–175
  vagal versus sympathetic response
    times, 57, 172–175
heart volume, 194, 198
heat stress and exercise. *See* cutane-
    ous circulation
Henry-Gauer reflex. *See* cardiorenal
    reflex
hepatic blood flow. *See* splanchnic
    circulation
humoral control, 82–113
  aldosterone, 96, 99–101
  angiotensin II, 96–102
  antidiuretic hormone. *See* vasopres-
    sin
  orthostasis, 96–113
  plasma renin activity. *See* renin
  vasopressin, 103, 104

hydrostatic indifferent point (HIP), 6, 37
hydrostatics, 6
    dynamic pressure, 6
    hydrostatic column, 6, 21, 40
    hydrostatic pressure, 6
    intracranial pressure, 8–10
    mean transit time, 20
    pooling, counteraction of, 20–25
    static pressure, 6
    transmural pressure, 6
    venostatic level, 8
    venous collapse, 8, 11, 12, 19, 44
    venous pressure, 6
hypergravity (acceleration), 44
hyperthermia and exercise. See heat stress and exercise
hypogravity. See weightlessness
hypothalamus, locomotor control, 379–382
hypoxemia
    central effects on sympathetic activity, 144, 145
    exercise, 170, 171
    orthostatic intolerance and, 139–149
    prejunctional effects, 141, 144

innervation
    alpha-adrenoreceptors, 69, 70, 84
    cutaneous veins, 69, 70
    skeletal muscle veins, 69, 70
    splanchnic veins, 69, 70
intermittent claudication, 429–430
interval-strength relationship. See ventricular function
intracranial pressure, 8–10
intramuscular pressure, orthostasis, 28
intrapleural pressure, 31, 178
ischemia
    cerebral, 245, 247
    Cushing reflex, 245–247
    muscle. See muscle chemoreflexes
isometric contractions, 302–323
    alternating motor unit recruitment, 310, 311
    arterial pressure and, 313–315
    cardiac output and, 312, 315, 316

    cardiovascular adjustments to, 302–323
    central circulatory responses to, 312–316
    femoral artery and vein flow, 308, 310
    heterogeneity of muscle blood flow, 309–311
    intramuscular pressure, 307, 308, 310
    muscle blood flow and, 304–311, 318
    muscle mass and arterial pressure, 314
    open-loop conditions and, 303
    regional blood flow and, 317–322
    skin blood flow, 318, 319
    stroke volume and, 312, 315
    sympathetic nervous activity, 320–322
    vascular compression, 304, 305, 307
    ventricular filling pressure and, 316

Krogh model, 46, 68
    distribution of blood volume, 46, 68
    heat stress, 228, 230, 233
    regional compliances, 68, 69, 217

Law of LaPlace, 194, 198, 262
length-tension relationship. See Frank-Starling relationship
limitations to oxygen uptake, cardiac output, 348–350
    muscle mass and, 348
    pericardectomy and, 348
    physical conditioning and, 349
limitations to oxygen uptake, muscle metabolism, 360–366
    arguments against, 361
    arguments favoring, 362–364
    blood flow versus metabolic limitation, 361
    enzyme kinetics, 366
    experimental constraints, 361
    free-fatty acid oxidation, 366
    glycogen sparing, 366

limitations to oxygen uptake,
        muscle metabolism (*continued*)
    mitochondrial volume and, 363
    muscle oxidative capacity, humans,
        364, 365
    physical conditioning and, 363, 365
    symmorphosis, 330, 335, 350, 364
    work capacity (endurance) and, 365
limitations to oxygen uptake, muscle
        oxygen extraction, 350–360
    arteriovenous oxygen difference
        and, 350
    blood flow inhomogeneities, 352,
        355, 356
    diffusion distance and, 351
    diffusion limitation and, 352–355
    Fick principle and, 350, 358, 360
    Fick's first law of diffusion, 354, 359
    hypoxemia and, 353, 354
    Krogh's cylinder model, 357, 358
    mean transit time and, 351, 354, 356
    muscle blood flow and, 351, 356,
        357
    muscle capillary density, 351, 358,
        360
    muscle capillary-mitochondrial
        gradient, 354, 355
    myoglobin, 355, 357, 358
    oxygen uptake : blood flow inequali-
        ties ($\dot{V}O_2/\dot{Q}$), 352, 355, 356
    physical conditioning and, 350, 360
    tissue diffusion capacity, 357–360
limitations to oxygen uptake, respira-
        tory, 326–348
    alveolar-arterial PO_2 difference and,
        332–348
    alveolar-capillary oxygen diffusion
        and, 341–347
    alveolar-to-arterial oxygen transfer
        and, 339–347
    alveolar ventilation, 331–335
    arterial oxygen desaturation, 332–
        335
    Fick principle and, 327
    hypoxemia and, 331–337, 341–343
    mean transit time and, 345
    postpulmonary arteriovenous
        shunts and, 341
    physical conditioning and, 330, 332,
        335

    pulmonary blood flow and, 345
    pulmonary blood volume and, 345
    respiratory system and, 330–348
    structural limitations, 327
    ventilation, 330–339
    ventilation : perfusion ratio ($\dot{V}_A/\dot{Q}$)
        and, 343, 346
    ventilatory limitations, human and
        equine athletes, 332–337
liver blood flow. *See* splanchnic blood
        flow
local control, vascular, 263, 271–273
local neural mechanisms, 273
    sympathetic venoarteriolar reflexes,
        64–66
lower body negative pressure. *See*
        lower body suction
lower body suction, 52, 53, 60–62,
        94–96, 100, 104, 109
low pressure baroreflexes. *See* cardio-
        pulmonary baroreflexes

maximal oxygen uptake
    classical concept of, 163, 165
    criteria, 165
    critical muscle mass and, 167
    determinants of, 163, 167–171
    endurance athletes, 164, 166, 170
    Fick principle and, 163
    "functional capacity" and, 162, 163
    hypoxemia and, 171
    limitations to, 326–367
    "maximal" versus "peak", 165–
        167
    muscle mass and, 165–167
    physiological basis for differences,
        169–171
    physiological definition of, 163
    range of, 164
    reproducibility of, 165
McArdle's Disease, 362, 404
mean transit time, 20, 190, 294, 345,
        351, 354, 356
    muscle capillary blood volume, 294,
        351, 360
    pulmonary capillary blood volume,
        345–347

metabolic capacity, muscle, 360–366
metabolic disease, 362
metabolic error signal. *See* muscle
    chemoreflexes
metabolic vasodilators, 263, 271–273
    adenosine, 263
    candidates, 272
    endothelial modulation, 272
    sites of action, 272
"metaboreflex". *See* muscle chemo-
    reflex
microcirculation. *See* skeletal muscle
    circulation
microcirculation and fluid exchange
    capillary pressures, 25, 62, 477
    edema and, 25
    hydrostatic pressure, 25
    lymphatics, 26
    net filtration pressure, 25, 26, 62
    oncotic pressures, 25
    Starling-Landis hypothesis, 25
    tissue pressure, 25, 26
microneurography. *See also* muscle
        sympathetic nerve activity, 85,
        88–96, 144, 145, 403
mitral stenosis, 166, 170
motor unit recruitment. *See* central
    command
muscle afferents. *See also* muscle
        chemoreflex
    chemosensitive, 398–403
    ergoreceptors, 399
    groups I and II, 398
    groups III and IV, 398–400
    mechanosensitive, 401–403
    "metaboreceptors", 400
    nociceptors, 399
muscle blood flow. *See* skeletal mus-
    cle circulation
muscle chemoreflex, 396–435
    arterial baroreflex, opposition to,
        430, 467, 475–477
    cardiac versus vasomotor control
        by, 400, 404, 414–417
    chemical stimuli, 399, 400
    critical tests of, 420–426
    exercise ischemia and, 420–428
    flow errors, 420–422, 428
    gain, open- and closed-loop, 420,
        422, 428–430, 434, 475
    groups III and IV afferents and,
        398–400
    hydrogen ion activity, 403, 428
    importance in dynamic exercise,
        408–435
    lactic acid and, 400–403, 405, 426–
        428, 430, 466, 475
    metabolic error signal and, 396,
        420, 428, 434, 466
    metabolites from muscle and, 400–
        403, 466
    muscle mass, roll of, 398, 404, 405,
        409–413, 430–432, 476
    muscle sympathetic nerve activity
        (MSNA), 403–405, 408, 466
    neurophysiological evidence, 398–
        403
    norepinephrine leakage and, 425,
        428, 433
    "open-loop" experiments, 408, 420
    oxygen delivery (critical), 427, 428,
        466
    positive feedback, 406, 408, 420,
        433
    postexercise ischemia and, 397,
        403, 414–420
    potassium and, 400, 401, 428
    pressor responses to, 400–402, 406
    pressure versus flow-raising reflex,
        406, 420
    response time, 410
    sensory blockade and, 417–420
    severe dynamic exercise and, 432–
        434
    sympathetic activity and, 468–475
    thermosensitivity, 399
    threshold, 422, 423, 426–429, 466,
        469
    tonic activity, 396, 417, 419–422,
        428, 429, 470
    vascular disease and, 429, 430
    ventilation and, 398, 400, 414
    voluntary contractions, activation
        by, 403–408
muscle mechanoreflexes, 396–403,
        414, 441, 454, 466
    aracidonic acid and, 400–402
    bradykinin, 401, 402
    cyclo-oxygenase, 401, 402
    discharge patterns, 402

muscle mechanoreflexes, (continued)
  golgi tendon organs, 398
  groups I and II afferents, 398
  groups III and IV afferents, 399,
      401, 402
  "muscle heart" reflex, 406
  muscle spindles, 398
  pressor responses, 400–402
  prostaglandin E$_2$, 401, 402
  sensory blockade and, 407
muscle pump, a second heart, 28–30,
    40, 130, 228, 229, 478
  antigravity muscles, 28
  arteriovenous pressure gradient
      and, 30, 184, 185
  elastic recoil of muscle veins, 30,
      184
  electrical stimulation of muscle and,
      185
  intramuscular pressures and, 28,
      184
  muscle perfusion, effect on, 183–
      185
  muscle venous transmural pressure
      and, 184, 185
  peripheral vascular volume and, 186
  pumping capacity, 29, 181
  stroke volume and, 29, 179–181
  transcapillary fluid exchange and,
      30, 477
  vascular conductance, 183–185
  venous valves, 29
  venous valves, absence and dam-
      age, 186, 187
  ventricular filling pressure and, 29,
      179–181
  "virtual" muscle vascular conduc-
      tance and, 183
  volume-flow dependency and, 186,
      187
muscle sympathetic nerve activity
    (MSNA), 59, 85, 91–96, 403–
    405, 408, 466
  arterial baroreflexes and, 94–96,
      142, 143, 147
  cardiopulmonary baroreflexes and,
      94–96, 142, 143, 147
  central command and, 405, 408
  central hypovolemia and, 55, 94,
      95, 142, 143, 147

  isometric contractions and, 321, 322
  lactic acid and, 404, 432
  microneurography, 85, 91–93, 144,
      145
  muscle chemoreflex and, 403–405,
      408, 422, 430–432
  muscle mass, role of, 404, 405,
      409–413
  orthostasis and, 94–96
  postexercise ischemia and, 405, 410
  regional differences in, 94
  relation to heart rate, 411, 412
  relation to norepinephrine, 91–93
  relation to vasoconstriction, 91–93
  response delay, 410, 451
  vasovagal syncope and, 133, 134,
      142, 143, 146
myocardial contractility. See stroke
    volume, exercise, and ventricu-
    lar function
myocardial function. See ventricular
    function
myocardial oxygen uptake
  determinants, 261–263
  inotropic state, 262
  pressure-rate product, 263
  time-tension index, 262
myogenic responses, 52, 65, 156, 274
myoglobin, 295, 355, 357, 358

natriuresis, 102, 104–108, 110, 112
  renal sympathetic nerve activity
      and, 105–107, 112
neural control, vascular, 82–85
  alpha-adrenergic, 85
  diffuse versus punctate, 85
neuropathies. See orthostatic intoler-
    ance
neuropeptide Y, 82, 239, 240
norepinephrine
  hypoxemia, 139–147
  modulation of release, 84
  neuronal leakage, 86, 87
  neuronal reuptake, 84, 87
  release, inhibition of, 141–144
  source in exercise, 287, 288
  spillover, exercise, 412, 425, 428,
      433, 471

norepinephrine (*continued*)
  spillover, orthostasis, 88
  spillover, regional, 86
  spillover, total, 84, 86, 87
  tritiated, radiolabeled, 87

obstructive arterial disease, 429, 430
open-loop experiments, 243–248
  arterial baroreflexes and, 451–460
  Cushing reflex and, 243–248
  isometric contractions and, 303
  muscle chemoreflexes and, 420
  open- and closed-loop gains, 248,
      420, 422, 428–430, 434, 475
organ blood flow. *See* splanchnic,
    renal, etc.
orthostasis
  arterial pulse pressure and, 51, 53,
      59
  abdominal cavity pressure, 18
  circulatory responses to, 39–74
  gravitational "pooling", counterac-
      tion of, 20–27
  humoral control, 96–113
  hydrostatics, 6–20
  mechanical adjustments to, 28–33
  muscle sympathetic activity and,
      94–96
  norepinephrine spillover in, 88
  passive effects of gravity, 3–33
  regional circulations and, 51, 52,
      59, 60
orthostatic hypotension, 3, 39
orthostatic intolerance, 20–29, 118–
    158
  autonomic dysfunction, 153–158
  autonomic neuropathy and, 155–158
  cardiac transplants, 152
  cardiovascular dysfunction, 139–
      152
  congestive heart failure, 150–152
  diabetes and, 156, 157
  heat-induced, 121–123
  local venoarteriolar mechanisms,
      66, 155–157
  maldistribution of blood flow and,
      120–139
  paraplegia and tetraplegia, 66, 154–
      156

postexercise, 121
spinal cord injury, 153
spinal reflexes in, 154–156
valvular heart disease, 148
weightlessness (hypogravity), 29,
    123–130
orthostatic reflexes, 52
osmoreceptors, vasopressin and, 103
oxygen cascade, 326, 328
  barriers to, 328, 339
oxygen dissociation curve, 189
oxygen transport. *See* limitations to
    oxygen uptake

pericardium, 42, 43
  constraints in exercise, 195–199
  pericardectomy and breathing, 42
peripheral vascular resistance. *See*
    total vascular conductance
physical conditioning, 190–199, 330,
    332, 335
  adjustments in skeletal muscle, 290
  arteriovenous oxygen difference
      and, 289, 349, 350
  blood volume and, 195, 196
  capillary blood volume, 294, 295
  capillary density and, 292–295
  capillary mean transit time and, 294
  cardiac volume and Law of La-
      Place, 194
  endurance, work capacity, 191, 192
  functional versus performance crite-
      ria, 190, 191
  maximal oxygen uptake and, 191–
      193, 290–293, 363, 365
  microcirculation and, 292–295
  muscle blood flow and, 290–292
  muscle oxygen extraction and, 292–
      295, 349, 350
  myocardial contractile state and,
      193
  myoglobin and, 295
  pericardial volume and, 198, 199
  pericardium, importance of, 195–
      199
  pulmonary oxygen transfer and,
      330, 332, 335
  regional blood flow and, 289, 290

physical conditioning (*continued*)
stroke volume and, 193–199
sympathetic control and, 291
ventricular afterload and, 193, 194
ventricular mass and, 194, 195
ventricular preload and, 194
plasma renin activity. *See* renin
plasma volume
exercise, 187, 196
gravity, effects of, 26, 33
physical conditioning and, 195, 199
postural hypotension. *See* orthostatic
hypotension
prolonged exercise, cardiovascular
drift, 230
pulmonary blood volume, 42
pulmonary circulation
alveolar pressure and, 10, 11
blood flow, exercise, 341, 342, 345,
346
capillaries, 11
compliance, 16
gravity, effects of, 10
hypoxemia, 347
pulmonary arterial pressure, 10
pulmonary mean transit time, 345
pulmonary venous pressure, 11
pulmonary ventilation
carbon dioxide production and, 332,
338, 339
hypoxemia and, 331–337
limits to, 332–339
mechanical limitations, 336–339
mechanoreceptive feedback and,
336–338
"minimum work hypothesis", 336
oxygen costs of, 265–268
putative transmitters
dopaminergic, 83, 239, 240
neuropeptide Y, 82, 239, 240
peptidergic, 83, 243, 273
purinergic, 83
vasoactive intestinal polypeptide
(VIP), 83, 220, 221

regional blood flow. *See* regional
circulations
regional circulations, 67–69

"cardiovascular drift" and, 228–233
distribution of cardiac output and,
67–69, 412, 413
exercise and, 204–249, 413, 471,
472
exercise and heat stress, 223–235
heat stress and, 219–222
isometric contractions and, 317–322
orthostasis and, 51, 52, 59, 60
regional vasoconstriction, importance of, 61, 62, 232–233, 470–
475
relative oxygen uptake, 169, 170
renal baroreflex, 98, 156, 157
renal circulation, 235–240
angiotensin II and, 237–240
autoregulation, 237
blood flow, 236
dopamine, 239, 240
epinephrine, 239
exercise, 238–240, 411, 412
humoral control, 237
measurement, 235
neural control, 236
neuropeptide Y, 239, 240
norepinephrine spillover from, 86,
238–240
orthostatic reflexes and, 51, 52, 55
reflex control, 51–55, 211, 238–240
renin, 239, 240
renal sympathetic nerve activity, 92,
104, 105, 139, 359
natriuresis and, 105–107, 112
renin
autonomic dysfunction, 154–158
autonomic neuropathy, 156–158
baroreflexes and, 101, 109
beta$_1$-adrenergic receptors and, 98
cardiorenal reflexes and, 101
control of release, 98, 101
exercise, 411, 412, 471
juxtaglomerular cells and, 98
macula densa and, 98
renal baroreceptor and, 98
spinal cord injury and, 154–156
renin-angiotensin-aldosterone system,
96–102, 237–240
cardiopulmonary baroreceptors
and, 97, 100, 101
orthostasis and, 96–102

respiratory muscle blood flow, 265–268
  exercise hyperpnea and, 268
  oxygen consumption and, 265–268
  voluntary hyperventilation and, 266
respiratory pump, 30–33, 178, 185
  intrathoracic pressure, 31, 178, 179
  liver volume, 32
  venous return, 30
right atrial pressure. *See* central venous pressure

sensory neuropathy, syringomyelia, 374, 375
skeletal muscle circulation, 268–295
  adjustments to physical conditioning. *See also* physical conditioning, 288–296
  autoregulation, 472
  blood flow, range of, 271
  blood volume, 271
  capillary fluid transfer, 477
  capillary pressure, 478
  cardiac output limitations and, 284–288
  catecholamines. *See* epinephrine
  cholinergic, 270
  endothelium and blood flow, 272, 276
  heterogeneity of flow, 271, 295, 309–311
  importance of vasoconstriction, 471
  inhibition of vasoconstriction, 472
  isometric contractions and, 304–311, 318
  local neural influences, 273
  "maximal blood flow", 260, 277–281, 286
  "maximal vascular conductance", 260, 281, 282, 286
  measurement, 268
  mechanical, 273
  metabolic control, 271–273
  microcirculation, 269, 292–295
  muscle pump and muscle perfusion, 184, 185, 281–284
  neural control, competition with metabolic, 274–277

norepinephrine spillover from, 85, 287
  orthostatic reflexes and, 51, 55
  oxygen extraction by, 292–295
  sympathetic vasodilators, 240
  vasoconstriction and exercise, 471–475
  veins, 69
skin blood flow. *See* cutaneous circulation
snakes
  hydrostatic force, 23, 24
  position of heart, 23, 24
  venous pooling, 24
spinal cord
  injury, 153, 156
  motor control, 390
  neuropathy, 374, 375
spinal reflexes, 154–156
splanchnic blood flow. *See* splanchnic circulation
splanchnic blood volume, 37, 67, 206, 207
  cirrhosis and, 32
  exercise, 206, 207, 213–216
  heat stress, 212
  measurement of, 213, 214
  respiratory pump and, 32
splanchnic circulation, 67, 88, 205–218
  epinephrine, 207
  exercise, 209–218, 411, 412
  exercise and heat stress, 209
  humoral control, 207, 208
  measurement of, 205
  neural control, 207, 214–216
  norepinephrine concentration and, 211, 212
  norepinephrine spillover from, 86
  orthostatic or postural hypotension and, 52, 214–216
  orthostatic reflexes and, 51, 55, 59, 60
  reflex control, 218
  veins, 208, 209
splanchnic veins, role of, 69–73
spleen, 72
Starling's Law. *See* Frank-Starling relationship

stroke volume, exercise. *See also* ventricular function, 175–182
afterload and, 176, 177
end-diastolic volume, 176, 177, 179, 180
end-systolic volume, 177, 179, 180
endurance athletes and, 166, 170
epinephrine and, 176
extrinsic factors, 175, 176
heat stress and exercise, 228–231
inotropism, 176
interval-strength relationship, 176
intrapleural pressure and, 178, 179
intrinsic factors, 176, 177
isometric contractions and, 312, 315, 316
mechanical limitations, 180, 181, 195–199
mitral stenosis and, 166, 170
muscle pump and, 179–181
pericardial constraints and, 180–182
physical conditioning, 193–195
preload and, 175, 177
range, 166, 170
ventricular filling pressure, 177, 178
ventricular transmural pressure, 178, 179
"symmorphosis", 330, 335, 350, 364
sympathetic axon reflexes. *See* sympathetic venoarteriolar reflexes
sympathetic nervous activity. *See also* muscle sympathetic nerve activity
activation, diffuse versus punctate, 85
exercise, 465, 467–475
heart rate and, 210–212, 411, 412
heat stress and exercise, 224–235
isometric contractions and, 320–322
measurements of, 85–96
microneurography, 85, 88–96, 144, 145
norepinephrine spillover, 86–88
orthostasis, 29
physical conditioning, 211, 291
regional blood flow and, 59, 60
tonic activity, 58
sympathetic nervous system
adrenergic, 82, 83
cholinergic, 83
cotransmitters, 82, 83
differential control, 83–85
neuropeptide Y, 82
peptidergic, 83
vasoactive intestinal polypeptide (VIP), 83
vasodilators, 83
sympathetic tone, 58
sympathetic venoarteriolar reflexes, 52, 64–66
orthostasis and, 52, 65
paraplegia, quadriplegia, (tetraplegia) and, 66, 154–156
syncope. *See also* vasovagal syncope and vasodepressor syncope, 22, 28, 29
systemic vascular compliance, 13

temperature regulation, heat stress and exercise, 224–227
thoracic blood volume. *See* central blood volume
time-tension index, 262
total peripheral resistance. *See* total vascular conductance
total (systemic) vascular conductance, 44, 182–185
exercise, 182–185
muscle pump and, 183–185
orthostasis, 44
physical conditioning and, 192
Starling resistor and, 183
"virtual" vascular conductance, 183–185
transmural pressure, gravity, 6
abdominal "water jacket" and, 17, 154
counterpressure and, 23
extravascular fluid pressure and, 17
venous, 17

upright posture. *See* orthostasis

vasodepressor syncope, 130
vasomotor control, 81–85
  active vasodilation, 83
  competition, neural versus local,
    274–277
  differential control, 83–85
  diffuse versus punctate activation,
    85
  generalizations, 82, 83
  homeostatic reflexes, 82
  local influences, 263, 271–274
  modulation of, 82–84
  neural influences, 82–85
  norepinephrine, 82
  sympathetic adrenergic, 83
  sympathetic cholinergic, 83, 270
  sympathetic tone, 58
vasopressin
  aortic pulse pressure, importance
    of, 103–107, 111–113
  arterial baroreflex, 103–107, 109–
    113
  cardiac denervation, 109, 110
  cardiorenal reflex and, 103, 106,
    107, 109, 110
  orthostasis and, 103, 104
  osmoreceptors, 103
  sinoaortic denervation and, 109, 110
  volume expansion and, 103, 105–
    108
vasovagal syncope, 130–139
  active neurogenic vasodilation and,
    131–133
  beta$_1$-adrenergic mechanisms, 137,
    138
  cardiac depressor reflexes and,
    137–139
  emotional stress and, 132, 133
  epinephrine and, 134, 136, 138, 142,
    143
  muscle sympathetic nerve activity
    and, 133, 134, 142, 143, 146
  norepinephrine and, 134, 136, 138
  pancreatic polypeptide and, 134,
    136
  passive vasodilation and, 133
  sympathetic cholinergic vasodila-
    tion, 131, 132
  vasopressin and, 134, 136

veins, reflex neural control, 66, 67
  measurement of, 70–73
  orthostasis and, 66, 67
  systemic compliance, 13
  venoconstriction, 66, 67, 70–73
venoarteriolar reflexes. See sympa-
    thetic venoarteriolar reflexes
venoconstriction, 66, 67, 70–73
  importance of, 66
  measurement of, 70
  splanchnic, 67
venostatic level, 8
venous innervation, 68–70
  alpha-adrenoreceptors, 69, 70, 84
venous pressures, 5–11
venous resistance, 47–50, 73
  pressure profile and, 48
  vasoconstriction, vasodilation and,
    47–50
  venoconstriction and, 73, 74
venous return, 30
  cardiac output and, 45
  muscle pump and, 30
  respiratory pump and, 30
  ventricular pacing and, 44
"venous return curve", 45, 46
venous system, physical properties
    of, 6–23
  capacitance, 16
  collapse, 8, 11, 12, 19
  compliance, 13
  delayed compliance and creep, 14,
    16, 27, 81
  distributed properties, 13, 15
  regional compliances, 15
  reservoir function, 20, 21
  resistance, 73
  specific compliance, 15, 16
  stress-relaxation, 14, 16
  "time constant", 20
  volume-pressure relationship, 13
  wall thickness, 21
venous valves, 21, 22, 29
  congenital absence of, 22
  incompetent, 22
venous volume
  active versus passive effects, 70–74
  arterial vasoconstriction and, 49,
    69

venous volume (*continued*)
  distribution of cardiac output and,
    48–51, 67–69, 213–217
  flow dependency and, 46, 68–70,
    186, 187
  venoconstriction, active, 70–74
ventricular filling pressure, 22, 29, 44
  isometric contractions and, 316
ventricular function. *See also* stroke
    volume, exercise
  afterload and, 176, 177
  beta$_1$-adrenoreceptors, 176
  cardiac sympathetic nerves, 176
  contractility, 176, 179, 193
  ejection fraction, 177, 179, 180, 193
  end-diastolic volume, 176, 177, 179,
    180
  end-systolic volume, 177, 179, 180
  extrinsic factors, 175, 176
  force-velocity relationship, 176, 193
  Frank-Starling relationship, 43, 175,
    176, 193
  interval-strength relationship, 176
  intrinsic factors, 176, 177
ventricular receptors, 53, 55, 56, 137–
    139

ventriculography, 177
  angiography, 177
  radionuclide scintigraphy, 177

water immersion. *See* central hyper-
    volemia
weightlessness. *See also* orthostatic
    intolerance
  baroreceptor resetting, 127
  baroreflex sensitivity and, 127–129
  blood volume, 124, 125
  depressed autonomic function and,
    126
  depressed cardiac function and, 126
  hypovolemic hyperadrenergic "pos-
    tural hypotension", 127
  increased venous capacitance and,
    126
  intramuscular pressures, 127
  physical conditioning and, 127–130
  skeletal muscle tone, 127
  venous transmural pressure, 127
work capacity versus functional ca-
    pacity, 190, 365

CPSIA information can be obtained at www.ICGtesting.com
Printed in the USA
BVOW060706100912

299627BV00005BB/8/P